Essential Immunology for Surgeons

Essential Immunology for Surgeons

Edited by

Oleg Eremin

Director of Research and Development
and Lead Clinician for Breast Services,
Research and Development Department,
United Lincolnshire Hospitals NHS Trust
Special Professor of Surgery,
Queen's Medical Centre,
University of Nottingham,
Nottingham, UK

and

Herb Sewell

Professor of Immunology,
University of Nottingham;
Honorary Consultant Immunologist,
Nottingham University Hospital Trust,
Nottingham, UK

OXFORD
UNIVERSITY PRESS

OXFORD
UNIVERSITY PRESS

Great Clarendon Street, Oxford OX2 6DP

Oxford University Press is a department of the University of Oxford.
It furthers the University's objective of excellence in research, scholarship,
and education by publishing worldwide in

Oxford New York

Auckland Cape Town Dar es Salaam Hong Kong Karachi
Kuala Lumpur Madrid Melbourne Mexico City Nairobi
New Delhi Shanghai Taipei Toronto

With offices in

Argentina Austria Brazil Chile Czech Republic France Greece
Guatemala Hungary Italy Japan Poland Portugal Singapore
South Korea Switzerland Thailand Turkey Ukraine Vietnam

Oxford is a registered trade mark of Oxford University Press
in the UK and in certain other countries

Published in the United States
by Oxford University Press Inc., New York

Previously published as *The Immunological Basis of Surgical Science and Practice,* 1992

This edition published 2011

British Library Cataloguing in Publication Data
Data available

Library of Congress Cataloging in Publication Data
Data available

Typeset in Minion by Glyph International, Bangalore, India
Printed in Great Britain
on acid-free paper by
CPI Antony Rowe

ISBN 978–0–19–958687–5

10 9 8 7 6 5 4 3 2 1

Foreword

Immunology has a reputation amongst clinicians for being difficult. Yet it is clearly relevant to many facets of disease. For surgeons, these include transplantation, cancer, inflammation and sepsis; all of major clinical importance. Contact with immunology is unavoidable. Patient management may involve potent biological therapies with antibodies such as herceptin or avastin. Many similar approaches are just around the corner, nearly a third of drugs under late stage development are 'biologicals'. Many new small molecule drugs target specific pathways in immune cells. Furthermore, expression profiling of gene expression in cancers can identify immunological targets. New imaging approaches may use antibodies to identify different cell types. In order to follow what is going on and what the clinical implications are, some understanding of immunology is becoming essential.

Why is immunology difficult? This book will tell you that it is not! Immunology before the 1980s was mired in phenomenology that could only be understood with mental acrobatics. However the advances in molecular biology and genetics in the last thirty years have changed this dramatically. Most of the phenomena have been explained, and validated, in quite simple molecular terms. For example, the old mysterious magic of adjuvants (such as alum) in enhancing immunizations is explained by the presence of pattern recognition receptors on macrophages and related cells, which set up inflammatory responses and release cytokines that activate antigen specific lymphocytes. Even the last of the unexplained 1970s phenomena, the suppressor T cell has yielded to more molecular approaches: production of immunosuppressive cytokines by a subset of T cells, called regulatory T cells, is controlled by a single protein, FoxP3, that regulates expression of their genes. Indeed, one no longer needs to try to understand the phenomenology until there is a molecular explanation; good journals now follow this principle. This book explains immunology on a base of secure and understandable molecular mechanisms.

Immunology also appears difficult because of the abbreviations and acronyms. This is an unnecessary hindrance that is addressed in this book by an index right at the front. However, the use of an abbreviation such as 'MHC' rather than 'major histocompatibility complex' is less cumbersome for both author and reader. Therefore, some limited 'language learning' may be necessary but it is not difficult, given a good dictionary.

Finally, immunology may be difficult because of the speed of change. It is very exciting because it moves so fast, but this can make it appear formidable to non-experts. Where there is already a clear molecular explanation of how things work, this rarely changes. What can happen is that further modulations of particular systems are found. These are of interest to those directly working in that area, but the rest of us can stand back a little and only really get excited by major paradigm shifts, which are rare. The apparent speed of change can make one wary of reading or buying textbooks, however books that are well grounded in the basics of the subject will not go out of date. This book is in this category and should form a secure platform on which to build an understanding of advances in the field.

Professor Sir Andrew J McMichael FMedSci, FRS

Professor of Molecular Medicine
MRC Human Immunology Unit
Director of the Weatherall Institute of Molecular Medicine
University of Oxford
UK.

Preface

Our knowledge and understanding of immunology has undergone major expansion and very significant changes over the last two decades. This has led to a much better understanding of the pathogenesis of various disease states and processes; in many diseases, to more effective management. Since the publication of our textbook, *The Immunological Basis of Surgical Science and Practice* in 1992, specifically targeted to a surgical readership, the scope of surgical immunology has broadened substantially, encompassing new aspects of practice in traditional areas (eg, new therapeutic approaches in transplantation rejection, novel vaccination strategies in cancer treatment as well as a better understanding of the beneficial effects of standard chemotherapy). In a range of diseases the immune response has been manipulated to lead to more targeted and effective humoral therapy – transplantation, cancer and musculoskeletal disorders. There have been major advances in our understanding of gut immune mechanisms and their importance to good health and state of well-being, the metabolic disturbances and associated dysfunction of host defences induced by severe trauma and sepsis and the resultant consequences to the critically ill patient. Anaesthesiologists and Intensive Care Physicians are recognizing the significant derangements of immune function in the critically ill patient and the possible therapeutic approaches to manage such patients.

This new textbook provides the reader with a concise and up-to-date account of immunology in general and its translation into key areas of clinical practice. This book aims to inform, educate, and provide the reader with a helpful biomedical template for a better understanding and management of important areas of clinical practice relevant to the surgeon and the critical care physician. Although targeted predominantly to the surgical trainee intending to sit the appropriate specialist examination, we hope that the more senior clinician in consultant practice, both surgical and non-surgical (gastroenterology, anaesthesiology), as well as undergraduate medical students, may find sections of the book informative, and a stimulant to further reading. Key references to more in-depth study are provided at the end of each chapter.

The two Senior Editors have been fortunate in having experts in their clinical disciplines and/or field of immunology from the UK, Spain, and the USA contributing to this book. All the contributors have been given the remit outlined above and all sections have undergone a rigorous editorial process to ensure a coherent volume and uniform style. We hope that our readers find the text interesting, informative, and stimulating. If you have comments/criticisms about the book, in particular suggestions about improvements in future editions, please write to the Editorial Team.

Lastly, the editors are very grateful to Professor Sir Andrew McMichael, world leading immunologist, for writing a Foreword to the book.

Oleg Eremin
Herb Sewell
October 2010

Acknowledgements

HS would like to acknowledge his debt and gratitude to the late Professor PGH. Gell FRS, and also to Dr M. Basu and Dr J. Rippon, Professor R. Thompson and Dr M. Haeney for their encouragement, stimulation and directions along his career road of travel in immunology.

OE is indebted to the late John Stevens, an enlightened surgeon who first introduced him to the concept of tumour immunology and, especially, to Professor Robin Coombs, who provided the crucial scientific environment and support in Cambridge that launched him on his career as a surgical oncologist and tumour immunologist.

We are very appreciative of everyone who has made this book possible, in particular the various authors and co-authors of all chapters, who have produced chapters of outstanding quality. Many of our colleagues in Nottingham were very helpful in reading and commenting on drafts of relevant chapters, flagging any weaknesses or occasional errors. HS thanks particularly Drs I. Todd, E. McDermott, A. Anwar, P. Vaitia and Professors W. Irving and Y. Mahida.

Heartfelt thanks to our secretaries: (For HS) Mrs Jane Renshaw (current) and Mrs Ann Marshall (previous) and (for OE), Mrs Sue Cooper. They were very understanding, patient and professional, putting up with our incessant demands and producing the goods! In particular, OE would like to thank Mrs Sue Cooper, who had overall responsibility for the production of the text before submission to OUP, and who dealt with all the enquiries and communications with the different contributors, here in the UK and the USA, as well as with OUP. She has done an outstanding job, and worked many unsociable hours and to numerous tight deadlines. My thanks also to my departmental personal assistant, Mrs Val Elliott.

Lastly, many thanks to our families, nearest and dearest friends who have been supportive and encouraging over many years, including throughout the production of this book. HS acknowledges Darreul, David, Marcia, Armand, Bronte, Deloris, Trev, Algie and Professors Owen Morgan and Eric Walker and others not listed due to space constraints – they know who they are and how they are appreciated. OE would like to acknowledge the great help and support provided by his wife, Jennifer.

Contents

Detailed contents

List of contributors

Mark Aloysius
Research Fellow,
Department of Surgery,
University of Nottingham,
Queen's Medical Centre,
Nottingham, UK

Alfred Ayala
Professor of Surgery (Research),
Division of Surgical Research,
Department of Surgery,
Alpert School of Medicine at
Brown University
and Rhode Island Hospital, USA

Anirban Bannerjee
Professor of Surgery,
Department of Surgery and Director,
Trauma Research Centre,
University of Colorado Denver,
USA

Eleanor M. Bolton
Assistant Director of Research,
Department of Surgery,
Addenbrooke's Hospital,
Cambridge, UK

J. Andrew Bradley
Professor of Surgery,
University of Cambridge;
Honorary Consultant Surgeon and
Clinical Director of Transplantation,
Addenbrooke's Hospital,
Cambridge, UK

Winston P. Choi
Surgery/Trauma Research Fellow and
Resident Physician,
Department of Surgery,
University of Colorado Denver, USA

Oleg Eremin
Director of Research and Development
and Lead Clinician for Breast Services,
Research and Development Department,
United Lincolnshire Hospitals NHS Trust
Special Professor of Surgery,
Queen's Medical Centre,
University of Nottingham,
Nottingham, UK

John C. Eun
Surgery/Trauma Research Fellow and
Resident Physician,
Department of Surgery,
University of Colorado Denver, USA

Manuel Garcia-Caballero
Professor of Surgery and Consultant
Surgeon,
Faculty of Medicine,
University of Malaga,
Malaga, Spain

Daithi Heffernan
Assistant Professor of Surgery,
Division of Surgical Research,
Department of Surgery,
Alpert School of Medicine at Brown
University and Rhode Island Hospital,
USA

Steven D. Heys
Deputy Head,
Division of Applied Medicine and
Consultant Surgeon,
University of Aberdeen,
and NHS Grampian,
Aberdeen, Scotland

Xin Huang
Research Associate,
Division of Surgical Research,
Department of Surgery,
Alpert School of Medicine at Brown
University and Rhode Island Hospital,
USA

Joanne Lomas-Neira
Instructor of Surgery (Research),
Division of Surgical Research,
Department of Surgery,
Alpert School of Medicine at Brown
University and Rhode Island Hospital,
USA

Ernest E. Moore
Bruce M Rockwell Distinguished Chair
of Trauma and Chief of Surgery,
Denver Health Medical Centre;
Professor and Vice Chairman,
Department of Surgery,
University of Colorado Denver, USA

Adrian Robins
Associate Professor/Reader in
Immunology,
School of Molecular Medical Sciences,
Queen's Medical Centre,
Nottingham, UK

Herb Sewell
Professor of Immunology,
University of Nottingham;
Honorary Consultant Immunologist,
Nottingham University Hospital Trust,
Nottingham, UK

Christopher Silliman
Senior Independent Investigator,
Research Department,
Bonfils Blood Centre,
Denver; Professor of Paediatrics and
Surgery,
University of Colorado Denver, USA

Rajan K. Thakkar
Division of Surgical Research,
Department of Surgery,
Alpert School of Medicine at Brown
University and Rhode Island Hospital,
USA

Paddy Tighe
Associate Professor in Immunology,
School of Molecular Medical Sciences,
Queen's Medical Centre,
Nottingham, UK

Chandan Verma
Research Scientist,
Department of Surgery,
University of Nottingham,
Queen's Medical Centre, UK

Klaus W. J. Wahle
Visiting Professor,
Department of Immunology,
University of Strathclyde,
Glasgow, and Division of Applied
Medicine,
University of Aberdeen, UK

Leslie Walker
Emeritus Professor of Cancer
Rehabilitation,
Institute of Rehabilitation,
University of Hull, UK

James H. Wood
Postdoctoral Research Fellow,
Department of Paediatric Surgery,
The Children's Hospital,
Aurora, USA; Resident Physician,
Department of Surgery,
University of Colorado Denver, USA

Abbreviations and acronyms

20-COOH-LTB4	20-carboxyleukotriene B4
20-OH-LTB4	20-hydroxyleukotriene B4
5-HPETE	5-hydroxyperoxyeicosatetraenoic
ABC	avidin–biotin complex
ACA	anticentromere antibody
ACTH	adrenocorticotropic hormone
ADCC	antibody-dependent cellular cytotoxicity
ADH	antidiuretic hormone
AFP	alpha-fetoprotein
AICD	activation-induced cell death
AID	activation-induced (cytidine) deaminase
AIDS	acquired immune deficiency syndrome
AIRE	autoimmune regulator
ALI	acute lung injury
ALPS	autoimmune lymphoproliferative syndrome
ANA	anti-nuclear antibody
ANCA	anti-neutrophil cytoplasmic antibody
ANNA	anti-neuronal nuclear antibody
AP	alternate pathway (complement)
AP-1	activator protein 1
AP100	alternate pathway 100 test
APA	antiphospholipid antibody
APAAP	alkaline phosphatase–anti-alkaline phosphatase
APACHE	Acute Physiology and Chronic Health Evaluation
APhC	allophycocyanin
APC	antigen-presenting cell
APECED	autoimmune polyendocrinopathy with candidiasis and ectodermal dysplasia
APrC	activated protein C
APTT	activated partial thromboplastin time
aPTT	partial thromboplastin time
ARA	arachidonic acid
ARC	AIDS-related complex
ARDS	acute respiratory distress syndrome
Arg	arginine
ART	antiretroviral therapy
AS	ankylosing spondylitis
ASC	antibody secreting (B) cell
AT	ataxia telangiectasia
ATG	antithymocyte globulin
ATP	adenosine triphosphate
αGal	galactose α-1-3-galactosyl-1-4-N-acetyl glucosamine
α-GALCER	α-galactosylceramide
α-MSH	alpha-melanocyte stimulation hormone
αβTCR	alphabeta T cell receptor
BAF	B cell activating factor
BAL	bronchoalveolar lavage
BALF	bronchoalveolar lavage fluid
BBB	blood–brain barrier
BCAA	branched chain amino acid
BCG	bacillus Calmette–Guérin
BCR	B cell receptor
BRM	biologic response modifier
β2-GP1	beta2-glycoprotein 1
β2M	beta2-microglobulin
C	complement
C/EBPβ	CCAAT/enhancer-binding protein beta
C1 INH	C1 inhibitor
C1q	first component of complement
CA	carbohydrate-associated
CALLA	common acute lymphoblastic leukaemia antigen
CAM	cell adhesion molecule
cAMP	cyclic adenosine monophosphate

CAPS	cryopyrin-associated periodic fever syndrome
CARS	compensatory anti-inflammatory response syndrome
CASP	colon ascendens stent peritonitis
CC	chemokine
CCL/CXCL	chemokine ligand
CCP	cyclic citrullinated peptide
CCR/CXCR	chemokine receptor
CD	cluster of differentiation
CDAD	clostridium difficile-associated diarrhoea
CDR	complementarity determining region
CEA	carcinoembryonic antigen
CFSE	carboxyfluorescein diacetate succinimidal ester
CGD	chronic granulomatous disease
CGH	comparative genomic hybridization
CGRP	calcitonin-gene-related peptide
CH	complement haemolysis (100, 50 test)
CINC	cytokine-induced neutrophil chemoattractant
CJD	Creutzfeldt–Jakob disease
CLA	conjugated linoleic acid
CLAA	cutaneous lymphocyte-associated antigen
CLIP	class II invariant chain peptide
CLP	caecal ligation and puncture
CMI	cell-mediated immunity
CML	cell-mediated lympholysis
CMV	cytomegalovirus
CNS	central nervous system
COPD	chronic obstructive pulmonary disease
COX	cyclooxygenase
CpG DNA	cytosine phosphate-guanine deoxyribonucleic acid
CR	complement receptor
51Cr	chromium^{51}
CRP	C-reactive protein
CSF-1	colony stimulating factor-1
CSR	class switch recombination
CSS	Churg–Strauss syndrome
CTL	cytotoxic T lymphocyte ($CD8^+$)
CTLA	cytotoxic T lymphocyte antigen
CTLA-4	cytotoxic T lymphocyte antigen-4
CTLA-4-Ig	cytotoxic T lymphocyte antigen-4-immunoglobulin fusion protein
CVID	common variable immune deficiency
CYP4F	cytochrome P450
CysLT	cysteinyl leukotriene receptor
DAF	decay accelerating factor
DAMP	danger (or damage)-associated molecular pattern
DC	dendritic cell
DDC	dermal dendritic cell
DHA	docosahexaenoic acid
DIC	disseminated intravascular coagulation
DMBA	7,12-dimethylbenz[a]-anthracene
DNA	deoxyribonucleic acid
DRC	dendritic reticulum cell
DTH	delayed type hypersensitivity
DTP	diphtheria, tetanus, pertussis (whooping cough)
EBV	Epstein–Barr virus
EC	endothelial cell
ECM	extracellular matrix
EFA	essential fatty acid
EGFR	epidermal growth factor receptor
ELISA	enzyme-linked immunosorbent assay
ELISPOT	enzyme-linked immunosorbent spot
EMS	emergency medical services
ENA	extractable nuclear antigen
EPA	eicosapentaenoic acid
EPCR	endothelial protein C receptor
ER	endoplasmic reticulum

ESR	erythrocyte sedimentation rate
FA	fatty acid
Fab	fragment antigen binding (immunoglobulin)
FAB	functional antibody
FADD	Fas-associated death domain
FasL	fas ligand
Fc	fragment crystallisable (immunoglobulin)
FCA	Freund's complete adjuvant
FCAS	familial cold autoinflammatory syndrome
FDC	follicular dendritic cell
FFP	fresh frozen plasma
FGF	fibroblast growth factor
FiO_2	fraction of inspired oxygen
FITC	fluorescein isothiocyanate
FKBP	FK binding protein
FLAP	5-lipoxygenase activating protein
Flt-3L	Fms-like tyrosine kinase ligand 3
FMF	familial Mediterranean fever
Foxp3	fork head box protein 3
FRC	fibroblastic reticular cell
GALT	gut-associated lymphoid tissue
GC	glucocorticoid
GCR	glucocorticoid receptor
GFAP	glial fibrillary acid protein
GFP	green fluorescent protein
GH	growth hormone
GI	gastrointestinal
GIT	gastrointestinal tract
GM-CSF	granulocyte-macrophage colony stimulating factor
GMP	good manufacturing practice
GPC	gastric parietal cell
GRE	glucocorticoid response element
GSH	glutathione (reduced form)
GSSG	glutathione disulphide (oxidized form)
GVH	graft versus host
GWAS	genome-wide association study
H1N1/H5N1	molecules associated with influenza virus H (haemagglutinin) N (neuraminidase)
H_2O_2	hydrogen peroxide
HAART	highly active antiretroviral therapy
HAE	hereditary angioedema
HAMA	human anti-mouse antibody
hCAP-18/LL-37	human cathelicidin-18
hCG	human chorionic gonadotrophin
HDL	high-density lipoprotein
HEV	high endothelial venule
HHV	human herpesvirus
HiB	Haemophilis influenza type B
HIDS	hyperimmunoglobulin D and periodic fever syndrome
HIV	human immunodeficiency virus
HLA	human leucocyte antigen
HMGB-1	high mobility group box-1 (protein)
HMVEC	human microvascular endothelial cell
HPA	hypothalamic–pituitary–adrenal (axis)
HPG	hypothalamic–pituitary–gonadal (axis)
HPT	hypothalamic–pituitary–thyroid (axis)
HPV	human papillomavirus
HS/R	haemorrhagic shock and resuscitation
HSP	heat shock protein
HSV	herpes simplex virus
hTERT	human telomerase reverse transcriptase
HTS	hypertonic saline
IBD	inflammatory bowel disease
IBS	irritable bowel syndrome
ICAM-1	intercellular cell adhesion molecule-1
ICOS	inducible costimulator
ICU	intensive care unit
IDC	indeterminate dendritic cell
IDO	indoleamine 2,3-dioxygenase
IEL	intraepithelial lymphocyte
IF	intrinsic factor

IFA	indirect fluorescent antibody assay
IFN	interferon
IFN-α	interferon-alpha
IFN-γ	interferon-gamma
IFs	intermediate filaments
IFNARI	component of type 1 interferon receptor
Ig	immunoglobulin
IGF-1	insulin-like growth factor-1
IKKB	I kappa/kappa B
IL	interleukin
IL-1β	interleukin-1-beta
IL-1ra	interleukin-1 receptor antagonist
IL-2 R	interleukin-2 receptor
ILXR	interleukin X receptor
IM	intramuscular
IMF	intermediate filament
iNOS	inducible nitrogen oxide synthase
INR	international normalized ratio
INTERSEPT	International Sepsis Trial Study Group
IP-10	chemokine ligand 10
iPSC	induced pluripotential stem cell
IRAK4	interleukin receptor-associated kinase 4
iRNA	interfering RNA
ISCOM	immunostimulatory complex
ISS	injury severity score
ITAM	immunoreceptor tyrosine activation motif
ITIM	immunoreceptor tyrosine inhibition motif
iTreg	induced T regulatory cell
IV	intravenous
IVIg	intravenous immunoglobulin
JAK	Janus kinase
JAK-STAT	Janus kinase-signal transducer and activator transcription
JAS	juvenile ankylosing spondylitis
JCA	juvenile chronic arthritis
JNK	c-Jun N-terminal kinase
JRA	juvenile rheumatoid arthritis
KC	keratinocyte-derived chemokine
KIR	killer inhibitory receptor/killer cell immunoglobulin receptor
KLH	keyhole limpet haemocyanin
KS	Kaposi's sarcoma
LAK	lymphokine-activated killer (cell)
LATS	long acting thyroid stimulator
LBP	lipopolysaccharide binding protein
LC	Langerhans cell
LCA	leucocyte common antigen
LCPUFA	long chain polyunsaturated fatty acid
LDL	low-density lipoprotein
LEMS	Lambert–Eaton myasthenic syndrome
LFA	lymphocyte functioning antigen
LGL	large granular lymphocyte
LIA	line immunoassay
LMP	low molecular weight polypeptide
LOX	lipooxygenase
LPS	lipopolysaccharide
LT	leukotriene
LTA	lipoteichoic acid
Lys	lysine
MAB	monoclonal antibody
MAC	membrane attack complex
MADCAM1	mucosal addressin cell adhesion molecule 1
MALDI-TOF	matrix-associated, laser desorbed/ionized, time-of-flight
MALT	mucosal-associated lymphoid tissue
MAP	mitogen-activated protein
MAPK	mitogen-activated protein kinase
MASP	mannose-associated serine proteinase
M-band	monoclonal band
MBL	mannan-binding lectin
MCA	methlycholanthrene
MCP	membrane cofactor protein

MCP-1/3	monocyte chemotactic protein-1/3
MDC/CCL22	macrophage-derived chemokine
mDC	myeloid DC
MDP	muramyl dipeptide
MDSC	myeloid-derived suppressor cell
MG	myasthenia gravis
MGUS	monoclonal gammopathy of uncertain significance
mHC	minor histocompatability complex
MHC	major histocompatibility complex
MIC	MHC class 1-like chain
MIC-A/B	MHC class 1-like molecules A and B
MIF	macrophage inhibitory factor
MIP-1	macrophage inflammatory protein-1
MIP-1β	macrophage inflammatory protein-1-beta
MLC	mixed lymphocyte culture
MLN	mesenteric lymph node
MLR	mixed lymphocyte reaction
MLTR	mixed lymphocyte tumour cell reaction
mM	millimole
MMP	matrix metalloproteinase
MMR	mumps, measles, and rubella
MODS	multiple organ dysfunction syndrome
MOF	multiple organ failure
mOsm	milliosmole
MPIVM	multiphoton intravital microscopy
MPL	monophosphoryl lipid A
MPO	myeloperoxidase
mRNA	messenger RNA
MSpec	mass spectrometry
MS	multiple sclerosis
mTOR	mammalian target of rapamycin
MUFA	monounsaturated fatty acid
MuSK	muscle specific tyrosine kinase
MWS	Muckle–Wells syndrome
NBT	nitroblue tetrazolium
NF-AT	nuclear factor of activated T (cell)
NF-κB	nuclear factor kappa light chain-enhancer of activated B cell
NHL	non-Hodgkin's lymphoma
NI-CAM	neural intercellular adhesion molecule
NK	natural killer (cell)
NKG2D	natural killer group 2 member D
NK T	natural killer T (cell)
NLR	NOD (nucleotide-binding domain)-like receptor
NMR	nuclear magnetic resonance
NO	nitric oxide
NOD-LRR	nucleotide-oligomerization domain leucine-rich repeat
NOMID	neonatal onset multi-system inflammatory disease
NORASEPT	North American Sepsis Trial Study Group
NOS	nitric oxide synthase
NS	normal saline
NSAID	nonsteroidal anti-inflammatory drug
nTreg	natural T regulatory cell
OPSI	overwhelming post-splenectomy infection
OSA	organ specific autoimmunity
PAF	platelet activating factor
PAI	plasminogen activator inhibitor
PAMP	pathogen-associated molecular pattern
PaO_2	partial arterial pressure of oxygen
PAP	peroxidase-antigen peroxidase
PAR	protease-activated receptor
PBL	peripheral blood lymphocyte
PBMC	peripheral blood mononuclear cell
PCR	polymerase chain reaction
PCV	postcapillary venule
PD-1	programme death molecule 1
pDC	plasmacytoid DC
PDGF	platelet derived growth factor

PE	phycoerythrin
PEM	protein energy malnutrition
PEP	postexposure prophylaxis (antiretroviral drug)
PFS	periodic fever syndrome
PG	prostaglandin
PGL	persistent generalised lymphadenopathy
PGT	post-genomic technology
PHA	phyto-haemagglutinin
PI	protease inhibitor
PI	prostacyclin
PI3	phosphatidylinositol 3
PICU	paediatric intensive care unit
pIgR	polymeric immunoglobulin receptor
PKC	protein kinase C
PLA_2	phospholipase A_2
PMA	phorbol myristate acetate
PML	progressive multi-focal leucoencephalopathy
PNS	peripheral nervous system
POMC	proopiomelanocortin
PP	Peyer's patches
PPAR-N	peroxisome proliferator-activated receptor-N
PR3	proteinase 3
PRBCs	packed red blood cells
PRL	prolactin
PROWESS	Recombinant Activated Human Protein C Worldwide Evaluation in Severe Sepsis Study
PRR	pattern recognition receptor
PSA	prostate specific antigen
PSML	post-shock mesenteric lymph
PT	prothrombin time
PTLD	post-transplant lymphoproliferative disease
PTPN22	protein tyrosine phosphatase N22
PUFA	poly-unsaturated fatty acid
R	receptor
R&D	research and development
RA	rheumatoid arthritis
RAE1	retinoic acid early transcript 1
RAG	recombination activating gene 1 and 2
RAGE	receptor for advanced glycation end-products
RAIGLR	retinoic acid-inducible gene-like receptor
RAOR/RORγ	retinoic acid orphan receptor
RAST	radioallergosorbent test
RBC	red blood cell
RFLP	restriction fragment length polymorphism
RF	rheumatoid factor
rh-G-CSF	human recombinant granulocyte colony-stimulating factor
RIA	radio-immunoassay
RIG-I	retinoic acid-inducible gene I
RLH	retinoic acid-inducible gene I-like helicases
RNA	ribonucleic acid
RNSs	reactive nitrogen species
RORr	retinoic acid orphan receptor
ROSs	reactive oxygen species
RPPA	reversephase protein array
RT	reverse transcriptase
RT-PCR	reverse transcriptase-polymerase chain reaction
SAM	sympathetic–adrenal–medullary (axis)
SeC	secretory component
SC	subcutaneous
SCC	squamous cell carcinoma
SCD1	delta-9 desaturase enzyme
SCID	severe combined immune deficiency
SCIg	subcutaneous immunoglobulin
SCLC	small cell lung cancer
SCNT	somatic cell nuclear transfer
SG	specific gravity
SHM	somatic hypermutation
SI	specific immunotherapy
SIgR	surface immunoglobulin receptor
siRNA	small interfering RNA
SIRS	systemic inflammatory response syndrome
SIS	self-initiated support
SIV	simian immunodeficiency virus

SLE	systemic lupus erythematosus
SMA	smooth muscle antibody
SMI	small-molecular inhibitor
SmIg	surface membrane immunoglobulin
SNP	single nucleotide polymorphism
SOD	superoxide dismutase
SP	substance P
SP-D	surfactant protein-D
sPLA2	secretory phospholipase A2
SPR	surface plasmon resonance
SPT	skin prick test
SPUR	serious, persistent, unusual or recurrent (infections)
SRID	single radial immunodiffusion
SS-A	anti-Ro antibody
SS-B	anti-La antibody
STAT	signalling transducer and activator of transcription
sTNFR	soluble TNF receptor
T reg	T regulatory cell
T/HS	trauma/haemorrhagic shock
TAA	tumour-associated antigen
TAFI	thrombin-activatable fibrinolysis inhibitor
TAM	tumour-associated macrophage
TAP	transporter-associated with antigen processing
TARC	thymus activation-regulated chemokine
TB	tuberculosis
TCR	T cell receptor (CD3/Ticomplex)
TF	tissue factor
TFPI	tissue factor pathway inhibitor
TGF-β	transforming growth factor-beta
Th	T helper (cell)
TI	thymus-independent
TIL	tumour-infiltrating lymphocyte
TIM	tumour-infiltrating macrophage
TIM-3	T cell immunoglobulin and mucin domain containing molecule 3
Tis	antigen-specific TCR
TLR	Toll-like receptor
TNFR	tumour necrosis factor receptor
TNF-α	tumour necrosis factor-alpha
TPA	12-O-tetradecanoyl-phorbol-13-acetate
t-PA	tissue plasminogen activator
TPN	total parenteral nutrition
TPO	thyroid peroxidase
TRADD	TNFR-associated death domain
TRAIL	TNF-related apoptosis-inducing ligand
TRALI	transfusion- related acute lung injury
TRAPS	TNF receptor-associated periodic fever syndromes
Treg	T regulatory cell
TSA	tumour-specific antigen
TSG	tumour suppressor gene
TSH	thyroid stimulating hormone
TSHR	thyroid stimulating hormone receptor
TSI	thyroid stimulating immunoglobulin
TSP	thrombospondin
tTG	tissue transglutaminase
TXA	thromboxane
UV	ultraviolet
VCAM-1	vascular cell adhesion molecule-1
VEGF	vascular endothelial growth factor
VEGFR	vascular endothelial growth factor receptor
VIP	vasoactive intestinal peptide
VLDL	very low-density lipoprotein
vWF	von Willebrand factor
WAS	Wiskott–Aldrich syndrome
WAT	white adipose tissue
WBC	white blood cell
WB-PLT	whole-blood derived platelet concentrate
WGD	Wegener's granulomatous disease
WT	wild type
X-SCID	X-linked severe combined immune deficiency syndrome
Zap70	zeta-associated protein of 70 kDa

Chapter 1

Basic immunology

Herb Sewell

Key summary points

- The evolutionary and physiological function of the immune system is to protect the host against infections and also to recognize and respond to mutated (potentially cancerous) and damaged cells. Immune defence mechanisms are conventionally described in terms of innate immunity and adaptive immunity. Innate immunity is seen as constituting the first line of defence against invading microbes; its responses are rapidly induced. Adaptive immunity, in contrast, develops more slowly and mediates delayed defence responses against infections.
- Innate immunity is made up of structural cellular physical barriers, components within soluble compartments (complement system proteins, cytokines), as well as specific cells (e.g. DCs, neutrophils, macrophages, etc.) widely distributed throughout the body which possess a group of germ-line-encoded (i.e. limited in numbers) receptors (e.g. TLRs). Pathogen recognition is mediated by the PRRs. Recognition by PRRs of PAMPs shared across groups of pathogens, DAMPs in damaged/stressed host cells, activate diverse cell signalling pathways and initiate proinflammatory responses (e.g. IL-1, IL-6, IFN-γ, TNF-α).
- Inflammatory reactions mediate, in large part, the beneficial effects of immune responses. The system requires tight regulation to avoid induction of damaging and progressive chronic inflammation which is recognized as contributing to a wide range of diseases, including autoimmune, cardiovascular, and neurological disorders as well as malignant transformations.
- Innate immunity and adaptive immunity integrate in bidirectional ways. Innate immune responses can also trigger and direct the development of particular forms of adaptive immunity.
- Adaptive immunity (specific acquired immunity) is stimulated when microbes have breached natural portals and/or have survived the initial innate responses. Adaptive immunity is mediated by T and B lymphocytes. The lymphocytes possess receptors which recognize specifically and individually non-self (antigens) using clonally (non-germ-line) distributed receptors (vast numbers). T lymphocytes recognize mainly protein peptide fragments linked to host self molecules encoded in the MHC region genes, namely the HLAs. T cells recognize

and respond to the peptide–HLA complex (signal 1) displayed predominantly on professional APCs (e.g. DCs). Additional costimulatory and accessory molecular interactions (signal 2) between the APC (e.g. CD80/86) and T cell (e.g. CD28) result in T cell signal transduction and gene(s) induction. T cells undergo cell activation, clonal proliferation, expansion, and differentiation into effector and regulatory cells, through local activation of TLRs and *in situ* secreted cytokines (e.g. IL-2, IL-12) (signal 3). There is also the generation of a pool of memory cells that can mediate secondary and subsequent better-quality responses (magnitude and duration) against the same antigen.

- Cytokines and chemokines and their respective receptors, along with cell–cell interactions, are the key drivers of immune cell signalling, activation, proliferation, and differentiation. Additionally, along with adhesion molecules, they are central to the ability of lymphocytes to recirculate and move through tissue, or home to particular anatomical sites.
- T cells develop from bone marrow precursors within the central lymphoid organ, the thymus, and emerge from that site as naive cells with the potential to develop along several effector and regulatory pathways on encounter in the periphery of peptide antigen–HLA presented by APCs. Bone marrow functions as the central lymphoid organ for B cell development; peripheral B cells generate effector (plasma) cells that produce and secrete antibodies, and also generate memory B cells.
- Two major subsets of T cells are defined, the $CD4^+$ Th cells and the $CD8^+$ CTLs. The $CD4^+$ T subset is further subdivided and defined by the effector functions the subsets mediate and the spectrum of cytokines produced, as well as by the signature transcription factors which help to regulate their cytokine profiles. $CD4^+$ Th types described are the $CD4^+$ Th1, secreting IL-1, IL-2, IL-6, IL-10, TNF-α, IFN-γ; Th2, secreting, IL-4, IL-5, IL-6, IL-9, IL-10, IL-13; and Th17, secreting IL-17, IL-22, IL-23. Other subtypes are being delineated. The main regulatory cell is defined as the $CD4^+$ $CD25^+$ $FoxP3^+$ T cell (Treg). Naive $CD8^+$ T cells recognize intracellularly derived peptide antigens presented by DCs and, upon appropriate stimulation, can become effector $CD8^+$ CTLs. $CD4^+$ T cells recognize peptides presented by HLA class II molecules on DCs. $CD8^+$ T cells recognize peptides presented by HLA class I-linked proteins, being defined by the cytosolic pathways used in antigen processing and peptide loading on to newly synthesized HLA molecules by the DCs. HLA class II present peptides generated mainly from extracellular protein antigens, HLA class I present peptides from intracellular sources. However, cross-presentation of peptides between these pathways has been demonstrated.
- B cell receptors recognize a wider range of antigens compared with T cells. They can recognize whole protein antigens or peptides (not linked with HLA), carbohydrates, lipids, etc. B cells and their derived plasma cells are responsible for the production of antibodies and humoral immunity. Antibodies are good at neutralizing extracellular pathogens; they also can activate the complement proteins, bind

to Ig Fc receptors on phagocytic and other cells, and induce, in turn, the activation of these cells. Many of these effector reactions generate controlled inflammatory responses. Secretory IgA antibodies represent a particular adaptation of protection at mucosal sites; they neutralize microbes and exclude entry of antigens across the mucosa without recruiting and exciting inflammatory responses.

- T and B lymphocyte responses of adaptive immunity, like innate immunity, also recruit, in large part, agents inducing controlled inflammation to eliminate or contain pathogens. T and B lymphocytes express a range of CD antigens which help to characterize the cells and which are also involved in the functions of these cells.
- Cells of innate immunity, e.g. DCs and macrophages, act as important APCs for adaptive immunity. Macrophages and other professional phagocytes, such as polymorphonuclear leucocytes, are also recruited by effector mechanisms of adaptive immunity. Within the central lymphoid tissues, namely the thymus and bone marrow respectively, the generation of clones of T and B lymphocytes occurs from bone marrow stem cell precursors. Following massive proliferation within those organs, relatively small numbers of the proliferating cells emerge as naive T and B cells which recirculate through the peripheral lymphoid tissues. Within the peripheral lymphoid tissues (lymph nodes, spleen, and MALT) T and B cells and APCs occupy defined anatomical sites, and are involved in regional cell migrations which facilitate their clustering, cooperation, and the triggering of the lymphocyte potential to respond to incoming antigens.
- Clones of T and B cells which meet their respective antigens in the peripheral lymphoid tissue become selected, activated, undergo proliferation, and differentiate into effector, regulatory, and memory cells. Some memory cells travel to peripheral tissues where they can respond rapidly to incoming antigens. Other memory cells recirculate, some showing selective preference for different anatomical compartments within the host. Much of the physiological benefit of the effector immune response is mediated by controlled inflammation; this is particularly exploited by antibodies activating the complement system of proteins. Effector $CD4^+$ T cells produce a range of cytokines and chemokines that mediate controlled inflammation, expressed largely as cell-mediated immune responses, and the $CD8^+$ T cell effectors generate cytotoxic responses. T cell effector responses are efficient at combating intracellular microbes or intracellularly derived peptide antigens.
- Other important effector and regulatory lymphocytes include NK T cells and $\gamma\delta$ T cells. These are considered unconventional lymphocytes as their biological properties reside somewhere between those of innate immunity and adaptive immunity.
- Other important mediators of immune defence reside in cells of the innate immune system, such as NK cells, mast cells, and basophils. NK cells have particular roles in recognizing and responding to mutated, potentially cancerous cells, as well as virally infected and other damaged cells.

- The success of the immune response in protecting against infections has, for more than a century, been successfully exploited by vaccination procedures. Better understanding of the immune system and of the nature of immunogens and antigens, and development of newer adjuvants, are contributing to new vaccine strategies and more effective long-term outcomes.
- The powerful immunological responses of innate and adaptive immunity, and their recruitment of inflammatory reactions, indicate the need for efficient regulation and modulation of the immune system to avoid serious immunopathological cell and tissue damage due to excessive and prolonged immune reactions and inflammation. There is also the need to avoid the immune system reacting against self and causing autoimmunity. Tregs play a key role (direct contact, secretion of IL-10, TGF-β), as well as expression of CTLA-4 by T lymphocytes (negative signalling and/or sequestration of CD80/86 costimulatory molecules on DCs).
- Control of the adaptive immune response is seen in the mechanisms of immune tolerance which operate mechanistically at the level of the central lymphoid organs (thymus and bone marrow), and also within the peripheral tissues against any clones with significant anti-self reactivity.
- A fundamental biological process, which is exploited by the immune system to control and/or destroy potentially self-reactive cells and to terminate clonal expansion after destroying microbes, is the process of apoptosis (programmed cell death—genetically controlled). This fundamental biological process is also key in many aspects of developmental biology and in the control of emergence of cancerous cells. Autophagy (controlled, autologous removal of intracellular components) is another important regulatory homeostatic process.
- Despite attempts at efficient immune regulation, damaging autoimmunity occurs in some individuals. These destructive anti-self responses are associated with clones of autoreactive T and B cells. These are associated with aberrant genes within individuals (many linked to the MHC); there is also linkage to aberrant immune responses to environmental agents (e.g. bacteria, viruses, chemicals).
- Detailed understanding of elements of the immune system has increased opportunities for immune modulation of deleterious autoimmune responses by way of use of biological response modifiers, including therapeutic MABs and cytokines and other immune suppressive agents, which target different aspects of signal transduction, cytokine responsiveness, and gene activation events.
- The nervous system (central and peripheral) with the HPA plays a major role in modulating responses of innate immunity and of subsequent downstream adaptive immunity. Conversely, the immune system can modulate brain cell development and plasticity. Cytokines (IL-1, IL-6, TNF-α) bind to receptors in the hypothalamus, glial cells express TLRs and respond to DAMPs by producing cytokines. $CD4^+$ Th1 and $CD8^+$ CTLs (and B cells) can enter the brain through a defective BBB (post infection, ischaemia) to induce CNS autoimmune diseases.

- Damaging reactions of the immune system have been classified in terms of the hypersensitivity reactions of Gell and Coombs (types I–IV). These mechanistic descriptions relate to damaging responses to drugs and anaesthetic agents; they are seen in cases of latex allergy, and are implicated in the damaging reactions, which are the expressions of autoimmunity (reactions to self antigens).
- Understanding of the allergic type I response has led to long-standing use of hyposensitization/desensitization approaches. Newer methods are being developed which exploit the targeting of elements of innate immunity (e.g. TLRs) as well as targeting clones of T and B cells in new immunotherapeutic approaches.
- The rapid development of molecular genetic techniques over recent decades has allowed the generation of a range of biological agents which are transforming aspects of clinical medicine. There is an ever-increasing range of MABs, many of the human type, which are finding their way into clinical practice, along with other biological constructs such as fusion proteins and Ig replacement therapy. They are being used in a wide range of diseases including cancers, autoimmune diseases, chronic inflammatory disorders, and certain infections.

Introduction

The seed of immunology took root in the fertile studies of infectious diseases in the 18th and 19th centuries. In the early 20th century it grew as a sturdy scientific sapling under the care of the immunochemists with continued input from microbiologists. The astute observations of Edward Jenner that recovery from cowpox protected against smallpox, together with his empirical immunization of James Phipps, laid the scientific basis of vaccination. This was an 18th-century validation of the observations made in ancient China and of the risky practice of variolation (using the fluid from smallpox vesicles). Mechnikov's studies of the engulfment of foreign (non-self) material by the leucocytes of the larvae of starfish defined the process of phagocytosis, a key element of the cellular components of innate immunity, preserved through evolution. His contemporaries, Erlich and von Behring, conceptualized, defined, and exploited the role of serum antibodies to protect individuals from diphtheria and tetanus by the use of antitoxins. These latter studies defined the key roles of antibodies in the evolutionary development of the much younger system of adaptive/acquired immunity.

By the 1970s, immunology emerged as a fully grown science, with extensive branches in immunochemistry, cellular immunology, immunobiology, immunogenetics, clinical immunology and immunopathology. Studies up to and beyond this period focused mainly on aspects of adaptive immunity with innate immunity being the junior partner. However, some 20 years ago, Charles Janeway put forward the concept that cells of innate immunity could sense and react to non-self molecules and, in so doing, elaborate responses against non-self and concomitantly influence and instruct the development of adaptive immune responses [1,2]. Thus, studies of the whole and integrated immune system became reinvigorated; the aim of this chapter is to present this modern, comprehensive, and integrated immunology.

In the latter part of the 20th century, immunology continued to extend its branches and develop new blossoms: the biotechnologies of hybridomas, T cell and gene cloning, peptide synthesis, and the use of transgenic and chimeric animal models enriched and expanded its development. An essential set of ingredients has continually contributed to the development of immunology. These are represented by original concepts, imaginative experimental research, astute clinical observations, and technological advances. The latter have continued with the sequencing of a range of whole genomes (including those of humans) and with the application of postgenomic technologies (proteomics, metabolomics, transcriptomics, and whole genome-wide sequencing) to detect polymorphisms; in particular, single nucleotide polymorphisms (SNPs) [3–5]. This has contributed to the establishment of modern immunology in the 21st century, commensurate with the developments in information technology (see Chapter 9). Computer search engines collect and collate information on the immune system. Descriptions are found of the complex interactions between the host's immune system and the myriad commensal microorganisms that populate the skin, gastrointestinal, and upper respiratory tracts, as well as the responses to potential pathogens. Hyperlinks describe the discovery of the *AIRE* gene in the thymus and its contribution to the generation of immune effector and regulatory cells. Other links outline the use of systems biology and mathematical modelling to predict intracellular signalling pathways, transducing information from outside the immune cell (responding to a microbe) to modify gene functions within the cell [6]. The systems-theoretical approaches are informed by data from the recent high-resolution sequence maps of the human genome (published 2001–2003), which identify more than 500 genes encoding enzymes involved in signal transduction. Laboratory experiments follow the modelling, which use recently defined small interfering RNAs (siRNAs) to block gene functions in cell lines, as well as *in vivo*, in chimeric and transgenic animal models. The experiments have yielded a plethora and a hierarchy of signalling pathways involved in immune cell functions and indicate potential new therapeutic targets to beneficially enhance or suppress immune functions in a wide range of diseases and disorders. The computer search exemplifies modern scientific discovery which is providing ideas and tools to enhance understanding, diagnosis, and treatment of a wide range of diseases, translating basic science into applications in clinical medicine. The clinician, on seeing the data on signalling pathways, is reminded of the recent surgical case that required emergency surgery. Postsurgical interactions with pathologists and other laboratory-based scientists indicate that the patient had a defect in a key signalling molecule which led to a defect in the immune system, and ultimately an overwhelming bacterial infection. Collaborative studies of the patient's cells and surgically derived tissues result in the precise molecular and genetic definition of the defect and a more fundamental understanding of the molecular interactions and possible novel therapeutic options for the future. This flow of activity indicates the bidirectional nature of modern translational research in immunology and, more generally, in biomedical research.

The immune system evolved as a defence against infectious diseases in order to maintain the homeostasis of the organism. Clinical observations of individuals with congenital or acquired defects of their immune system strongly support this postulate.

Furthermore, classical experiments performed with laboratory animals, resulting in controlled deletion and replacement of elements of the immune system and, more recently, with the knock-in and knock-out of genetic elements, further illustrate the basis of an efficient immune system. Humans or experimental animals who are immune deficient experience a combination of serious, persistent, unusual, or recurrent microbial infections. It is also noted that in some situations they have an increased incidence of certain tumours, particularly lymphomas and carcinomas, and these tumours often show more aggressive behaviour than in the normal population.

Immunology also provides significant knowledge and understanding regarding transplantation and malignancy. Historical studies of transplantation and, more recently, the use of nonautologous stem cell therapy for treating human diseases, have indicated that the major barrier to successful use of transplantation is the host immune system (see Chapter 3). New modalities for treating cancers have emerged from our better understanding of the events that induce, amplify, coordinate, and control immune responses. Attempts at cancer immunotherapy are proving to be more than abstract and indeed are now becoming a reality (see Chapter 4). The outstanding success of vaccinations to bacterial and viral pathogens (note the worldwide elimination of smallpox and also the imminent eradication of poliomyelitis), together with a deeper understanding of the cellular interactions in the immune system, has led to reinvigorated attempts to develop new vaccines for more complex infectious diseases, such as those associated with HIV and the malaria parasite (see 'HIV, AIDS, and the surgeon', below). A better understanding of these diseases, and of the cell and molecular mechanisms of immunology, is suggesting that useful vaccines will emerge in the near future. Another area that is being explored is the generation of vaccines against noninfectious diseases, such as multiple sclerosis (MS) and type 1 diabetes. These so-called autoimmune diseases occur where the immune system acts against self, as opposed to non-self, antigens. The clones of immune cells that are identified and thought to mediate these diseases are being targeted as if they were pathogens. Therapeutic vaccines for allergic diseases are being used and evaluated. There are currently useful, albeit limited, specific immunotherapeutic vaccines for house dust mite, grass pollen, and a few other allergens (see 'Allergy, immunotherapy, and new vaccines', below).

Immune cells and their products can now be expanded and obtained routinely in large quantities by *in vitro* and *ex vivo* cell culture systems and by generation *de novo* in the laboratory by molecular genetic approaches—monoclonal antibodies (MABs) from human, mouse, and other sources. These approaches have already yielded, and continue to yield, very useful new agents to aid in the diagnosis and treatment of a range of diseases (see 'Monoclonals and other biological therapies', below). These new immunotherapies continue to expand exponentially; indeed, currently they represent the largest number of new medicines (so-called biologicals) being introduced into clinical use.

Essential understanding of immunology requires knowledge of its nomenclature and the principle components of the immune system, and an understanding of the general responses elicited. This helps to define the types of immune responses which protect against infections by pathogenic microbes and non-self antigens, and the mechanisms involved. Similarly, pathology-inducing aberrant immune responses, such as allergy to seemingly innocuous environmental agents and autoimmunity against self molecules, are better understood (see Chapter 8).

Overview of immunology

Introduction

Historically, immunity has been classified as innate and adaptive immunity. Innate immunity uses recognition mechanisms encoded directly by the host genome, necessitating the use of a limited repertoire of recognition structures that identify generic features shared by major groups of pathogens and non-self molecules. Adaptive immunity, in contrast, uses randomly generated recognition structures expressed as soluble molecules (antibodies) or as surface antigen receptors on B or T cells (BCRs and TCRs, respectively) that recognize their target (antigen) with exquisite specificity. The innate and adaptive components of the immune system complement and interact with each other to achieve an effective and integrated defence of the body.

Innate and adaptive immunity

Innate immunity

Innate or natural immunity is encountered as the initial, early phase, first line of defence by the host. It is made up of the host physical barriers, consisting of epithelial linings of the body such as skin, respiratory tract, and gastrointestinal tract (GIT), together with soluble factors and various bone-marrow-derived leucocytes (including phagocytes) found in blood and body fluids, and widely distributed in tissue sites. When foreign, non-self agents, such as microbes and their toxins, breach the epithelial defences they encounter molecules and cells of innate immunity which recognize them as non-self. Microbes have molecular structures that are conserved across a broad range of organisms and are not generally found associated with the host/mammalian cells. These structures are referred to as pathogen-associated molecular patterns (PAMPs). They are recognized by various receptor molecules present on and within a wide range of host cells, including cells of innate immunity (see Chapter 5). These receptors (predicted by Janeway) are referred to as pattern recognition receptors (PRRs) [2]. Toll-like receptors (TLRs), nucleotide-binding domain (NOD)-like receptors (NLRs), and retinoic-acid-inducible gene 1 receptors (RLRs) are well-documented PRRs that bind a range of Gram-positive and Gram-negative bacteria, fungi, protozoa, viruses, DNA, and RNA (Table 1.1). PRRs have also been shown to (directly or indirectly) recognize products of damaged, injured, or stressed host cells. Such compromised cells are said to release so-called 'danger signals' or alarmins (see Chapter 2). They are also called danger (or damage)-associated molecular patterns (DAMPs), in accord with Matzinger's 'danger signal' hypothesis (see Chapter 4).

Innate immunity mechanisms provide rapid defence against non-self microbes (antigens), preventing or eradicating early infection. Adaptive immunity responds more slowly; it is mediated by lymphocytes and their products. Antibodies are effective at eliminating or blocking extracellular microbes and antigens. T lymphocyte responses are effective in dealing with many intracellular microbes and antigens.

Table 1.1 Cells, receptors, and soluble factors of innate and adaptive immunity

	Innate immunity	Adaptive immunity
Cells	Phagocytes-macrophages, monocytes, polymorphs, DCs (APCs), mast cells, basophils, platelets, NK and NK T cells, γδ T cells	Lymphocytes, T and B cells
Cell receptors for microbes/ antigens	Limited numbers of receptors encoded in the germ line (inborn): TLRs, scavenger receptors, NLRs, complement receptors, mannose receptors, dectin receptors, Fc receptors	TCRs BCRs Vast numbers of receptors generated by somatic recombination events (non-germ line).
Soluble factors	Complement, cytokines, chemokines, IFNs (type 1 and type 2), acute phase proteins, lysozyme, collectins, mucins	Antibodies—IgM, IgG, IgA, IgD, IgE Interleukins (cytokines).
Other factors	Natural barriers, epithelial lining cells of the GIT, respiratory and urogenital tracts and skin; natural antibiotic peptides (defensins); normal commensal microbiota	
Kinetics of response after exposure to microbes	Rapid, immediate—minutes to hours	Over several days

APCs, antigen-presenting cells; BCRs, B cell receptors; DCs, denditic cells; GIT, gastrointestinal tract; IFN, interferon; NLRs, NOD-like receptors; TCRs, T cell receptors; TLRs, Toll-like receptors.

There are significant bidirectional interactions between elements of innate and adaptive immunity.

When encountered in abnormal amounts or in nonphysiological sites internally, DAMPS are believed to trigger inflammatory responses and, in some cases, downstream adaptive immune responses. Examples of such molecules include uric acid, heat shock proteins (HSPs), S100 proteins, serum amyloid A, DNA, human mobility group box protein 1 (HMGB1), and probably interleukin-33 (IL-33). HMGB1 is usually sequestered within the nucleus, but in damaged and stressed cells it can leak from the nucleus into the cytoplasm and escape from the cell. Indeed, DNA linked with HMGB1 has been shown experimentally to stimulate significant inflammatory and immune reactions, contrary to the concept that DNA is an inert molecule. These observations are helping to define inflammatory and immune reactions that are induced by abnormal amounts or abnormal locations of self molecules [7–10]. Recent research has demonstrated that, following major trauma, release of mitochondrial DNA and other DAMPs triggers severe, widespread inflammation—the systemic inflammatory response syndrome (SIRS) (see Chapter 2). Following the recognition of PAMPs/DAMPs by PRRs, the activation of intracellular signalling pathways often follows, resulting in gene activation and the production of molecules such as cytokines and chemokines (see 'Cytokines, chemokines, and signalling', below).

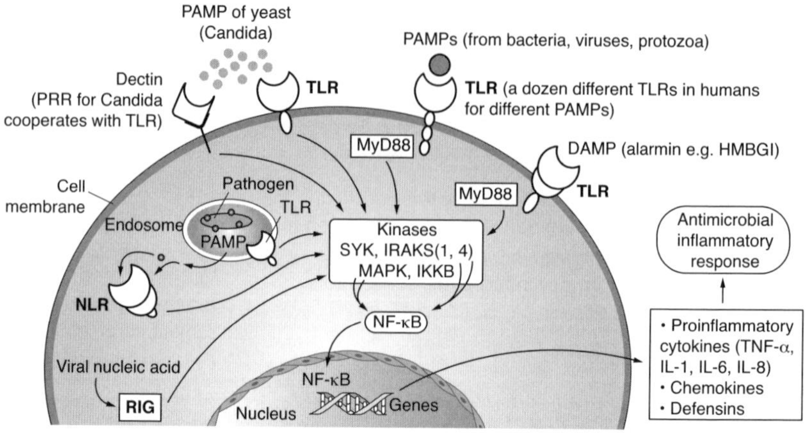

Fig. 1.1 Cell-associated PRRs (TLRs, NLRs, RIG, dectin) bind extra and intracellularly to various PAMPs or DAMPS (alarmins, e.g. HMGB1). Binding leads to signal transduction using key adaptor molecules such as MyD88 which facilitate downstream kinase (IRAK, TRAF, MAPK) phosphorylation leading to activation of the transcription factor NF-κB which translocates to the nucleus to activate/induce its target genes. Gene activation results in production of proteins (e.g. cytokines, chemokines, defensins) that mediate antimicrobial inflammatory responses. These innate responses are rapid in onset and aim to localize, control and/or eliminate the infection. Excessive PRRs systemically can contribute to shock, e.g. in sepsis or severe trauma. DAMPS, danger/damage-associated molecular patterns; NLR, NOD (nucleotide-binding domain)-like receptor; PAMPs, pathogen-associated molecular patterns; PRRs, pattern recognition receptors; RIG, retinoic acid-inducible gene; TLR, Toll-like receptor.

These pathways ultimately generate reactions which are expressed as inflammation aimed at destroying or containing the microbe in a controlled and localized reaction. The early events recognizing non-self and other 'danger signals' lead to signal transduction, the engagement of intracellular adaptor proteins, such as MyD88, and the activation of enzyme cascade systems, particularly tyrosine kinases and phosphatases. Subsequently, activation of transcription factors, such as nuclear factor kappa light-chain-enhancer of activated B cell (NF-κB) and their interaction with nuclear genes, results in the production of activated gene products such as cytokines and chemokines which induce inflammatory responses (Figure 1.1). The interleukin-1 receptor (IL-1R) belongs to the superfamily of TLRs, sharing a common molecular feature called the Toll-IL-1R domain. IL-1 is a key cytokine in innate and adaptive immune responses, and in integrating the two.

Kinases and phosphatases are responsible, respectively, for the attachment of phosphate groups to proteins and their removal, the major mechanism used by cells to regulate and coordinate intracellular processes and protein function. This reversible intracellular protein phosphorylation is at the core of the mechanisms involved in a range of diseases where inflammation (especially chronic inflammation) is now recognized as a major contributor. Diseases such as cancer and autoimmune diseases are being targeted in pharmaceutical R&D strategies aimed at developing drug inhibitors, particularly of protein kinases. In the past decade, some ten orally active anticancer drugs, mainly broad-acting kinase inhibitors, have been approved for clinical use, in the treatment of leukaemia and lung cancer (see Chapter 4). Many others are being clinically investigated in immune and inflammatory disorders, including new immunosuppressants for use in transplantation and autoimmune diseases (see Chapters 3 and 8, respectively).

The acute inflammatory response is a primary outcome of innate immunity. Many of the endstage effector protective responses which characterize adaptive immunity are also expressed in inflammatory processes. Damage to host cells and perturbation of homeostasis by microbes or their products and the downstream enzyme cascade signal transduction events result in the release of cytokines as well as other proinflammatory molecules. These include histamine, leukotrienes (LTs), and prostaglandins (PGs), which aim to contain the microbe, preventing the spread of infection and also, subsequently, promoting the healing and repair of tissues. The inflammatory response is characterized by classical clinical features in tissues—localized increased blood flow, redness, swelling and, in some situations, pain associated with the vasodilatation induced by the proinflammatory mediators and cytokines released. The localized, protective inflammation induced by the immune response often occurs without being clinically noticeable.

Cytokines, produced by many cells, are small polypeptides which regulate immunity and inflammation. Following their induction by the immune response to microbes and antigens, they act over a short range, have short half-lives, and are highly biologically active, being effective at very low concentrations. They are also seen as hormones of the immune and inflammatory response—some cytokines enter the vasculature and can act at distant sites, e.g. liver and brain. These properties of cytokines help to limit and regulate the expression of inflammation they induce. Cytokines act by binding to their specific membrane receptors that transduce signals into cells causing gene transcription and expression of their encoded products. Cytokines with chemotactic activity, attracting blood leucocytes into sites of tissue infection and/or damage along a concentration gradient, are called chemokines.

The term cytokine is generic, covering historical nomenclatures for molecules including lymphokines (cytokines produced by lymphocytes), ILs (cytokines produced by leucocytes and facilitating their interactions), and monokines (produced by monocytes). Nearly all cells can produce cytokines in response to appropriate stimuli. Cytokines show autocrine actions by acting on the same cells that produce them; their action on other nearby cells is termed paracrine activity. In this chapter, reference will be made to various cytokines, including tumour necrosis factor alpha (TNF-α), ILs (IL-1, IL-6, etc.), and chemokines (CC and CXC chemokines)—see later. The cytokines and other mediators released by responding innate immune cells such as epithelial cells, tissue resident macrophages, dendritic cells (DCs), and mast cells act on local endothelial cells lining the vasculature. They induce the expression and up-regulation on these endothelial cells of adhesion molecules, such as selectins and integrins. Adhesion molecules are proteins/glycoproteins that bind cells to each other and also mediate cellular interactions with the extracellular matrix. Similar adhesion molecules, some of which act as counter-ligands (L) for the endothelial molecules, are also induced or up-regulated and activated on leucocytes within the vasculature. The release of mediators and cytokines thus promotes fast responses, including vasodilatation, the activation of leucocytes, their margination and binding to the endothelium, and their transmigration from the vasculature into the site of tissue infection and/or damage. The leucocytes (resident and newly arrived) within the tissues phagocytose the microbes, become activated, and release their intracellular toxic granules into endophagosomal vacuoles to destroy or contain the phagocytosed organisms. Leucocytes also release mediators, cytokines, and chemokines which further amplify the inflammatory response. The recognition events (via various cell receptor systems) and signal transduction associated with proinflammatory cytokines and chemokine production also enhance phagocytosis and microbicidal killing within the endophagosomal compartments by way of lysosomal enzymes, reactive oxygen species (ROSs), hydrogen peroxide (H_2O_2), and inducible nitric oxide synthases (iNOSs) (see Figure 1.2). Recently, an additional and important cytoplasmic complex that contributes to the inflammatory response has been defined. A cytoplasmic multiprotein

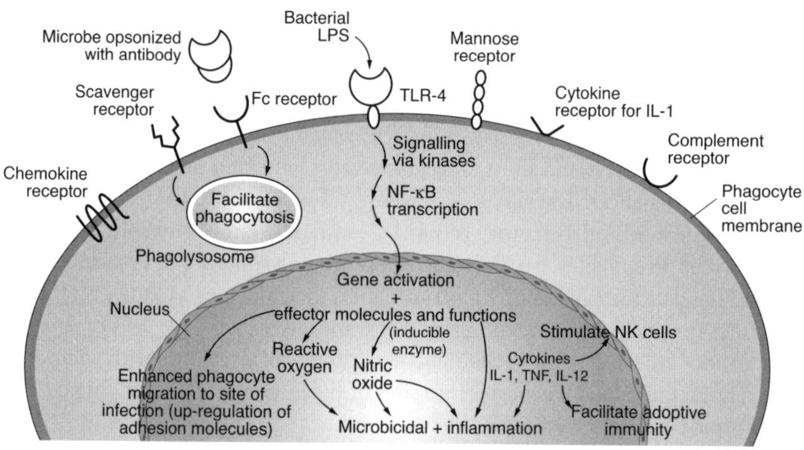

Fig. 1.2 Phagocytes have a range of receptors for recognition of microbes and their products, as well as for molecules produced in the inflammatory response such as chemokines and cytokines. Ligands binding to these various receptors signal and activate cellular responses in phagocytes to stimulate inflammation and prevent infection or eliminate the microbes. Phagocyte receptors shown are the mannose receptor (detects terminal mannose sugars on microbes), TLR4 which binds bacterial LPS, IL-1R, scavenger receptor, Fc receptor for immunoglobulin (Ig) and chemokine receptors. The receptors use varying signalling pathways and activate several transcription factors including NF-κB. The effector molecules and functions generated include reactive oxygen species (ROSs), nitric oxide (NO), cytokines (e.g. TNF, IL-1, IL-12), all of which contribute to killing or containing microbes by way of inflammatory responses (innate immunity). They also help to prime the host for adaptive immune responses, e.g. the role of IL-12 acting on DCs and lymphocytes. DC, dendritic cell; IL-1R, interleukin-1 receptor; LPS, lipopolysaccharide; TLR4, Toll-like receptor 4.

complex, termed the inflammasome, is an enzyme system which leads to the processing and secretion of the key proinflammatory cytokine IL-1, generated from its precursor molecule pro-IL-1 [8]. The multiprotein complex inflammasome interacts and synergizes with TLRs and NLRs in combating pathogens. Inflammasomes have also been shown to be activated by nonmicrobial substances such as uric acid (associated with gout), silica, aluminium salts, and asbestos. Clearly, there is a need for tight control to avoid excessive damage to the host. Indeed, diseases have now been described, some of which are called autoinflammatory, which involve spontaneous, inappropriate, and recurrent activation of the inflammasome (see Chapter 8).

Poorly controlled and persistent chronic inflammatory responses can also contribute to the induction of neoplasia (see Chapter 4). Clinical and epidemiological evidence has established the increased risk of developing colon cancer in patients with long-standing inflammatory disease of the GIT, especially ulcerative colitis (see Chapter 8). Chronic inflammatory skin diseases, such as lichen sclerosus and lichen planus, are known to be associated with an increased risk (up to 5%) of developing squamous carcinoma. Recent experimental studies have documented, at the molecular level, mechanistic models explaining the links between inflammation and cancer induction. A central link is the transcription factor NF-κB which is activated in innate immune responses to generate proinflammatory mediators [11]. Persistent activation of NF-κB induces antiapoptotic gene functions and also induces excessive ROSs, both of which have been shown to favour the emergence of cancers in model systems (Figure 1.3). More recently, persistent NF-κB activity has been shown directly to inhibit the gene *TP53* (encoding protein p53) (the master antitumour gateway tumour suppressor gene) and chronically to elevate IL-6 which is thought to favour continual cell proliferation leading to possible mutated premalignant cells. Targeting inflammation is a therapeutic option being pursued in the prevention of oncogenesis.

Concomitant with the migration of leucocytes to extravascular sites there is a leakage of soluble factors from the blood compartment to the site of tissue invasion by microbes/antigens. Among the soluble mediators released are components of the complement system and C-reactive protein (CRP), both synthesized mainly in the liver and in some leucocytes, which have inherent potent antimicrobial activity. Clinically, they are characterized as part of the acute-phase protein response, along with serum amyloid A, α_1-acid glycoprotein, and fibrinogen. Activation of the complement system amplifies immune responses. Activated components bind to the surface of microbes (opsonization) and enhance their ingestion by the phagocytic leucocytes which have receptors for these complement components. CRP, used in clinical practice to monitor acute inflammation (trauma, surgery, burns, etc.) and infection, also has a direct role as an antimicrobial agent by recognizing and binding to PAMPs of a range of microbes; CRP is an example of a soluble form of a PRR. Phagocytes also have receptors for parts of the CRP molecule not bound to the microbe to further enhance phagocytosis and inflammation. Additionally, CRP complexed to microbes can activate the complement system via the binding of the first component of the complement system (C1q) to further amplify inflammation. Recent evidence has linked chronic elevation of serum CRP levels in the apparently clinically well

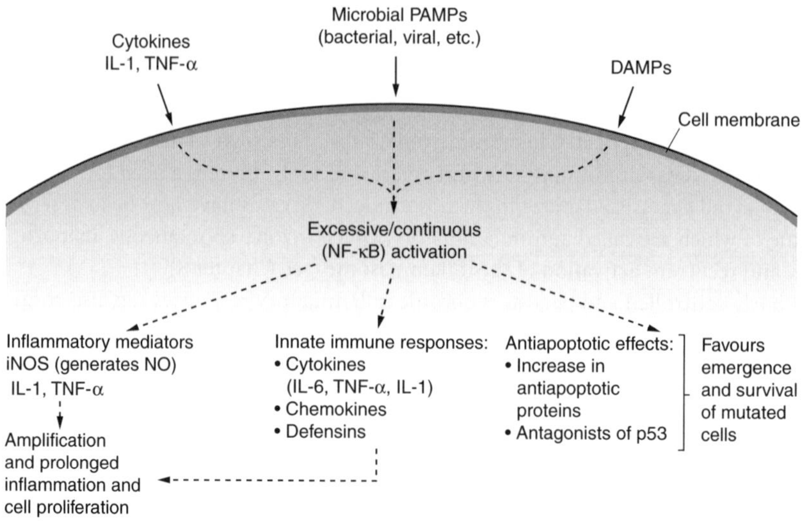

Fig. 1.3 Multiple and persistent cell stimuli (e.g. from cytokines, microbes) activate the transcription factor NF-κB, a key molecule linking excessive prolonged inflammatory responses with the process of oncogenesis. Prolonged inflammatory responses favour cellular proliferation that together with concurrent induction of antiapoptotic processes by NF-κB stimulation, favours the emergence and survival of mutated cells—a prerequisite for the development of neoplasia. DAMPs, danger/damage-associated molecular patterns; iNOS, inducible nitric oxide synthetase; PAMPs, pathogen-associated molecular patterns.

individual with an increased risk of cardiovascular disease, independent of the well-established factors such as hypertension and smoking.

The early recognition events—signal transduction and cytokine–chemokine production responses of innate immune cells—which generate controlled and protective inflammation, are crucial for host survival. Indeed, it has been suggested that (contrary to long-held views) innate immunity may be as important as adaptive immunity in terms of survival, if not more so. It is known that defects of innate immunity are associated with severe morbidity and mortality. If the innate immune response does not completely eliminate pathogens, it nevertheless gives time and instruction (direct cell–cell interactions of DCs with lymphocytes, and by the actions of cytokines produced by innate cells on lymphocytes) to develop an effective adaptive (T and B cell) immune response [12].

Adaptive immunity is also responsible for protective immune responses against non-self antigens (e.g. microorganisms). However, induction of the adaptive response is considerably slower (days) than that of innate immunity, which tends to elicit immediate or very early inflammatory responses. Furthermore, adaptive immunity shows qualitative and quantitative changes following subsequent encounters with the same antigen. This is in contrast with innate immune responses, which are stereotypical and essentially nonchanging generic responses. Innate immunity does not confer long-lasting immunity, unlike adaptive immunity which exhibits the property of immunological memory for previously encountered antigens.

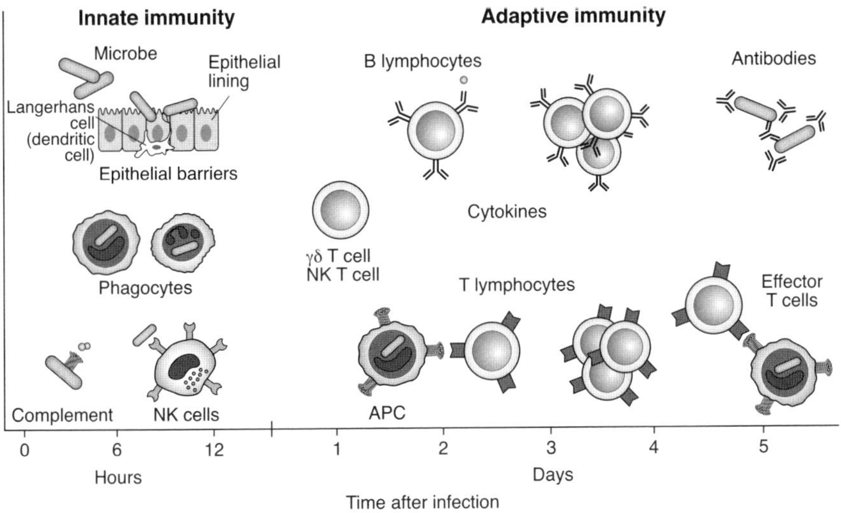

Fig. 1.4 Cells and the kinetics of innate and adaptive immunity. The cells and mechanisms of innate immunity provide a very rapid, immediate response against infections involving cytokines, phagocyte killing of engulfed microbes, and features characteristic of acute inflammation. T and B lymphocytes mediate the slower responding adaptive immune response (over days) involving T cell effector responses, generation of memory T cells, antibody production by B lymphocytes and also generation of memory B cells. γδ T cells and NK T cells have responses intermediate in time between innate and adaptive immunity (hours) and they generate a range of cytokines. NK T cells also exhibit some cytotoxicity. APC, antigen-presenting cell.

Figure 1.4 schematically represents the key elements of innate and adaptive immune responses to a microbe (antigen) and the kinetics involved in the response.

Figure 1.5 illustrates the role of adhesion molecules and cytokines (chemokines) in the attraction of polymorphonuclear leucocytes to the site of infection in an innate immune response. Similar mechanisms are used by lymphocytes in adaptive immunity to migrate from blood vessels into tissues to interact with antigens [13]. Different families of adhesion molecules and chemokines/receptors are used in lymphocyte–endothelial interactions (see 'Clusters of differentiation and monoclonal antibodies', below). The functional roles of adhesion molecules (e.g. the heterodimeric integrins with α/β-chains), apart from cell migration, include cell survival, differentiation, and proliferation. These molecules are becoming attractive targets for therapeutic strategies for cancer, autoimmunity, and other inflammatory diseases, and in enhancement of wound healing (see 'Immunopathology and tissue damage, immune deficiency, and immunotherapeutics', below).

Immune reactions use controlled inflammation to beneficial effect, facilitated by the properties of many cytokines and chemokines acting at the local site of microbial/antigen invasion. However, certain cytokines, in particular IL-1, IL-6, and TNF-α, produced by localized innate immune responses, also act at sites distant from the

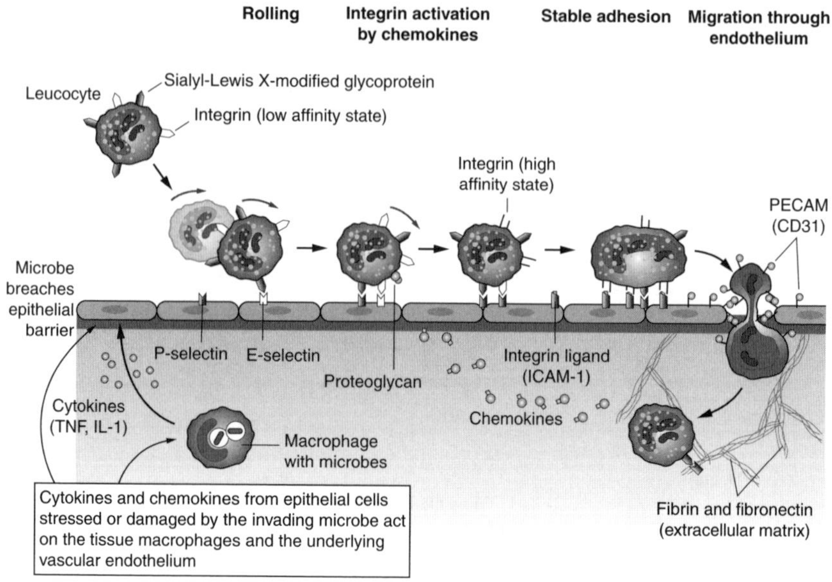

Fig. 1.5 Recruitment of the acute inflammatory response by innate immunity to combat microbes that breach the first line of defence, the epithelial cell lining. The activation of cells produces cytokines and chemokines, resulting in increased vascular permeability and the migration and activation of leucocytes that enter the extracellular site of microbial invasion. ICAM-1, intercellular cell adhesion molecule-1; PECAM, platelet endothelial cell adhesion molecule.

local site. They can enter the bloodstream in small quantities, travel to the liver, and there induce activation of hepatocytes. These hepatocytes produce acute-phase proteins, such as CRP, α_1-antitrypsin, and serum amyloid A, which in turn target a wider range of tissues. They can be detected in blood after the induction of innate responses to microbes. IL-1, TNF-α and other bioactive proteins from the liver account for the many systemic manifestations of infection. Thus, TNF-α acts on the hypothalamus, inducing fever, and is partly responsible for cachexia by stimulation of catabolism in fat and muscle cells.

Innate–adaptive inmmune interactions

Both types of immunity (innate and adaptive) interact in synergistic and bidirectional modes in protecting the host. Hence, cytokines and cells active in innate immunity (macrophages, DCs, neutrophils, mast and epithelial cells), apart from their direct antimicrobial actions, also send signals that help adaptive immunity to respond in a way best suited to eliminate microbes, wherever they are encountered in the host. Some microbes (e.g. bacteria and fungi) can be found in extracellular sites and in blood. Others are found intracellularly (e.g. viruses and some bacteria—mycobacteria, salmonella) and are dealt with by differing adaptive immune responses which are partly shaped by elements of innate immunity (see later).

Cells of the mononuclear phagocyte system, apart from their ingestion and intracellular destruction of microbes, play a key role between innate and adaptive immunity as antigen-presenting cells (APCs). APCs, best exemplified by DCs, sample and take up antigens in peripheral tissues, process them and then migrate, transporting antigens to lymph nodes and other aggregates of immune cells in sites such as the GIT and respiratory tract. APCs, thus, communicate directly with lymphocytes in helping to initiate adaptive immunity. Cells of the phagocytic lineage—macrophages and neutrophils—are also active as effectors in destroying microorganisms when recruited by products of responding T and B lymphocytes. Products of complement activation can enhance B lymphocyte responses in their production of antibodies. The cytokines TNF-α and IL-1 have direct effects on T and B lymphocyte responses. The details of these interactions of innate and adaptive immunity are expanded in subsequent sections.

The protective mechanisms of innate and adaptive immunity can, in certain situations, become dysfunctional and induce significant tissue damage. These maladaptions may be facilitated by host genetic factors, by the portal of entry and virulence of microbes, or by the presence of comorbid condition of individuals. The consequences of severe trauma or sepsis are due in part to widespread uncontrolled activation of elements of innate immunity. This results in nonphysiological high levels of production of cytokines, chemokines, and other proinflammatory mediators, with marked perturbations *in vivo* of inflammatory and coagulation pathways (see Chapters 2 and 5). This 'cytokine storm' has been documented to result in the release of more than 100 inflammatory mediators whose multiple interactions are often lethal. Primary contributors to this serious pathological state are TNF-α and IL-6. Not surprisingly, both these cytokines (along with others) are being investigated as therapeutic targets for these severe disorders. Real and potential pandemics associated with influenza viruses such as H1N1 and H5N1 are believed to be particularly serious. This is because of the virus's potential to markedly dysregulate innate cytokine responses in the lungs from protective to pathological levels in individuals without background protective adaptive immunity, who may succumb to the severe inflammation and/or secondary bacterial pneumonias. Maladapted adaptive immunity is seen in the immunopathological lesions associated with allergic diseases and autoimmune disorders, defined mechanistically in the Gell and Coombs nomenclature of hypersensitivity reactions, types I–IV (see 'Immunopathological processes: hypersensitivity (types I–IV) and tissue damage', below).

Fundamental to all immune responses in the host is a marked proliferation of cells induced by perturbations of immune homeostasis caused by invading antigens or microbes. There is a need for mechanisms to restore that homeostatis after the microbe or antigenic insult is eliminated or contained. A crucial process to ensure maintenance of physiological homeostasis is apoptosis—a process of controlled, genetically regulated cell death. Apoptosis is central also in lymphocyte development, in controlling and regulating immune responsiveness to non-self, and, in some situations, to self molecules. It ensures the death and clearance of cells without exciting destructive inflammation, in contrast with necrotic cell death which sends 'danger' signals that trigger inflammation. Failure of apoptotic mechanisms is considered a significant contributor in the development of many cancers and some autoimmune disorders (see 'Autoimmunity', below). Accordingly, manipulation of apoptotic mechanisms is being utilized to control pathological inflammation and to enhance cancer therapy and immunotherapy.

Adaptive immunity

The characteristic features of adaptive immunity are its specificity, its memory, and its diversity. The cells responsible for these features within the immune response are the T and B lymphocytes. They provide the basis whereby entry of non-self components (e.g. microbes, proteins, chemicals, collectively termed antigens) will lead to specific recognition via the TCRs and BCRs. Most importantly, if a member of the original group of antigens is encountered again it will be recognized specifically, and a second encounter will lead to the enhanced response. This implies that after the first encounter a definite and predetermined perturbation occurred in the homeostasis of the organism and its immune system which resulted in the generation of a 'memory' for that non-self substance. Following the primary response and the secondary memory-based response, both of exquisite specificity for the exciting antigen, specific augmentation of the effects of the responses occurs, leading to the destruction or containment of the antigen. These augmenting effectors, recruited by and interacting with the specific immune factors from lymphocytes, include complement and phagocytic cells, as described for innate immune responses (see 'Innate immunity', above). These interactions result in the features of an inflammatory response induced by adaptive immunity. Inflammation is thus a common final pathway for eliminating antigens, as described in the section on innate immunity. Some antibody responses can block and neutralize microbes directly, without recruiting elements of innate immunity.

Hence, inflammation, when induced in a controlled and regulated manner, can be seen as the beneficial final pathway of an efficient and responsive immune system. The products of T and B lymphocyte reactions in adaptive immunity and the effector mechanisms they generate are responsible for cell-mediated immunity (CMI) and humoral immunity, respectively.

CMI is associated with and is transferable by intact T lymphocytes (classified generally as having two major subsets, $CD4^+$ and $CD8^+$ T cells) which recognize and respond predominantly to peptide antigens complexed with self HLA molecules on host cells.

Humoral immunity results in the production of fluid-phase antibodies (generated from B cells and derived plasma cells) which interact specifically with antigens in extracellular locations.

CMI and humoral immune responses of adaptive immunity are directed against non-self molecules, i.e. antigens. Pre-eminent antigens are components of potential pathogens (bacteria, viruses, fungi, and protozoa) which attempt to enter the host by breaching the epithelial lining of portals of entry in the GIT, respiratory tract, and the skin; or antigens injected for medical interventions such as vaccinations. Complex antigens, such as those of attenuated microbes or intact inactivated pathogens or their protein products (e.g. toxoids), are commonly used in vaccines such as the MMR (for mumps, measles, and rubella), DTP (diphtheria, tetanus, and pertussis), and BCG (bacillus Calmette–Guérin; for tuberculosis), and pneumoccocal, and haemophilus immunization regimens.

Antigens are typically proteins of high molecular weight which induce immune responses and are recognized by and interact with the products of immune responses, in particular, those associated with T and B lymphocytes of adaptive immunity. Less commonly, antigens can be sugars/polysaccharides of microbes, lipids, or other chemical groupings. These latter antigens, along with the protein antigens, tend to induce and be recognized by B lymphocyte antibody responses. In contrast, T lymphocyte responses are induced predominantly by peptide antigens from proteins (from extracellular and intracellular sources). These are recognized by those T cells in complexes with self molecules encoded in a chromosomal region in humans called the major histocompatibility complex (MHC) (see 'Major histocompatibility complex', below). The encoded products of the MHC, which bind the peptide antigens (ingested and processed in APCs and other cells), are called human leucocyte antigens (HLAs). The key HLA molecules that present peptides to T cells are termed HLA class I and class II, which interact with $CD8^+$ and $CD4^+$ T cells, respectively. As in many areas of science, exceptions are found to these general principles of antigen recognition. Some so-called 'unconventional' T cells, such as NK T cells and $\gamma\delta$ T cells, can recognize and respond to lipid/glycolipid antigens presented by non-classical HLA molecules, such as the CD1 molecular complex (see 'Effector cells and receptors', below).

The central role of lymphocytes in adaptive immunity was demonstrated by classic experiments which depleted animals of lymphocytes by various manoeuvres such as chronic thoracic duct drainage, surgical extirpation of lymphoid organs, or transfer of lymphoid cells. Those experiments showed that the lymphocytes contained the information for making antibodies and for transferring the elements of CMI, as recognized by and embodied in biological processes—rejection of skin grafts and killing of virus-infected cells which display viral peptide antigens on their surfaces bound to HLA molecules. The reactions of CMI are mediated by T lymphocytes—$CD4^+$ T helper (Th) and $CD8^+$ T cytotoxic lymphocyte (CTL) subsets. Observations of rare immune deficiency states in humans, such as the Di George syndrome associated with congenital thymic aplasia/hypoplasia, as well as experimental surgical removal of the thymus in birds and in mammals, led to the definition of the thymus-dependent lymphocytes or T cells. The T cells that are generated and educated to interact with HLA–peptide complexes and that emerge from the thymus (a central lymphoid organ) are seen as naive (uncommitted) T cells. These T cells have a competence to respond to peptide antigens although they have not, as yet, encountered antigens outwith the thymus in the peripheral (secondary) lymphoid system. The developmental expression of receptors for antigens and the effective functions of T cells are dependent on an intact and functioning thymus. Compared with the normal counterparts, athymic animals were also observed to have significantly fewer lymphoid cells in blood and at various secondary lymphoid tissue sites, and showed significant defects of cellular and humoral immunity. These observations indicated that T lymphocytes represented the major lymphoid population in blood and that the T cells, although not directly involved in antibody synthesis, affected cells responsible for antibody production. Hence, T lymphocytes were communicating with B lymphocytes and helping in the latter's production

Table 1.2 The role of T and B lymphocytes—the agents of specific (adaptive) immunity

T cells ($CD4^+$ and $CD8^+$) (cell-mediated immunity)	**B cells (and derived plasma cells) (humoral immunity)**
Resistance to intracellular microbes	Neutralization
Rejection of transplant grafts (acute)	Cell lysis of microbes
Delayed type hypersensitivity	Opsonization of microbes
Contact dermatitis	Hyperacute graft rejection
Resistance to some tumours	Types I–III hypersensitivity

of antibodies. Birds were shown to have a discrete central lymphoid organ called the bursa of Fabricius which was responsible for the development of B lymphocytes. Mammals do not possess this organ, but the bone marrow throughout life and, to some extent the foetal liver, subserve similar functions in generating recognizable and immunocompetent but naive B lymphocytes. B cells; their progeny, the plasma cells, are responsible for the synthesis and secretion of antibodies into blood and other body fluids. Tables 1.2 and 1.3 summarize the role of T and B lymphocytes as agents of adaptive immunity.

T lymphocytes are the pivotal cells in the recognition/early phase of all adaptive immune responses. Apart from the effector functions associated with CMI, they also provide additional important Th, effector, and immunoregulatory T cell functions in the initiation, control, and expression of a wide range of immune responses. Figure 1.6 gives an overview of humoral and CMI and illustrates that the $CD4^+$ Th/effector subset can currently be defined (by their functions, pattern of cytokine production and transcription factor expression) into at least three well-characterized subgroups: Th1, Th2, and Th17 (see 'T cells, receptors, and effectors: $CD4^+$ Th1, Th2 and Th17; $CD4^+$ Tregs and $CD8^+$ CTLs', below).

It is evident that inflammation, as harnessed by immune responses (innate and adaptive) in a controlled manner, is very effective and essential for survival of the host. Evolutionary adaptations have ensured tight checks to contain potentially damaging inflammatory processes. If the acute inflammatory response is persistent it can

Table 1.3 Effects of lymphocyte loss on adaptive immunity

	Cell-mediated immunity	**Humoral immunity**
Intact animal (no loss)	+++	+++
Loss of T cells		
◆ Thymectomy	-	+
◆ Di George syndrome	-	+
Loss of B cells		
◆ In bone marrow	++	-
◆ Hypogammaglobulinaemia	+++	- (±)

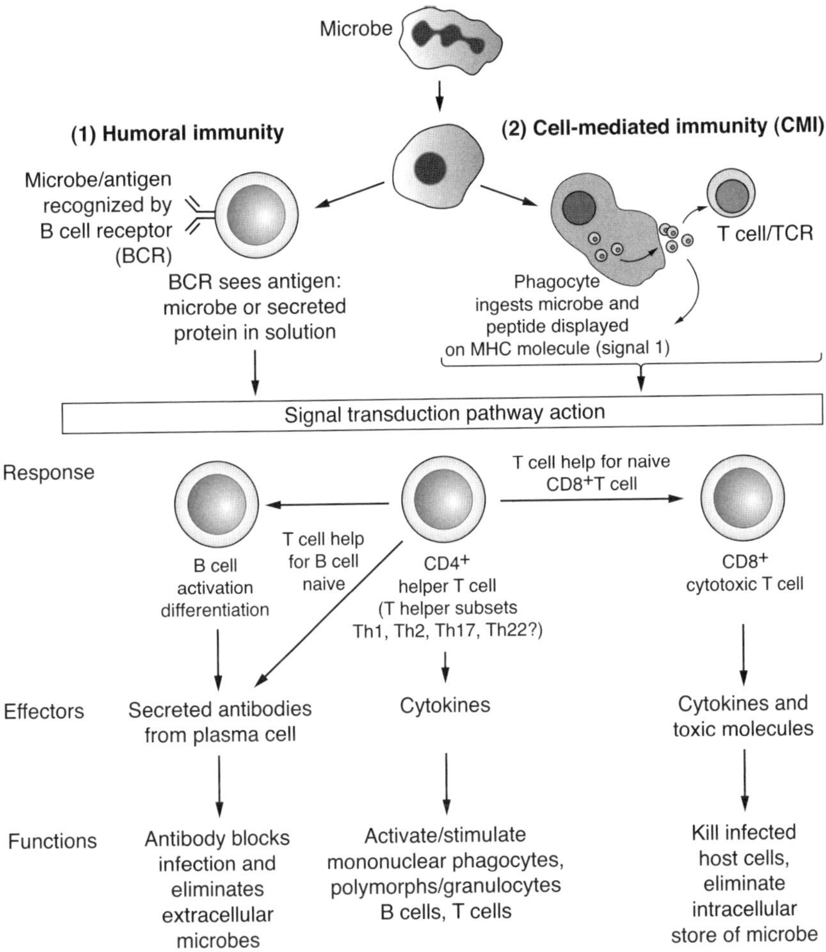

Fig. 1.6 Overview of humoral and cell-mediated immunity (CMI): Adaptive immunity is made up of (1) humoral immunity mediated by antibodies produced from B cells and their plasma cell progeny which neutralizes and eliminates extracellular microbes/antigens; (2) T cells are responsible for CMI ($CD4^+$ and $CD8^+$ T cell subsets) which destroy intracellular microbes/antigens either directly ($CD8^+$ T cells) or indirectly by T cell secretion of cytokines which can activate phagocytes to effectively kill ingested microbes. Various effector $CD4^+$ T cell subsets (Th1, Th2, and Th17) have been defined based on cytokine profiles and associated functions. BCR, B cell receptor; TCR, T cell receptor.

transform into chronic inflammation, characterized by lymphocytes and macrophages replacing the neutrophils that dominate the acute responses. Acute inflammation is, in part, controlled by the limited range and action of most cytokines and chemokines, as well as the loss of stimulating signals when the microbe/antigen is destroyed, and by the death of leucocytes. Recent evidence has indicated alternate pathways of phagocyte activation that result in the release of anti-inflammatory mediators (e.g. IL-10).

This contrasts with the predominant proinflammatory mediators (TNF-α, IL-1, and IL-6) that are released from phagocytes in the early innate immune response. Ultimately, the inflammatory response must be tightly controlled to prevent the emergence and persistence of chronic inflammation which characterizes diverse disorders including autoimmune diseases, e.g. rheumatoid arthritis (RA) or systemic lupus erythematosus (SLE)—see Chapter 8; cardiovascular disease, (atheroma formation has major elements of inflammation involved); chronic obstructive pulmonary disease (COPD); asthma; elements of neurodegenerative diseases (MS and Alzheimer's); and induction of malignancy (see Chapter 4). A great deal of research has now established that these diverse diseases have common pathophysiological pathways associated with chronic inflammation. Mononuclear phagocytes and lymphocytes, which characterize this inflammation, when persistently stimulated release a range of cytokines, chemokines, and other mediators which target cells of epithelial and mesenchymal origin in the different organ-based systems. Common responses elicited in the organs include cell proliferation, adhesion molecule induction and activation, additional leucocyte recruitment, angiogenesis (formation of new vessels), and fibrosis. Figure 1.7 shows the relationship between immune responses and inflammatory outcomes.

As a reuslt of our increased understanding of immune–inflammatory interactions new and important therapeutic agents have come into clinical use, including MABs or

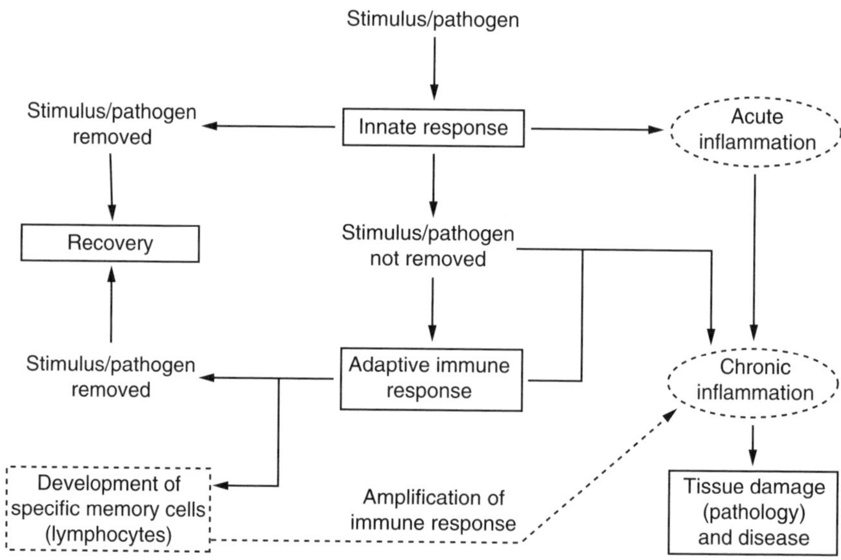

Fig. 1.7 Innate and adaptive immunity use inflammatory responses as key effectors for defence against microbes. Innate immunity exploits acute inflammation; if the inflammation persists because the microbe is resistant there is a risk of developing chronic inflammation and significant host tissue damage and disease (immunopathology). Similarly, persistent adaptive immunity against extrinsic antigen or intrinsic antigen (autoantigens) without resolution and recovery can also generate damaging chronic inflammation and disease.

other biologicals that block or antagonize the reactions of cytokines central to the inflammatory reactions. Examples of important targets include TNF-α, IL-1, IL-6, and their respective receptors (see 'Monoclonals and other biological therapies', below).

Dendritic cells

The classical studies of Steinman and others in the 1980s firmly established innate system DCs (their nomenclature, describing their morphology) as the key third cell needed in *in vitro* clusters with T and B cells to trigger adaptive immune responses. More recently, these observations have been confirmed *in vivo* using dynamic and elegant imaging technology which have documented the antigen-presenting roles of DCs in real time (videos available online—see 'Further reading') showing the kinetics of DC–lymphocyte interactions.

DCs are found in most tissues, particularly in those that form an interface with the environment—skin, intestinal, respiratory, and urogenital tracts—where they are intertwined with the epithelial lining cells, as well as being represented in the subepithelial compartment of the mucosa. They are sparsely represented in the central nervous system (CNS) and are absent in the corneal epithelium of the eye. Their locations make them particularly suitable for sampling and capturing potential non-self molecules and antigens that may breach natural portals. Within lymphoid organs and lymphoid aggregates they are abundant in T cell areas (e.g. paracortex of lymph nodes) and are also present in the B cell zones (primary follicles and germinal centres). Small numbers of DCs and their progenitors can be found circulating in blood.

DCs have a large array of surface receptors and molecules which allow then to detect many molecules including PAMPs/DAMPs, complement components, CRP, regions of antibody molecules (Fc receptors), HLA molecules, etc. Functional DCs in different locations can perform, with varying degrees of efficiency, phagocytosis, endocytosis, and pinocytosis of environmental extracellular material; they also show migratory ability such as moving from peripheral tissues to secondary lymphoid organs. Tissue DCs are replenished by the movement and differentiation of DC precursors from the bone marrow to blood and thence to tissue sites. The originally defined DC is the well-known Langerhans cell (LC) which is associated with skin epithelium; other related DCs are found just below the epithelium and have been termed dermal DCs (DDCs) and indeterminate DCs (IDCs). The LC and related cells are derived from bone marrow and relate to the mononuclear phagocyte lineage. They have many features in common with macrophages and monocytes and also some significant differences. They sample antigens from the local environment adjacent to and between epithelial cells. They are part of the family of generic DCs which we associate with particular functions of antigen presentation to lymphocytes. The functions of LCs and IDCs, and macrophages, have qualitative and quantitative differences with regard to endocytosis, phagocytosis, intracellular killing, and processing of internalized protein molecules to peptide antigens to be bound to HLA for the presention of antigens to T cells. Macrophages are very efficent at phagocytosis and intracellular killing but much less efficient at antigen presentation; mature DCs have the converse properties. Essentially, the DCs capture antigen, either in its complete form on their surface receptors or as phagocytosed/endocytosed material, for partial digestion and processing for presentation, complexed with DC self-HLA molecules. The cells then have the ability to migrate as well as to mature. During the migration and maturation stages from the epithelial and subepithelial areas to the regional lymph nodes the cells change their functional ability, becoming less endocytic/phagocytic and more firmly committed to processing and presenting antigens to T cells. The stages of DC maturation and activation are correlated with changes in cell markers and DC function. In migration from the periphery to lymphoid tissues, DCs show loss of adhesive properties, lowered endo/phagocytosis, increased surface expression of HLA and costimulatory molecules (CD80/86), together with increased synthesis and secretion of cytokines (e.g. IL-12). These maturation events clearly correlate well with the DCs' ability to present peptide antigen complexed with HLA to naive T cells in the lymphoid tissues and to provide the necessary costimulatory and cytokine signals for full T cell activation (Figure 1.8).

DCs present a peptide antigen bound to its HLA class II molecule to a $CD4^+$ T cell (signals 1, 2). For full T cell activation a third signal is required (presence of a TLR agonist or cytokine) (Figure 1.9). Newer studies are also revealing that DCs can down-regulate

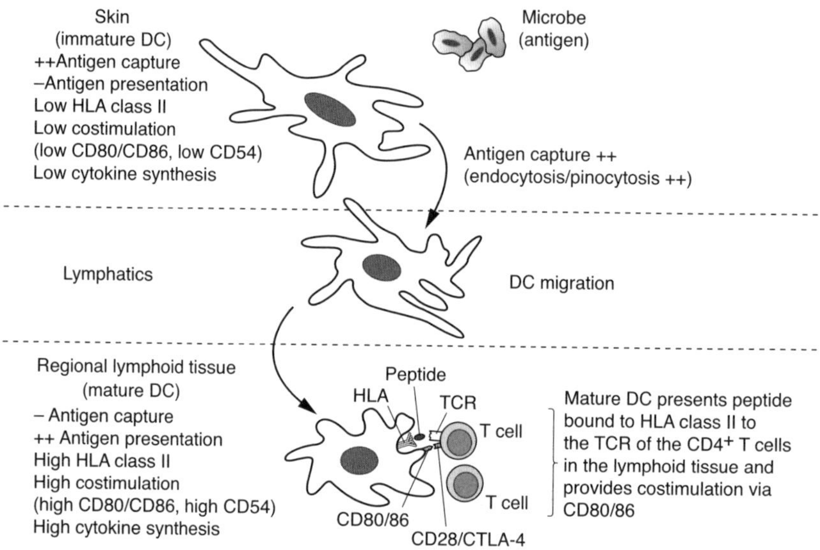

Fig. 1.8 Phenotypic and functional changes in immature DCs (e.g. LCs and IDCs) as they migrate from the skin site to regional lymphoid tissues to become mature APCs. In the lymphoid tissues they present peptide complexes either with HLA class II molecules to the TCR of $CD4^+$ T cells or with HLA class I to $CD8^+$ T cells. The DCs also provide costimulatory signals by way of their CD80/CD86 molecules engaging CD28 molecules on the T cells (and subsequently CTLA-4). The peptide presentation to TCRs of the T cells by the DC is termed signal 1, the costimulatory function is termed signal 2. Mature DCs can also produce cytokines such as IL-12, IL-18, IL-23 which can help in T cell differentiation. These signals are sometimes termed signal 3. APC, antigen-presenting cell; CTLA-4, cytotoxic T lymphocyte antigen-4; DC, dendritic cell; HLA, human leucocyte antigen; TCR, T cell receptor.

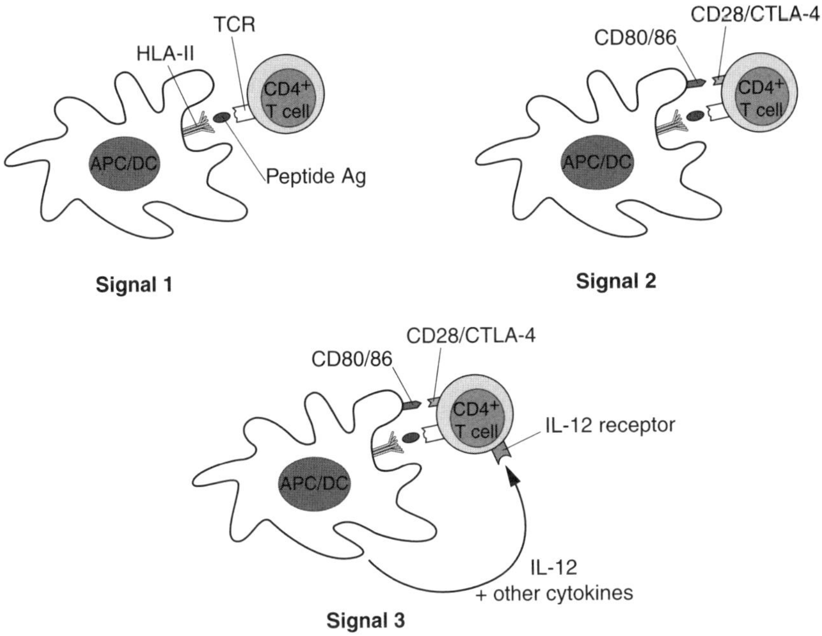

Fig. 1.9 Antigen-presenting DC presents processed peptide antigen bound to its HLA class II molecule to the specific TCR on the CD4$^+$ T cell (*signal 1*); the maturing DC expresses the CD80/CD86 molecules which bind to the CD28 family of molecules on the activating T cells: this costimulation interaction is deemed to be *signal 2*. For full T cell activation a further signal (*signal 3*) is provided by cytokines produced by and secreted from the mature DC. The cytokine binds to the specific cytokine receptor on the T cell. Different cytokines may direct varying functionality in the responding T cells. APC, antigen-presenting cell; CTLA-4, cytotoxic T lymphocyte antigen-4; DC, dendritic cell; HLA, human leucocyte antigen; TCR, T cell receptor.

immune responses acting in concert with T regulatory cells (Tregs), with both cell types producing the suppressive cytokines transforming growth factor-beta (TGF-β) and IL-10. DCs also have been shown to suppress activated T cells and facilitate the appearance of Th2 cells in favour of Th1. This is part of the physiological control of immunity. However, in some areas such as cancer immunotherapy using DCs, these suppressive interactions may be amenable to positive modulation to enhance antitumour responses (see Chapter 4). These suppressive DCs have been shown to facilitate survival and growth of cancer cells by promoting an immune-tolerant environment; the DC enzyme indoleamine 2,3-dioxygenase (IDO) appears to be responsible for the suppressive function [14]. Inhibitors of IDO are being investigated in antitumour therapeutic strategies. In contrast, suppressive DCs may be harnessed where down-regulation of responses may prove desirable, in autoimmunity and allergic responses.

The major DC subtype is termed the myeloid DC (mDC); this is CD11c$^+$ and requires the cytokine granulocyte–monocyte colony stimulating factor (GM-CSF) for survival. Experimentally, mDC-like cells can be generated from blood mononuclear cell precursors by culturing *in vitro* with a cocktail of cytokines including GM-CSF, IL-4, and TNF-α (see Chapter 4). A less frequent and more recently defined DC subtype derived from lymphoid progenitors is called the plasmacytoid (p) DC (CD11c$^-$); this cell appears to have particular roles in detecting and responding to viral PAMPs and producing large amounts of type 1 antiviral interferon (IFN)-α/β. Some experiments suggest pDCs are efficient in cross-presentation of peptide antigens, a property which may be exploited in immunotherapy strategies using T cell (CD4$^+$ and CD8$^+$) mediated responses. Other minor subsets of DCs have been defined in tissue sites based on phenotypic markers; whether they have discrete functional roles is currently being investigated.

Overall, DCs can be seen to play crucial roles in the initiation of immune responses and probably in the termination of such responses, as well as in maintenance of physiological tolerance to self molecules, to commensal flora, and to ingested potential food antigens. DCs are the key bridge between innate and adaptive immunity. Their role in initiating and maintaining different types of CD4$^+$ Th cells (Th1, Th2, Th17), CD8$^+$ T effector cells, and Tregs are examined in the section 'T cells, receptors, and effectors: CD4$^+$ Th1, Th2 and Th17; CD4$^+$ Tregs and CD8$^+$ CTLs', below.

Natural killer cells

Natural killer (NK) cells are so named historically because of their observed ability to kill certain target cell lines (e.g. K562, a leukaemia cell line) without any prior sensitization (natural cytotoxicity). NK cells are derived from bone marrow and are widely distributed in lymphoid and nonlymphoid tissues. They are considered as cells of innate immunity. They are found within the small population of morphologically defined large granular lymphocytes (LGLs) which account for approximately 1–10% of blood lymphoid cells. In keeping with other cells of innate immunity, they express a series of germ-line-encoded receptors. They do not undergo somatic gene rearrangement, as is the case for immunoglobulin (Ig) and TCR genes, in B and T lymphocyte development. Experimentally, and with some clinical evidence, NK cells have been shown to have definitive effector and regulatory roles. They have been shown to recognize and respond to stressed autologous cells, as a result of infection, particularly with intracellular organisms (e.g. viral infections), and malignant transformed cells. On detecting stressed cells, they can induce cell killing by the process of apoptosis using one of two pathways—the Fas-ligand (L) system and/or the release of their intracellular granules comprising perforin and granzymes (see 'Effector cells and receptors', below). When responding to stressed cells, in some situations NK cells have also been shown to rapidly secrete very high levels of proinflammatory cytokines such as TNF-α, IFN-γ, and IL-17, which in turn rapidly recruit and regulate other inflammatory cells. Importantly, by their rapid and high secretion of IFN-γ, NK cells can drive APCs and assist the development of adaptive immune responses of CD4$^+$ Th cells and CD8$^+$ CTLs. They can also have an effect on B lymphocyte production of antibody.

Phenotypic markers used to characterize NK cells include expression of CD56 and CD16, but lack of expression of CD3 (CD3 is a positive marker present on all peripheral naive and effector T cells). CD56 can occur on a subset of T cells, hence it is important to show CD3 negativity with respect to LGLs which are $CD56^+$ and $CD16^+$. Similarly, NK cells lack B lymphocyte markers (CD19, CD20) and the surface immunoglobulin receptor (SIgR). In recent years, some highly specific phenotypic markers have been defined for NK cells which are also functional receptors; they are represented by CD335–CD337. The most specific is CD335, known as NKP46. It represents one of the so-called natural cytotoxic receptors on NK cells.

Because of their potentially very potent and destructive effects, NK cell reactions need to be tightly controlled and regulated to ensure avoidance of damage to normal tissues while acting against target tissues. This is partly achieved by a complex of different receptor systems found in NK cells. Among the lymphoid cells they possess a unique combination of inhibitory and activating receptors (with ITIM and ITAM motifs, respectively, on the intracellular receptor domains) which control their cytotoxic functions. The inhibitory receptors, typified by the killer inhibitory receptors (KIRs), have a dominant role, recognizing HLA class I self molecules (different from $CD8^+$ T cells, which recognize HLA class I with bound peptide). The KIRs recognize HLA class I products expressed on all nucleated cells of the body. Surveillance, detection, and receptor interaction with conserved residues of the class I molecules result in a dominant inhibitory ITIM-mediated intracellular signal to the NK cell, preventing it from killing normal self cells. However, if tissue cells become compromised by stressors (intracellular infection or neoplastic transformation) this results in the loss of HLA class I molecules; these cells then become recognized by the activating NK cell receptor systems. Biologically, this recognition of abnormal cells (with loss of HLA class I) complements the activity of $CD8^+$ CTLs which recognize HLA class I antigen peptide complexes generated from intracellular microbial infections or from transformed malignant cells expressing tumour-associated antigens (TAAs). NK cells will respond very quickly to such stressed cells. This is in contrast to $CD8^+$ T cells, which need to be induced and undergo clonal expansion. To escape CTLs some intracellular microbes, e.g. cytomegaloviruses (CMVs) and other herpesviruses, use the strategy of down-regulating or overcoming HLA class I expression with decoy molecules, thus avoiding their viral peptide presentation. Hence, by the down-regulation of class I molecules, although they escape $CD8^+$ CTLs, they become susceptible to NK cell cytotoxicity. Clinically, patients with the rare deficiency of NK cells and/or NK cell function have been shown to have problems with recurrent and serious infections associated with herpesviruses.

NK cells have been shown to have a marked antileukaemic effect in allogeneic bone marrow transplantation, while not inducing potentially damaging graft versus host responses, as occurs with antileukaemic T cells. NK cells are also considered to be significant contributors to transplant tolerance (see Chapter 3). Although NK cells are accepted as innate immune cells, they are best considered as cells at the interface of, and bridging, innate and adaptive immunity. Recent experiments have indicated that they can show some degree of immunological memory (a property hitherto considered to be restricted to T and B lymphocytes). Some authorities are accordingly questioning the usefulness of maintaining the descriptive divide between innate and adaptive immunity [15,16]. In this author's view it remains a useful biological and clinical mechanistic paradigm.

Further details of NK cell inhibitory and activating receptor molecules and functions can be found in the section 'Effector cells and receptors', below.

Another functional NK receptor is related to the CD16 molecule, which is a low-affinity receptor for the IgG Fc region. This receptor functions in antibody-dependent cellular cytoxicity (ADCC) and can be mediated by NK cells. The specific IgG antibody binds to its target antigen via its specific Fab region whilst the Fc region binds to the NK CD16 receptor, thus, bringing the NK cell into close juxtaposition with the target antigen. This NK-mediated ADCC is believed to be one of the components operative in rituximab therapy, using anti-CD20 IgG MABs to target B cell tumours and some autoimmune and inflammatory diseases (see 'Monoclonals and other biological therapies', below).

For some years now, NK cells have been used in cancer immunotherapy (e.g. against renal cell carcinoma and melanoma), as well as in attempts to modulate transplantation rejection and tolerance induction (see Chapters 4 and 3, respectively).

Many aspects of NK cell physiology are still undergoing investigation, including their possible role in autoimmunity, and their role in self-surveillance and not damaging other NK cells. In humans, there is still a lack of knowledge regarding their physiological recirculation in peripheral lymphoid tissues. They can also be found in human central lymphoid organs where they are considered to be trafficking through rather than being matured in sites such as the thymus and the bone marrow, although their progenitors are bone marrow-derived. Current research supports their bone marrow origin but with major maturational events occurring in secondary lymphoid tissue sites. Key cytokines central to human NK cell development include IL-15 together with stromal stem cell factor/Kit L, and to a lesser extent IL-2.

Cocktails of these cytokines can be used *in vitro* to expand pure populations of NK cells. Rare human immune deficiency states indicate that NK cells are derived from a common lymphoid precursor cell before that precursor gives rise to cells that migrate to the thymus to produce T cells and to the bone marrow to produce B cells. This is confirmed by the occurrence of patients with a form of severe combined immune deficiency (SCID) which is known to be induced by mutations in *RAG1* and *RAG2* genes. These genes are responsible for the somatic gene recombination events crucial for the development of TCRs and BCRs. These SCID patients have no T or B cells, but they have normal numbers of functional NK cells. NK cell functional deficiencies are well described in the rare Wiscott–Aldrich syndrome (WAS). In WAS there is a gene mutation of the WAS protein; this interferes with cytoskeletal dynamic processes, including those needed mechanistically for NK cell cytotoxic function. The natural history of patients with WAS indicates that up to one-third die from severe herpesvirus infections, and one-third succumb to blood cell malignancies—observations that highlight the *in vivo* biological importance of NK cells.

NK cells recognize danger signals produced by stressed and damaged host cells. They complement the range of other receptors found on phagocytes such as scavenger receptors, TLRs, and NLRs. They are able to detect damaged cells even without recognition of DAMPs. Interestingly, NK cells have also been shown to express receptors that recognize molecules on stressed cells referred to as MIC-A and MIC-B, which are produced from genes in the MHC class I region (see 'Major histocompatibility complex', below). These MIC-A/B molecules appear not to be recognized by standard innate immune phagocytic cells, although there is evidence that they can also be recognized by sets of unconventional T cells such as γδ T cells and NK T cells (see 'Effector cells and receptors', below). Other important receptors on NK cells recognize and respond to type 1 IFNs which are rapidly produced and secreted by virally infected cells and are susceptible to NK cell killing. NK cells responding to type 1 IFNs enhance their killing functions and produce IFN-γ, which stimulates other innate immune cells to generate additional inflammatory reactions against the virally infected cells. The NK cell-generated IFN-γ can also link to adaptive immunity by stimulating T cell activation/proliferation (directly and indirectly via DCs) and by facilitating class switching of B cells in antibody production (see 'B cells, receptors, and antibodies', below). NK cells have receptors for IL-1, IL-12, IL-15, and IL-18, all produced by macrophages, monocytes, and APCs. Thus, NK cells play an important role at the interface of innate and adaptive immunity.

Clusters of differentiation and monoclonal antibodies

Introduction

Hybridoma technology, developed by Kohler and Milstein more than 30 years ago, has resulted in the production of many MABs that have significantly increased our knowledge and understanding of the immune system [17]. Such reagents have also contributed significantly to defining leucocyte development, lymphocyte physiology, and interaction, as well as the immunopathology of various diseases. Over the past 10–15 years, an increasing number of MABs have been used as primary therapeutic agents in a range of human diseases. Some well-known agents used in clinical practice include avastin, rituximab, and herceptin (see 'Monoclonals and other biological therapies', below, and Chapters 4, 7, and 8).

MABs specific for cell-associated molecules have, by international workshop agreement, been placed into groupings according to their reaction with specific antigens. These antigens are termed clusters of differentiation (CD). At the present time, there are more than 300 approved CD antigens.

CD molecules define the antigen, generally of known molecular weight, against which a series of MABs have been derived. Currently, by common usage, the antibodies against the CD antigens are also referred to as CD antibodies (grouping together various synonymous reagents produced by different researchers and companies). Documented below are some selected examples of CD groupings which will prove useful in subsequent sections of this and other chapters.

Common CD antigens

- CD1 (a, b, c, d, and e)—a series of molecules involved in antigen presentation, particularly of lipid/glycolipid antigens to 'unconventional' T cells (e.g. γδ T and NK T cells). CD1a, b, and c are found on cortical thymocytes, LCs, and some APCs. CD1d is expressed on intestinal epithelial cells, B cell subsets, and other APCs.
- CD2—An antigen (50 kDa) present on all normal T lymphocytes (pan-T cell marker); also detectable on a population of morphologically defined LGLs, which have demonstrable NK cell function. The CD2 antigen (also named lymphocyte

functioning antigen 2, LFA2) functions as the receptor for an adhesion molecule CD58 (LFA3) which is widely distributed.

- CD3—Defines a multimolecular protein complex (including molecules of 19, 21, and 26 kDa) restricted to T lymphocytes. The CD3 molecules are closely associated on the T cell membrane with the antigen-specific TCR molecule termed Ti. The complex is often referred to as CD3/Ti or the T3/Ti complex, or simply as TCR. It is the TCR that binds peptide antigens associated with HLA molecules, the so-called signal 1 complex. If the TCR recognition is also accompanied by additional signals to the cells, known as signal 2, then a specific response is likely to be triggered.
- CD4—The 55-kDa antigen is detected on the major subset of peripheral T lymphocytes (Th subset). Also, the CD4 antigen, which is known to function as a key receptor for HIV, forms an integral part of the membrane of monocyte-macrophage cells. In addition, CD4 is expressed on developing thymocytes within the thymus. CD4 also functions as a coreceptor in TCR recognition of peptide antigens associated with MHC class II molecules.
- CD5—Another pan-T cell antigen, but also found on a rare subset of normal B cells and commonly on neoplastic B cell clones of chronic lymphocytic leukaemia, and some non-Hodgkin's lymphomas. CD5-expressing B cells may have an important role to play in the production of so-called natural autoantibodies.
- CD8—An antigen detected on a subset of peripheral T lymphocytes (CTLs). CD8 is also expressed on developing thymocytes. It functions as a coreceptor during TCR recognition of MHC class I peptide complexes.
- CD11—Antigens (~180 kDa) that define a family of adhesion molecules associated with cell–cell interactions and functions. There are varying names associated with this series of antigens, such as LFA1 (a heterodimer of CD11α with β-chain integrin CD18). The CD11 series is detectable on a wide range of leucocytes, including monocytes, granulocytes, and subsets of T and B cells. They are also called leucocyte integrins, where CD11 identifies the α-chains and CD18 the β-chains of these adhesion molecules.
- CD14—Antigen (50–55 kDa) known to be specifically expressed on the membrane of blood monocytes, although it can be detected in the cytoplasm of granulocytes. It has an important function as part of the receptor for bacterial lipopolysacharide (LPS) protein complexes recognized by TLR-4.
- CD15—Antigen (50–180 kDa) present on the myeloid-monocytic series of cells, on some epithelial cells and corresponding carcinomas, as well as on the Reed–Sternberg cells associated with Hodgkin's disease.
- CD16—Defines an antigen on the cell membrane (50–80 kDa) which functionally interacts at low affinity with the Fc portion of the IgG class of Igs. CD16 is found on neutrophils, eosinophils, NK cells and on lymphokine-activated killer (LAK) cells within the morphologically defined LGL population. LAK cells continue to be investigated in strategies of adoptive immunotherapy of cancer. CD16 mediates phagocytosis and also ADCC.

- CD18—β2 integrin, which is broadly distributed on all leucocytes; it associates with the various CD11 (a, b, c) molecules, to function in cell adhesion interactions. CD18 is the common β-chain of the heterodimeric adhesion molecule (e.g. LFA-1, CD11a/CD18).
- CD19—Defines an antigen restricted to the B lymphocyte lineage (pan-B cell antigen). CD19 MABs are extremely useful for qualitative and quantitative enumeration of B cells in research and clinical analysis of lymphocyte markers.
- CD20—B lymphocyte-specific antigen, but more restricted on B cells than CD 19. It is the target for the therapeutic antibody rituximab which is used to treat some human cancers (lymphomas). Rituximab is also being increasingly used to treat autoimmune diseases (see Chapter 8).
- CD21—Defines an antigen on some B cells and APCs of the lymph node known as dendritic reticulum cells (DRCs). The CD21 antigen functions as a receptor for the Epstein–Barr virus (EBV). Some epithelial cells (e.g. of the uterine cervix) have been demonstrated to express CD21. CD21 is known to be a functional receptor also for fragments of an activated complement component termed C3d. CD21 is also referred to as complement receptor 2 (CR2).
- CD25—Antigen (50–55 kDa) which defines a marker expressed on activated T cells (cells that have been stimulated either by the TCR or by nonspecific mitogenic stimuli). CD25 represents part of the IL-2R and is referred to as the TAC antigen. Physiologically, T cell-derived IL-2 binds to CD25 which is part of a trimolecular receptor complex. Interaction of IL-2 with this receptor initiates important signal transduction events for T cell activation and proliferation in cell-mediated reactions. The expression of CD25 is also a key marker of Tregs, which are $CD4^+$ $CD25^+$ and express the transcription factor FoxP3 (Forkhead box protein 3) (see 'T cells, receptors, and effectors: $CD4^+$ Th1, Th2 and Th17; $CD4^+$ Tregs and $CD8^+$ CTLs', below).
- CD28—Located on T cell subsets and some activated B cells. It plays a key role in activation of naive T cells as a receptor for costimulatory signals (signal 2). CD28 binds to molecules defined as CD80 (B7.1) and CD86 (B7.2) expressed by APCs.
- CD34—Present on haematopoietic precursors (including the pluripotential bone marrow stem cell). It is also found on capillary endothelial cells.
- CD40—Located on B cells, on APCs (macrophages and DCs) and on some basal epithelial cells. CD40 binds to its ligand (L-CD154) which is found on activated T cells. The interaction induces B cell proliferation and activation.
- CD45—Present in various isoforms (CD45 RO, RA, RB) of haematopoietic cells. The different isoforms are correlated with different types of T cell properties, defining respectively naive, memory, and other functional correlates of T cells.
- CD52—Distributed on lymphocytes, monocytes, and granulocytes. CD52 is the target for one of the earliest therapeutic MABs (CAMPATH-1) which has been used to deplete T cells from bone marrow for transplantation (see Chapter 3).
- CD54—Intercellular cell adhesion molecule-1 (ICAM-1) present on endothelial cells, monocytes, and lymphocytes; functions as a receptor/counter-ligand for CD11a/CD18 (LFA-1) and CD11b/CD18 (Mac-1) integrins.

- CD56—Antigen (~220 kDa) expressed on most NK cells and a subset of T cells which exhibit cytotoxic function and are part of a pool of cells referred to as unconventional T cells, in particular the NK T cells. CD56 is known to function as a neural intercellular adhesion molecule (N-CAM).
- CD69—Inducible on a wide range of bone-marrow-derived haematopoetic cells. It is one of the earliest activation markers detectable on, and characterizing, T cells stimulated by antigen or mitogen. CD69 is involved in further activation and proliferation of lymphocytes, acting as a signal-transducing molecule.
- CD80/CD86—Previously called B7.1 and B7.2, found on macrophages-monocytes and DCs; also expressed by activated T and B lymphocytes. CD80/CD86 function by binding to CD28 and CD152 in T cell costimulatory activity.
- CD152—Found on activated T cells; engages the ligands CD80 and CD86 (similar to the interaction for CD28). However, the interaction of CD152, also called CTLA-4, results in the negative regulation of T cell activation. CD152 has been employed in immunotherapeutic approaches to switch off immune-driven and mediated chronic inflammatory disorders.
- CD154—See CD40 above.
- CD 161—Lectin-like molecule found on NK cells and subsets of $CD4^+$ and $CD8^+$ T cells. It is thought to function in NK cytotoxicity; CD161 is being correlated with differentiation, cytokine production, and functions of $CD4^+$ and $CD8^+$ T cell subsets.
- CD207—Langerin, found on and in LCs, and functions as an endocytic receptor. It is used as a specific marker for LCs.
- CD228—Defines molecules that are found predominantly in human melanomas. They have been used as TAAs for immunotherapy of melanomas.
- CD254—RankL is the major effector of bone resorption; it is produced by osteoblast lineage cells and is expressed on the surface of T and B lymphocytes. Its physiological receptor RANK is expressed on the surface of osteoclasts. CD254 is a key player in the bone loss associated with metastatic cancer (e.g. breast, prostate); it is also implicated in the immune-inflammatory destructive lesions of RA.

The above summary of some important CDs is mainly restricted to their expression on cells—their phenotypic demonstration. The exploitation of phenotypes to enumerate cell numbers and subsets, cell development, and functional properties is illustrated throughout the remainder of this chapter. The molecules defined by the CDs have specific biological functions associated with the cells possessing them. These functional aspects of CDs, e.g. the important functional roles of CD28, CD25, and CD40 in lymphocyte interactions, are becoming better understood. This elucidation has been greatly helped by exploiting biological techniques allowing isolation and cloning of genes encoding the CDs and the subsequent transfection (direct DNA insertion), and expression of the genes in *in vitro* cell lines. Thus, the *in vivo* biological role of the T cell CD4 antigen, for instance, was shown to be its interaction with MHC class II molecules on APCs. Similarly, the CD3 molecular complex has been defined as playing an important role in signal transduction from the CD3 Ti (TCR) on the cell surface through the cell membrane via the cytosol and ultimately to the nucleus of the cell. This signal transduction represents critical biochemical information which flows from the interaction of the foreign antigen peptide–MHC complex with the TCR to ultimately result in effectors which will destroy or contain the foreign antigen. Many steps in the transduction process have now been well defined [18] and are proving useful as potential new targets for immunotherapy. The characterization of patients with rare deficiencies associated with lack of expression of parts of the CD3 complex, and of patients with deficiencies of parts of other signalling molecules such as CD25, have helped to closely define the components involved in signal transduction within lymphocytes.

Cytokines, chemokines, and signalling

Cytokines

In parallel with the explosion in knowledge and exploitation of CD antigens and antibodies, there has been an equally remarkable expansion in our knowledge of cytokines and their roles, together with exploitation of such knowledge in clinical medicine.

The generic term 'cytokine' covers the IFNs (originally discovered with respect to their antiviral function), lymphokines, ILs, chemokines, and monokines, as well as other important haematopoietic factors and other growth factors. Outlined below are some details of key cytokines—with emphasis on ILs—that are of particular importance in understanding the science of immunology and immune reactions.

Cytokines are mainly generated in response to various stimuli and act as signalling molecules binding to specific receptors in an autocrine or paracrine fashion. They are central in controlling inflammation and immunity and are drivers of cellular differentiation and proliferation. They also have important regulatory roles in immune and inflammatory responses. Importantly, they play key roles in immune homeostasis, and in tissue healing and repair. Modulation of the immune response by cytokines occurs at multiple levels. They may affect lymphocyte proliferation (IL-2, IL-4), cell survival (IL-7, Fas L), cell differentiation (IL-4, IL-12), antigen presentation to lymphocytes (IFN-γ, GM-CSF, IL-10), cell trafficking (chemokines), etc. [19]. Cytokines are, therefore, key in linking the immune response to the inflammatory response; note the role of IL-1, TNF-α, and IL-6, especially in innate immune responses. Cytokines can also have major immune suppressive roles; IL-10 and IL-13 can inhibit macrophage production of proinflammatory cytokines. Gene cloning and the subsequent production of recombinant cytokines, together with the use of cell culture systems and transgenic animal models, including gene knock-out mice studies, have all been crucial to help isolate and elucidate the roles of cytokines.

Structurally, some cytokines are single-chain proteins while others are homodimers (identical polypeptide chains), heterodimers (nonidentical polypeptide chains), or trimers (e.g. TNF-α). Some cytokine family members are integral membrane proteins such as Fas L and CD40 L. Cytokines bind to specific receptors; although they are structurally different and discrete molecules, they may, in part, utilize the same receptor. Such cytokines will often have a common polypeptide chain which will access the common receptor. Cytokines can often be grouped into families on the basis of structural homologies (see later). The overlapping functions of many cytokines have suggested a system that has significant in-built redundancy. However, experimental methods adopted to monitor responses of cells following inductive signals for cytokine production have yielded very interesting data. Thus, in an environment where multiple cytokines can be demonstrated, it can be shown that some cytokines have the dominant functional role. Techniques that have been used include tracking the production kinetics of cytokines at the gene transcriptional level by analysis of mRNA, using the polymerase chain reaction (PCR), or tracking the intracellular storage and movement of proteins to the extracellular compartment by techniques such as Western blotting, flow cytometry, and enzyme-linked immunosorbent assay (ELISA). Furthermore, cellular techniques documenting cytokine binding to target cell receptors and functional readouts are used (see Chapter 9). From such experimental approaches it has been demonstrated, for instance, that TNF-α is a master controller cytokine within an acute inflammatory response. This was well defined in surgical specimens from patients with RA and subsequently in cell culture and in *in vivo* animal models, and led to the pioneering and successful use of anti-TNF-α immunotherapy which has revolutionized the management of this disease (see 'Monoclonals and other biological therapies', below and Chapter 8). The dominant role of TNF-α is due, in part, to the kinetics of its production (very rapid) and the fact that TNF-α itself induces the production of other potent proinflammatory cytokines (e.g. IL-6). Additionally, other important studies *in vivo* using animal models, including gene knock-out mice, as well as *ex vivo* use of human tissue and organ culture systems, together with the use of specific anti-cytokine MABs or cytokine receptor antagonists, have helped to further elucidate the role of key cytokines in other immune-mediated inflammatory diseases and in certain cancers. Rare 'experiments of nature', namely human cytokine deficiencies due to gene mutational events, have also helped to define the *in vivo* biological roles and relevance of certain cytokines. For example, patients with deficiencies of IL-12 or IFN-γ, and/or deficiencies of the corresponding receptors, have been shown to develop severe infections with intracellular microbes. This has established the major role played by these cytokines in the development of CMI in combating intracellular microbes.

An overview of some key cytokines with regards to their source, target cells/receptors, and functions is outlined in Table 1.4. The cytokines chosen are those that will inform the context and content of this and the following chapters. An extensive listing of cytokines can be found at http://www.copewithcytokines.de/

Chemokines

Chemokines are the most abundant cytokines in the body. In recent years they have been systematically classified on the basis of structurally conserved cysteine amino acid residues, being denoted as CCL, CXCL, or CXXXCL chemokines. X denotes amino acids other than C (cysteine), and L denotes ligand. Corresponding chemokine receptors have the nomenclature CCR, CXCR, or CXXXCR. Historically, many chemokines were named descriptively on the basis of their functional targets or actions; for example, monocyte chemotactic protein-3 (MCP-3) is now CCL7, and IL-8 is now CXCL8. The new structural nomenclature is much less haphazard and more precise in defining these most abundant of molecules.

Table 1.4 Selected cytokines and their functions in humans

Cytokine	Producing cell	Target cell	Function
TNF-α	Macrophages, mast cells, NK cells	Macrophages	CAM and chemokine expression
		Tumour cells	Cell death
TNF-β	Th1 cells and CTLs	Phagocytes	Phagocytosis, NO production
		Tumour cells	Cell death
GM-CSF	Th cells	Progenitor cells	Growth and differentiation of monocytes and DCs
IL-1α IL-1β	Monocytes Macrophages B cells DCs	Th cells	Costimulation
		B cells	Maturation and proliferation
		NK cells	Activation
		Various	Inflammation, acute phase response, fever
IL-2	Th1 cells	Activated T and B cells, NK cells	Growth, proliferation, activation
IL-3	Th cells NK cells Mast cells	Stem cells	Growth and differentiation
		Mast cells	Growth and histamine release
IL-4	Th2 cells Basophils Mast cells	Activated B cells	Proliferation and differentiation of IgG1 and IgE synthesis
		Macrophages	MHC class II antigens
		T cells	Proliferation; Th2 polarisation
IL-5	Th2 cells Mast cells	Activated B cells	Proliferation and differentiation, IgA synthesis; eosinophil activation
IL-6	Monocytes Macrophages Th2 cells Stromal cells	Activated B cells	Differentiation into plasma cells
		Plasma cells	Antibody secretion
		Stem cells	Differentiation
		Various	Acute phase response
IL-7	Bone marrow stroma Thymus stroma	Stem cells	Differentiation into progenitor B and T cells.
IL-8 (CXCL8 chemokine)	Epithelial cells Macrophages Endothelial cells	Neutrophils Endothelial cells	Chemotaxis
IL-9	Th2 cells	T and B cells	IgM, IgG, and IgE products (stimulate mast cells)
IL-10	Monocytes Macrophages Th2 cells CD8^{+} T cells Mast cells	Macrophages	Cytokine production inhibited
		B cells	Activation

(Continued)

Table 1.4 Selected cytokines and their functions in humans (*continued*)

Cytokine	Producing cell	Target cell	Function
IL-12	DCs Macrophages B cells	Activated T cells	Differentiation into CTLs (with IL-2); Th1 polarisation
		NK cells	Activation IFN-γ
IL-13	Th2 cells Mast cells NK cells	Th2 (autocrine) B cells Macrophages	Growth and differentiation of B cells (IgE production) Inhibition of Th1 cells Inhibition of macrophage production of proinflammatory cytokines IL-1, IL-6, IL-8, IL-12
IL-15	Macrophages Monocytes	T cells Activated B cells	Induces production of NK cells
IL-17	Th17	Epithelium Endothelium	Inflammatory cytokines IL-1, IL-6, TNF-α. Attracts neutrophils Stimulation of angiogenesis and oestoclasts
IL-18	Macrophages	Th1 cells NK cells	Increased production of IFN-γ Increased NK cell activity
IL-21	Activated T cells NK T cells	Lymphocytes DCs	$CD8^+$ T cell cytotoxicity NK cell killing B cell antibody production Th17 cell differentiation
IL-22	Activated $CD4^+$ T cells	Epithelial cells	Regulation of differentiation and proliferation
IL-23	Monocytes Macrophages DCs	Th17 cells Endothelium Extracellular matrix Intestinal innate cells	Inflammatory response Angiogenesis in peripheral tissue and autoimmune disease $CD8^+$ T cell tissue infiltration
IL-25	Th2 cells Mast cells Eosinophils Basophils	Th17 cells Th2 memory cells Fibroblasts	Production of IL-4, IL-5, IL-8, and IL-13. Eosinophil proliferation Inflammatory responses. Allergic responses
IL-33	Endothelial cells Smooth muscle cells Keratinocytes (epithelial cells) Fibroblasts (nuclear location of IL-33)	Mast cells Th2 cells Various	Enhanced Th2 responses 'Danger signal' activation (alarmin) in innate immunity
IL-35	Tregs	Th17 Th cells	Suppression of Th cell activation (including Th17 cells), anti-inflammatory

(*Continued*)

Table 1.4 Selected cytokines and their functions in humans (*continued*)

Cytokine	Producing cell	Target cell	Function
MIP-1α (CCL3)	Macrophages	Monocytes T cells	Chemotaxis
MIP-1β (CCL4)	Lymphocytes	Monocytes T cells	Chemotaxis
TGF-β	T cells Monocytes	Th1 cells Monocytes Macrophages	Suppresses Th1 responses Chemotaxis
		Activated macrophages	IL-1 synthesis
		Activated B cells	IgA synthesis
		Various	Proliferation inhibited
IFN-α	Leucocytes	Various	Viral replication inhibited MHC class I expression increased
IFN-β	Fibroblasts	Various	Viral replication inhibited MHC class I expression increased
IFN-γ	Th1 cells, CTLs, NK cells	Various	Viral replication inhibited weakly
		Macrophages	MHC expression
		Activated B cells	Ig class switch to IgG1
		Th2 cells	Proliferation inhibited
		Macrophages	Pathogen elimination

CAM, cell adhesion molecule; CTL, cytotoxic T lymphocyte; DC, dendritic cell; NO, nitric oxide.

Chemokines, together with adhesion molecules, guide massive leucocyte migration out of the vasculature into areas of inflammation. Physiologically, they guide blood lymphocytes into lymphoid tissues via high endothelial cells in venules (HEVs) and their subsequent segregation into T and B cell zones. They move effector cells into peripheral tissues and sites of antigen or microbe invasion. Chemokines guide immature DCs from peripheral tissue sites to secondary lymphoid tissues (e.g. lymph nodes), where the DCs act as APCs. Chemokines bind promiscuously to chemokine receptors showing much redundancy in the system. The roles of these interactions are being studied in many diseases. For example, the CCR5 receptor present on T cells and monocytes is known to be highjacked and used as a coreceptor along with CD4 for HIV binding and infection of those cells (see 'Monoclonals and other biological therapies', below). Antagonists are being urgently explored. Cancerous cells can produce large amounts of chemokines, some of which are angiogenic, thus favouring growth, survival, migration, and metastasis of cancer cells. Chemokines produced by cells in the vicinity of tumours (e.g. stromal cells) can enhance the attraction of immune cells to the site. Clearly, manipulation of the tumour–chemokine microenvironment presents a potential therapeutic strategy.

Table 1.5 Chemokines and chemokine receptors: physiological and pathological functions

Chemokines	Receptor	Target cells	Physiological functions	Pathological functions
CCL3, CCL5 (Rantes), CCL7 (MCP-3)	CCR1	T cells Monocytes Eosinophils	Facilitates innate and adaptive immunity	Increases the pathological lesions of RA and MS
CCL2, CCL7, CCL8	CCR2	Monocytes DCs Memory cells	Combats intracellular microbes	Increases the pathological lesions of RA, MS, and type 2 diabetes Increases atheroma formation
CCL11 (eotaxin), CCL5, CCL8	CCR3	Eosinophils Basophils Th2 cells	Enhances defence against helminth parasites	Increased activity in allergic asthma and rhinitis
CCL17, CCL22	CCR4	T cells DC macrophages	T cell homing	Increases incidence in graft rejection
CCL3, CCL4, CCL5	CCR5	T cells Monocytes	Mucosal immune responses	HIV-1 coreceptor molecule (CCR5)
CCL19, CCL21	CCR7	T cells DCs	Transport of T cells and DCs to T cell areas of peripheral lymphoid tissue	
CCL25	CCR9	T cells B cells and secretion of IgA	Homing of T cells and IgA+ B cells to MALT	Involved in IBD
CXCL8, (IL-8)	CXCR1	Neutrophils Monocytes	Early innate immune responses at epithelial surfaces	Involved in IBD
CXCL12	CXCR4	Many cell types Monocytes T cells	Haematopoiesis lymphopoiesis	HIV1 coreceptor CXCR4 for T-trophic forms of HIV
CXCL13	CXCR5	Follicular helper T cells, B cells.	Formation of B cell follicles	

DC, dendritic cell; IBD, inflammatory bowel disease (Crohn's and ulcerative colitis); MALT, mucosal-associated lymphoid tissue; MS, multiple sclerosis; RA, rheumatoid arthritis.

Table 1.5 summarizes some chemokine–chemokine receptor interactions, target cells, physiological actions, and diseases or pathological processes where the interactions are deemed significant and potentially targetable.

Both CC and CXC chemokines are involved in recruiting leucocytes to sites of inflammation. Additionally, CXC chemokines play important roles in wound healing and in angiogenesis. Chemokine receptors show significant promiscuous binding for various chemokines.

Cytokines and signalling

Certain heterodimer cytokines (e.g. IL-2, IL-4, IL-7, IL-9, IL-13, and IL-15) bind using a common signal-transducing receptor chain. These cytokines use the common IL-2R γ-chain, which is a component common to each of their respective receptors. The γ-chain was first identified as part of IL-2R trimolecular complex. Patients with SCID have profound defects in T and B cell immunity. The largest subgroup of X-linked SCIDs have been shown to have a molecular defect (mutation) in the gene encoding the γ-chain. This nonfunctional receptor signalling subunit compromises all cytokines in this grouping, hence, the global defects in T and B cells (note the role of these cytokines on lymphoctyes in Table 1.4). The use of a common chain as part of different cytokines is also seen with other molecules; for example, IL-12 and IL-23 share a common polypeptide chain designated P40. In contrast, IL-10 and IL-22 share a common receptor subunit (chain of the IL-10R, designated IL-10R2).

As indicated above, cytokines can be grouped into families or superfamilies based on their overall molecular form and structure, including usage of shared chains or common receptor units for signalling. Some examples are:

- IL-1 superfamily—IL-1, IL-8, IL-33
- IL-6 family—IL-6, IL-11, IL-27
- common γ family—IL-2, IL-4, IL-7, IL-9, IL-13, IL-15, IL-21 (as outlined above)
- IL-12 family—IL-12, IL-23, IL-27, IL-35

Cytokines are often produced in cascades with varying kinetics. One cytokine will often stimulate cells to make additional cytokines. Some of these molecules may act synergistically, thus amplifying responses, or they may act antagonistically, opposing or suppressing the induction of other cytokines. Figure 1.10 presents an overview of a dominant cytokine signal transduction pathway, the well-defined JAK/STAT system. Unravelling the details of such pathways is providing the potential for new therapeutic targets for diseases where cytokine signalling and/or the activation pathways involved in gene expression can be used to treat chronic inflammatory or autoimmune diseases and some cancers. Figure 1.10 shows the cytokine receptor signal transduction pathway that is used by IL-2 and IL-2R (trimer; common γ family). It also shows the heterodimer cytokines (IL-12 and IL-23) sharing the common p40. Following the interaction of the cytokine with the receptor the latter becomes phosphorylated and acts as a docking site for signalling molecules called Janus kinases (JAKs), which in turn phosphorylate and activate the members of a family of transcription factors referred to as STATs (signal transducers and activators of transcription), which induce their STAT-dependent genes. Activated STATs translocate from the cytoplasm to the nucleus, binding to DNA sequences to regulate the expression of genes within cells that have been stimulated by the cytokine (note the similarity with TLR and NLR signalling which targets transcription factors such as NF-κB and MAPK). There are several JAKs and STATs; three JAKs have been defined in humans and, at present, seven different STATs. Different JAKs and STATs have shown variation in their distribution and functions in different leucocytes and other cell types, and varied profiles in different diseases. These differential expressions give a rationale for therapeutic targeting for molecules which have been considered historically as ubiquitous in cellular signalling [20].

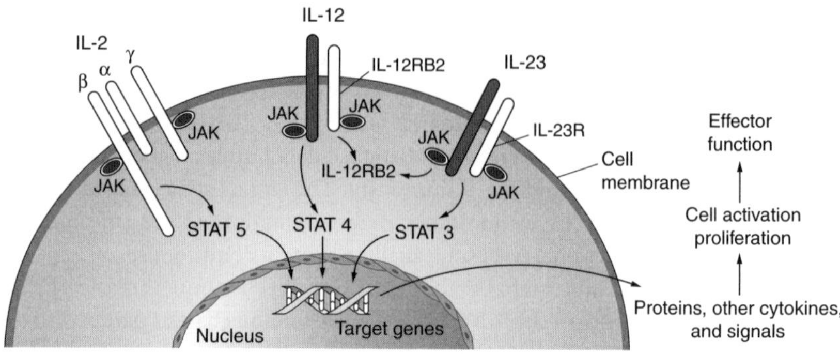

Fig. 1.10 Cytokine/cytokine receptor interactions and signal transduction via JAK/STAT. IL-2 is shown binding to the IL-2R which has three chains, CD25 (α-chain), CD122 (β-chain), and CD132 (γ-chain). The γ-chain is also used for signalling by other cytokines in the superfamily—the common γ-chain grouping. The other cytokines shown (IL-12 and IL-23) are heterodimers. IL-12/IL-23 share a common p40 chain which binds to the IL-12RB1 chain common to both of their receptors. The cytokine–receptor interactions lead to the phosphorylation of JAKs which in turn provide docking sites for STATs which become phosphorylated, dimerize, and translocate to the nucleus to induce activation of genes and their products, along with other cellular changes. The result commonly is cell activation, proliferation, and generation of effector functions. Dominant STATs used by each cytokine signal are shown; in reality, other STATs are involved in each of these signalling pathways. IL-12R/23R, interleukin-12 receptor/23 receptor; JAK, Janus kinases; STAT, signal transducers and activators of transcription.

In lymphoid cells, knocking out genes for JAK3 induces markedly impaired T cell development and down-regulates their functions, although other cell types are left largely unaffected. Drug antagonists of JAK3 are being developed to use as possible therapeutic agents to treat diseases associated with excessive or unwanted T cell function (autoimmune diseases or acute transplant rejections). Similarly, different STAT molecules have been shown to be associated with different cytokine-driven differentiation pathways of various Th subsets (IL-4 uses STAT6 to develop Th2 subsets). Again, researchers are trying to define antagonists which may have specificity for STATs within particular disease situations.

Central and peripheral lymphoid organs; lymphocyte recirculation

Introduction

Classical anatomical studies, together with histological staining methods supplemented by immunohistological specification of cell types and molecules, have provided a more detailed background of the organization of lymphoid tissues (see Figures 1.11, 1.12 and 1.13). Subsequent studies, using fresh slices of tissues *ex vivo* with labelling of living cells, have provided some insight into the dynamic interaction of cells and/or molecules (e.g. integrins with their ligands). Additionally, the use of MABs or antibody

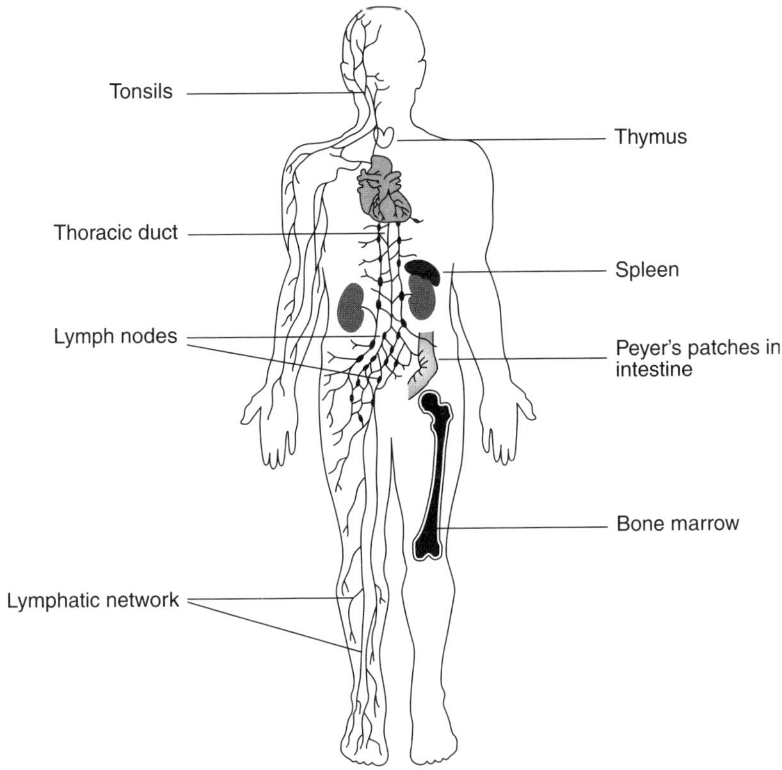

Fig. 1.11 The human lymphoid system. T and B lymphocytes can be defined in compartments within various tissues, as well as undergoing continuous recirculation between lymphatics, blood, and lymphoid organs. Thymus and bone marrow function as central (primary) organs for development of T and B cells.

fragments to inhibit such interactions has helped to define the importance and hierarchy of different molecular interactions. These latter approaches have helped to define in great detail the interactions of leucocytes with normal endothelial cells or those derived from inflammatory tissue. The interactions that have been well defined include T cell integrin LFA-1 binding to its ligand ICAM on endothelial cells.

The integrated working of the whole immune system has specific requirements and unique demands, including the following:

- T lymphocytes need to recognize their antigens linked to self HLA, to respond appropriately to the foreign peptide antigen and, at the same time, not to respond detrimentally.
- T and B cells with specific receptors for antigen are relatively rare cells (1 in 10^4 to 1 in 10^6 cells). The appropriate receptors must find their target antigen, which may enter at any site in the body.
- The encounter with the antigen must occur in a form and at a density to allow a productive interaction.

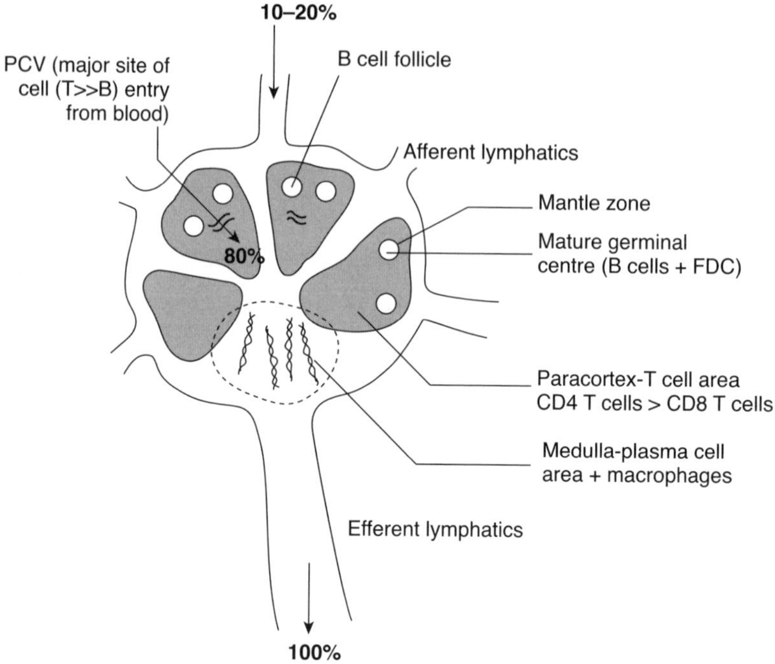

Fig. 1.12 Organization of the lymph node structure facilitates entry of antigen and its specific interaction with the appropriate T and B cells. FDC, follicular dendritic (antigen presenting) cell; PCV, postcapillary venule; %, estimate of lymphocyte traffic. > greater than; >> substantially greater than.

- Naive T and B cells in the peripheral lymphoid tissues need to meet innate cells, in particular DCs, that sample antigens from the peripheral tissues.
- Effector T cells need to access nonlymphoid peripheral tissues for activation by cells (APCs and non-APCs with cognate antigen), particularly in sites of inflammation.
- Tregs need to recognize and interact with responding T and B effector cells to regulate peripheral immune responses.
- Additionally, the effector cells and their regulation need to occur at sites interfacing with pathogens, as well as with potentially malignantly transformed cells, wherever they are found in the body.

These demanding and stringent requirements for immune functions (innate and adaptive immunity) are integrated through complex interplays of diverse cells. Such diverse cells must have the appropriate anatomical and physiological requirements to satisfy the stringent criteria above. This includes such cells as DCs, epithelial cells, $CD4^+$ Th (Th1, Th2, Th17) lymphocytes, $CD8^+$ CTLs, Tregs, B cells, NK cells, NK T, and many other cells of innate immunity, together with the stromal cells associated with the extracellular matrix in lymphoid tissues. Gaining an insight into these complex interactions has required significant advances in technological expertise.

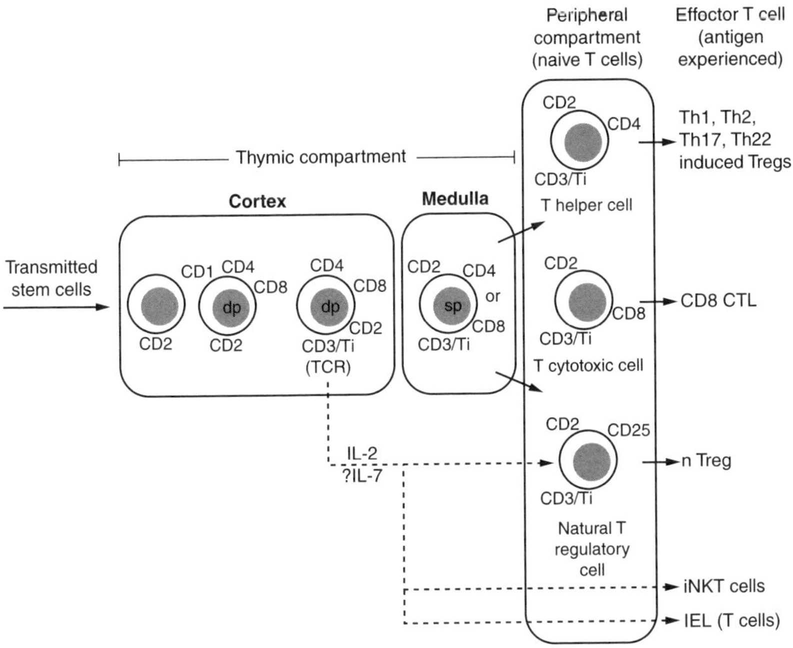

Fig. 1.13 T cell development within the thymus and emergent immunocompetent but naive T cells in the peripheral compartment are shown. Antigen-responsive naive T cells develop into effector cells. The precise pathways to development of invariant (i) NK T cells and IELs are still being unravelled. CTL, cytotoxic T lymphocyte; Dp, double positive thymocytes with CD4$^+$and CD8$^+$ expression on single cells; IELs, intraepithelial lymphocytes; nTreg, natural T regulatory cell; Sp, single positive thymocytes, CD4$^+$ or CD8$^+$ on single cells; TCR, T cell antigen receptor (Ti/CD3 complex).

In the past 10 years, major developments have enabled the use of dynamic real-time techniques, including video imaging of leucocyte interactions. Additionally, there have been advances in confocal microscopy and, more recently, the use of multiphoton intravital microscopy (MPIVM) coupled with the use of MABs and recombinant cytokines. These approaches are giving an unparalleled view and insight into interactions within the central and peripheral lymphoid tissues. This has facilitated direct observation of cell mobility and migration, for example:

- naive T and B cells compared with T and B effector and memory populations (see 'Effector cells and receptors', below)
- cell–cell contact dynamics of T cells (CD4$^+$ and CD8$^+$) with DCs
- cell migration and accumulation at sites of peripheral inflammation
- lymphoid development and interactions in central lymphoid organs [21].

An overview of the knowledge gained from these various approaches, together with particular features of the human central and peripheral lymphoid system, is presented below.

Thymus

This central lymphoid organ, located in the upper anterior mediastinum in humans, is known to be the primary site for the development of T lymphocytes from immigrant bone marrow lymphoid stem cells, which migrate into the thymus from as early as the eighth week of gestation. The inductive factors in the thymus responsible for the differentiation of stem cells to thymic lymphocytes (thymocytes) include a number of small polypeptide hormones. Several such hormones have been isolated, including thymosin (~12 kDa) and thymopoietin (~7 kDa). Organ culture experiments have clearly indicated that direct cell–cell contact between the bone-marrow-derived cells and the mesenchymal/stromal, dendritic, and epithelial elements of the thymus are also crucial for cell proliferation and differentiation, as is the need for cytokines (e.g. IL-2, IL-7).

A scheme for thymocyte development is shown in Figure 1.13, indicating recognized T-cell-associated CD antigens. These CD differentiation antigens are acquired at various stages within the thymus, the most undifferentiated cells being found in the outer cortex and the most mature in the medulla. From the medulla a small percentage of cells migrate out of the thymus, to become the antigen-responsive immunocompetent naive T lymphocytes recognized in the peripheral secondary lymphoid T cell compartments. Thus, peripheral T cells are found in the paracortex of lymph nodes; in the systemic circulation; as intraepithelial lymphocytes (IELs) and lamina propria T cells; and as lymphoid aggregates in the GIT and other mucosal sites. The naive T cells emerging from the thymus are immunocompetent but have not reacted with antigens outside the thymus. Some Tregs are also produced within, and emerge from, the thymus. These are referred to as natural (n) Tregs and have the predominant phenotype $CD4^+$, $CD25^+$, and the Fox P3 transcription factor. The thymic developmental pathway of cells found in the periphery, such as $\gamma\delta$ T cells, NK T cells, and $CD8^+$ IELs are not yet fully elucidated.

It has been well established that both massive proliferation and death of cells occurs in the thymus. These events have been demonstrated by classic histological methods, as well as by labelling cells with radio-isotopes and following the fate of labelled cells. Experiments in mice have demonstrated that within the thymus more than 10^8 lymphocytes are produced per day, but only about 10^6 cells are exported to the periphery. Hence, less than 10% of the cells produced within the organ survive and exit from the gland. This apparent 'mysterious' behaviour within the thymus has been unravelled by modern cellular and molecular biological techniques.

The *raison d'être* of the thymus encompasses three important biological functions:

1. The generation and selective maturation of individual $CD4^+$ and $CD8^+$ immunocompetent T cells, which exit from the thymus. The cells possess specific TCR complexes which will recognize a vast array of possible foreign antigens—complexed with self MHC molecules—to mount an efficient immune response. The TCR repertoire is generated by a random process of somatic gene rearrangements in the TCR genetic loci controlled by *RAG1* and *RAG2* genes.

2. The destruction within the thymus of developing cells which, during proliferation and differentiation, develop TCRs with the potential to react strongly solely against self antigens (rather than against foreign antigens—linked to self MHC). Intrathymic

destruction of such cells (by apoptosis) is seen as a crucial mechanism in the development of central self-tolerance and, thus, a lack of tissue-damaging responses to self antigens, as occurs in autoimmunity.

3. The generation in the thymus of nTregs which migrate to the periphery and there regulate (suppress) other lymphocyte functions. This suppression is thought to occur by direct and indirect mechanisms orchestrated by nTregs. Additionally, induction in the periphery of Tregs has been demonstated; these induced (i) Tregs have a similar phenotype to the nTregs from the thymus, namely they are $CD4^{+}CD25^{+}FoxP3^{+}$ Tregs; some subsets are $CD25^{-}$ but appear to still function as regulatory cells.

The first key biological role (1) is thought to occur by a process termed *positive selection.* Developing cortical thymocytes (possessing both $CD4^{+}$ and $CD8^{+}$ T cells) with TCR binding to particular molecules on thymic epithelial cells (with self antigens including self MHC) are *selected* for survival. The future TCR recognition of foreign antigens (outside the thymus) by these cells will also require them to 'see' the self molecules responsible for their survival. This positive selection is used to explain thymic education of T cells—the process where they must recognize peptide antigen in the context of self HLA. Thymocytes which do not bind to the self molecules at this stage of development undergo apoptosis (programmed cell death). There is strong experimental evidence indicating that in this second key biological role (2) a process of *negative selection* occurs, whereby cells with strong binding TCRs for self molecules (perhaps encountered at the corticomedullary junction) are deleted, again by apoptosis. The CD4 and CD8 molecules on thymocytes are believed to play direct and contributory roles in the processes of positive and negative selection, but these mechanisms require further clarification.

Thus, the T cells trafficking from the thymus have the following properties:

- *unresponsiveness* to self MHC antigens alone
- ability to react to MHC antigens of other members of the species (the basis of recognition of MHC antigens in transplantation, leading to acute rejection; see Chapter 3)
- ability to react with foreign antigens, associated with self MHC (termed MHC restriction).

The massive cell proliferation in the thymus will generate many different families of cells (clones) with TCRs to recognize and interact with the many millions of antigens that may be encountered in life. The price of such diversity could be the development of TCRs with anti-self specificity. Such clones would, however, be largely deleted in the massive death of cells by apoptosis that occurs in the thymus. The thymic selection processes are less than 100% efficient, however; some potentially tissue-damaging reactive anti-self T cells escape deletion and can be found in peripheral lymphoid tissues of most individuals. Additional mechanisms have been described in the periphery to control such potentially self-reactive clones of cells. Some thymic emergent Tregs and other peripheral Tregs act to suppress these potential anti-self responses in secondary lymphoid tissues. This is one form of peripheral tolerance (see 'Immune tolerance: central and peripheral tolerance', below).

An important question regarding deletion of self-reactive T cells in the thymus is: How can the myriad of self antigens, many anatomically and physiologically active outside the thymus, be presented to CD4$^+$/CD8$^+$ T cells in the thymic microenvironment to allow deletion? This conundrum was in part explained by the discovery of the *AIRE* (autoimmune regulator) gene which is functionally associated with thymic cells. This gene encodes a transcription factor which causes a promiscuous transcription of a range of organ-specific genes and translation of their protein products that are usually only present in peripheral tissues. The correctness of this finding is proved by a situation where the *AIRE* gene is nonfunctional either by natural causes (mutational events), or experimentally. Humans with nonfunctional mutations in *AIRE* develop a range of autoimmune disorders and syndromes due to failure of elimination of self-reactive T cells which were not eliminated by negative selection as a result of lack of presentation of the antigens (see 'Autoimmunity', below). The best-characterized autoimmune disorder is called APECED (autoimmune polyendocrinopathy with candidiasis and ectodermal dysplasia).

Bursa equivalents

B lymphopoiesis, like T lymphopoiesis, takes place in a primary lymphoid organ. In birds, a discrete organ found near the cloaca (the bursa of Fabricius) has been shown to be responsible for the development of B cells from bone marrow lymphoid stem cell precursors. In mammals no bursa exists, but there is experimental evidence that the bone marrow and the foetal yolk sac and liver serve a similar function. Modern techniques using MABs and radionuclide tracing have clearly defined differentiation pathways of B cell development (see Figure 1.14), analogous to T cells in the thymic environment.

A feature common to both T and B primary organs is that the cells in their early development in those sites are relatively immunoincompetent; they will not react positively and generate immune responses against classic non-self antigens. Indeed, encounter with antigens at this time can result in deletion or inactivation of such cells.

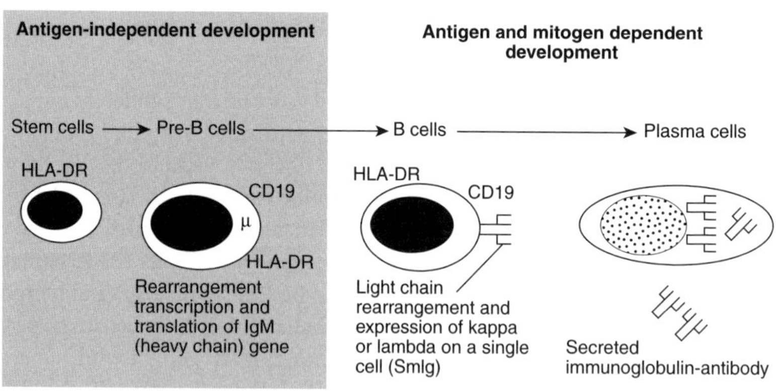

Fig. 1.14 B lymphocyte development. Surface membrane immunoglobulin (SmIg) on the B cell functions as the antigen-specific receptor.

Naive but immunocompetent T and B lymphocytes, by contrast, are found in the secondary lymphoid organs and other sites.

Secondary lymphoid organs

The common feature of all these sites (lymph nodes, spleen, tonsils, etc.) is that T and B cells can be found in fairly identifiable compartments and are closely juxtaposed anatomically to members of the APC family. Figure 1.12 shows a cross-section of a lymph node with the predominant collection of T cells in the paracortex and B cells in the follicular areas. Plasma cells, which are derived from B cells and secrete antibody molecules, can be found in the medullary region. In all of these areas of the node, appropriate APCs can be demonstrated along with a stromal network of fibroblastic reticular cells (FRCs) associated with the extracellular matrix. These FRCs are now known to be a major source of IL-7 which is critical for the survival of lymphoid cells within the secondary lymphoid organs.

Lymphatic network; recirculation pathways

The lymphoid cells detectable in a blood differential count consist of T cells (~50–90%), B cells (~5–15%), and a minor population (~1–10%) of LGLs which contain NK cells. The blood T and B cells enter the substance of lymph nodes through the postcapillary venules (PCVs) via the HEV cells. The cells then traffic through the respective T and B areas of the node and, together with a smaller percentage of cells that enter via the afferent lymphatics, leave the node via the efferent lymphatics. Figure 1.12 shows this traffic, based on experiments using fine needle cannulation of the lymphatics and blood vessels. Ultimately the lymphatics empty into the circulating blood, where the thoracic duct joins the left subclavian vein, from whence the lymphocytes recirculate (Figure 1.11). Lymphocyte migration in tissues is, in part, dependent on three-dimensional anatomical arrangements associated with sinuses, capsular canals (trabeculae), and interactions of the follicular T cells and of the proteins that constitute the extracellular matrix. Additionally, lymphocytes express receptors for various chemokines (CC and CXC) which show variable segregation on different functional and phenotypic groups of cells. Chemokines produced by stromal and other cells, and found in solution or bound to the surfaces of cells such as endothelial cells, direct trafficking of lymphocytes in and out of tissues. Furthermore, certain lymphocyte–integrin interactions (with their ligands) will segregate and help to activate cells in various tissues. Integrin–ligand interactions form the basis of the selective homing of some cell types to certain sites. The best-known example is the recirculation and homing of IgA-committed B lymphocyte populations to mucosal-associated lymphoid tissues (MALT—see below). Some key features of cell recirculation, trafficking, and homing in physiological and pathological states are as follows:

- Naive T cells in their quest to find their cognate antigens constantly recirculate during their lifetime between blood and the lymphatic tissues making up the secondary lymphoid organs. Naive T cells adhere to the endothelial cells of the HEVs within the secondary lymphoid organs by engagement of their CCR7 receptors with the corresponding ligands CCL19 and CCL21. The migration of these naive T cells is further enhanced by T cell LFA-1 integrin interaction with the endothelial ICAMs to facilitate the T cell migration into T cell areas at these sites—paracortex of lymph nodes and white pulp of spleen. In these sites, if the T cells meet the appropriate DCs expressing HLA–peptide antigen complexes for which the T cells express specific TCRs, dynamic and strong interactions occur resulting in the formation of anatomically defined immunological synapses. This facilitates the interactions of TCRs with the HLA–peptide complexes, which is further enhanced by costimulatory and other adhesive interactions and cytokine signalling within that local synaptic area. The sum total of these interactions will provide the necessary first signal and potential for subsequent full activation of the cell.

- Effector and memory T cells generated from activated and differentiated naive T cells express different signalling chemokine and adhesion receptors (compared with the naive cells) which facilitate their functional properties, imparting to effector T cells their ability to enter peripheral tissues and respond in sites of inflammation and/or pathogen/antigen entry [22]. Concommitant with the induction of effector T cells and associated new receptors to underpin their new functions, they lose the ability to recirculate like naive T cells through secondary lymphoid organs—they lose the expression of CCR7. Additionally, well-differentiated effector T cells use the key integrin $\alpha 4\beta 1$ to react with MADCAM 1 on endothelial cells in peripheral tissues.
- Central memory cells retain the ability to recirculate, and continue to express CCR7 and L selectin, along with other CD markers, which help to characterize them as memory cells. Physiologically, wherever they re-encounter their inducing antigen they are capable of inducing a more efficient secondary/memory-based immune response.
- The discrete segregation of T and B cells into defined areas within secondary lymphoid tissues is largely explained by their differential expression of ligand and receptor pairs for various chemokines. The use of antichemokine receptor agents is currently being tested in some early clinical studies: for instance, the differential expression of CCR5 and CXCR3 on T cells which enter the CNS of patients with MS. This raises the potential for new targets and opportunities to destroy these tissue-damaging T cells and modulate the course of the disease.
- Visualization by MPIVM of the interactions of $CD8^+$ T cells and Tregs in the vicinity of malignant cells allows concepts of immune modulation to be placed on firmer grounds to enhance antitumour responses *in situ*. Dynamic experiments have already demonstrated that individual cancer cells can be simultaneously or sequentially attacked by multiple cytotoxic T cells.
- Tregs have been shown to operate by direct or close physical associations with DCs to modulate their function for supporting or, in some situations, suppressing, effector T cell responses [23]. Tregs have also been shown to directly interact with T effectors without an intermediary. Tregs exert their effects by elaboration of suppressive cytokines such as IL-10 and TGF-β. These mechanisms are not mutually exclusive. Tregs have been shown to direct DCs to secrete large amounts of TGF-β.

The lymphatics, which also transport antigens in solution or associated with migrating APCs, as well as facilitating the recirculation of lymphocytes, provide a most efficient system for immune cells to encounter and interact with non-self antigens, irrespective of where such antigens have managed to breach the integrity of the host.

Clonal selection

The concept of specificity within the immune system, coupled with its evident ability to react against huge numbers of different antigens, is best explained and crystallized in the *clonal selection theory* of immunology. This original concept, elaborated in various forms by Burnet, Jerne, and Talmage to explain antibody production, is now equally applicable to T lymphocyte responses.

Apart from its specificity and memory, the other striking feature of the immune system is its diversity. The T and B lymphocytes within an individual can react to a great number (calculated to be many millions) of non-self antigens. How does such enormous diversity come about, and how is it harmonized with the salient features of immunological specificity and memory which characterize adaptive immunity? This is best explained and encapsulated in the clonal selection theory.

Figure 1.15 represents the essence of the theory, the basis of which is as follows:

- A lymphocyte and its identical progeny, termed a *clone* (identical with respect to their genes) possess on their cell membranes receptors with specific binding sites for only one or a very limited number of antigenic determinants. The number of cells comprising a single clone (e.g. clone A3) has been calculated as ranging from 10^3 to 10^5 in the B and T cell compartments. It has been estimated that the

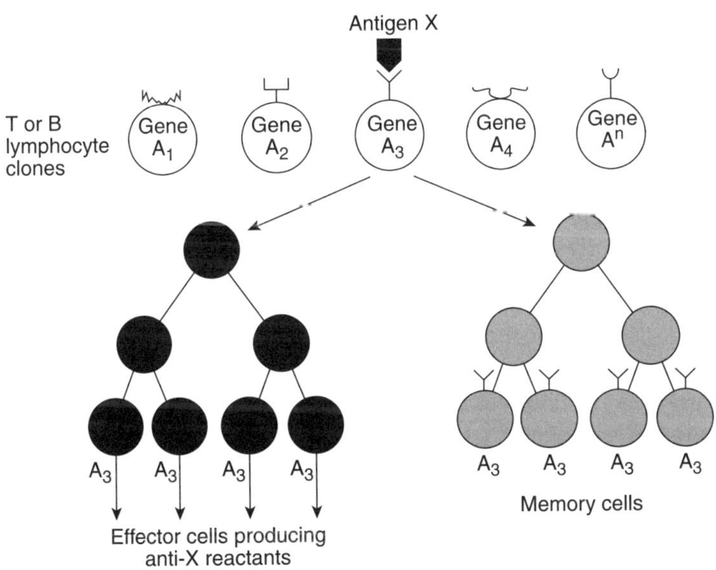

Fig. 1.15 Clonal selection: antigen X selects and interacts with the clone expressing the 'best fit' (complementarity) receptor. The clone responds by proliferation and differentiation to generate anti-X effector and memory cells.

total number of lymphocytes in humans is more than 10^{14} cells. Thus, by simple arithmetical analysis, there are over 10^6 different individual clones (A1, A2, . . ., A^n). The mechanisms of receptor specificity for antigens are explained in terms of the genetics and molecular events that occur during the development of B and T cells and are outlined in the sections on B and T cells (see 'Recognition elements, cells, and receptors in adaptive immunity', below).

- Implicit in the clonal selection theory is the idea that the specificity of a clone antedates any experience or encounter with classical non-self antigens. Hence, lymphocyte clones possess specific receptors, each precommitted to a single antigen. Thus, ultimately, when antigen is encountered, *selection* of a precommitted clone with the 'best-fitting receptor' for that antigen occurs.

The shape of the receptor expressed on the surface of A_3 (see Figure 1.15) gives the basis of the specificity. The events following receptor–antigen interaction involve cell proliferation and differentiation, resulting in the exponential expansion of the responding clone, some of the clone members proceeding to endstage effector cells, which will act against the inciting antigen. In the case of B cell clones, some of the cells differentiate into plasma cells and secrete antibodies with the same specificity as that expressed by the BCR originally selected by the antigen. Similarly, for CMI some T cells differentiate into effector cells, such as CTLs. It is noteworthy that with clonal expansion not all the progeny become endstage effectors. Some reach an intermediate point of differentiation and proliferation, and such cells form the cellular basis for the immunological property of memory. Thus, if the same antigen is encountered on a subsequent occasion, the memory bank of cells undergoes a quantitatively greater and more rapid response against the antigen. Clonal expansion gives four memory cells each with the specific A_3 receptor for antigen, compared with only one cell in the original primary response. Furthermore, the clonal expansion events also qualitatively result in changes in the affinity (strength of binding) of the lymphocyte receptor for antigen, although maintaining the same specificity.

Most experimental evidence to date supports the tenets of the clonal selection theory. 'Suicide' experiments using high dose radiolabelled antigens have resulted in radiation-induced deletion of specific clones; rechallenge with the same antigen gives no response, yet challenge with a different antigen elicits an appropriate response. Recent experiments have indicated that certain sites, such as the germinal centres of lymph nodes, provide the appropriate microenvironment for generating 'memory' B lymphocytes and for long-term retention of small amounts of antigen on specialized APCs within the germinal centre.

In summary, immunocompetent lymphocytes express glycoprotein receptors on their cell membranes. Lymphocytes undergoing activation and differentiation retain the same specificity of their receptors for antigens as that of their progenitors. Hence, in the case of the B lymphocyte, its antibody receptor V region specificity (see 'B cells, receptors, and antibodies', below) is the same as the binding specificity of antibodies secreted from plasma cells derived from the B cells. Each immunocompetent B or T cell (representing a member of a clone) bears receptors of unique specificity, when compared with receptors on lymphocytes from another clone.

Immunogens, antigens, and adjuvants

Antigens and immunogens

The term antigen strictly defines substances that will react specifically with preformed immune effector molecules. If they induce the production of such immune effectors, they are termed immunogens. All immunogens can be antigens but the converse is not always true. Through imprecise usage over many years the term immunogen and antigen are now often used interchangeably. Large proteins are usually the most efficient antigens but polysaccharides, synthetic polypeptides, and simple polymers can also be antigenic. Pure nucleic acids have been shown experimentally to be nonimmunogenic, yet it is known that, in old age and in autoimmune disorders, humans and other animals can produce antibodies that will react with nucleic acids. Hence, patients with SLE may have antibodies against different nucleic acids, including those reacting with double-stranded DNA. It is possible that antibodies arise against large nucleoproteins (or cross-reacting substances) and that some antibodies have the ability to react specifically with the associated nucleic acid. It has been shown that danger signalling molecules, such as HMGB-1, can complex with DNA molecules to form an immunogen that induces anti-DNA antibodies.

There are several well-defined properties of molecules which render them good immunogens. Foremost of these properties is their *'foreignness'*, which the immune system discriminates from self. The size of the molecule is important and, as a generalization, molecules more than 10 kDa in size tend to be strongly antigenic, especially if they are polypeptides. The actual *genetic background* of the animal exposed to a non-self substance may dictate whether the substance functions as an antigen. Careful experiments with inbred strains of mice, rats, and guinea-pigs have clearly documented the existence of so-called *immune response genes*, which determine whether an introduced non-self substance will function as an antigen in the animal. The immune response gene effect has most often been shown to be expressed as an autosomal dominant trait. Many of the immune response genes are contained within the MHC region and are products of genes found in and around that region.

The apparent antigenicity of a substance will also depend on the *dose* and its *route* of administration. In some situations, a non-self substance known to be extremely antigenic can fail to elicit an immune response. This effect is produced by manoeuvres such as intravenous injections of very small or very large doses of antigen, i.e. either side of the standard antigenic dose. With a very large dose, a definite negative influence is exerted on the immune system such that a *tolerant* state (acquired immunological tolerance) to that foreign antigen is induced.

Classic experiments by Landsteiner defined the properties of substances called *haptens*. These are molecules (usually very small) which by themselves are unable to induce an immune response. Nevertheless, they are capable of being recognized by, and interact with, antibodies or effector T cells induced by another means. The experimental method of inducing the immune response is usually to link the small hapten to a larger carrier molecule (usually a protein). This provides the necessary information for the combined molecule to be recognized as part of an immunogen. Processed peptides derived from the carrier molecules are recognized by T cells, and antibodies produced by the B cells will recognize and bind the hapten. The study of 'haptenization'—attachment of the small agents to large protein carrier molecules—provides an explanation of how diverse substances, including very small metallic ions (e.g. nickel), anaesthetic gases such as halothane, and antibiotics such as penicillin, can, in individuals of the appropriate genetic background, induce demonstrable immune responses, often of a pathological nature. It is suggested that the small molecules complex to normal readily accessible self proteins, such as albumin and prealbumin (which are widely distributed extra- and intravascularly). More recent evidence also indicates that binding of small molecules to self DAMPs induced by cell stressors also results in immunogenic complexes. The complexing presents 'altered' self determinants which can appear as non-self to immune cells and thus induce humoral and cell-mediated responses, some of which are directed to the haptens of the complex.

Concept of complementarity

The interaction of antigen with antibody or with the specific receptor on the membrane of T and B lymphocytes is often expressed in terms of a 'lock and key' interaction. It can best be thought of in terms of the overall three-dimensional shape, which is recognized by the receptor or antibody regions that interact with the complementary shape of the antigen. The binding affinity of the specific immune elements with the antigen can be thought of in terms of their degree of closeness of fit or complementarity. Apparent antigen *cross-reactions* may thus be accounted for in regard to overall complementarity, rather than likeness in terms of overall charge or size. Hence, cross-reactions result from the closeness in overall shape of the two molecules and their complementarity with the antibody's '*antigen combining regions*' or complementarity determining regions (CDRs). A well-documented example involves certain streptococcal antigens that induce antibodies which can cross-react and bind to other human cardiac antigens that are very dissimilar in terms of size and charge.

A further consequence of considering the overall shape of antigens and the corresponding binding regions of antibodies and lymphocyte receptors is the realization that, even though antigens may be very large molecules, it is only a few sites (usually accessible surface sites) of a large folded protein structure that are recognized by B lymphocytes and antibodies. The sites are termed the *antigenic determinants* or *epitopes* of the antigen molecule. It is calculated that four to six amino acids or sugar residues may contribute to an epitope of a protein or polysaccharide antigen, respectively. T lymphocytes do not recognize native conformational (folded) protein antigen epitopes, as described for B lymphocytes. Instead, T cells recognize peptide fragments of antigens (eight to nine amino acids) presented on self HLA, after having undergone significant intracellular '*processing*' and transport to the surface membrane of APCs and other cell types.

A single large antigen may, therefore, induce both T and B cell responses, usually elicited to different epitopes on the same molecule.

T cell requirement for optimal B cell response

Efficient humoral immune responses require the dual function of T and B cells. In fact, the B cell antibody response (for optimal results) requires T cell recognition of the same molecule—albeit different epitopes—to provide 'help' for an efficient antibody response. The B cell itself can function as an APC, presenting processed peptide bound to HLA to the cognate Th cell. These types of antigens are often referred to as *thymus (T cell)-dependent antigens*. Contrastingly, there is a group of substances termed *thymus-independent (TI) antigens*, which have the property of eliciting B lymphocyte and antibody responses with minimal or no requirement for T cell involvement. Such TI antigens are exemplified by bacterial polysaccharides, which have the structural feature of many identical repeating molecules and epitopes. They tend to induce IgM antibodies and some IgGs, especially of the IgG2 subclass in humans. TI antigens can be made more antigenic by linking them to protein carrier molecules (exploiting the principle of hapten–protein complexes). This approach has in recent years led to successful new vaccines against encapsulated bacteria and prevention of much mortality and morbidity, especially in the paediatric setting. Noted successes are vaccination programmes against pneumococcus and haemophilus where microbial polysaccarides are linked to proteins, such as tetanus toxoid, to generate strong immunogens.

Tailor-made antigens

The recent advances in the isolation and molecular cloning of genes have led to the possibility of generating large amounts of pure antigens for vaccination programmes. This is particularly so in the case of complex microbial antigens. Parasites, such as those causing malaria or schistosomiasis, are very complex organisms with potentially hundreds of epitopes, some of which may induce protective immune responses. Using molecular biological techniques, researchers are now defining and cloning specific genes, to produce a single or a few dominant antigens and their epitopes in the hope of generating vaccines to the latter in order to combat such pandemic infections. Furthermore, the acquired knowledge concerning the generation of processed peptides as antigens is also resulting in attempts to synthesize tailor-made peptide antigens for vaccination programmes. Both approaches—gene cloning and peptide synthesis—are currently being employed in the fight against AIDS, seeking to define and produce noninfectious peptide antigens of HIV to use in possible vaccination programmes (see 'Vaccination', below). The need for effective adjuvants is key to the potential success of using these newer antigens.

Adjuvants

Adjuvants are a wide range of compounds which act in a nonspecific immunostimulatory fashion to enhance the immunogenicity and/or antigenicity of weak antigens. The classic example is *Freund's complete adjuvant* (FCA), which is a combination of mycobacterial products, organic oils, and a detergent. FCA is commonly mixed with a solution of antigen to form an injectable emulsion. The resultant antigen–adjuvant complex is a very potent stimulator of the immune response. FCA, however, is so potent that it is not used in humans as it induces extensive granulomatous reactions at the injection site. Adjuvants in general have been shown experimentally to nonspecifically increase the action of macrophages and other APCs and to enhance T and B lymphocyte functions.

In humans, the most commonly used adjuvants are aluminium compounds (alums), which form precipitates with antigens in common usage, such as tetanus and diphtheria toxoids. Newer adjuvants are being evaluated for human use, especially those designed for increasing the antigenicity of synthetic peptides and the newer DNA recombinant antigens. Two examples of newer adjuvants investigated over the past decade are muramyl dipeptide (MDP), a relatively nontoxic extract of mycobacterial membranes, and the potent immunostimulating complexes (ISCOMs) composed of a glycoside extracted from the bark of an Amazonian tree which readily forms micelles containing entrapped peptide or polypeptide antigens. However, *in vivo* ISCOMs have proved disappointing, and MDP is still being evaluated.

Alum-based adjuvants (still the most widely used) are known to be effective in generating strong Th2-biased antibody responses. Their effectiveness is extensively exploited in vaccines used worldwide—DTP and parenteral polio vaccines. Their immunostimulatory role has now been largely defined and includes activation of inflammasomes and induction of inflammation, as well as recruitment and stimulation of APCs such as DCs. Alum, however, shows limited potentiation of $CD8^+$ CTLs and Th1 responses. These immune mechanisms are deemed desirable for vaccines against 'life-limiting' infections (especially associated with intracellular microbes, viruses, and bacteria such as *Mycobacterium tuberculosis*). Similarly, $CD8^+$ CTLs and Th1 responses are seen as crucial for effective anticancer vaccines. Newer adjuvants, therefore, are urgently needed (see Chapter 4).

Many of the antigens currently being explored to combat microbial agents causing HIV/AIDS, malaria, tuberculosis, and other less well known infectious diseases, are generated by genetic engineering techniques in the form of recombinant protein molecules, or subunits of pathogens. Also, DNA vaccine constructs, along with synthetic peptides, are being produced by state-of-the-art molecular biological approaches supported by informatics and predictive algorithms on antigenicity. These newer antigens all have the common drawback of relatively poor immunogenicity; hence the urgent need for powerful and safe new adjuvants to enhance their immunostimulatory properties. Knowledge gained over the past 20 years of the integration of innate and adaptive immune responses has reinvigorated vaccine/adjuvant studies. The knowledge of innate receptors—TLRs, retinoic-acid-inducible gene 1-like receptors (RAIGLRs), NLRs—responding to microbial PAMPS, as a key event for antimicrobial inflammatory responses and, concurrently, inducing the development of T and B cell adaptive immunity, has led to new thinking and ways of producing adjuvants that will exploit innate receptors to enhance immunogenicity. Examples of very promising adjuvants that act as TLR agonists include a modified form of lipid A, a PAMP isolated from some species of salmonella. Modification of lipid A is necessary as it is too toxic for human use. A derived modified product called monophosphoryl lipid A (MPL), retains the property of lipid A, thus allowing it to act on TLR-4 as a potent agonist. MPL has been incorporated into vaccines licensed for human use against hepatitis B and human papillomavirus. The vaccine constructs incorporating this new adjuvant induce very good T cell CMI and antibody responses. Other TLRs targeted by newer adjuvants exploit the PAMP molecule CpG which is a ligand targeting the endosomal TLR-9 molecule.

Consideration of all vaccine strategies must balance efficacy with safety concerns. One of the perceived potential risks of using TLR agonists is the possibility of stimulating too prominent an inflammatory response. This is an important reason why FCA is so potent a stimulator of excessive inflammation; the mycobacterial-associated PAMPs within the oil and water complex. Another concern regarding possible excessive TLR stimulation is the possibility of the development of damaging autoimmunity. Currently, large studies of the licensed vaccines that are targeting TLR-4 indicate no significant problems with inflammatory disease or autoimmunity. However, vigilance will be required for all new constructs.

Another exciting area of adjuvant development is aimed at enhancing and exploiting the mucosal route and MALT immunity. Attenuated microbes have long proven the value of exploiting the mucosal route, as seen with the relatively successful use of oral polio, typhoid, and cholera vaccines and, more recently, an oral live attenuated rotavirus vaccine. Many pathogens or potential pathogens cause human infections via the mucosal route and not parenterally. Increased understanding of mucosal immune responses (innate and adaptive) is allowing the development of safe and efficacious adjuvants to enhance a broad range of mucosal-directed vaccinations (see 'Mucosal-associated lymphoid tissue' and 'Vaccination', below). Major efforts are being pursued in the use of the modified cholera toxins and of the heat-labile *E. coli* enterotoxin. They are proving good candidate adjuvants to enhance mucosal immunity. Some forms of these modified toxins are in advanced clinical trials with careful monitoring of efficacy and safety. Another intriguing approach to the development of good adjuvanted vaccines, aiming to induce all-round good Th1, Th2, $CD8^+$ CTL, and antibody responses, is based on a promising construct known as a virosome. This approach essentially takes an envelope virus, such as influenza, and by the use of detergent solubilization, ultracentrifigation, and extraction of infectious nucleic acids, together with functional reconstitution of the envelope, provides an empty body. This is the virosome, which can then be loaded internally with vaccine antigens; adjuvants and molecules can also be incorporated within the envelope itself. The elegance of the virosome is that its envelope still retains the noninfectious haemagglutinin of influenza, which allows it to bind to surface receptors of many cells, including APCs and DCs. It is then effectively taken up and processed in class I and class II antigen-processing pathways. Virosomes have been shown to induce $CD4^+$ Th, $CD8^+$ CTL, and antibody responses.

The field of adjuvant research is undergoing a renaissance fuelled by our increased knowledge of the details of integration of innate and adaptive immunity. Coupled with international coordination and funding from organizations in the USA (such as the National Institute of Allergy and Infectious Diseases) and the European Union, and the ongoing efforts in the biotechnology industry, there is much optimism that we will have significant new novel and effective adjuvants to help advance vaccines to combat the major morbidity and mortality of infections and cancers, in both the developing and developed world.

Recognition elements, cells, and receptors in adaptive immunity

Major histocompatibility complex

Structure, location, and function

The MHC is a discrete, chromosomally assigned region where genes are located that encode the information for the production of molecules (glycoproteins) that are

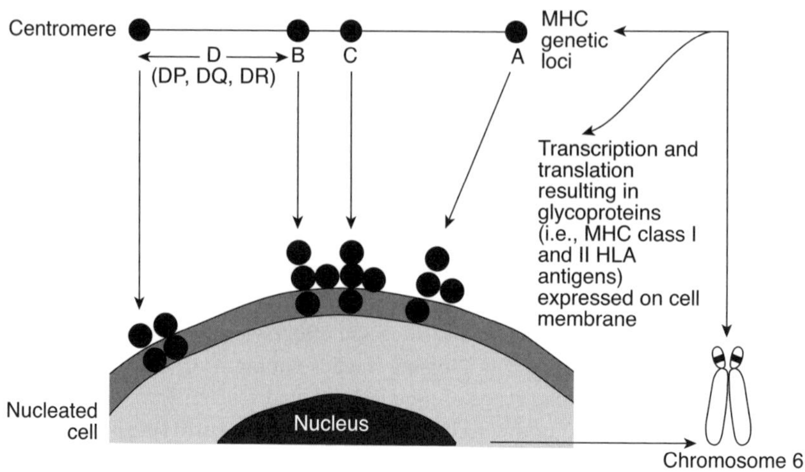

Fig. 1.16 The human major histocompatibility complex (MHC) and expressed human leucocyte antigens (HLAs) at the cell membrane.

expressed phenotypically on and in cells. The MHC is located on the short arm of chromosome 6 in humans, and on chromosome 17 in mice. Located within the MHC region are discrete loci (points) of defined genes. The classic products of human MHC genes are the HLA glycoproteins; the original demonstration of the products was in leucocytes. Other genes within the MHC code for non-HLA glycoproteins.

Figure 1.16 outlines the events from the level of the genes to the cell expression of HLA (some texts also use the term MHC antigens to define the HLA) (see Chapter 3).

The classical HLAs are termed class I (for the collective HLA loci A, B, and C) and class II (loci HLA-DR, DQ, and DP). They are good examples of an allelic system; i.e. many alternative forms of any one particular gene (gene variant) or its products can be found in different members of the same species.

The many alleles encoded within the MHC genes, together with the potential for many differing combinations of A, B, C, DR, DQ, and DP, lead to a system which can also be defined as very polymorphic. The collection of MHC genes on a single chromosome is termed the haplotype; the genotype is determined by the paternal and maternal chromosomes. The MHC genes of maternal and paternal alleles are codominantly expressed. The inheritance of the MHC genes follows classic mendelian rules (see Chapter 3).

Linkage disequilibrium defines the situation where certain MHC genes are found associated together (linked) on a chromosome at a frequency far in excess of the predicted/expected occurrence of these genes associating, if the association events were a completely random process through evolutionary time. From an evolutionary perspective, the occurrence of linkage disequilibrium suggests that such a nonrandom association must have some selective advantage to the organism. The effects of linkage disequilibrium are further discussed in the chapters on transplantation (Chapter 3) and autoimmunity (Chapter 8).

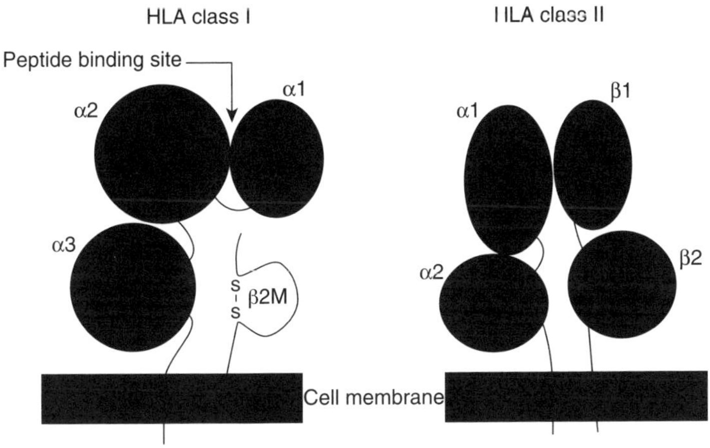

Fig. 1.17 HLA class I (with associated peptide binding site) and class II molecules expressed at the cell membrane. β2M, β2-microglobulin; α1, β1, etc., domain units; HLA, human leucocyte antigen; S–S, disulphide bonds.

The polymorphisms (between individuals in DNA sequences in which the differences are present at a frequency >1% in the population) are mostly represented by SNPs, with many fewer deletion/insertion polymorphisms. Details of the identification, cataloguing and typing of the alternative genes in the MHC class I and II regions are given in Chapter 3.

The overall forms of HLA class I and II products have been determined and are shown diagrammatically in Fig 1.17. The figure illustrates the concepts of 'domains'; segments of the protein where defined lengths and sequences of amino acids can be seen as folding into a particular three-dimensional conformation. The HLA class I antigen has α1, α2, and α3 domains, which on the cell membrane are associated with the small polypeptide called β_2-microglobulin (β2M). The latter is not encoded by a gene in the MHC; in humans the β2M gene is on chromosome 15. The evolutionary reason for the close association of class I antigen with β2M is not clear, but functionally it appears to be necessary for the full expression of the HLA class I. The HLA class I antigen molecules thus are made up of two chains, α and β, although α is the true class I HLA chain. In contrast, both α- and β-chains of the HLA class II antigens are coded for by MHC genes. Class II molecules are expressed mainly on macrophages, DCs, and B lymphocytes. The class I molecules, however, are expressed on all nucleated body cells. Although class II expression is restricted physiologically, at times of significant inflammation and/or immune activation, class II can be induced on a much wider range of cell types—on epithelial and endothelial cells in association with inflammation.

Within the HLA class III region are found genes for complement components and regulatory proteins of the complement system, and also genes for inflammation-associated cytokines (TNF and lymphotoxin α and β).

Since the discovery of the MHC in the 1970s, much research has focused on its role in transplantation and, subsequently, more broadly in adaptive immune responses to infections (initially focusing on viral infections). The classical Nobel prize winning experiments of Zinkernagel and Doherty and others demonstrated that for T cells to recognize an antigen that antigen had to be complexed with self MHC, i.e. with the HLA products. This biological property was termed MHC restriction. Subsequent biochemical, molecular biological, and x-ray crystallographic studies demonstrated HLA-bound peptide–antigen complexes in great detail. The size of the peptides, their affinity for binding to HLA class I and class II molecules, their precise amino acid interactions (e.g. via various residues), and the kinetics of peptide binding have all been studied in great detail.

It is clear that the biological and evolutionary role of the MHC is to provide protection against infection, rather than a system persisting to frustrate the transplant surgeon! As outlined below, pathways have been defined by which HLA class I molecules can present bound endogenous peptides to $CD8^+$ T cells, while HLA class II can present exogenous antigen-derived peptides to $CD4^+$ T cells. The polymorphism associated with the MHC appears to be advantageous for the individual and the species in optimizing the opportunity to potentially respond to the vast array (diversity) of antigenic peptides that are associated with the universe of microbial proteins. Variations in MHC allow opportunities for binding such peptides and presenting them to the T cell system. Thus, no matter how novel or pathogenic the microbe (e.g. a new pandemic influenza virus), peptides can be derived that would be seen by some members of the species to facilitate immunity, protection, and survival.

Over the past several decades, studies of the MHC have focused on its involvement in adaptive immunity. However, it has become increasingly clear that the MHC also has a crucial role in innate immunity. Indeed, the MHC appears to have a key role in integrating these two arms of immunity. This is most evident with the better understanding of the extended mapping of the MHC since 2003, as part of the successful project to sequence the entire human genome [24]. The extended MHC map has confirmed the clusters of genes in the classical class I and II regions and in class III (see Fig 1.18). Moreover, it has provided more detailed information on additional genes in all of these regions (defining so-called superclusters). Many of these genes are clearly linked to functions in innate and adaptive immunity. For example, the HLA class I supercluster now includes, along with the classical HLA-A, B, and C, the nonclassical

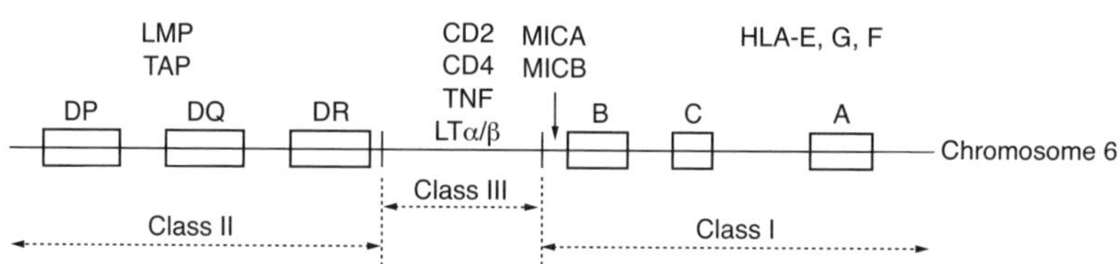

Fig. 1.18 Extended MHC map: MHC loci products are expressed codominantly in the alleles inherited from both parents as HLA molecules on or in each cell. The entire MHC-linked genes tend to be inherited as an intact complex. Nonclassical MHC genes are shown in the class I region (MICA and B, HLA-E, G, and F); class II (LMP and TAP); and class III (TNF, LTα/β, C2, C4A). MHC, major histocompatibility complex; MIC, MHC class I-like chain.

class I genes for HLA-E, F, and G. The products of these genes are recognized by receptors on innate immune cells, such as the NK cell inhibitory and activating receptors. Additionally, some class I like-genes, *MICA* and *MICB*, are also found in this class I supercluster. These latter genes appear to be activated particularly by stressed host cells. Their products are considered to represent self danger signals or DAMPS and are switched on by cells perturbed by infectious agents, malignant transformations, or nonphysiological trauma. The MIC products expressed on stressed epithelial cells are recognized not only by innate NK cell receptors but also by unconventional T cells, such as γδ T cells and NK T cells, which are able to produce rapid responses mainly through the secretion of IFN-γ and IL-17. These cytokines enhance innate inflammatory responses as well as augmenting downstream adaptive responses of T and B cells. Interestingly, the MHC class I region also encodes genes for HSPs. HSPs have long been known to be up-regulated by cellular stressors; they have been implicated as danger signals for the innate immune system.

The HLA class II supercluster contains the classical class II (HLA-DR, DQ, and DP) and nonclassical HLA-DM and DO. The latter two gene products are not expressed on the cell surface but form intracellular complexes involved in peptide exchange and loading on to classical class II molecules for antigen presentation by class II expressing cells to T cells (see Chapter 3).

Overall, the MHC is seen to contain genes involved in a whole range of innate and adaptive immune responses. Table 1.6 shows a selective set of genes in the MHC involved in different aspects of immunity.

The importance of the MHC is underlined by the fact that from the sequencing of the whole human genome, it has been calculated that 5–6% of the genome is committed to functions involved in immune defences. Moreover, rare human deficiencies of MHC class I and class II are associated with severe morbidity or mortality (e.g. stillbirth) indicative of the profound loss of immunity as a consequence of loss of these genes.

MHC and disease associations

At present, MHC association has been documented for several hundred diseases, including most autoimmune diseases (see 'Autoimmunity', below and Chapter 8).

Table 1.6 MHC genes associated with immune functions

MHC genes	Functional areas
HLA class I and class II TAP genes (transporter for antigen presentation)	Antigen processing and presentation
TNF, LTA, LTB	Inflammation
BF (factor B), C2, C4a, C4b	Complement cascade
HLA E, F G	Nonclassical MHC class I presentation to NK cells, γδ T cells, and NK T cells
MIC A, MIC B, HSP genes	Stress responses (innate and adaptive immunity)

In most diseases, MHC is associated rather than proven or shown to be causative. In rare situations, gene mutations in MHC genes have been firmly established as causative, e.g. the bare lymphocyte syndrome (a form of immune deficiency associated with loss of MHC class I or II) and some forms of haemochromatosis. Defining direct correlation or cause and effect between disease and an MHC allele is difficult because most MHC-associated diseases are multifactorial and they have genetic and environmental contributions. The latter are usually proven by epidemiological studies, as well as by sibling association and twin studies. Further difficulty arises because of linkage disequilibrium in the inheritance of MHC genes, the inheritance occuring across a whole haplotype. Thus, it is difficult to be certain whether a defined association is the precise or the most important gene involved in the association, or if it is linked to a more relevant but not recognized gene. Those reservations notwithstanding, some strong and well-known MHC associations, such as HLA-B27 with ankylosing spondylitis (AS), have allowed detailed studies of subtypes of B27. This has revealed precise binding of different amino acids to these HLA subtypes which result in differential T cell repertoire responses against self peptides. This sort of information infers that subtle differences in antigen presentation associated with different MHC alleles may play a significant role in our understanding of MHC disease association. Detailed studies of coeliac disease have given one of the best-defined mechanistic models of MHC and disease association (see Chapter 8). In the case of HLA-B27 there is also the suggestion that protein misfolding may contribute to its role in pathological processes.

Antigen processing and presentation: adhesion molecules and costimulation

Introduction

An essential requirement in the study of immunology is to understand how adaptive immunity generates the responses (humoral and/or cell-mediated) best suited to combat microbial agents that have survived, bypassed, or overcome the first line of innate immunity and associated inflammatory responses. The understanding has come, in part, from animal experimental models of infection and immunization over the past 60 years along with careful documentation of clinical cases, especially of individuals with defined lesions in their adaptive immune system. A substantial body of evidence indicates that microbes that are found in extracellular sites are best dealt with by B cell-generated antibodies (helped by CD4$^+$ T cells) and by phagocytosis by a range of leucocytes. Both of these defence mechanisms are very efficient. In contrast, viruses and certain bacteria (e.g. mycobacteria, listeria) that gain access to intracellular niches are not susceptible to antibodies. In general, antibodies do not readily enter living cells or are directly susceptible to phagocytosis. Evidence from animals with induced lesions of their immune system and humans with genetic mutations (e.g. primary immune deficiencies) have clearly shown that CD8$^+$ T cells, in particular primed CD8$^+$ cells with cytotoxic properties, are essential for defence against intracellular/cytosolic-located microbes and antigens. Cumulative evidence indicates that help from subpopulations of CD4$^+$ T cells enhances the efficiency of CD8$^+$ CTLs.

Detailed studies by immunologists, cell biologists, biochemists, and ultrastructural microscopists have unravelled the pathways of microbial antigen processing and presentation to T and B cells which helps to give mechanistic explanations for the observations and conclusions above: namely, that antibodies and phagocytes are best for dealing with extracellular pathogens and antigens while CD8$^+$ CTLs are best for dealing with intracellular pathogens and cytosolic antigens.

Extracellular pathogens and antigens

Extracellular pathogens and antigens are taken up by many mechanisms associated with phagocytic cells. This includes DCs, macrophages, and B lymphocytes. Although the primary role of B cells is the generation of antibodies, they can also act as APCs and constitutively express membrane HLA class I and II molecules.

Phagocytic cells sample the external environment in many ways. They may use sensing receptors such as PRRs, receptors for components of the complement system and for the Fc region of antibodies. Microbes which are opsonized (coated) with bound molecules such as complement components or antibodies are efficiently taken up by phagocytes, including APCs. Other nonspecific (non-receptor-mediated) mechanisms such as pinocytosis (macro- and micropinocytosis—cell sampling/drinking from the extracellular environment) are also used by phagocytes. Essentially, the material taken up (including microbes) is engulfed in the acidic environment contained within the endosomal vesicles of the phagocytes. The vesicles essentially keep the engulfed microbial material within the cell but segregated from the cytoplasmic compartment of the cell. The endosomes fuse with the lysosomal vacuoles of the phagocyte. The lysosomes contain many proteolytic enzymes and reactive chemical radicals which contribute to the breakdown of microbial proteins to many peptide forms.

Simultaneously, in the endoplasmic reticulum (ER) of the same cell, there is continuous generation of MHC-encoded HLA class II molecules which have associated, in their potential peptide-binding groove, a molecule called CLIP (a component of the class II invariant chain peptide). The HLA class II with its blocked peptide-binding groove is transported from the ER to the endophagolysosome for transport to the cell surface. Within that new location, by the action of a molecule called DM (encoded in the MHC class II region—see above), the CLIP peptide is removed from the HLA class II binding site. The now empty HLA class II groove is then occupied by the best-fitting peptide within the environment (generated from the ingested external microbes and antigens). The peptide with the best fit (determined by its amino acid sequence) then binds firmly to the HLA class II groove. This binding protects the HLA class II molecule from cellular proteases. The complex is then transported to the cell membrane and expressed there. Evidence shows that the peptides that are bound by HLA class II molecules are commonly of approximately 12–20 amino acid residues in length. The APC membrane-expressed HLA class II peptide complex is recognized and sampled by CD4$^+$ T cells. Importantly, this interaction is restricted to CD4$^+$ T cells because the CD4 molecule itself binds to the nonpolymorphic areas of the HLA class II molecule, well away from the peptide-binding area, while the TCR of the CD4$^+$ T cell binds to residues of the microbial peptide antigen and to some residues on the closely opposed aspect of the HLA class II binding groove; these tend to be polymorphic residues. The responding CD4$^+$ T cells can ultimately provide help to B cells which are responding to other antigenic determinants of the same microbe from which the peptides were derived. The help from the CD4$^+$ T cells assists the B cell to switch on genes to produce the most efficient antibody responses (antibody class switching—see 'B cells, receptors, and antibodies', below). The responding CD4$^+$ T cells also produce cytokines and accessory molecules that enable the phagocytes to more efficiently kill phagocytosed microbes. This processing and presentation of extracellular antigens by the innate immune system APCs, via their class II pathway, directs the adaptive responses best suited for these extracellular microbes, i.e. responses associated with antibody formation and phagocyte killing.

Intracellular pathogens and antigens

Most types of cells in the body can be infected by an appropriate virus. Additionally, most cells can also be the target for mutational changes associated with cancer development. These intracellular viral and cancer antigens have proteins as their major components. Such proteins generated in the cytosol have been shown experimentally to be represented in peptides found associated in the binding grooves of HLA class I molecules. Elegant experiments involving eluting and sequencing of peptides from cell surface HLA molecules and identifying them in protein databases have confirmed the intracellular origin of the parent protein. The cytosolic proteins of intracellular microbes, mutated (potential) cancerous self protein, or the many self proteins that are degraded daily during cell turnover, are all broken down by a proteolytic mechanism in the cytosol by the proteosome. The target proteins generally become unfolded and tagged in a process called ubiquitination. In the proteosome enzyme complex the ubiquitinated (tagged) proteins are recognized as such and are enzymatically degraded to peptides of various sizes. These peptides then need to be moved in 'reverse flow' from the cytosol to the ER (to meet the newly and continuously generated HLA class I molecules in that site). This reverse flow is facilitated by an active pumping process involving molecules termed TAP (transporter-associated with antigen processing). By energy-dependent mechanisms they transport the cytosolic peptides into the ER where the newly synthesized HLA class I molecules have empty grooves (contrast this to the CLIP-blocked groove of HLA class II), and must quickly find an appropriately fitting peptide newly arrived via TAP. If a peptide is not bound, the HLA class I molecule degrades. Peptides which bind tightly to the class I groove have been found on average to have about eight amino acid residues. The HLA class I–peptide complex is transported to, and expressed in, the membrane of the cell. HLA class I molecules are found on all nucleated cells (not restricted to APCs, like HLA class II). Hence, presentation by this HLA class I pathway will allow the presentation of viral peptides or cancer protein peptides on any cell. This class I–peptide complex is seen by, and interacts with, CD8$^+$ T cells. The CD8 molecule itself binds to the nonpolymorphic region of the HLA class I molecule while the TCR binds to amino acid residues of the peptide antigen or to some polymorphic residues of the HLA class I binding groove. This pathway of peptide presentation explains why CD8$^+$ CTLs are generated to deal with intracellular/cytosolic antigens. The HLA class I and II pathways of peptide antigen processing and presentation are well established. However, more recent findings indicate additional mechanisms of antigen presentation. There is new evidence of cross-presentation mechanisms for both pathways. Endosomal and phagosomal molecules that are normally processed for the HLA class II pathway can, in some situations, be demonstrated to leave those vesicles—by leakage, by pathogen circumvention, or by other active processes—entering the cytosol and becoming processed and transported by TAP into the HLA class I pathway. Thus, a peptide from an extracellular antigenic source may be presented by HLA class I to $CD8^+$ naive T cells. There is evidence that plasmacytoid DCs (a type of APC) are particularly prone to using this cross-presentation mechanism. Less robust but growing experimental evidence suggests that the physiological process of autophagy, responsible for cellular degradation/recycling of ubiquitinated self (housekeeping) cytosolic protein turnover can, in some circumstances, deliver cytosolic protein-derived peptides to the HLA class II pathways. It should be stressed that cross-presentation of peptide antigens appears to be physiologically very much the minor player in antigen processing and presentation. However, these latter processes provide opportunities to enhance beneficial immune responses in vaccination against cancer cells and some microbes, where vaccine stratagems are currently not successful.

B cell recognition

Antigen presentation to B cells needs to be considered in the context that antibodies can see a much wider range of antigenic determinants than T cells, which, with a few exceptions, are restricted to recognizing protein-derived peptide antigens. Exceptions are found in the minor T cell types (e.g. $\gamma\delta$ T and NK T cells) which are able to recognize some glycolipid antigens presented by nonclassical HLA class I-like molecules, such as those of the CD1 complex CD1d.

BCRs, which are membrane-expressed antibody molecules, can recognize conformational epitopes of intact protein molecules; they can also recognize lipids, small chemical entities, and some peptides, as well as carbohydrate and nucleic acid antigens. This wide recognition by B cells of various types of antigens is useful. For instance, T cells may respond to the peptides generated from a microbe's protein but the B cell can respond to many other associated antigens of the same microbe while receiving significant help from the $CD4^+$ T cell that is responding to the peptidic epitopes. Note that the B cell itself can act as an APC to present the peptide to the $CD4^+$ T cell on its associated HLA class II molecules.

Table 1.7 summarizes the main features of the HLA class I and II pathways for antigen processing and presentation to T cells.

Essential signalling (1, 2, and 3)

Effective triggering of adaptive immune responses requires more than the lymphocyte receptor specific recognition of presented antigen. The initial recognition by $CD4^+$ and $CD8^+$ TCRs of HLA class II and I peptide complexes, respectively, is seen as the necessary but not sufficient signal 1 for effective triggering of T cells. Similarly, B cell antigen recognition (via its BCR) also represents signal 1. Additional signals, now termed signals 2 and 3, are deemed necessary for the full cellular activation and

Table 1.7 Main features and properties of the HLA class I and II pathways of antigen processing and presentation

Property	HLA class I pathway	HLA class II pathway
Peptide–HLA complex	Peptides of ~8 amino acids, bound in groove formed by α1 and α2 domains of HLA class 1 molecules	Peptides (12–20 amino acids) bound in groove formed by α1 and β1 domains of the HLA class II molecules
Cell type presenting the HLA–peptide complex	All nucleated cells of the body	Class II-restricted cells, mainly APCs (DCs, macrophages, B cells); at site of immune inflammation epithelial and endothelial cells can present peptides via class II pathway
Source of protein antigens for peptides	Cytosolic proteins produced within the cell (some cross-presentation by endosomal peptides entering cytosol)	Endosomal/phagosomal peptides derived from extracellular phagocytosis and degraded proteins; some evidence of cross-presented peptides from autophagic digestion of cytosol protein entering endosomes and class II pathway
Site of peptide loading to HLA groove	Endoplasmic reticulum (also site of newly synthesized HLA molecules)	Specialized endosomal phagosomal compartment
Molecules involved with peptide transport or loading to HLA molecules	TAP	CLIP with the invariant chain, HLA DM molecules
Responding T cell	$CD8^+$ naive T cells generating CTLs	$CD4^+$ Th cells

APCs, antigen-presenting cells; CLIP, class II invariant chain peptide; CTLs, cytotoxic T lymphocytes; DCs, dendritic cells.

proliferation that characterizes effective T and B cell immune responses. Figure 1.19 illustrates some of the key molecular interactions involved in the costimulatory events between T cells and antigen-presenting DCs, and also between T cells and endothelial cells. The mediators/inducers of signals 2 and 3 are defined by sets of costimulatory molecules and cytokines. Signal 2 molecules are provided directly by the microbe or by the APCs reacting with the microbe. Thus, signal 2 molecules include microbial PAMPs reacting with APC PRRs (e.g. TLRs), which results in the up-regulation of more signal 2 molecules, such as CD80/CD86 on the DCs (and the induction of cytokines such as TNF-α, IL-1, and IL-6, as part of innate responses). For adaptive T cell responses, the mechanism of signal 2 is best defined by the molecular interaction between CD80/CD86 on the APCs with the activation-induced molecules of T cells known as the CD28 family of proteins (these also include negative regulators of cell

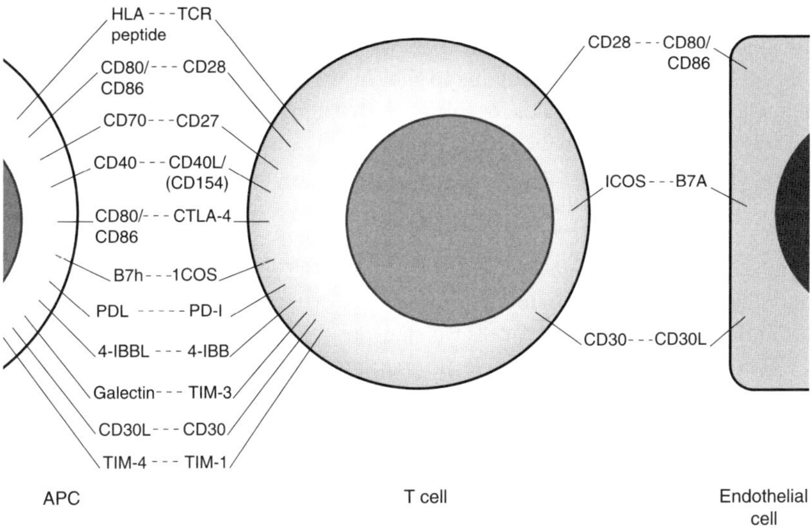

Fig. 1.19 A range of costimulatory molecules and their ligands on a T cell interacting with an antigen-presenting cell (APC), and the T cell interacting with an endothelial cell. Endothelial cell activation occurs in many inflammatory reactions and up-regulates the molecules shown which interact with the T cell. The molecules on the T cells show varying levels of expression and kinetics on naive, activated, memory and effector T cells. APC, antigen-presenting cell; B7h (a B7 family member); ICOS, inducible costimulator; PDL, programmed death ligand; TIM-1/4 : T cell immunoglobulin and mucin protein receptors-1/4; 4-IBBL (CD137L).

activation such as CTLA-4). These key interactions, referred to as costimulation, result in clonal expansion of the specific T cells responding via signal 1 and facilitate cellular differentiation and the generation of effector cells and memory cell precursors. The requirement for at least two signals is a means of ensuring good activation and focused responses against potentially damaging microbes and antigens (which themselves can provide signal 2) while safeguarding against signal-1-induced responses against self antigens on normal cells, which generally do not produce signals 2/3. One of the mechanisms of maintenance of tolerance to self molecules is seen in the property of anergy induction. Experimentally, it has been shown that strong signalling to T cells via signal 1 alone tends to switch the cell off (i.e. makes the cell anergic and refractory to stimulation).

Signal 3, as provided by IL-12 and IL-23 produced by activated DCs, is important in the development of $CD4^+$ Th1 cells.

Costimulation and adhesion molecules

The signal 1 reaction of the TCR with the HLA–peptide complex is facilitated and enhanced by adhesion interactions typified by ICAM-1 (CD54) on the APC interacting with the integrin LFA-1 on the T cell. Other adhesion pairs are formed by CD58

(LFA3) on the APC and the CD2 molecule on the T cell. The microanatomic result of this adhesion interaction, which synergizes with the signals 1/2, is the formation of an immunological synapse (analogous to that in the nervous system) which focuses interactions to reach thresholds for full T cell signalling and activation.

B cells via their BCRs bind the antigen (signal 1) and gain additional signals (signals 2/3) from specialized APCs such as follicular DCs (FDCs) found in B cell areas of lymphoid tissue. The FDCs trap and display immune complexes coated with complement activation products, such as C3b and C3d, which faciltate B cell signalling via interaction with the complement receptors CR1and CR2 on the B cells (see 'B cells, receptors, and antibodies', below). There is now strong evidence that some committed B cells receive costimulation from activated T cells which express the CD40 L (CD 154). This binds to CD40 on B cells and drives their differentiation and antibody class switching to produce antibodies of various classes. Additional data have recently shown that cells such as basophils (and by implication tissue mast cells) can produce cytokines (e.g. IL-4) which can act as signals 2/3 to T cells to commit them to Th2 responses, and to B cells to trigger the production of IgE antibodies.

Biologically costimulatory interactions have been defined which, rather than enhancing T cell activation, have been shown to down-regulate or block activation. The best-defined interaction is that between the T cell expressed CTLA-4 (also known as CD152), which belongs to the same family of molecules as CD28, which competitively engages (apparently at higher affinity) the APC-associated molecules CD80/CD86. CTLA-4 expression on activated T cells appears after that of CD28, and is considered a major means of limiting ongoing T cell immune responses. More recently, other costimulatory molecules have been defined on T cells which result in down-regulation of T-cell-mediated immune responses. Recent targets defined on mouse and human T cells that have this property include PD-1 and TIM-3; when ligated they send negative signals. Not surprisingly, TIM-3 and PD-1 are being targeted, along with CTLA-4 ligation, in immunotherapeutic regimens to overcome unwanted T cell responses in situations such as acute transplant rejection as well as combating autoimmunity (see Chapters 3 and 8, respectively) [25]. They are also being explored as a means of enhancing tolerance induction in the field of transplantation. Other targets, such as adhesion molecules (e.g. CD54), are also being considered in similar immunotherapeutic approaches.

In addition to the interactions described, a number of other receptor–ligand pairings have been defined as contributing to costimulation with varying importance in primary and established immune responses. A plethora of such interactions are summarized in Figure 1.20 along with the molecules previously described. Several of these interactions are being explored as targets in immunotherapeutic strategies in the fields of transplantation rejection and tolerance induction and in cancer and autoimmune disease therapy (see Chapters 3, 4, and 8, respectively).

The concept of a signal 3 is now supported by experimental evidence. It is based on our understanding that APCs of innate immunity can influence the class of T cell response that is induced, i.e. Th1, Th2, Th17, Tregs, or CD8$^+$ CTLs. The most studied model has defined how IL-12 produced from responding APCs, which binds to the IL-12R on naive T cells, can drive those cells towards the Th1 phenotype characterized

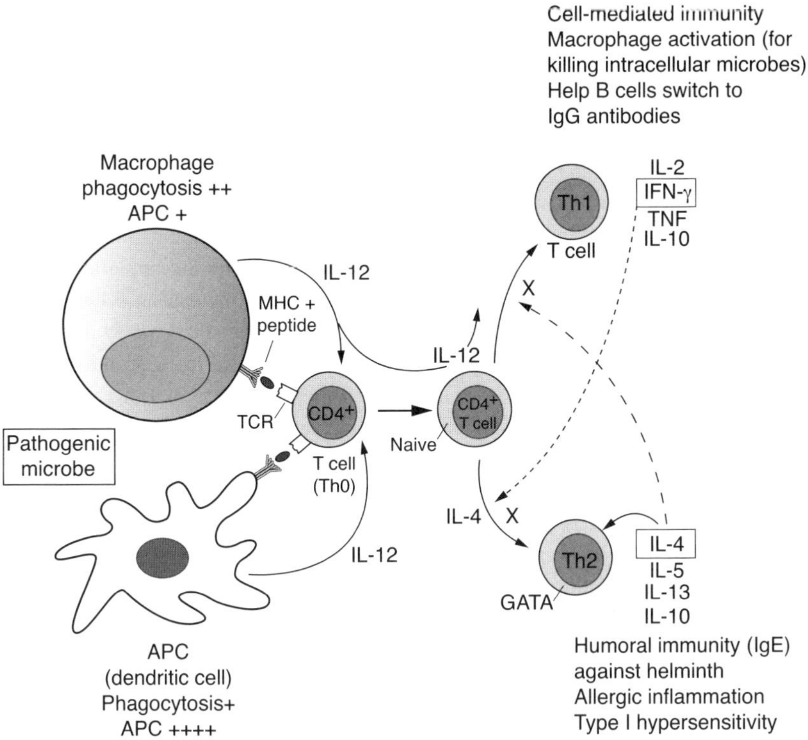

Fig. 1.20 Presentation of antigen peptide–MHC complexes to naive CD4$^+$ T cells by professional antigen presenting cells (APCs) and development of T effector subsets, Th1 and Th2. APCs present processed microbial peptide–antigen complex with self MHC class II molecules to naive CD4$^+$ T cells with the specific TCR (signal 1). APCs also produce cytokines, e.g. IL-12, which facilitates activation, proliferation, and differentiation of the naive T cell along the Th1 pathway. Sources of IL-4 (e.g. defined for basophils and mast cells) contribute towards Th2 differentiation. Once the cell is committed to Th2, the differentiated Th2 cells also produce IL-4 which acts in an autocrine fashion. Note the signature cytokines (boxed), characterizing the particular helper-effector subset for Th1 (IFN-γ) and Th2 (IL-4); IL-4 and IFN-γ negatively regulate the reciprocal development of each helper subset. Note that IL-10 (an immunosuppressive cytokine) is also produced by both subsets; it plays an important role over time in the control of the immune responses generated. APC, antigen presenting cell; GATA, guanine, adenine, thymine, adenine (DNA sequence); MHC, major histocompatability complex.

by the induction and secretion of IFN-γ. IL-12 signalling has also been shown to favour the induction of CD8$^+$ CTLs. Similar recent data in mouse and human cells has shown that IL-4 from basophils can act as signal 3, committing naive T cells to the Th2 helper phenotype. Undoubtedly, more evidence will emerge of different signal 3 inducers for Tregs and other cell types.

T cells, receptors, and effectors: CD4$^+$ Th1, Th2 and Th17; CD4$^+$ Tregs, and CD8$^+$ CTLs

T cell receptors

Thymus-derived T lymphocytes can rightly be considered the conductors of the adaptive immunological orchestra. These cells play central roles as effectors of T cell-mediated immune responses and as regulatory cells in T and B cell immune responses. As outlined in 'Antigen processing and presentation; adhesion molecules and costimulation' above, T cells possess clonally distributed receptors generated by massive gene recombination (controlled by *RAG1* and *RAG2* genes as in the case in B lymphocyte development), thus, generating the vast T cell repertoire from a limited number of germ-line gene segments. The TCR recognizes peptides derived from protein antigens displayed on self HLA molecules. A second small subset of TCRs (γδ TCRs), expressed by less than 10% of peripheral T cells, can also recognize peptide antigens as well as some glycolipid antigens presented by CD1d molecules and other antigens (see 'Effector cells and receptors', below).

The antigen-specific TCRs, sometimes referred to as Tis, to distinguish them from the complex of TCR with the CD3 molecule which makes up the fully functional and signal-transducing receptor, are glycoprotein heterodimers. The major TCRs consist of α and β chains linked by a disulphide bond in a functional receptor. Experiments, using gene transfection of isolated α and β genes, indicate that a composite conformation formed by α and β chains 'sees' the appropriate and matching conformation of the foreign antigen–MHC complex. The Ti on a CD4$^+$ Th cell will bind to the antigen-MHC class II molecule complex on an APC. In contrast, the Ti on a CD8$^+$ CTL will bind to the antigen–MHC class I complex on the appropriate target cell. It is established that the CD4 and CD8 molecules on the respective peripheral T cells play an important role in increasing the affinity of the T cell antigen recognition and binding reactions, particularly in primary T cell responses. The CD4 molecule binds to nonpolymorphic determinants of the MHC class II on the APC, at some distance from the antigen–MHC class II complex site. CD8 performs a similar role, enhancing the binding to comparable determinants on the MHC class I molecule.

The Ti is not immunoglobulin, as is the case for the BCR. Nevertheless, Ti has a comparable molecular genetic arrangement, whereby the separate genetic loci, designated V, D, J, and C gene segments, are found in the germ-line of cells committed to a T lymphoid lineage (early in the thymus environment). The genes undergo somatic rearrangement events (similar to those described for the BCR in 'B cells, receptors, and antibodies', below) resulting in the transcription and translation of protein 'messages' for the Ti receptor molecule, which becomes expressed on the T cell membrane closely linked with the CD3 molecule. The CD3/Ti complex (TCR) is essential for proper triggering of T cells following interaction with the antigen–MHC complex. Specificity is the property of the Ti α/β heterodimer and can be shown to be associated with the V domain determinants. Diversity is due to V regions associating with different D, J, and C combinations. Like BCRs, idiotypic determinants can be shown to be associated with the V domain of the Ti of the TCR.

The second, phylogenetically older, TCR has been described with a functional receptor complex (Ti) comprising a γ and δ heterodimer, distinct from α/β and encoded by separate genes. Within the thymus it precedes the gene rearrangements for the α/β receptor and may play a role in the thymic selection events associated with T cell development. The majority of TCRs found on most peripheral T cells in blood and secondary lymphoid organs, however, are the classical α/β Ti, associated with CD3.

Experimental data over the past 20 years has documented the intimate association of $\gamma\delta$ T cells with epithelia lining the GIT, the respiratory tract, and skin in mammalian species. These T cells, compared with the classical α/β T cells, have more limited diversity and have limited reactions with HLA–peptide complexes. Evidence indicates that they see lipids/glycolipids presented by the CD1 molecules. It is suggested that they can also recognize molecules induced/expressed by epithelial cells which are stressed either by microbial infections or by mutational changes. They will respond to these stressed cells while remaining tolerant to normal unstressed epithelia. The stressed molecules recognized by these T cells have been documented to be products of the *MICA* and *MICB* genes found in the MHC class I region. Another unconventional T cell described more recently, called the NK T cell, expresses the CD56 antigen found on NK cells along with T cell α/β receptors of very limited diversity. The NK T cell also appears to recognize antigens presented by the CD1 family of molecules. The overall suggestion is that the unconventional $\gamma\delta$ and NK T cells have functions similar to cells of the innate immune system. Their receptors show limited diversity, they can respond very quickly to detected antigens, and they are believed to act in a form of surveillance at epithelial sites, thus detecting and responding rapidly to cells damaged by infection, injury, or mutational events. They are known to be high secretors of IFN-γ, therefore, influencing other innate immune cells such as phagocytes, as well as the adaptive immune responses of T and B cells downstream, which also respond to IFN-γ. Interestingly, significant numbers of NK T cells can be found among tumour infiltrating lymphocytes (TILs) in human cancers.

T cell effectors: CD4$^+$/CD8$^+$ subsets

Many of the functions mediated by and attributable to T cells are due to their production of cytokines (IFN-γ, IL-2, TNF-α, IL-17) which in turn target receptors on responding cell types. Some T cell effects are notably due to their cell–cell contact reactions involving various ligand–receptor bidirectional interactions.

Effector T cells are found in the CD4$^+$ and the CD8$^+$ subsets. Classic experiments in mice in the 1990s, using highly polarized, nonphysiological generation of immune responses to microbes and to protein antigens, led to the seminal discovery that CD4$^+$ T cell subsets could be described and classified on the basis of the cytokines they produced. These cytokines correlated with their biological effects in adaptive immunity. The studies of Coffman and Mosmann defined the Th1 and Th2 subsets [26,27]. The Th1 cells produce the signature cytokine IFN-γ along with IL-2, which promote the activation of macrophage/phagocytic cells, especially in CMI. In contrast, Th2 cells are defined by the production of the signature cytokine IL-4 along with IL-5, which promotes B cell differentiation with Ig heavy chain class switching and, particularly, IgE-mediated antibody inflammation with eosinophilia. Clones of murine Th1 and

Th2 cells were readily isolated and strongly supported the paradigm. They also revealed that certain transcription factors including the STAT molecules, segregated and correlated with the subsets. Thus, Th1 cells expressed the T-bet transcription factor, which is known to be the master genetic regulator for Th1 development as well as selective STAT molecules (e.g. STAT 4) along their developmental pathways.

Definition and acceptance of $CD4^+$ Th1 and Th2 initially proved more difficult in the human system, for several reasons. Most investigations of human T cells use readily accessible blood lymphocytes. We now know these consist mainly of the naive recirculating pool of T cells and some memory T cell subsets: they are not comparable to the highly stimulated and polarized cells excised from the responding secondary lymphoid organs (spleen and lymph nodes) as used in mouse experiments. This realization, coupled with some investigations using human cells obtained from experimental lesions (e.g. highly challenged repeated skin tests to subcutaneously injected microbial antigens) or rarer biopsy samples from patients with severe immune-induced inflammatory lesions (skin of patients with lepromatous or tuberculoid leprosy) essentially showed the correctness of the Th1 and Th2 subset paradigm in humans. As in the mouse system there was also a correlation with the transcription factors and the use of various STAT molecules. Human Th1 is also associated with the T-bet transcription factor and the Th2 subset with a GATA transcription factor and, respectively, with some STAT molecules. Additionally, it was noted that the signature cytokines produced by the Th1 and Th2 cells could have reciprocal suppressive effects on the development of each cell type.

Figure 1.21 summarizes the findings of Th1 and Th2 subsets in humans showing the signature cytokines, the biological/immune functional correlates, and the transcription factors associated with their development from naive T cell precursors designated Th0.

Many clinical pathological associations have held up well with the Th1 and Th2 paradigm. However, with time the designation has become inadequate; it is unable to explain some clinical pathological states and, importantly, could not explain the occurrence of the diseases seen in some clinical immune-deficient patients. Ultimately, experiments with mice and human cells led to the definition of an additional Th subset termed Th17, which has been implicated in the defence reactions against certain extracellular pathogens. Th17 cells act directly by producing cytokines such as IL-17, IL-21, and IL-23 that attract polymorphonuclear phagocytes to sites of tissue invasion by microbes and activate them. Th17 have also been linked to the destructive inflammation associated with various autoimmune disorders. More recent experiments are apparently defining other subsets of $CD4^+$ Th cells. These include Th follicular cells, which are believed to produce signature cytokines and play a discrete functional role in secondary lymphoid follicles, facilitating microanatomical interactions between T and B cells and APCs. Most recently, a Th22 cell has been proposed which can be distinguished from Th17 cells and which produces almost exclusively IL-22, and has the propensity to home to epithelial sites [28]. Th17 cells can also produce IL-22, but along with several other cytokines.

Useful as the Th subset definitions are, caution needs to be exercised regarding their definition as fixed irreversible entities. Biologically, such cells may have some inherent

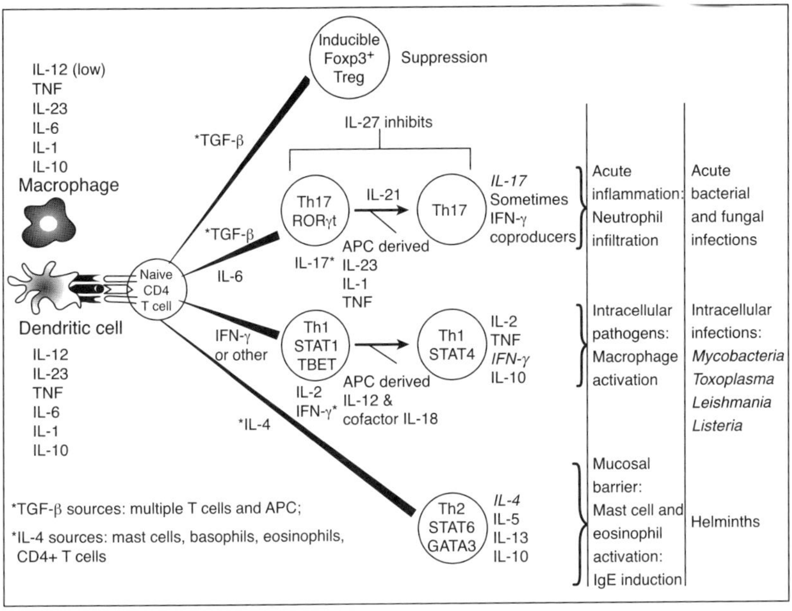

Fig. 1.21 Extended CD4$^+$ T helper-effector subsets with cytokines produced and associated transcription factors. Extended CD4$^+$ T helper subsets are shown with their signature transcription factors and cytokines produced. Their main functional and protective responses are also shown. The suppression from Tregs is considered to help re-establish homeostasis in the immune system following responses against microbes and also to protect against the development of autoimmunity or other immunopathological damage. The transcription factors shown related to the subsets are T-bet, GATA3, RORγt, and Foxp3—they control and promote the secretion of the associated cytokines; T regs Foxp3 (forkhead box protein 3) cell; Th17 RORγt (retinoic acid-related orphan receptor gamma t); Th1 Tbet (T-box expressed in T cells); Th2 GATA 3 (transcription factor 3 binding the DNA sequence GATA)

plasticity, their dominant phenotype merely reflecting essentially an expression of the dominant cytokines within the microenvironment at the time of analysis [29]. Movement of such cells *ex vivo* into changed environments may yield changing cytokine profiles and different phenotypic expressions. Recent research has firmly established that human CD4$^+$ Th17 cells can be derived from Th17 precursors which produce both IL-17 and IFN-γ (the supposed signature cytokine of Th1); some mature Th17 cells can continue to produce IFN-γ. However, they have not been demonstrated in any situation to be capable of producing IL-4 (the signature molecule of Th2 cells). CD161, which is an NK cell marker/receptor, is proving useful in defining the Th17 precursors (CD161$^+$CD4$^+$Th17, IL-17/IFN-γ producers). CD161 is also found on subsets of CD8$^+$ T cells. Treg plasticity has been documented by their transformation to Th1 and Th17 subsets under particular experimental conditions. The plasticity shown for the human CD4$^+$ Th subsets may have some biological advantage for a species that is relatively long-lived, providing flexibility to deal with myriad antigens within a system which, over time, shows marked immune senescence (see Figure 1.21).

Nevertheless, even with the caveat regarding plasticity, at present the accepted designations of Th1, Th2, and Th17 (and probably of Th22) is useful with regard to therapeutic targeting of such cells in clinical diseases (e.g. autoimmunity), where different $CD4^+$ Th effector subsets have been shown to express different chemokine receptors that may offer new therapeutic targets. For instance, this is occurring within the setting of MS where the T cells that enter the CNS have been shown to be a particular subset (Th17) and to express particular chemokine receptors involved in their ingress into the CNS.

Figure 1.21 summarizes the various $CD4^+$ Th subsets and Tregs, with their correlated functions and markers. Figure 1.22 gives an overview of the linkages between $CD4^+$ T cell subsets of adaptive immunity with cells of innate immunity, indicating their bidirectional interactions.

$CD8^+$ effector CTLs predominantly target cells expressing the HLA class I–peptide complex as a way of eliminating intracellular sources of microbial infections (microbial reservoirs), or of eliminating mutated (potentially cancerous) cells, which present the mutated peptide fragments at the surface of the cell; the latter can be killed by the $CD8^+$ T cells. $CD8^+$ T cells, like NK cells, use at least two pathways of cell

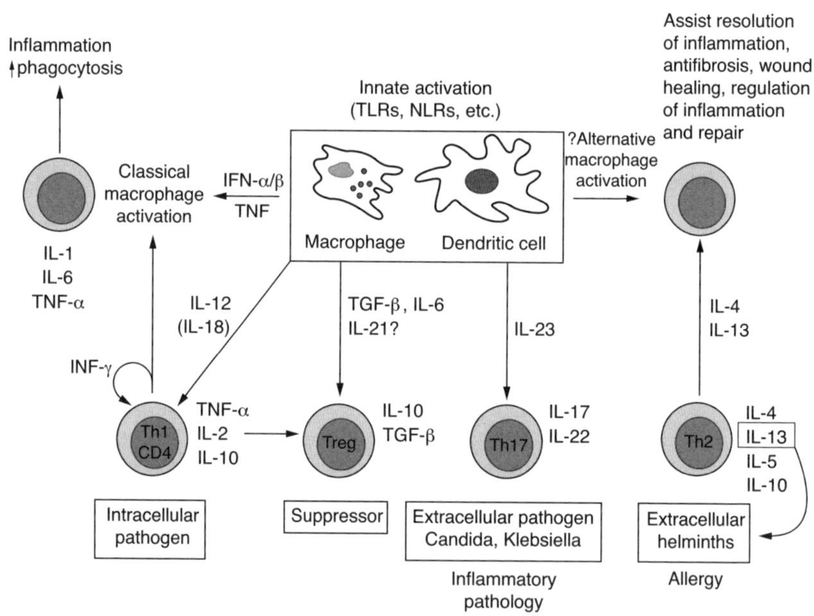

Fig. 1.22 The dynamic interactions between cells of innate immunity (shown as macrophages and DCs) and of adaptive immunity ($CD4^+$ Th cell subsets), illustrating key cytokines and functions linked to each cell type. Note the innate cells can direct the development of various adaptive immune effector responses. NLR, NOD (nucleotide-binding domain)-like receptor; TLR, Toll-like receptor.

killing: granule-associated perforins and granzymes, and/or cell membrane-associated Fas–Fas L interactions.

For effective $CD8^+$ CTL killing *in vivo*, there is good evidence showing that $CD4^+$ T cell help is important by way of cell–cell contact and by cytokines generated to optimize $CD8^+$ CTL movement to sites for killing of target cells *in vivo*.

T cell effectors: $CD4^+$ Tregs

$CD4^+$ T cells with regulatory effects on T and B cell responses and on antigen-presenting DCs are now firmly established. Predominant among these cells are the so-called natural (n) Tregs produced in the thymus, from which they exit to the periphery. The nTregs are mainly $CD4^+$, $CD25^+$ Tregs which express the Foxp3 transcription factor. Tregs can be induced in the periphery also and are called, not surprisingly, induced (i) Tregs, which may express the same set of markers as nTregs, but some populations may be $CD25^-$, although they still suppress T and B cell responses. There is recent evidence showing that Tregs are generated in the very early phases of the induction of the adaptive immune response and that IL-2 is central to their development and survival. Tregs appear to exert their suppressive function, in part, by direct cell–cell contact with responding DCs, T effectors, and B cells, as well as by the secretion in the local environment of the suppressive cytokines IL-10 and TGF-β [30]. These cytokines can be secreted by the Tregs themselves, or the Tregs can induce other local cell types to secrete them, especially IL-10. Much effort is being directed at ways of inducing/enhancing Treg function *in vivo* to control disorders such as autoimmune diseases or destructive immunity associated with type I IgE-mediated allergic responses. Recent experiments have documented the expansion of Tregs *ex vivo* and their reinfusion *in vivo* to beneficially suppress ongoing transplantation rejection (rejection associated with Th1 cells and with $CD8^+$ CTLs). Experimental mouse systems have recently demonstrated expansions of Tregs by engagement of their CD40 L with CD40 expressing B cells and immature DCs. *In vivo* expansion of Tregs has been demonstrated in experiments using injected immune complexes of IL-2 and anti-IL-2 antibody.

B cells, receptors, and antibodies

B cells and receptors

As an integral part of their membranes, mature B lymphocytes express Ig glycoproteins which function as the specific antigen receptors (BCRs). These B cells, following binding to the receptor and appropriate activation, can proliferate and differentiate into plasma cells producing and secreting Ig. Some B cells fail to reach the endstage of plasma cell development, but after mitotic division may revert to surface membrane immunoglobulin (SmIg) receptor-bearing memory B cells. The basic structure of the Ig receptor is shown in Figure 1.23. This is also the structure of secreted Ig found in blood and other body secretions. Ig molecules of known antigen-binding specificity are called antibodies. The terms are often used synonymously.

Plasma cells produce and secrete all classes and subclasses of antibodies: IgM, IgG (1–4), IgA, IgD, and IgE. The latter are associated with either kappa (κ) or lambda (λ) light chains on individual molecules. Single heavy chains of immunoglobulin are

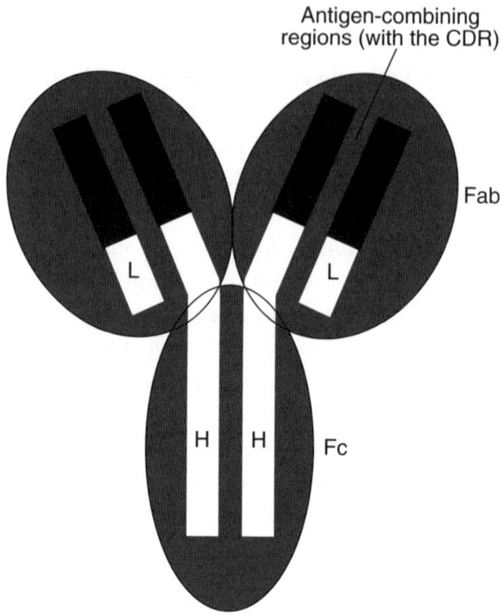

Fig. 1.23 Basic structure of an immunoglobulin antibody molecule and the surface immunoglobulin antigen receptor on B lymphocytes. CDR, complementary determining regions; Fab, fragment antigen-binding domain; Fc, fragment crystallizable domain; H, heavy chain; L, light chain; variable region, ■; constant region, □.

never found with mixed κ and λ chains. Table 1.8 summarizes some definitions and properties of Ig antibody molecules. In their development from the lymphoid stem cell, the earliest B lineage cells do not have antibody receptors on their membrane, but can be defined by the presence of other differentiation molecules, such as CD19 (see 'Clusters of differentiation and monoclonal antibodies', above). The cell designated the pre-B cell has restricted to its cytoplasm the heavy chain (μ) of IgM with no associated light chain. Figure 1.14 shows the normal sequence of development of the B cell, with some of the important markers recognized on the cells and some of the genetic events occurring during this development.

Apart from their specific antigen receptors, B cells also express other important phenotypes which can be correlated with their function. Thus, the HLA class II DR molecules on B cells have been shown to function as presenters of antigen to $CD4^+$ T cells. B cells react to antigens and produce antibody, but may also present other epitopes of the antigen to T cells for their reactivity. Similarly, receptors have been defined on B cells which bind secreted products of activated T cells (IL-2, IL-4, IL-6, and IFN-γ) (see 'T cells, receptors, and effectors: $CD4^+$ Th1, Th2 and Th17; $CD4^+$ Tregs and $CD8^+$ CTLs', above) which in turn assist in B cell differentiation and/or proliferation events leading to antibody production and secretion. CD40 on B cells interacts with the CD40 L on activated T cells, the interaction being a major determinant of B cell class switching from IgM to the other classes of immunoglobulins.

Table 1.8 Characteristic properties of the immunoglobulin classes

Properties	**IgG**	**IgM**	**IgA**	**IgD**	**IgE**
Heavy chain	γ	μ	α	δ	ε
Subclass chains	γ1, γ2, γ3, γ4	–	α1,α2	–	–
L chain	κ or λ	κ or λ	κ or λ	κ or λ	κ or λ
Molecular mass	150 000	900 000	160 000 monomer 400 000 dimer	180 000	190 000
Serum half-life	28 days	4–5 days	4–5 days	2–8 days	1–5 days
Complement fixation	++	+++	±	–	–
Placental transfer via Fc region	Yes	No	No	No	No
Binding to mast cells via Fc region	γ4(?)	No	No	No	+++
Antibacterial	+	+++	+	±	±
Antiviral	+	++	+++	–	–
Fc binding to phagocytes	+++	±	+	–	+ (eosinophils, macrophages) Some DCs

$CD40^+$ B cells have recently been demonstrated in model systems as important for the development and expansion of Tregs. Newly defined cytokines such as B cell activating factor (BAF, also called Blys) produced by mononuclear phagocytes can also influence B cell class switching and proliferation independent of the CD40 pathway. Hence, a two-way cooperation between B and T lymphocytes is becoming more apparent. Some of the other molecules defined on the surface of B cells include HLA class I antigens, various TLRs, and receptors for complement components termed CR2 and CR3.

Diverse ligands such as Gram-negative bacterial LPS, *Nocardia* extracts, viruses such as EBV, T cell lymphokines, chemicals such as phorbol esters, and antibodies directed against the B cell Ig can all act as mitogens (stimulators) for B cells. Following the binding of these various ligands, singularly or in various combinations, triggering of membrane-associated enzyme systems (involving turnover of inositol phospholipids and Ca^{2+} ion mobilization) results in cell cycle changes in DNA and protein synthesis in B cells. Mitogens have largely been exploited in research to dissect the details of B cell physiology; knowledge of their activity has also helped to explain clinical and laboratory observations, such as the marked proliferation of B cells, lymphocytosis, lymphadenopathy, and hypergammaglobulinaemia associated with EBV infections. Most of the clinical and laboratory findings can be explained by the mitogenic effects of EBV on B cells together with T cell responses against EBV-infected B cells. Furthermore, the interaction of EBV with normal cell-growth-controlling gene elements (e.g. the c-*myc* proto-oncogene) offers a molecular explanation for the origin of some B cell lymphomas. The translocation of the c-*myc* oncogene from chromosome 8 to the reactive regions of the Ig genes on chromosomes 14, 2, and 22, together with the mitogenic drive of EBV for B cells, result in disorders such as Burkitt's lymphoma and other B cell non-Hodgkin's lymphomas.

B cells are produced continuously in the human bone marrow throughout life and it is estimated that more than 10^8 cells are formed every day. It is calculated that such production provides in excess of 10^6 clones of B cells (each clone expressing an antibody receptor with a unique antigen specificity—clonal selection theory), ample provision for the diversity of human antibodies necessary to counteract the potential universe of antigens.

Immunoglobulins and antibodies

The immunogenetics of Ig (receptor and secreted antibody) production provides evidence to support the clonal selection theory and to explain specificity and diversity. The genes for Ig heavy chains are found on chromosome 14, while the genes for κ and λ light chains are found on chromosomes 2 and 22, respectively. In all nucleated cells these genes can be demonstrated to be in what is termed a '*germ-line*' configuration. In a given cell only the maternal or paternal genes (not both) are selected for expression by a process termed *allelic exclusion.*

Some important definitions regarding antibodies are outlined below. The characteristic properties of antibodies are summarized in Table 1.8.

- Basic antibody unit (see Figure 1.23)—The heavy chain pairs define the classes of antibody.
- V and C regions—V (variable) regions contain marked variability of amino acid sequences between different antibody molecules; C (constant) regions contain very little variability.
- Antigen-binding sites—Formed by small numbers of amino acids in the V regions of heavy (H) and light (L) chains.
- Antibody classes—Five classes of immunoglobulins in man—IgG, IgM, IgA, IgD, and IgE—defined by determinants in the H chains which are respectively denoted as γ, μ, α, δ, ε. Subclasses are found in the IgG and IgA immunoglobulins.
- Antibodies react mainly against antigens located in extracellular sites. Exceptions have been described whereby antibodies attached to viruses which enter cells interact with a cytosolic Fc binding protein called TRIM 21; the resulting complex is rapidly directed to the intracellular proteasome for desctruction, thus, providing a novel and useful antiviral effect.
- Polymer forms of antibodies—Composed of more than one of the basic monomer units linked by a J chain produced in the plasma cell. Thus, IgM in blood is usually pentameric (five basic units linked by disulphide bridges to the J chain). IgA occurs as a J-chain-linked dimer in body secretions, linked by disulphide bonds to an additional polypeptide called secretory component (also called the polymeric Ig receptor) produced by epithelial cells.

- Genes encoding H chain V regions are VDJ and those encoding L chain V region are VJC; encode the corresponding H and L chain constant regions.

The term 'gene' applies to discontinuous segments (sequences) of nucleotide bases. The stretches of bases containing the information that will be transcribed to mRNA and translated to Ig-antibody protein are termed *exons* and the intervening nonencoding sequences are termed introns. The exons encoding for different parts of the antibody molecule are named V, D, J, and C for the heavy chains, and V, J, and C for the light chains. The critical point to note is that cells which are committed along the pathway of B lymphoid development change their germ-line configuration of the Ig 'gene' elements (V, D, J, C exons) by undergoing so-called *somatic rearrangement and recombination*—bringing together the gene exons by the removal of the intervening introns. The process involves various nuclear enzyme systems and subtle nucleic acid curling, splicing, and recombining events. Two genes (recombination activating genes) have been defined, *RAG1* and *RAG2*, whose products have been shown to regulate the process. The end result is the product of a final mRNA transcript which is translated into an Ig protein. In pre-B cells only the IgM-V, D, J, C-genes are rearranged and expressed as μ heavy chain protein in the cytoplasm. In the immature B cell the μ gene element is present along with genes for V, J, and C for either κ or λ. Mature B cells rearrange and express IgM and IgD heavy chain genes, both of which are associated with the same rearranged light chain on the cell membrane. Thus, the antigen receptors on mature B cells is composed of IgM and IgD, but both Igs use the same light chain for association and have the same antigen binding specificity, i.e. the same V region.

At the gene level there are many alternative V, D, and J gene segments which can combine in various combinations during rearrangement, and can then be translated into many alternative V region proteins for both heavy and light chains. These numerous combinations of V-D, J, or V-J provide the major part of the genetic basis for diversity implicit in the clonal selection theory. Each combination contributes to a novel receptor; similarly, each individual combination provides part of the unique specificity of the individual clone. Interestingly, patients (newborns and infants) have been described with mutations in *RAG1* and *RAG2*; they present with clinical SCID. They have no detectable B cells (or T cells) in blood. It is now recognized that *RAG* genes which are activated in early immature lymphocytes (before commitment to T or B lineage) are also responsible for controlling similar somatic recombination to generate TCR diversity in cells destined for that lineage.

The basis of diversity and specificity can also be seen in the amino acid sequences of antibody proteins. The V regions of heavy chains show segments of extreme amino acid variability between the N-termini of differing antibodies of the same class. Different Igs with different antigen-binding specificities show marked amino acid differences in their V regions which correspond with the points of contact and binding of antigen. These so-called *hypervariable regions* (three to four in number) correspond to the CDRs which interact with antigens. The term *idiotope* is used to define the unique sequence of amino acids associated with the unique specificity of a single hypervariable region. Antibodies recognizing and defining the unique conformation contributed by the combination of CDRs in heavy- and light-chain V regions are called *anti-idiotypes*, i.e. the idiotype is the summation of the epitopes derived from the combination of

CDRs of heavy and light chains. TCRs are not Igs, but their heterodimer receptors (α/β and γ/δ) have similar molecular organization in terms of CDRs and defineable idiotypes.

Additional diversification occurs in B cells and their BCRs (but not in TCRs) by the processes termed somatic hypermutation (SHM) and class switch recombination (CSR). SHM results in the accumulation of point mutations in the V region, especially in the antigen-binding regions (i.e. CDRs), increasing diversity of antigen recognition and binding. CSR results in the exchange of the constant region of IgM for the constant region of the downstream heavy chains of IgG, IgA, or IgE in differentiating plasma cells, thus diversifying antibody effector functions. SHM and CSR genetic mechanisms are under the control of a gene called *AID* (activation-induced cytidine deaminase) which also regulates the generation and maintenance of memory B cells in germinal centres.

The molecular rearrangements of Ig genes, together with the definition of light chains and idiotypes on the BCR, have been readily exploited in clinical medicine to characterize lymphoid neoplasia. The surgeon who is called on to remove lymph nodes during the clinical investigation of lymphadenopathy may find that the B cells in the removed specimen all express one type of light chain, thus, indicating a 'clonal' neoplastic proliferation. In a normal or reactive node, analysis reveals approximately 60% κ and 40% λ positive cells. Anti-idiotypic MABs have been used in the immunotherapy of clonal B cell malignancies.

In more difficult and complex analyses, the neoplastic nature of the B cells is defined by demonstrating the presence of the predominant and most widespread idiotype. When necessary, these sophisticated examples of phenotyping can be complemented

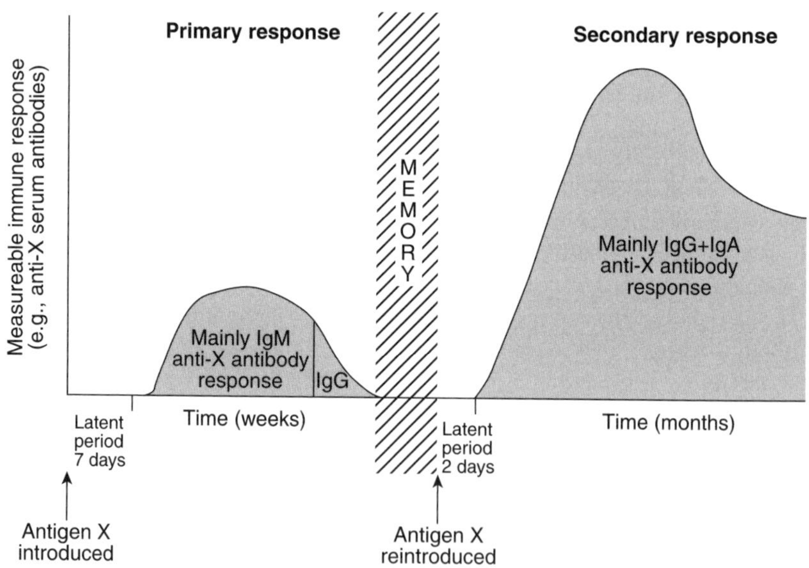

Fig. 1.24 Kinetics of primary and secondary immune responses following injection of an antigen.

by genotypic analysis using DNA probes to define gene rearrangement events in clonal B cell proliferation.

Primary and secondary antibody responses

Figure 1.24 shows the classic kinetics and features of the *primary* and *secondary* antibody responses following injections of an antigen. The secondary response has a shorter lag period, the antibody response is quantitatively greater and lasts longer, the quality of the antibody is better—it has a stronger binding 'affinity' for the antigen—and the classes of antibody change from predominantly IgM to IgG and IgA. It is important to appreciate that, although the antibody classes (heavy chain) have changed, the antigen-binding specificity is the same (i.e. anti-X, V-region specificity is maintained). The effect of the secondary response, therefore, is to generate antibodies that will bind the antigen strongly and rapidly and recruit effector mechanisms, such as complement and phagocytic cells, which will contribute to efficient elimination of the antigen. The molecular basis for these properties of antibodies is outlined above under the SHM and CSR mechanisms (see 'Immunoglobulins and antibodies', above). More recent molecular findings on recombination, SHM, and CSR events have further illuminated our scientific understanding of B cells and antibody responses.

As discussed previously, the clonal selection theory of the cellular aspects of lymphocyte responses following receptor–antigen interaction antedated and predicted the cell basis of immunological 'memory' of the secondary antibody response. The kinetics and qualitative changes of primary and secondary responses are equally applicable to T cells.

The basis of the change in antibody class is hence defined at the molecular level in the CSR events. The antibody-producing cells in the secondary response rearrange and select IgG and IgA (γ and α C-region) rather than IgM C-region exons, while essentially maintaining the same V, D, J exons for the heavy chains and the V, J exons for the light chains, thus ensuring the same specificity. The molecular messages and signals responsible for isotype switching are now clear. Newer evidence indicates that cell–cell contact between the switching B cells and activated T cells is required, via their respective CD40L molecules. Additional cytokine signals involved in antibody class switching have emerged: for example, the need for IL-4 for IgE and molecules such as BAF and APRIL (cytokine members of the TNF superfamily), derived mainly from non-T cell sources [31]. They target various receptors and provide signals that favour B cell survival and class switching. Indeed, anti-BAF MABs are currently being used in clinical trials as a new therapy for SLE.

A resurgence in studies of antibody independent functions of B cells has emerged, as a result of the use of B-cell-depleting anti-CD20 MAB therapy (rituximab) in human diseases (including B cell neoplasia and a range of organ-specific and systemic autoimmunity—RA, SLE, pemphigus vulgaris), and in mouse model systems. These studies document profound non-antibody-associated actions of B cells as modulators of CD4$^+$ T effector and regulatory cells. Mechanisms of B cells shown to operate include their role as APCs, as costimulatory cells, and as cytokine producers, all influencing T cell responses and linked immunopathology.

Memory T and B lymphocytes are the cellular drivers responsible for the secondary and subsequent specific adaptive immune responses. They are key targets of research aimed at enhancing and exploiting their functions for vaccination programmes. Additionally, studies of these cells are giving deeper insights into diseases affecting cells of the immune system, especially lymphoid tumours and immune deficiency diseases. Phenotypic markers which characterize and segregate with functional B and T memory cells have proved very useful to study, isolate, and functionally manipulate such cells. For B lymphocytes, their cell surface marker profile of $CD19^{+}C20^{+}$ $CD27^{+}$surface Ig^{+} defines approximately 30% of the circulating peripheral blood B cells in humans, that are memory B cells; half of that subset are the surface IgG^{+} long-lived memory B cells. Additional markers, such as $CD38^{+}$, differentiate the antibody-secreting B cells (ASC) in blood, which differentiate within days as a response to infection or vaccination [32]. The ASCs home to peripheral lymphoid sites to differentiate into plasma cells secreting high titres of antibody. Populations of long-lived (over decades) plasma cells have also been defined secreting low levels of antibody (e.g. antitetanus specificity).

Memory T cells have for decades been phenotyped with respect to their expression of isoforms of the CD45 molecule; the $CD45RO^{+}$ marker characterizes $CD4^{+}$ and $CD8^{+}$ T memory cells.

Recognition events and functionality of the integrated immune system *in vivo*

Introduction

Having an overview of the immune system and its major recognition elements and receptors, it is possible to achieve an understanding of the system's connectivity and functionality *in vivo*. Consider two scenarios of antigen challenge to the host. One is via a natural portal of entry by a potentially pathogenic microbe and the other by the systemic (parenteral) presentation of antigen, as used in many experimental approaches or vaccination programmes (using intramuscular, subcutaneous, or intravenous routes). The two scenarios will reveal elements of commonality and differences in the induction of the immune response.

Antigen entry and responses via the natural portal of the GIT

GIT innate defences

Consider an ingested or resident potential pathogen in the host GIT. It will encounter soluble factors and cells of innate immunity and, in varying parts of the tract, the resident commensal microflora. The human commensals are known to be in their hundreds of millions, some providing vital substances (e.g. key vitamins) for the host. They also produce nutrients such as short-chain fatty acids and other substances that antagonize potential pathogens. Recent evidence also indicates they may induce a basal state of activation of epithelial lining cells via microbe PAMPs interacting with the PRRs (TLRs and NLRs) of the host cells. This basal state may assist homeostasis with commensals while priming the system for additional signals from and reactions against potential pathogens. This suggestion gains credibility if we consider colitis induced by *Clostridium difficile*. This Gram-positive organism is known to reside in the GIT of many people without any resultant morbidity; it is also known, however, to cause severe inflammation in some individuals on antibiotic therapy. It is surmised that the commensal flora normally suppresses *C. difficile*. A simplistic quantitative model suggests that antibiotic depletion of sensitive commensals creates room for the antibiotic resistant *C. difficile* to dominate, attach to, and disrupt the epithelial barrier. With the aid of its two toxins (A and B) it is able to enter deeper tissues and intracellular sites, dysregulating and amplifying inflammatory mediator pathways/responses, leading to a highly damaging acute inflammation. Alternative models, supported by some experimental evidence, indicate that some commensals induce the production of bactericidal molecules from intestinal cells which suppress *C. difficile*; antibiotic therapy thus provides an indirect advantage for propagation of *C. difficile*. Clearly, these models are not mutually exclusive.

Within mucosal secretions are found various molecules such as mucins, lectin-like glycoproteins (collectins), enzymes (e.g. lyzozyme), and complement components together with antimicrobial peptides, such as defensins, which are produced and secreted by epithelial lining cells and closely related Paneth cells. These soluble factors have important antimicrobial activities, including binding to and disrupting microbial membranes and preventing microbe attachment to receptors on the epithelial cells. The increasing understanding of the role of commensals and their interactions with the gut immune system is providing new insights into the use of nonpathogenic bacteria and yeasts as probiotics to treat or augment the treatment of microbial or nonmicrobial inflammatory disease/disorders of the intestines. Probiotics can be perceived as resetting appropriate basal interactions in the gut (see Chapter 6). The common disorder irritable bowel syndrome (IBS) is considered to have an underlying low-grade inflammation and perturbation of commensal flora as key factors in its pathology. Current IBS treament recommendations involve the use of pre/probiotics, as well as anti-inflammatory agents.

If pathogens survive the initial defences, as well as the interactions with the natural ecosystem of commensal microflora, and gain a foothold on or in epithelial cells, then additional mechanisms are activated. The barrier function of epithelial cells via their tight intercellular junctions is well known. However, the epithelial cells themselves have functions beyond that of a pure physical barrier. When stressed or damaged by microbes, such cells can switch on genes after PAMP–PRR and other receptor interactions to produce cytokines and chemokines to signal and enhance a localized inflammatory response. Key cytokines and chemokines produced by epithelial cells include IL-1, IL-8, and other CC and CXC chemokines. From the early epithelial cell recognition events and responses, defence mechanisms are triggered which attempt to eliminate the microbes. Microbes that survive these defences encounter other cells that contribute to early defence, synergizing with epithelial cells found in close anatomical association. Predominant among these and intertwined between epithelial cells are morphologically recognized DCs.

Dendritic cells

The best-known DC is the LC, which is associated with epithelia. Other related DCs are found just below the epithelium and have been termed DDCs and IDCs. The Langerhans and related cells are derived from bone marrow and develop from the mononuclear phagocyte lineage. They have many features in common with macrophages and monocytes and also some significant differences. They sample antigens from the local environment around and between epithelial cells. They are part of the family of generic DCs which we associate with particular functions of antigen presentation [33]. The functions of LCs and IDCs and macrophages have qualitative and quantitative differences with regards to endocytosis, phagocytosis, intracellular killing, processing of internalized protein molecules, and peptide antigen presentation, bound to HLA molecules, to T and B cells found in GIT lymphoid aggregates and regional lymph nodes. Essentially, the DCs capture antigen either in its complete form via their surface receptors or as phagocytosed/endocytosed material for partial digestion, processing, and subsequent presentation complexed with DC self HLA molecules. The cells then migrate to lymphoid compartments and, in the process, mature. During the migration and maturation the cells change their functional characteristics, becoming less endocytic/phagocytic, and become more firmly committed to processing and presenting antigens to T cells (see 'Innate and adaptive immunity', above). The DCs ultimately move to areas of secondary lymphoid tissues. In lymphoid aggregates in the GIT, respiratory tract and other mucosal sites, lymph nodes, and the spleen, they present the antigens to the relevant T and B cells with the appropriate receptors (i.e. the specific receptors for those antigens). The DC presentation of peptide antigens, bound to HLA class II and I molecules that are recognized by the TCRs of $CD4^+$ and $CD8^+$ T cells, respectively, provide the signal 1 needed for induction of the protective immune response. However, signal 1 is not sufficient on its own. Indeed, if only signal 1 predominates it has been shown to switch off and to tolerize immune responses by inducing T cell anergy. In the responding MALT, the required signals (signals 2 and 3—see 'Costimulation and adhesion molecules', above) for inducing positive immune responses are provided by products from the pathogens and by the cytokines generated from the PAMP–PRR interactions of epithelial DC/APC cell types. The overall functions of the families of DCs can be summarized as follows:

- DCs produce proinflammatory cytokines and chemokines following early recognition events—PAMPs via PRRs. Dominant among the cytokines produced are IL-1 and TNF-α. They are the main mediators, along with chemokines, for the recruitment of leucocytes and soluble mediators to the site of infection and/or inflammation. DCs enhance the intracellular killing processes of leucocytes upon contact with microbes and their antigens. This occurs within the intracellular endosomal lysosomal compartments.
- DCs migrate from the site of microbial entry to regional lymphoid tissues, taking with them microbial products which they can present either in native form (recognized by BCRs) or associated as processed peptides bound to self HLA (recognized by TCRs). During DC movement from superficial tissue sites to regional lymphoid tissues to interact with T and B cells, the DCs undergo maturation characterized by increased expression of surface molecules such as CD80/CD86 (B7.1 and B7.2),

which function as costimulators in triggering immune responses. DC maturation/activation is also characterized by the cytokines they produce, in particular key cytokines such as IL-12 and IL-23. Costimulators and cytokines have tended to be grouped as signal 2, necessary for full triggering of lymphocyte responses. However, recent data is now indicating a separation, whereby, molecules such as CD80/86 are regarded as producing signal 2 and the cytokines secreted as providing signal 3 needed for full triggering, especially of T cells. These considerations are important in cancer immunotherapy which uses *in vitro* manipulated (e.g. antigen-pulsed) DCs to induce antitumour responses. This indicates the importance of having the right maturation and activating protocols for DCs to promote T cell antitumour responses (see Chapter 4). This is in addition to having optimal tumour peptide antigen presentation by DCs, utilizing the standard antigen-processing HLA class I and II pathways or the alternatively described cross-presentation pathways.

- The GIT immune system has some particular adaptations that favour functionality against antigens entering via that route. This includes specialized antigen sampling and capture by the M cells, found interspersed among the epithelial lining cells of the lower intestine. M cells engulf antigens by endo/pinocytosis and transfer them to lymphoid aggregates such as the Peyer's patches (PP) to start the induction of T and B cell responses. The PP themselves drain via the equivalent of afferent lymphatics to regional mesenteric lymph nodes for full induction and dissemination of immune responses. Other important GIT adaptations include a range of cell types (innate and adaptive) and molecules found associated within the epithelium: namely, interepithelial effector lymphocytes (e.g. T cells and NK T cells) and lamina propria-associated DCs, T and B lymphocytes, plasma cells, and macrophages, along with scattered mast cells and rarer NK cells and eosinophils.

Mucosal-associated lymphoid tissue

Introduction

Another key adaption in the GIT, including the oral site, and other mucosal sites such as the respiratory and urogenital tracts (collectively termed mucosal-associated lymphoid tissue or MALT), is the selective homing of effector T and B cells to MALT using specific adhesion molecule–ligand interactions and chemokine/receptor pairings. Interestingly, recent data suggest a new functional CD4$^+$ Th22 subset (reflecting the predominant production of IL-22 by the cells) that home selectively to skin and MALT. A memory T cell subset, which when activated expresses the molecule CLAA (cutaneous lymphocyte-associated antigen), is known to home selectively to normal and inflamed skin. CLAA interaction with E-selectin on cutaneous endothelium is the main pathway for this selective homing. Different integrins associated with oral and GIT mucosa also favour the homing of some CLAA$^+$ CD4$^+$ T cells. The CD4$^+$ Th17 subset also shows preferential homing to MALT and skin, and is implicated in immune defences, as well as in immunopathological states. IgA-committed B cells and IgA-secreting plasma cells have been known for some 50 years to have a selective predisposition to home to MALT, as a result of specific adhesion-integrin–ligand interactions between lymphocytes and specialized endothelial cells in MALT sites.

Intestinal IgA antibodies are produced as dimers linked by a J chain in MALT plasma cells (in contrast with IgA in blood, which is a monomer), when secreted from the cells near the basal area of epithelial cells. The dimeric IgA binds with high affinity to the polymeric Ig receptor (pIgR), a molecule produced by epithelial cells that facilitates the transport of IgA antibodies to the GIT lumen. At the apex of the enterocyte the pIgR is enzymatically cleaved, releasing the IgA into the gut lumen with a bound major fraction, termed the secretory component (SeC). The SeC protects IgA from intestinal enzymes and confers mucophilic properties to the antibody. The IgA–SeC complex thus has some relative resistance to proteases in the GIT; the antibody is efficient at excluding antigens from GIT uptake, and neutralizes some microbes by preventing their binding to epithelial cells. Most importantly, IgA acts as an anti-inflammatory molecule as its immune complexes with antigen tend not to activate complement and other phagocytic proinflammatory actions. This is in marked contrast to other Ig antibodies such as IgG and IgM (see 'B cells, receptors, and antibodies', above).

Intestinal $CD4^+$ and $CD8^+$ T cells, which preferentially migrate to MALT, express the integrin molecule $\alpha 4/\beta 7$ and the chemokine receptor CCR9, which bind selectively to respective counter-ligands on intestinal vascular endothelium and intestinal epithelial cells: MADCAM1 (mucosal addressin cell adhesion molecule 1) and CCL25. Some IgA-committed B cells express the receptor CCR10 which interacts with the ligand CCL28, produced by GIT epithelial and lamina propria cells. The potential overlapping functions of these homing molecular pairings are the subject of ongoing research and are being targeted as a means to modulate trafficking of cells involved in disease induction and/or perpetuation in the GIT. They are also being studied in the context of vaccination strategies aimed at mucosal vaccines and exploitation of the homing of effector and memory T and B cells (see 'Effector cells and receptors', below).

Figure 1.25 summarizes the interactions for GIT immune responses and the effectors generated. Antigens are taken up via M cells and delivered by a process of transcytosis to subepithelial DCs, or taken across the epithelium in solution or associated with other DCs (some sample antigen directly from the gut lumen by their dendrites); they are delivered respectively to the PPs or the MALT lymph nodes where immune responses are induced, if appropriate costimulation occurs (signals 1, 2, and 3). Activated and proliferating T cells with effector and regulatory properties (Th1, Th2, Th17, and Tregs) then express the integrin and chemokine receptors that allow them to migrate selectively throughout MALT.

MALT and GIT diseases

The balance between the different lymphocyte subsets in the GIT varies with physiological homeostasis and with inflammation. Th17 and Th1 cells dominate in inflammatory environments, whereas Th2 and Treg functions appear to maintain a more suppressive/homeostatic GIT setting. The homing properties of GIT resident, effector, and memory lymphocytes distinguish them from the naive T cells from which they are derived and from other naive and effector T and B lymphocytes (in sites such as spleen and peripheral lymph nodes) with no predilection for the MALT environment.

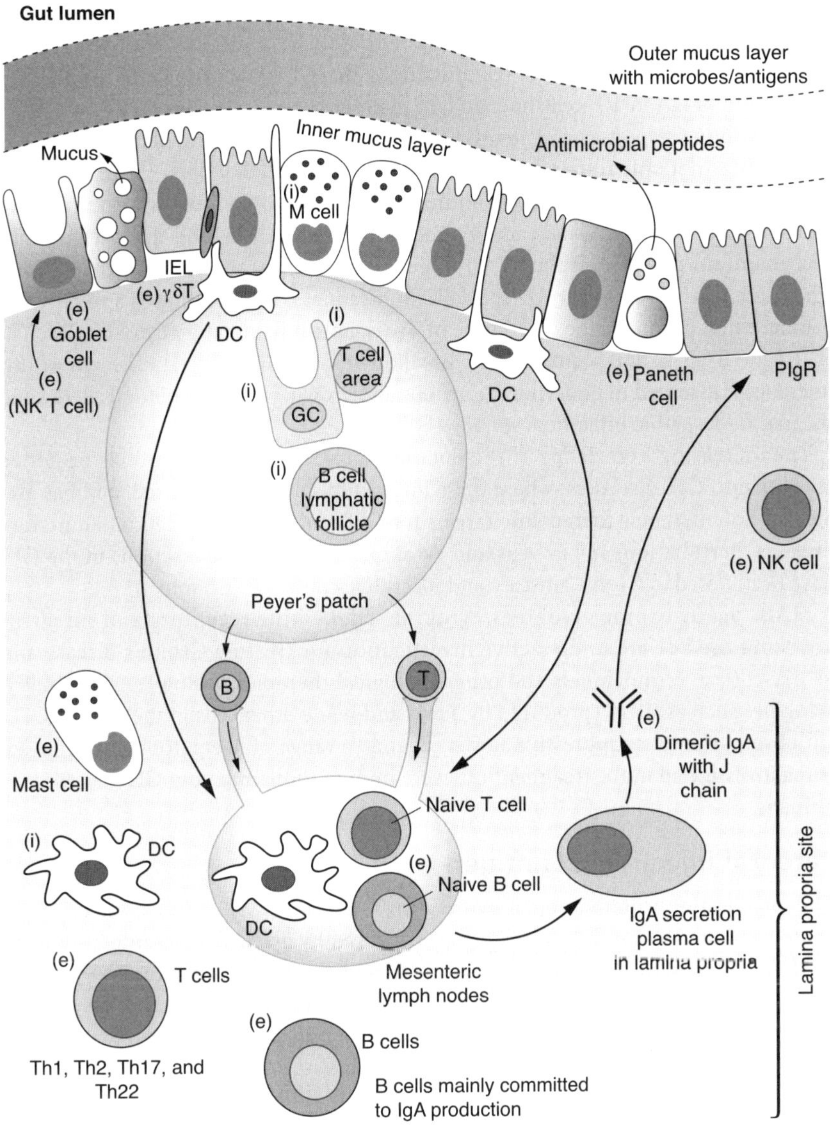

Fig. 1.25 Relationship between induction and effector immune response sites in the gastrointestinal tract (GIT). The lamina propria, effector, and memory T and B lymphocytes selectively home to the GIT and other MALT sites. i, induction role; e, effector role. GC, germinal centre; IEL, intraepithelial lymphocyte; MALT, mucosa-associated lymphoid tissue; PIgR, polymeric immunoglobulin receptor.

There is recent evidence indicating that MALT DCs can imprint GIT homing on activated lymphocytes by a process involving retinoic acid (a metabolite of vitamin A). Interestingly, this metabolite in conjunction with TGF is also known to induce GIT production of IgA in a T-cell-independent manner from B cells [34–37].

The immune response generated via the GIT faces some additional challenges. The system must not only respond effectively to pathogens, as described above, but must also not over-react to its myriad commensal flora and to the very large numbers of antigens (proteins, lipids, and carbohydrates) ingested daily in food. The mechanisms that maintain physiological non- or hyporesponsiveness (oral tolerance) to these agents are considered to involve specialized intestinal DCs operating in a microenvironment that promotes the emergence of Tregs, anti-inflammatory cytokines such as IL-10 and TGF-β, and secretory IgA. Breakdown or failure of establishment of this tolerance is assumed to underpin the serious and growing problem of food allergy and the major idiopathic inflammatory bowel diseases.

The increasing knowledge of the detailed interactions in the gut has provided insights into GIT disorders, where these interactions are compromised, and has also yielded potential new therapeutic targets for GIT and skin-associated inflammatory diseases. Pertubations in key cells and cytokine (e.g. IL-21) interactions in the GIT have been noted in Crohn's disease and ulcerative colitis (see Chapter 8).

MABs against some cytokines/cytokine–chemokine receptors and integrins are being used or are under active investigation for treating Crohn's disease and psoriasis (see 'Monoclonals and other biological therapies', below). Additionally, cytokines such as IL-10 (produced by Tregs and many other cells in the normal GIT) with broad immunosuppressive activity against a range of haematopoietic cells, are being investigated in the treatment of severe immune/inflammatory GIT disorders in humans.

Parental injection of antigen

The injection of protein antigen by the intramuscular (IM) or subcutaneous (SC) route bypasses the important responses triggered by epithelial cell interactions in MALT. Furthermore, the pure protein antigen is likely to be a poor stimulator of PRRs on subepithelial DCs/APCs. Nevertheless, the protein antigen is likely to be endocytosed and processed by the DCs/APCs and will be transported for presentation to T and B cells in lymphoid tissues with the capability of providing signal 1. However, because of the lack of signals 2 and 3 (lack of PAMP–PRR interactions as found with antigen entry via the mucosa), this injection of pure protein antigen could lead to immune unresponsiveness/tolerance rather than active immune responses. Indeed, immunologists have been aware of this situation for many decades; it is referred to as the immunologists' 'dirty' little secret, alluding to the fact that they need to use adjuvants ('dirty' materials such as FCA, containing mycobacterial products and mineral oils) to ensure induction of immune responses against the injected protein antigen in experimental animal systems (see 'Immunogens, antigens, and adjuvants', above). Aluminium salts are another important, though less potent, adjuvant (see 'Adjuvants', above). Currently, much effort is being focussed on production of adjuvants that may target PRRs in various tissue sites to increase vaccine efficacy to treat a wide range of human diseases. The systemic immune response generated following protein antigen–adjuvant immunization by the IM or SC route is dominated by the production of IgG antibodies, with lesser amounts of other Ig classes characteristic of Th2-driven humoral immunity; additionally, some cell-mediated ($CD4^+$ and $CD8^+$ T) reactions can also be demonstrated.

Parenteral administration of antigens via the intravenous (IV) route (clearly without adjuvant) generates immune responses dependent particularly on splenic function. Discrete T and B cell areas and APC populations are defined in the spleen, as in other peripheral lymphoid tissues, but that organ has some particular features. There is an anatomic marginal zone with a population of B cells that respond particularly to carbohydrate/polysaccharide antigens; it is important for antibacterial responses to encapsulated organisms such as pneumoccoci. Splenectomized patients are at particular lifelong risks from such organisms; vaccinations against them are important for patients undergoing elective or emergency splenectomy (see Chapter 7). The immune response induced by the IV route is dominated by humoral immunity with IgM and IgG antibodies with a relatively poor cell-mediated response.

The IV route of antigen administration is also known to be a convenient way (by giving very low or very high doses of protein antigens) to induce experimental models of peripheral tolerance, which is also dependent on an intact and functioning spleen.

Superantigen

T cell activation

The term superantigen refers to microbial products, often protein toxins (exotoxins, enterotoxins), which mainly enter the host via MALT or skin and that have profound immune stimulating effects simultaneously on large numbers of T cells and APCs. This stimulation is associated with the toxin binding to the APC/HLA class II molecule, outside the peptide-binding groove, and stimultaneously binding to multiple TCR V β regions. Superantigens bypass normal antigen-processing pathways and are often relatively resistant to heat and proteases. Unlike standard peptide antigens within the HLA class II groove, which stimulate a small number of specific T cells (at best, 1 in 10 000 or 0.001% of the total T cells with the specific TCR), superantigens can stimulate of the order of 1% up to 20% of all T cells (binding to multiple TCRs). That reaction represents a massive polyclonal (or oligoclonal) T cell stimulation which, in large part, accounts for the serious diseases and morbidity associated with exposure to superantigens in humans. Superantigens from group A streptococci are considered the main agents causing necrotizing fasciitis and streptococcal toxic shock syndrome associated with hypotension and multiple organ failure. Staphylococcal and viral superantigens have also been associated with serious pathological disorders, including toxic shock syndrome and Kawasaki disease. There is evidence of their involvement in upper and lower chronic inflammatory airways diseases, such as chronic rhinosinusitis with nasal polyps and COPD.

Superantigen polyclonal activation of T cells cross-linked with APCs results in massive systemic release of proinflammatory cytokines from both cell types. Documented cytokines include TNF-α, IL-2, IFN-γ, IL-6, and many chemokines. These molecules can account for much of the local and systemic disturbances (fever, hypotension, diffuse skin rashes, and shock) which occur with the severe acute and ultimately chronic inflammatory lesions, if the individual survives and the stimulus persists. Superantigens can have profound effects on other elements of the immune system. Recent experiments have documented their severe impairment of iTregs and nTregs ($CD4^+/CD25^+/Foxp3^+$ T cells), which suggests that superantigens may contribute to some forms of autoimmune inflammatory diseases. The many T cells activated by superantigens can subsequently be shown, after releasing their cytokines, to undergo apoptosis; if the T cells survive they become anergic. This results in the individual being functionally immunocompromised, at least for some period of time. By the very nature of superantigen binding to, and stimulation of, a large number of T cells, there results a marked skewing of the T cell clonal repertoire. This again limits the individual's clonal diversity and, therefore, potentially the ability to react to some antigens.

B cell activation

B cells, by virtue of their expression of HLA class II molecules, can also be engaged by superantigens directly (as APCs) and bridged to T cells; the excessively activated T cells, in turn, induce marked polyclonal stimulation of B cells. Chronic inflammatory disorders associated with superantigens commonly have polyclonal increases in serum Ig levels (raised levels of IgM, IgG, IgA, and IgE). Superantigens have been shown to favour the emergence of Th2 responses; this helps to explain the level of raised Th2-associated B cell responses linked to B cell heavy chain class switching and thus panhypergammaglobulinaemia.

Physiological benefits of the effector immune response

Introduction

Previous sections of this chapter have provided an overview of the basis of immunology as it pertains to protection of the host against infection. The cells, recognition events, and molecules that define interactions of innate and adaptive immunity, and their actions and interactions to protect the host, while maintaining homeostasis, have been outlined. In this section, the cells and soluble proteins operative in innate and adaptive immunity will be described with regard to how they confer the physiological benefits of immunity in an integrated way. The complement system of proteins of innate immunity interacts bidirectionally with elements of adaptive immunity. Some components of complement assist B cells in their production of antibodies. Antibody molecules of particular isotypes directly recruit and activate complement. Leucocytes that generate innate or adaptive immunity function as major effectors of antimicrobial responses in peripheral tissue sites.

$CD4^+$ and $CD8^+$ T effector cells of adaptive immunity, NK cells of innate immunity, and the 'unconventional lymphocytes' (NK T and $\gamma\delta$ T cells, which operate at the interface of innate and adaptive immunity) function in discrete, coordinated, and cooperative ways in delivering highly efficient effector functions. T cells and CMIs deal particularly with intracellular microbes. T cells recruit and enhance the functions of mononuclear phagocytes to deal with the intracellular phagocytosed microbes. $CD8^+$ CTLs kill infected cells which express processed peptides of intracellular microbes bound to HLA class I at the cell surface. T cells also help B cells to generate antibodies of the best isotype suited to dealing with a range of extracellular microbes, including the extracellular phases of viruses, some bacteria, and protozoa which colonize cells intracellularly.

The physiological benefits of the innate and adaptive immune responses become very evident when investigating nature's experiments—natural deficits of elements of both systems which result in immune deficiency. Delineation of such disorders indicates mutational events affecting proteins, secreted molecules, and receptors associated with immune reactions. These observations are supported by experimental animal model systems where discrete elements of adaptive and innate immunity can be genetically disrupted or more global effects can be induced by surgical manoeuvres (e.g. thymectomy). These approaches have clearly indicated that the effector elements of immune responses (cells and protein components in soluble compartments) are directly responsible for the reactions that lead to the elimination of microbes. The effector molecules of the innate system, in many circumstances, are able to eliminate the microbes directly. However, they additionally play important roles in augmenting the functional effectors of adaptive immune responses, such as the products of B lymphocytes (antibodies).

One of the major elements of the innate immune system that functions as a powerful effector in immune response is the complex of proteins that makes up the complement system.

Complement system of proteins

The complement system is a series of some 30 protein enzymes and cell membrane-associated components essential for defence against non-self antigens/microbes. Complement is part of the innate immune system, its elements acting rapidly and directly against antigens. The system is also recruited by elements of adaptive immunity, especially antibodies, to enhance their protective effector antimicrobial reactions. Historically, the term 'complement' is a recognition of the system's role in assisting or complementing antimicrobial antibodies. Invading non-self antigens (e.g. viruses, bacteria, fungi, mismatched transfused red blood cells, or organ transplants) can interact with, and lead to their destruction and elimination by, the complement series of blood proteins. Most of these proteins are synthesized in the liver and can function as major components of the acute-phase response. Molecules and PAMPs on the surfaces of some microbes can lead to a direct activation of the complement system. Microbes and mismatched tissues, which are coated (opsonized) with antibody molecules, especially of IgM and IgG class, are very effective at activating the complement system. Activation of complement involves sequential proteolytic cleavage of members of the system. This leads to the generation of effector molecules and by-products that ultimately results in the destruction of the activating antigen by way of inflammatory responses. Complement activation, as is common with enzyme systems, results in the amplification of the responses downstream. Some products of this activation bind covalently to surfaces in the vicinity of the activation process. This is represented by binding to the opsonized microbes as well as to self cells in the environment. Biologically, the self cells have, as part of the human genome, a series of encoded proteins known as complement regulatory proteins which protect against damage induced by complement activation. These protective components are not found in microbial genomes, hence the microbes are damaged by the activation products. Because the amplified complement activation system is potentially very powerful, other regulatory mechanisms exist to protect self cells. Some of these mechanisms involve components of activation with very short half-lives and/or acting over very short ranges *in situ*. Some fluid-phase regulatory molecules also exist which limit the complement enzymatic activation pathways.

Three major pathways are known to lead the complement activation: two of them, the alternative pathway and (the relatively recently described) lectin pathway, are considered 'old' in evolutionary terms. The lectin pathway is antibody independent and occurs when mannose-binding lectin, a serum protein, binds to mannose or fructose groups on microbial cell walls. This then attracts the activity of the mannose-associated serine proteinase (MASP) which drives the activation process. The alternative and lectin pathways are activated directly by binding to microbes (without the need for antibody), functioning as soluble PRRs recognizing microbial PAMPs. The third and most studied system is called the classical pathway.

Figure 1.26 gives an overview of the three pathways and the key molecules generated by the activation process. The initiating molecules for activation in these pathways are respectively C3b, mannose-binding lectin, and C1q for the alternative, lectin, and classical pathways. Activation proceeds in a precise sequence; key in the early parts of the complement activation system is targeting of the most abundant and central component, the plasma protein C3. Breakdown of C3 is brought about by the enzyme system complex termed the C3 convertase. The generation of their respective C3 convertases is a common feature of all three pathways (see Figure 1.26). The C3 convertase enzymes cleave C3, generating two products. The first, C3b, attaches covalently to the surfaces of microbes directly and/or to antibody-coated (opsonized) antigens. The other product is a soluble fluid-phase entity, termed C3a. It has biological activity; it is sometimes called anaphylatoxin as it binds to receptors on leucocytes, especially neutrophils and mast cells, and can result in chemotaxis (a movement of neutrophils along a concentration gradient) towards the sites of microbes/antigens responsible for activation of complement. C3a binding also mediates the release of potent inflammatory mediators from both cell types.

The bound C3b element helps in all three pathways towards generating another downstream convertase enzyme called C5 convertase. This enzyme, which cleaves C5, is responsible for the late stage of activation of complement. Cleaved products of C5 are analogous to those of C3; C5b becomes covalently bound to the activating complex and the fluid-phase C5a acts as a chemotactic agent and mediates cellular release of inflammatory mediators.

The late steps of complement activation (C6–C9) generate products which can result in the lysis of some bacteria, such as neiserria. These late activation products can also lyse incompatible transfused red blood cells and leucocytes. The activated complex of C5b with C6, 7, 8, and 9 is termed the membrane attack complex (MAC). The MAC inserts into susceptible cell membranes in the manner analogous to the evolutionarily related protein perforin, involved in $CD8^+$ T cell and NK cell cytotoxicity (see 'T cells, receptors, and effectors: $CD4^+$ Th1, Th2 and Th17; $CD4^+$ Tregs and $CD8^+$ CTLs' and 'Innate and adaptive immunity', respectively). The insertion of the MAC complex facilitates osmotic cell lysis. It should be noted that the alternative pathway is initiated by the binding of low levels of C3b. Interestingly, plasma C3 before complement activation undergoes a small degree of continual and spontaneous hydrolysis (autolysis), generating small amounts of C3b. This fluid-phase C3b is

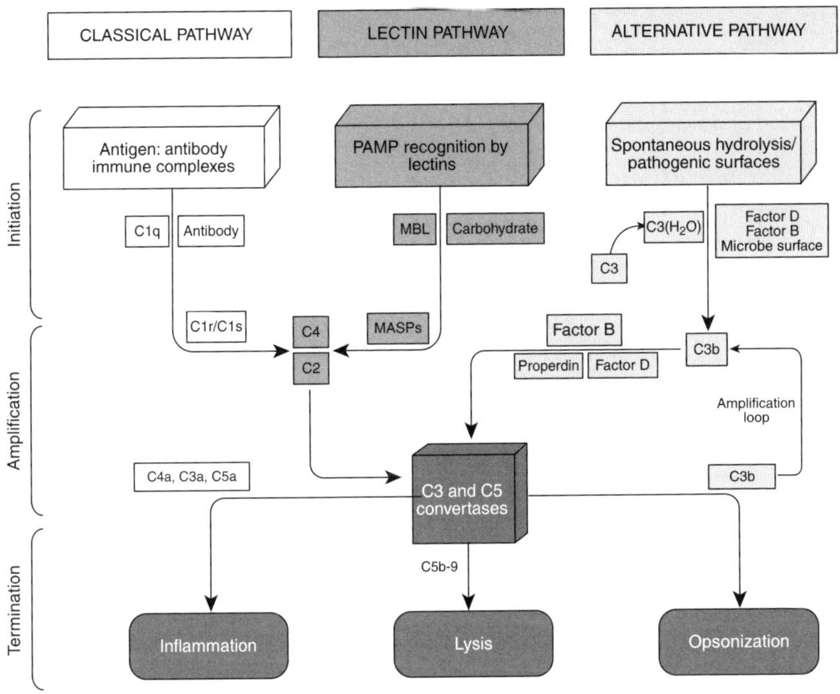

Fig. 1.26 The three pathways of complement activation: the classical, lectin, and alternative pathways. The phylogenetically youngest and most studied classical pathway is activated by C1q binding to antibody complexed with antigen, which in turn activates C1r and C1s. The generated esterase enzyme cleaves C4 and C2. Activation of the lectin pathway occurs when MBL, a soluble PRR, binds to conserved carbohydrate motifs on microbes that leads to activation of the MASPs which also cleave C4 and C2. The cleavage products of C4 and C2 from both pathways form the C3 convertase, C4bC2a. This key molecule targets C3 resulting in its cleavage into C3b and C3a. Some C3b binds to nearby activating surfaces, while other C3b molecules associate with the C4bC2a to form the C5 convertase of the lectin and classical pathways. The alternative pathway (AP) is activated when C3 undergoes spontaneous hydrolysis generating an AP C3 convertase which is facilitated by factors B and D. An AP C5 convertase is also generated. Properdin supports alternative pathway activation by stabilizing both convertases. The three pathways of complement activation can be seen to result in the formation of the key C3 and C5 convertases. The reactions result in the generation of the major effectors of complement activation namely the anaphylatoxins (C4a, C3a, and C5a), the MAC (C5–C9), and the major opsonin C3b. The biological readout of complement activation is the induction of inflammation, the lysis of target cells, and the opsonization of microbes and antigens. The anaphylatoxins are potent proinflammatory molecules activating polymorphs and mast cells as well as acting as chemotatic agents for leucocytes. The terminal MAC complex is responsible for direct lysis of some target cells. The C3b opsonin facilitates phagocytosis of opsonized targets; it is also a key amplifying molecule for the alternative pathway. MAC, membrane attack complex; MBL, mannan-binding lectin; MASP, MBL-associated serine protease; PRR, pattern recognition receptor.

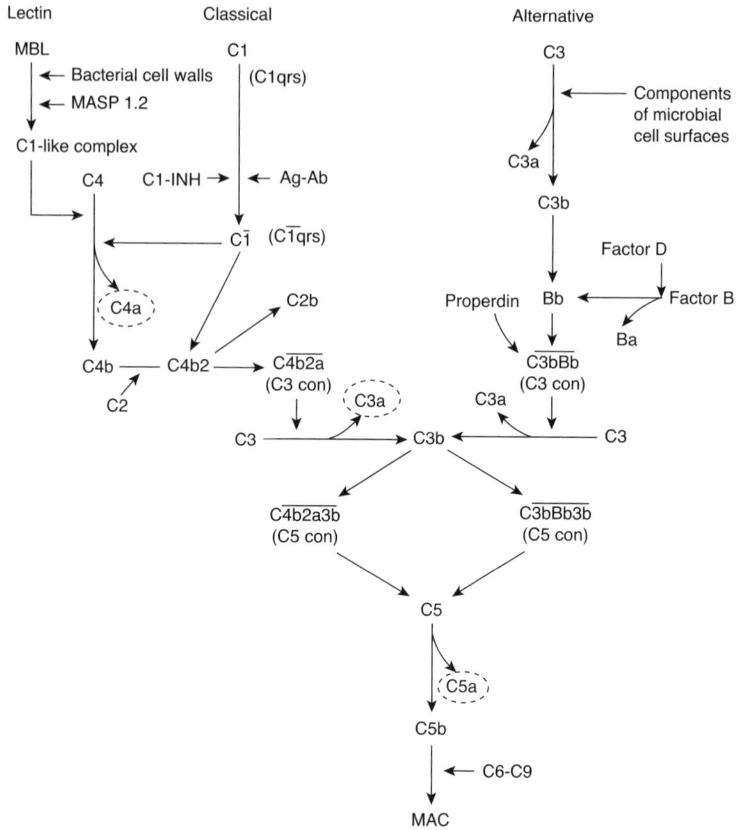

Fig. 1.27 The alternative, lectin, and classical complement activation pathways converge into the final common pathway when C3 convertases cleaves C3 into C3a and C3b. Overbar indicates activation. C4a, C3a, and C5a act as anaphylotoxins and as chemotactic factors.The main outcomes of complement activation are induction of inflammation,target cell lysis and opsonization of microbes/antigens. Ab, antibody; Ag, antigen; C1-INH, C1 inhibitor; MAC, membrane attack complex; MBL, mannose-binding lectin; MASPs, MBL-associated serine proteases; P, properdin.

unstable and rapidly decays. However, if it binds to the surface of an invading microbe it is stabilized and acts as a substrate for further activation and generation of the alternative pathway C3 convertase. That pathways reaction is assisted and controlled by other proteins called factors B and D, and properdin. Figure 1.27 gives a more detailed overview of the three pathways of complement activation.

Such a potentially powerful inflammation-inducing system needs to have very sensitive and tight control and regulation. This is brought about in various ways including the following. Mammalian cells lack terminal mannose residues, hence are not susceptible to the lectin pathway of activation. Additionally, mammalian cells possess complement regulatory proteins such as CD55 (decay accelerating factor, DAF) and CD46 (membrane cofactor protein, MCP) which antagonize C3 convertases/complement activation and potential damaging reactions at the surfaces of human cells. Patients with deficiencies of CD55 and CD46, due to a genetic lesion that leads to loss of anchorage of the proteins to the human cell surface, have marked complement-induced lysis of their red blood cells. Experimental models have also demonstrated increases in inflammatory and autoimmune disorders linked to loss of those regulatory molecules.

Interestingly, the cells and organs of animals (pigs) being considered for use in xenotransplantation lack human CD55 and CD46. Such animals have been genetically engineered (transgenics) to express these human complement components, as one of the means of protecting against complement activation *in vivo* in the context of xenotransplantation. Other means of regulating complement activation include the protein C1 inhibitor (C1IN) which regulates the early activation events beyond C1q by inhibiting the esterase activity associated with cleavage/activation of the C4 and C2 components. C1IN is the only known inhibitor of C1r and C1s, the activated proteases of C1; it is also a major inhibitor of activated coagulation factor XII and of plasma kallikrein, a protease that cleaves kininogen and releases bradykinin. The importance of this C1IN protein is seen in patients with the autosomal dominant disease hereditary angioedema, or with acquired deficiency of the C1 inhibitor. These patients present with severe and often life-threatening acute inflammatory responses associated with excessive complement activation; the inflammation also involves the kinin/kallikrein enzyme pathways.

Box 1.1 provides a vignette of patients with C1 inhibition deficiency.

Box 1.1 Patients with C1 inhibition deficiency

These patients can have life-threatening acute angioedema, e.g. affecting the upper airways. They also present with an 'acute abdomen' with pain and vomiting, associated with jejunal involvement and diarrhoea with colonic acute (sterile) inflammation. Management of the disease has improved in recent years, with the availability of newer therapeutic agents for disease prophylaxis and for treatment of acute episodes of oedema. Preventive therapies use several anabolic steroids to induce hepatic production of C1IN. More recently, a C1IN protein concentrate from pooled plasma has become available for intravenous administration. A recombinant DNA produced form of the protein is also being evaluated. Therapy for acute, potentially life-threatening attacks, in addition to emergency care (intubation/ventilation, etc.), ranges from immediate replacement of the inhibitor using fresh frozen plasma (previous practice) to the present, preferable options including C1IN protein infusions, to newer agents directed at physiological targets including enzyme systems involved in the pathological disturbances. A bradykinin B2 receptor antagonist (icatibant) and an inhibitor of kallikrein enzymes (ecallantide) have recently been added to the treatment regimens. Diagnosis of C1IN deficiency involves quantitative measurement of the protein and of its function (see section 'Immunopathology and tissue damage, immune deficiency, and immunotherapeutics', below, and Chapter 9). The simple and rapid measurement of serum C4 is most helpful as it is invariably low at the time of an acute attack, due to unchecked cleavage of C4 consequent on the lack of inhibition of the esterase activity by the low level of, or nonfunctional form of, the C1IN protein.

At present, clinical deficiencies of most proteins in the complement system have been documented. These deficiencies have helped to clarify the overall functions of the system, which can be summarized as follows:

- Complement plays a key role in eliminating microbes in innate and adaptive immune responses. Figure 1.28 demonstrates the principles of opsonization and the efficiency of the process regarding phagocytosis and destruction of microbes, when coated with complement activation products and with antibody molecules.
- Some components of complement have been shown to augment the development of humoral immunity. The binding of the activation products C3b (and a further degradation product called C3d) to complement receptors on B lymphocytes termed CR1 and CR2, respectively, amplifies B cell responses. For instance, this reaction is demonstrated in germinal centres of lymph nodes to assist B cells in what is called affinity maturation—a process for the selection of high-affinity BCRs to generate high-affinity antibodies. The CR2 receptor (CD21) for C3d also functions as a receptor for EBV, known to infect B cells and to dysregulate B cell Ig production. EBV is used experimentally to derive B cell lines *in vivo*. The virus is linked to the development of certain B cell neoplasms in some immunosuppressed transplant recipients, in HIV/AIDS, and in some primary immunodeficient patients (e.g. Duncan's syndrome). Burkitt's lymphoma was one of the first human tumours shown to be caused (at least in part) by EBV. The C3d augmentation of B cell responses acts as the equivalent of a signal 2, analogous to that described for T cell activation. Signal 1, in the case of B cells, is the BCR binding of antigen and intracellular signalling.
- Complement is believed to be important for the physiological removal *in vivo* of immune complexes and of apoptotic cells. Such cells have molecules that are

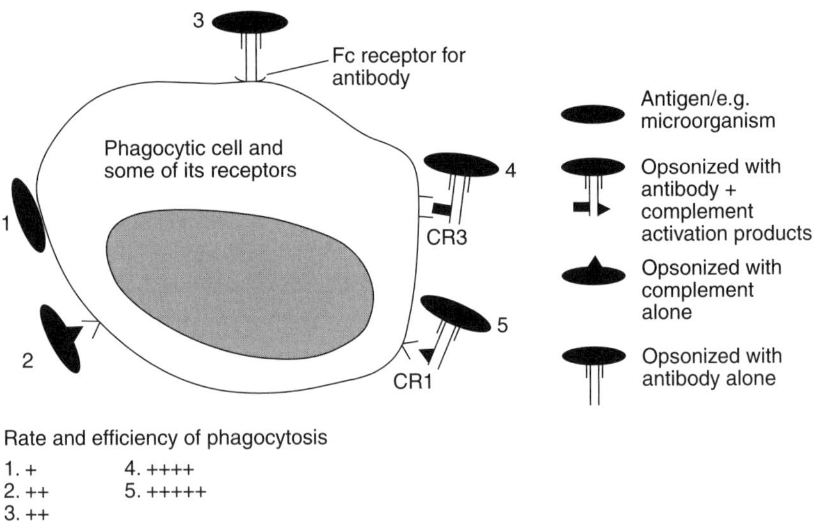

Fig. 1.28 Opsonization of microorganisms and the role of phagocytic cells, CR1, and CR3 receptors for complement activation products C3b (▲) and C3d (■).

recognized directly by some complement components. Such complexes are envisaged as occurring in normal cell turnover events associated with apoptosis and by the actions of natural low-affinity polyreactive IgM antibodies (some with autoantibody specificity). Additionally, immune complexes generated in the removal of microbial invaders are facilitated by the complement system. Patients with deficiencies of early components of complement (e.g. C1q, C2, C4), have been described with typical clinical immune complex problems resembling serum sickness syndrome or lupus-like syndromes, with complexes deposited in skin and renal tissue.

- Many complement-deficient patients present with various microbial infections; some complement deficiencies are rapidly fatal, e.g. deficiency of C3, the major component targeted by all three activation pathways.

In summary, it can be seen that the alternative and lectin pathways act as important immune effectors in innate immunity, while the use of antibodies, as exemplified by classical complement pathway activation, is seen as a key effector of adaptive immunity. Overall, the complement system plays a key role in the elimination of microbes during innate and adaptive immune responses. The system also helps to maintain physiological homeostasis by facilitating the removal of immune complexes and of apoptotic cells. Importantly, the complement system is being understood as playing a major role in the integration of innate and adaptive immunity.

Effector cells and receptors

CD4$^+$ and CD8$^+$ T cell effectors

To appreciate the mechanisms used in developing efficient effector CD4$^+$ and CD8$^+$ T cells, it is helpful to consider them in terms of their maturity, anatomical location, and physiological recirculation. Some key points to note regarding CD4$^+$ and CD8$^+$ T cells are as follows:

- Naive, non-antigen-experienced, peripheral T cells recirculate between blood and secondary lymphoid tissues. In these latter sites they may encounter and interact with their cognate peptide antigen–HLA complex displayed on APCs. Following TCR–peptide–HLA interaction, signalling events occur which facilitate naive T cell activation, proliferation (clonal expansion) and differentiation to effector T cells, some of which also generate memory T cells. This sequence of events occurs for both CD4$^+$ T cells and CD8$^+$ T cells.
- The primed (antigen experienced) effector T cells generated from naive T cells migrate from their peripheral lymphoid sites of induction and circulate through all secondary lymphoid tissues, including dispersed lymphoid elements as found within the GIT and other MALT sites. They also migrate into nonlymphoid tissues. If the effector T cells re-encounter their cognate antigen they can undergo further episodes of activation, together with more marked proliferation and differentiation to become well-defined and polarized effector subpopulations. These subpopulations for CD4$^+$ T cells are the Th1, Th2, and Th17 effectors. Similarly, CD8$^+$ T cells respond and develop as fully functional CD8$^+$ CTLs. After executing their effector functions many of the proliferating clones of lymphocytes undergo apoptosis, thus, maintaining the

homeostatic cellular pool. A proportion of $CD4^+$ and $CD8^+$ T effector cells survive and differentiate to become long-lived memory T cells. Some of the memory $CD4^+$ and $CD8^+$ T cells recirculate while other subsets remain within peripheral tissue sites, ready to respond rapidly to any incoming microbial antigens. The physiology of recirculation of the primed and differentiated effector T cells provides an excellent surveillance system ready to respond rapidly to incoming microbes/antigens to which they have had previous experience.

T cells respond to intracellular microbes endeavouring to colonize the host and to persist as intracellular, protected reservoirs of infection. The range of potential intracellularly located microbes includes viruses (such as herpesvirus, CMV, EBV), bacteria (such as *Mycobacterium tuberculosis*, *Listeria monocytogenese*, legionella) and protozoa (such as *Leishmania major*). Some microbes phagocytosed by macrophages and other APCs can be detected in intracellular vesicles (endosomes and lysosomes) where they can survive having developed mechanisms to subvert intracellular killing. Additionally, components of such microbes may leak from the vesicles into the cytoplasmic compartment. Viruses can infect APCs (macrophages and DCs) but also many other cell types; they are the most successful parasites. After hijacking the genetic machinery of the host cells they produce, intracellularly in the cytoplasm, components such as proteins for assembly of new viruses. In some situations, virus-infected host cells may be recognized and phagocytosed by macrophages, some viral antigens will then be present in endosomal compartments.

Microbial proteins in endosomal compartments and proteins in the cytosolic compartment are degraded to peptides which become associated with the HLA class II and HLA class I pathways of antigen presentation, respectively.

- APCs transport microbial antigens from peripheral sites to the regional/secondary lymphoid tissues. In these sites, the APCs provide the opportunity for the recirculating naive T cells to recognize processed peptide–HLA complexes. Within the recirculating pool of naive T cells are the relatively rare clones with specific TCRs for any given peptide antigen displayed on the APCs. The recirculating naive T cells in blood leave the vessels in the lymphoid tissues via the HEV, using their integrin and L selectin adhesion molecules, and are directed to the T cell areas within the lymphoid structure by their chemokine receptor CCR7. This moves directionally toward the ligands CCL19 and CCL21 which are produced by stromal cells within the paracortical T cell areas. The rare specific T cell (estimated at $\sim 1:10^5$) with the specific TCR has the opportunity to interact with the recently arrived APC displaying the appropriate peptide–HLA complex. $CD4^+$ T cells interact with HLA class II-associated peptides while $CD8^+$ T cells interact with the HLA class I–peptide complex.
- Initial interactions assist in increasing the strength of the antigen-specific interaction, i.e. the signal 1 interaction. Thus, the integrin LFA1 present on the T cells binds to the ICAM-1 on the APC and, additionally, the CD4 molecules of the T cell bind to the invariant part of the class II molecules; similarly, for $CD8^+$ T cells, the CD8 molecule reacts with the nonpolymorphic residues of the HLA class I molecule. Key interactions also occur between the specific T cell and the APC, most

notably by the binding of the CD28 molecule on the T cell which interacts with the costimulatory molecules CD80/CD86 on the APC.

- The above interactions cause a clustering of molecules around the primary signal 1 complex of TCR with the antigenic peptide–HLA on the APC. The clustering results in the microanatomical formation of a synapse between the APC and the T cell membranes. This is referred to as the immunological synapse and is believed to be the main means for focusing reactions at that site, including aggregation of several TCR complexes. The interactions within the synapse facilitate biochemical signals (including calcium ion fluxes) which rise above a particular threshold and lead to further signals resulting in T cell activation (this reaction occurs for $CD4^+$ and $CD8^+$ cells responding to different peptide antigens derived from the same microbe).
- The biochemical signals are well described for T cells and are summarized in Figure 1.29. The essence of the signalling is due to the CD3 component of the TCR. The CD3 molecule is made up of three chains, one of which contains in its cytoplasmic domain an ITAM motif, phosphorylation of which along with a molecule called the zeta (ζ) chain attracts the intracellular kinase termed Zap-70. The Zap-70 is in turn phosphorylated as it contains ITAM residues and it attracts downstream adaptor proteins. They, in turn, activate additional downstream biochemical pathways which are linked to further active enzyme systems. Ultimately, the signalling pathways target transcription factors located in the cytoplasm. On interaction, modified transcription factors translocate and enter the nucleus of the T cell to target their particular genes, inducing the production of their encoded proteins. Key enzymes and the transcription factors targeted are (1) the calcium-dependent enzyme calcineurin which acts on the transcription factor nuclear factor of activated T cells (NFAT), (2) PKC targets NF-κB, and (3) ERK/JAK targets the transcription factor activator protein-1 (AP-1).
- The molecules produced during T cell activation characterize activated T cells and include membrane-associated molecules and cytokines. Among the earliest activation molecules detectable (present within hours of TCR full signalling) is CD69. This is followed in turn by FasL (CD95L) and, subsequently, by the key functional molecule CD40L (CD152). Most of these molecules are expressed over hours rather than days. However, 24–48 hours after activation the production of the cytokine IL-2 can be demonstrated, with concomitant production and expression on the cell membrane of the high-affinity IL-2R complex. This series of events then favours autocrine binding of the cytokine IL-2 to its receptor and drives proliferation of the specific T cells (clonal expansion). The proliferative events are characterized by DNA synthesis and ultimately cell mitosis. The dividing cells are evident and measurable from approximately 3 days onwards (see Chapter 9).
- The proliferating cells have the ability to differentiate into various effectors (primed T cells). The differentiation events are facilitated by the CD40L on the activated and proliferating T cells; thus can bind CD40 expressed on APCs, macrophages, and B cells. Cytokines and their receptors induced on various cells also contribute to proliferative outcomes. Thus, for responding $CD4^+$ T cells, along with the CD40L/CD40

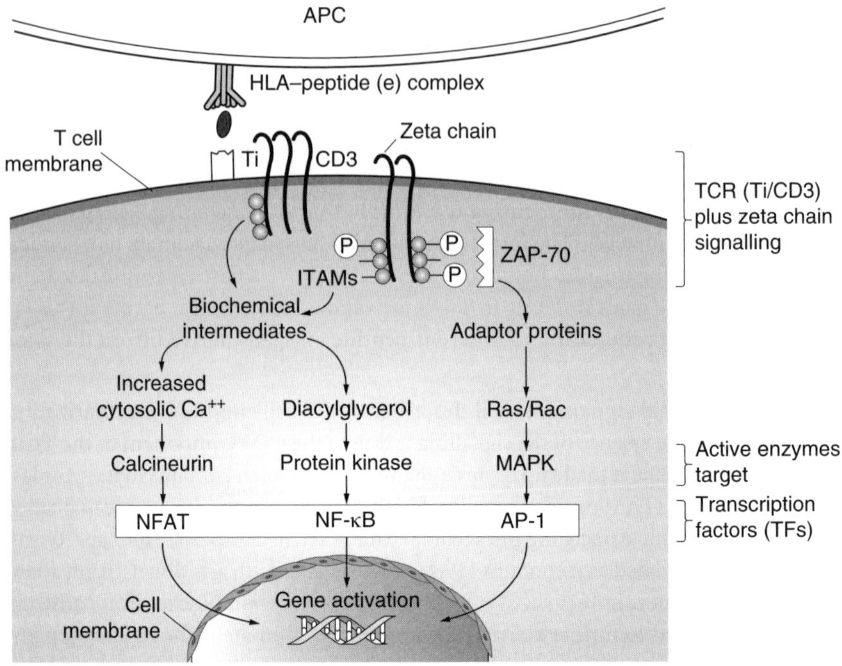

Fig. 1.29 T cell signalling pathways: TCR complex (Ti/CD3) recognizes and binds peptide–HLA complex display on the APC. The ITAM motifs of CD3 molecules and of the zeta chains become phosphorylated and bind the ZAP-70 protein. Further adaptor proteins dock into the complex and various biochemical intermediates and pathways are activated, including key enzyme systems (e.g. calcineurin) which target and activate TFs. The TFs move into the nucleus and stimulate various genes whose products characterize and mediate the T cell responses, e.g. cytokines, chemokines and their receptors and other activation markers. AP-1, activating protein 1; MAPK, mitogen-activated protein kinases; NFAT, nuclear factor of activated T cells; P, phosphorylation site; TF, transcription factor; ZAP-70, zeta-associated protein of 70 kDa.

interaction, if the cells bind the IL-12 (produced abundantly by APCs and macrophages), the cells receive additional biochemical stimuli (signal 3) which favour their differentiation as CD4 $^+$ Th1 effectors. Their differentiation is under the control of the transcription factor T-bet along with STAT4. These Th1 cells produce a signature cytokine IFN-γ along with IL-2 and TNF-α. Th2 effectors develop under the control of the transcription factor GATA, along with STAT 6, with signals induced by the binding of the cytokine IL-4. Sources of IL-4 in the tissue sites have recently been defined in innate cells such as tissue mast cells and basophils (see later). The differentiated Th2 cells produce in turn more IL-4, its signature cytokine, which can act in an autocrine manner to drive further differentiation. Additional cytokines produced by Th2 cells include IL-5, IL-9, and IL-13. Analogous reactions occur to facilitate the differentiation of Th17 cells. Current evidence in humans shows that this latter differentiation is driven by IL-6, IL-21, and TGF-β; also, IL-23 is seen as important for the maintenance of differentiated Th17 cells. The related transcription factor for Th17 is retinoic acid orphan receptor (RORγ).

For naive CD8$^+$ T cells, their development to primed effector cells generally needs help from CD4$^+$ T cells by way of the latter cells' production of IFN-γ and IL-2 which bind to receptors on the naive CD8$^+$ T cell and stimulates biochemical signals for proliferation and differentiation. The differentiated CD8$^+$ T cell effectors can be shown to have prominent intracytoplasmic granules which contain the molecules perforin and the enzyme granzyme B.

The differentiated primed effector CD4$^+$ and CD8$^+$ T cells develop changes in cytokine/chemokine receptors and adhesion molecules that favour their movement from their site of induction in the lymphoid tissues. They become recirculating cells that have the ability to move into tissue sites including sites of inflammation. This physiological change gives them the opportunity of re-encountering their cognate antigens, wherever those antigens may enter the host. This recirculating surveillance by effector T cells moving into and through tissues is not antigen specific. However, if the specific antigen is encountered, the T cells undergo rapid expansion and execute their effector function to destroy the antigen. For CD4$^+$ Th cell effectors (Th1, Th2 or Th17) the effector readouts are summarized in Figure 1.21. CD8$^+$ T cells, which develop into efficient CD8$^+$ CTLs, effectively kill cells harbouring the intracellular microbes, whose peptides are displayed on the cell surface associated with HLA class 1. This is a crucial response because viruses can infect a wide range of cell types and the recirculating effector CD8$^+$ T cells must be able to recognize such cells to execute their function. Importantly, once CD8$^+$ T cells are primed, in most situations they require little or no CD4$^+$ T cell help to carry out their effector killing functions. The killing mechanism of the CD8$^+$ T cell is associated with the formation of yet another immunological synapse. It can be shown that CTLs within this location secrete their perforin and granzyme complexes toward the target cell. The molecules are taken up by receptor-mediated endocytosis. Within the endosomes of the target cell the perforin induces a pore in the membrane, allowing, in turn, entry of the granzyme into the cytoplasm and also in to the nucleus of the target cell. The granzyme mediates the apoptotic death of the cell by activating caspases (see 'Apoptosis and autophagy', below). CD8$^+$ CTLs can also kill targets by FasL (CD95) binding to the death receptor CD95 on the target cell. That pathway also leads to apoptosis of the target cell. The FasL pathway of CD8$^+$ T cell killing is believed to represent a minor pathway. The CD8$^+$ CTLs also produce and secrete IFN-γ. Th1 cells produce IFN-γ which stimulates macrophages with phagocytosed microbes to enhance their intracellular killing mechanisms. The IFN-γ from CD8$^+$ T cells also acts in a similar manner.

Following the antimicrobial effector lymphocyte responses, there is a contraction of the responding clones by the process of apoptosis, induced by loss of cell survival factors such as cytokines and up-regulation of proapoptotic genes. The apoptotic mechanism is referred to as activation-induced cell death (AICD; see 'Apoptosis and autophagy', below), and ensures homeostatic maintenance of the peripheral lymphocyte pool. Some effector T cells survive and differentiate to generate long-lived antigen-specific memory lymphoctyes. Two distinct subsets of human memory T cells have been documented based on their differential expression of the receptors CD62L and CCR7. These memory cells are termed effector memory and central memory cells. They show differential recirculation patterns and homing to tissue sites; they have been shown to mediate early and effective recall responses against previously encountered antigens. Such responses are much more rapidly induced than those generated by responding naive T cells. Memory cells are seen as key protectors at sites of natural portals of microbial entry such as the GIT, respiratory and urogenital tracts, and the skin. Understanding the induction, recirculation, and tissue-specific homing of memory T cells is seen as crucial to enhancing vaccine strategies against microbes, particularly against currently intractable targets, such as HIV and the malaria parasite.

B cells expressing CD40, which are engaged by the CD40L on activated T cells, are induced to undergo class switching. These cells move from IgM production toward other heavy-chain Ig isotypes. B cell differentiation to antibody-secreting plasma cells uses various cytokines along with the CD40/CD40L interaction to drive different class switch Ig heavy-chain outcomes. Thus, Th1 cells produce IFN-γ favouring B cell differentiation to plasma cells producing complement-fixing antibodies, such as IgG1 and IgG3. In contrast, Th2 cells produce IL-4 favouring the production of IgE and IgG4 non-complement-fixing antibodies, while IL-5 in MALT sites favours the production of IgA antibodies. Th17 cells produce cytokines including families of IL-17, IL-21, and IL-22 and favour the attraction of neutrophils and monocytes to sites of tissue inflammation and their activation.

Regulation of beneficial effector T and B cell responses is important to avoid host tissue damage. It is achieved in part by removal of the exciting antigen by the immune response and by apoptosis of effector cells after execution of their beneficial role. Another major contribution is from nTregs and iTregs, found in peripheral tissue sites and secondary lymphoid tissues. They regulate immune responses at various levels, including direct suppression of DCs, T cells, and B cells, by direct cell–cell contacts and by their secretion of suppressive cytokines.

The early phases of T cell activation and differentiation toward effector T cells involves the cytokine IL-2. It is now recognized that Treg proliferation and differentiation is also supported by the early IL-2 interactions. Thus, the cytokine IL-2 appears to play a dominant role in driving Treg biology. The kinetics and signals for $CD4^+$, $CD25^+$, $Foxp3^+$ Tregs induction, and control of effector $CD4^+$ Th, $CD8^+$ CTL, and B cell responses is an area of ongoing intense investigations.

NK cells

The innate NK cells function as effectors in cell cytotoxicity; they also produce significant amounts of IFN-γ which can activate macrophages and APCs, as described for T cell IFN-γ action. NK cells destroy virally infected cells and transformed/mutated, potentially malignant, cells [38]. As mentioned previously, NK cells have activating and inhibitory receptors. The latter are seen as dominant, and both types of functions are found in the family of KIR molecules and in heterodimers comprising CD94, along with a lectin molecule (NKG2A or NKG2B). These latter molecules function as inhibitory receptors; in contrast, NKG2D is an activating receptor. The inhibitory receptors, on binding to self HLA-C molecules on host cells, activate their cytoplasmic

ITIM motif which on phosphorylation, activates phosphatases which suppress the ITAM motifs on the activating receptor such as NKG2D. When viruses, as part of their evolutionary escape mechanism, try to avoid CD8$^+$ T cell killing by down-regulating or, in other ways, subverting or destroying HLA class I molecules (preventing presentation of viral peptides to CD8$^+$ T cells), the biological advantage of the NK cells' dual receptor system becomes apparent. The now naked (missing self HLA class 1) virally infected host cell cannot be engaged by the inhibitory NK cell receptor. The activating receptor now has the opportunity to recognize the infected cell and sends positive biochemical signals into the NK cell, which results in the death of the target cells using perforin and granzyme, similar to that described for CD8$^+$ CTLs above. The target cells undergo death by apoptosis.

NK cells express the molecule CD16 (the low-affinity FCγRIII that binds to the Fc of IgG molecules). Cells coated with IgG antibodies via their Fab region have Fc portions that undergo conformational changes and become attractive to receptor binding by CD16. The interaction forms a bridge between the target antibody-coated cell and the NK cell, which is brought into close juxtaposition. The NK cell can then contribute to the destruction of the antibody-coated target cell via ADCC.

NK T cells

These populations are currently considered in the category of 'unconventional T cells' even though they contain somatically rearranged TCRs. In the case of NK T cells, these are of very limited diversity.

NK T cells are defined as cells which recognize antigen presented by the non-MHC molecules termed CD1. NK T cells are said to be CD1-restricted cells. They have an invariant α-chain which is linked to a very limited number of β-chains. In humans, they can be CD4$^+$ or CD8$^+$ and some subpopulations have been defined which are CD4$^-$ and CD8$^-$. The term NK T cells also indicates that such cells express some NK cell molecules, including CD56 and the activating NK receptor NKG2D. The characteristic effector role of NK T cells is that, on recognizing their antigens (lipid and/or glycolipid antigens presented by CD1d on transformed/stressed cells), they respond very rapidly—within hours. That contrasts with standard naive T cell adaptive immune responses that evolve over days. The rapid kinetics of NK T cell responses is much more in keeping with that seen for innate immune cells rather than that of cells of adaptive immunity, hence their classification as unconventional T cells.

A dominant lipid antigen presented by CD1d to NK T cells is α-galactosylceramide (α-GALCER). This specific antigen has allowed the production of CD1d tetramers (analogous to MHC tetramers—see Chapter 9). The CD1d complexed with α-GALCER in the tetramer has been used to enumerate and isolate NK T cells. Although these cells are seen to represent a small population in human peripheral blood and other secondary lymphoid tissues, it is evident that there exist several subsets. A dominant subset is termed the classical type I invariant (i) NK T cell. Experimentally, NK T cells have been shown to enhance Th1 responses and they also modulate DC and B cell responses, as well as enhancing NK cell functions. NK T cells are seen as important effectors with regard to antimicrobial responses and also they have the ability to respond against stressed and/or mutated or overt cancerous cells. There is growing evidence that they also have potentially important immunoregulatory roles with regards to autoimmunity and allergy. NK T cells are being used currently in anticancer immunotherapeutic studies. They can be shown to expand T and B cell immune responses and appropriate strategies are being pursued to exploit NK T cell functionality within the design of various vaccine candidates [39,40]. NK T signalling can also enhance TLR responses occurring in innate immunity. These wide-ranging effects of NK T cell subsets are, in part, associated with their rapid production of a range of cytokines including IFN-γ, TNF-α, IL-17, and IL-22. The range of cytokines produced by NK T cells indicate they can be proinflammatory. However, they also have a suppressive role and can induce cell apoptosis. They are clearly seen as cells bridging innate and adaptive immunity. Anatomically, apart from the low populations in blood and secondary lymphoid tissues, NK T cells can be found in mucosal sites near or in epithelia; they are also present in TILs associated with some tumours. It is surmised that they are responding to the stress molecules expressed by mutated cells; similarly, they recognize stressed/infected epithelial cells at mucosal sites.

γδ T cells

As described in 'T cells, receptors, and effectors: $CD4^+$ Th1, Th2 and Th17; $CD4^+$ Tregs and $CD8^+$ CTLs', above, these T cells express the phylogenetically older γδ heterodimer. They represent a small population (<10%) in peripheral blood, compared with conventional αβ T cells. They can be $CD4^-$ and $CD8^-$ or they can be $CD4^+$ and $CD8^+$ γδ T cells. Anatomically, they can be shown to be abundant in epithelial sites where they are believed, like NK T cells, to act as essential sentinels capable of inducing rapid effector responses against microbial invasion and against damaged/stressed cells. Like NK T cells, γδ T cells can recognize glycolipid antigen presented by CD1 molecules. Interestingly, they have been shown to have specificity for lipids and glycolipids presented by other members of the CD1 family, namely CD1b and CD1c found on DCs. Unlike NK T cells, γδ T cells appear to have the ability to recognize not only lipids but also protein antigens; they have also been demonstrated to recognize directly various microbial metabolites. Thus, γδ T cells appear to be able to recognize various antigens in a more flexible way than other T cells. Such flexibility may relate to their key sentinel role at natural portals of entry of microbes, where the ability to recognize various constituents of antigens, whether lipid, protein, carbohydrate, or glycoprotein molecules, can be deemed beneficial. Like NK T cells, the evidence indicates that γδ T cells, on recognizing antigen, respond quickly (within hours), with the production of a range of cytokines including IFN-γ. They are believed to be responsible for killing early infected or stressed epithelial cells. γδ T cells have been documented to show potent actions against intestinal parasite infections, as well as against viral infections.

Mast cells and basophils

Mast cells and basophils have long been studied with regard to their inflammation-potentiating roles in allergy and parasitic diseases. In the latter situation, the inflammation induced by mast cells and basophils is seen as protective, helping in parasite expulsion, e.g. from the GIT. In human allergic disease (asthma and other type I IgE-mediated disorders), these cells are seen as key instruments in the undesirable inflammation-inducing immunopathology. Within the most serious condition of life-threatening anaphylaxis, mast cells and basophils are key players. Their role in mediating type I hypersensitivity is known to be induced by the cross-linking of their high-affinity IgE receptors by bound IgE leading to mast cell and basophil activation, with release of their preformed mediators along with the generation of new mediators. Among the well-known preformed mediators are histamine, proteoglycans, and a spectrum of neutral proteases. Released histamine acts on its various defined receptors (H1, H2, H3) to mediate its effects. Among the proteases released from mast cells is tryptase. Measurement of blood tryptase is one of the assays used in the investigation of suspected anaphylactic reactions, IgE or non-IgE mediated (see 'Immunopathology and tissue damage, immune deficiency, and immunotherapeutics', below). It is also used in investigating possible diagnosis of mastocytosis. Among the newly generated mediators from mast cells and basophils are arachidonic acid metabolites, including the LTs and PGs D series. Importantly, it is recognized that a significant number of cytokines can also be produced by both cell types.

Detailed studies of mast cells and basophils indicate they can have much more diverse roles in several aspects of innate and adaptive immunity. Mast cells are strategically located in connective tissue sites. They are sessile cells derived from bone marrow precursors; the precursors enter the tissues and mature *in situ*. They are strategically placed below key sites of possible microbial entry. The microbes or their antigens, which get through the epithelial barriers, are likely to encounter mast cells. In contrast, basophils remain in blood as a minor population of circulating granulocytes, but they are readily mobilized and recruited into sites of tissue inflammation.

The physiological effector functions of mast cells and basophils have become clearer with the definition of a wide range of membrane receptors associated with both cell types. These receptors relate to their cell function and to their site of location. Both cell types have a range of chemokine receptors including CCR3, which can be activated by the ligand CCL11 (eotaxin) produced by epithelial cells. A range of other CXC and CC chemokine receptors have been demonstrated on both cell types. Mast cells, unlike basophils, have also been shown to have membrane receptors for PAMPs, namely TLR-2 and TLR-4, indicating that in tissue sites they can respond to PAMPs as part of the innate early antimicrobial effector reaction. Indeed, LPS stimulation of mast cells via TLR-4 demonstrates another important role of mast cells as producers and secretors of cytokines. In response to such stimulation, mast cells produce IL-4, IL-13, and other Th2-associated cytokines. This illustrates that mast cells of innate immunity can harness and direct the development of adaptive immune effector responses. The responses favour the production of IgE, which in turn can enhance mast cell effector reactions via its binding to mast cell Fc receptors. Such augmenting responses between mast cells and Th2 cells in sites such as the GIT may be seen as very positive [41]. However, in sites such as the lung of atopic individuals this may be counterproductive. TLR activation of mast cells results not only in cytokine production but also in increased release of LTs. The knowledge that microbial stimulation can directly stimulate mast cell production of cytokines and other inflammatory mediators may well relate to the long-known clinical association of some respiratory tract infections triggering or exacerbating allergic asthma.

Basophils have recently been shown, in several model systems, to be very significant producers of IL-4 and IL-13 when attracted to tissue sites via chemotactic reactions associated with their CCR3 receptors. Several bacterial and viral proteins have been shown to induce/up-regulate CCR3. The efficient production of IL-4 and IL-13 by basophils is now placing these cells as key *in vivo* effectors for generating Th2 cells from Th0 precursors. Other very recent findings are again illustrating some new potential functions of mast cells and basophils with relation to signalling molecules. The recently identified cytokine IL-33 (a member of the IL-1 family) is produced by many cell types—endothelial, epithelial, and fibroblast cells. IL-33 is also believed to be released from damaged or dying cells, and is seen to be active as a DAMP. Mast cells have been shown to have high levels of receptors for IL-33 [42]. Thus, in areas of significant tissue damage mast cells can be stimulated to enhance proinflammatory reactions within such sites. Another key cytokine, IL-25, has been shown to be produced both by mast cells and by Th2 cells. Both cells also possess receptors for the cytokine, suggesting a powerful augmenting stimulus for allergic reactions. Indeed, IL-25 is being investigated as a potentially major target to modulate the allergic response.

Key insights that have been gained into the role of mast cells and basophils in innate and adaptive immunity, along with their well-established role in type I IgE-mediated responses, makes both cell types important entities to consider for immune manipulation.

Vaccination

Introduction

Vaccination procedures have been demonstrated, for more than a century, to be the most beneficial means of protecting humans and animals from infections. From the early 20th century vaccine efficacy and effectiveness has been unrivalled in utilizing effector immune responses for beneficial outcomes. Noteworthy examples include use of attenuated microbes, e.g. BCG, which induces partially effective immunity; the use of the inactivated toxins of diphtheria and tetanus (highly effective vaccines); and the recent successful use of polysaccharide protein conjugates (for haemophilus and strains of meningococcus bacteria). Over this period, limited numbers of adjuvants have also been used to enhance vaccination responses (see 'Immunogens, antigens, and adjuvants', above).

Striking decreases in the incidence of a range of infectious viral and bacterial diseases have been documented worldwide. Vaccination programmes have led to the worldwide elimination of smallpox and the imminent elimination of poliomyelitis—truly universal medical triumphs. When vaccination programmes become compromised, as occurred with the MMR vaccine in the UK in the late 1990s, mumps and measles infections re-emerged with resultant associated morbidity. This highlights the need for constant vigilance and use of robust vaccination programmes.

Most successful vaccines are based on preventive pre-exposure challenge; very few vaccines are available for postexposure treatment (therapeutic vaccines). Use of passive immunity by way of Ig/antibody therapy is helping to control postexposure risks. The success of vaccines has most often been correlated with protective humoral (antibody) immunity. Correlation of protection by serological analysis is relatively straightforward using various techniques such as ELISA, complement fixation, and agglutination methods (see Chapter 9). Implicit in many antibody responses to vaccines, which are mainly of the IgG class, is the understanding from basic immunology that CD4$^+$ Th cells have contributed to the protective immune response. The CD4$^+$ Th cells induce B cell class switching, antibody affinity maturation, and generation of memory cells. With some antiviral vaccines protection is correlated with antibody production, and again the involvement of the CD4$^+$ Th subset is important. In some situations, using rare attenuated virus vaccines, there is also a likely contribution by CD8$^+$ CTLs as effectors and memory cells. Successful as vaccination has been, there is nevertheless a range of viral, bacterial, and protozoal diseases that are currently proving intractable to various attempted vaccine strategies. Problem areas include attempts at developing vaccines against tuberculosis (TB). BCG is only partially protective, in limited patient groups and with waning immunity over the years. Other major challenges are HIV/AIDS and malaria. The concepts highlighted throughout this chapter need to be borne in mind in vaccinology. Examples of such considerations are as follows:

- Microbes that have a predominant extracellular effect, either prior to infecting host cells or occupying that space at key times in their natural history, should be targeted by antibodies. The antibodies may directly neutralize the microbes or recruit effector mechanisms such as complement activation and ADCC. Particular antibody isotypes may be needed to be invoked for particular infections. A successful antihelminth vaccine should stimulate good Th2 responses with the production of effector IgE antibodies targeting the large extracellular helminth pathogens. The immune response may harness ADCC via eosinophils, which are activated and recruited to sites of infection by IL-5 produced by Th2 cells. Activated eosinophils have high-affinity Fc receptors for IgE and can execute ADCC reactions. The actions of chemokines that attract eosinophils, via their corresponding receptors, can also focus reactions against helminths in the local tissue sites. Eosinophils, by release of their basic cytoplasmic granules, can damage directly the parasite or favour the generation of an inflammatory microenvironment that is disadvantageous for parasite survival and/or nutrition.
- Microbes that exist mainly intracellularly (viruses, some bacteria such as mycobacteria) require vaccine strategies that can present antigens to the HLA class I pathway for CD8$^+$ T cells. Additionally, to get effective and robust CD8$^+$ T cell effector and memory cells, CD4$^+$ T cell help is required; therefore, the vaccine strategy also requires engaging the HLA class II antigen presentation pathway. To achieve access to both HLA class I and II pathways, may require strategies to exploit cross-priming—cross-antigen presentation (see 'Antigen processing and presentation; adhesion molecules and costimulation', above). Consider the case of the TB microorganism; over time it remains within a granuloma, remaining alive in the endosomal compartment of macrophages. The strong host anti-TB CD4$^+$ T cell response, which has been documented *in vitro* by the ELISPOT assay or by the tuberculin (Mantoux) skin testing (DTH responses *in vivo;* see 'Type IV hypersensitvity', below), appears

to be insufficient to remove the microbe. Strategies to facilitate leakage of the TB antigen from the protective endosomal compartment into the cytosol and thus to the class I presentation pathway would be a rational way forward. Indeed, some ongoing experimental vaccines are exploiting certain bacterial cytolysins as a means of helping to induce CD8$^+$ CTL responses against the TB organism. The bacterial cytolysins are used to create pores in the endosomes, thus, allowing mycobacterial antigens to enter the cytosol and ultimately be presented on HLA class I molecules for CD8$^+$ T cell recognition.

- Attempts to get wide CD4$^+$ T cell, CD8$^+$ T cell, and antibody responses against difficult targets (HIV and malaria) have used novel immunization methods including the so-called prime-boost strategy. Essentially, DNA constructs encoding target antigens (often antigens too dangerous to be used in whole live or attenuated microbial vaccines), such as the HIV *env*, *pol*, and *nef* genes, are administered by a gene gun. Within the tissues the incorporated genes become transcribed and translated to their protein products to stimulate immunity. After some time, a booster vaccine is given, commonly using one of the viral proteins as a recombinant molecule in a nonpathogenic viral vector (such as adenovirus). Laboratory analysis, by use of MHC tetramers, ELISPOT, and serology, has documented that prime-boost vaccines can induce good CD8$^+$ T cell responses, followed by CD4$^+$ T cell responses and some antibody production, with the responses noted in that order of quantitative positivity. Unfortunately, trials of such prime-boost vaccines have so far not proved protective or efficacious in clinical trials of HIV vaccines in the field.
- Strategies using the bridge between innate and adaptive immunity have targeted DCs. This has been done particularly in attempts at anticancer immunotherapy (see Chapters 4 and 7). These approaches involve antigen pulsing, DNA transfection, and other means of exploiting HLA class I and II peptide cross-presentation antigen-processing pathways. Caution is needed to ensure that the DC approach uses the right type/subset of DCs (proinflammatory rather than suppressive DCs; see 'Innate and adaptive immunity', above), as well as using appropriate additional costimulatory signals ensuring good signal 2 and/or 3 delivery.
- Newer strategies, enhancing and exploiting links between innate and adaptive immunity, are targeting TLRs on other innate cells as a form of novel cellular adjuvant. A particular innate cell that is being used in such strategies is the NK T cell. Additionally, the TLR molecules expressed as intrinsic membrane molecules on T and B lymphocytes are being investigated as pathways to enhancing possible vaccination responses.

A crucial and, in this author's view, under-investigated area to enhance vaccination strategies is the use of mucosal administration of vaccines to generate responses against microbes and environmental antigens. Exploitation of the MALT system has proved to be highly successful in the past, as with the oral attenuated polio vaccine. Increased knowledge of the induction of mucosal immunity, coupled with the concomitant knowledge of tolerance (hyporesponsiveness) induction by that same route, suggests the potential for the wide exploitation of vaccines administered orally or intranasally. At present, investigational mucosal vaccines are being explored for allergic diseases and for human autoimmunity, including oral vaccines for MS.

Vaccines at the extremes of life

Incisive studies of the integrated immune system at the extremes of age are needed to inform the best approaches for immunization for the very young and the elderly population. Infectious diseases worldwide still cause considerable mortality and morbidity. This is seen particularly at the extremes of life. Observations in humans and studies in model systems have indicated elements of the innate and adaptive immunity that are compromised with age; some salient observations are as follows:

- In infants (<2 years of age) the immune system responds poorly to polysaccharide antigens. Such antigens are major components of the capsule of significant numbers of bacterial pathogens. Knowledge of that situation has led, over the past decade, to the introduction of children's vaccines where polysaccharide antigens are conjugated to proteins, exploiting the protein hapten biological process (see 'Immunogens, antigens, and adjuvants', above). The conjugated vaccines, e.g. against haemophilus and pneumococcus bacteria, have had major beneficial effects in decreasing infant mortality and morbidity.
- Observations of the aged immune system (referred to as immune senescence) have documented the following:
  - (i) T cell, quantitative and qualitative, immunity declines with advanced age (>65 years). This is partly explained by the involution of the thymus which shows minimal function beyond the age of 60. Additionally, aged T cells have significant telomere shortening and lose the ability to undergo repeated cell divisions (a prerequisite for generating effector and memory T cells). Interestingly, NK cells appear to be much better preserved in older people.
  - (ii) T cell responses in older people have been shown to be oligoclonal, especially for $CD8^+$ T cells. The loss of polyclonality restricts the diversity of T cells able to respond to incoming antigens.
  - (iii) Similarly, B cell responses in older people show increased oligoclonality. From the age of 55 years onwards, significant monoclonal Igs can be found in blood. They are not malignant myeloma and are referred to as monoclonal gammopathy of uncertain significance (MGUS). It is known, however, that when MGUS patients are followed over decades a significant proportion is found to develop true malignant myeloma.
- Other observations in older people show a reduction in the MALT system of secretory IgA levels and responses.
- With regards to the innate immune system, macrophages in older people show less efficient intracellular killing of bacteria. This may be due, in part, to lack of T cell cytokines to stimulate the macrophages.
- Immune senescence is also characterized by the detection of increased levels of autoantibodies. This arises, in part, because of diminished Tregs and their function. Often, the autoantibodies detected are not associated with clinical disease and are of low titres.

All of the above observations would predict poor responses to common vaccines in older people. Indeed, studies looking at patients aged 65–90 years, using conventional non-adjuvant-containing influenza vaccines, have documented very poor or no vaccine responses in the very old. In contrast, other studies using influenza vaccines with adjuvant, compared with standard vaccines, clearly demonstrated boosting of the immune response in those given the adjuvant, with little significant increase in adverse effects. It is speculated that the immune stimulus given by the adjuvant, acting via TLR stimulation and cytokine/chemokine induction, helps to overcome the poor lymphocyte immune responses characteristic of older people. Overall, more research is needed to address the observations documented in cases of immune senescence. The findings may inform appropriate and novel vaccine strategies for the elderly population. It must be remembered that this age group has the heaviest mortality and morbidity associated with seasonal influenza infections. Additionally, bacterial pneumonias, especially community-acquired pneumonias, are also very serious in older people, causing much morbidity and death.

In summary, our ever-increasing knowledge of the early and subsequent responses of immunity and the links between innate and adaptive responses is proving enlightening. Concurrent advances in technologies for generating recombinant antigens and novel adjuvants and using systems biology (see Chapter 9) to model host–microbial interactions provide new therapeutic strategies.

Indeed, transformational research using synthetic biology to generate and express a synthetic genome, as published by the J. Craig Venter Institute in 2010, signals a potential exponential advance in new ways of generating vaccines for a range of diseases [43].

Immune regulation and modulation

Introduction

Innate and adaptive immune responses normally exhibit excellent self-regulation. They provide protection against homoeostatic perturbations threatened by pathogens (non-self) and their associated antigens. The immune system is characterized by sequential and integrated responses. These reactions involve receptor ligand interactions, signal transduction, gene induction, cell activation, proliferation, and differentiation. The effects of these responses generate reactions that can contain or destroy the potential non-self invaders. The system then resets its components back to the basal state. A qualitative difference is noted, however, with adaptive immunity, whereby the responding clones of lymphocytes exhibit memory status after the first encounter.

An often-quoted tenet of immunology is that it is an efficient self-regulatory system that does not react against self. That statement requires qualification; it is evident that in generating protective immune responses there is some inevitable reactivity against self, albeit within physiologically tolerable limits. Thus, innate immunity, which exploits controlled inflammation to deal with non-self, causes limited collateral tissue damage although the system initiates rapid downstream responses to facilitate repair. Adaptive immunity fundamentally displays reaction against self as part of the basal response. T cells need to recognize and respond against peptide antigens linked to self HLA molecules. This signal 1 event requires recognition of antigen peptide amino acid residues as well as self HLA polymorphic amino acids. Within humoral immunity it is recognized that physiological levels of autoantibodies exist with specificity for self components. Efficient immune regulation can thus be seen in terms of responses and mechanisms to prevent excessive pathological anti-self reactions while tolerating and facilitating some physiologically useful anti-self reactions, which in themselves contribute to effective immune responses.

Evidence for these regulatory processes and mechanisms has been obtained by animal experiments, in particular the use of gene knock-out mice and transgenic mouse strains. Similarly, the recent use of cell culture systems, using dynamic inhibitory RNA (siRNA) in systems biology approaches, has added useful information. Importantly, careful and detailed studies of rare 'experiments of nature' (humans with associated gene mutations) have contributed significant knowledge with respect to immune regulation. Immune regulatory mechanisms have been much studied in adaptive immunity, but over the past decade increased attention has been paid to such studies in the field of innate immunity. More recently, integrated views of regulation within, and bidirectionally between, adaptive and innate immune systems are being studied and published.

Immune regulation and innate immunity

Within this expanding field some salient examples of regulation are as follows:

- At the level of TLR and NLR responses (see 'Innate and adaptive immunity', above) natural antagonists have been described to the TLR/IL-1 pathway, evident in the existence of the inhibitory IL-1Ra molecule.
- TLR/NLR cell signal transduction events are mediated predominantly by intracellular phosphorylation of kinases (e.g. JAK, MAPK), ultimately targeting primarily the transcription factor NF-κB. These kinase responses are regulated by phosphatases responsible for dephosphorylation and inactivation of kinases. Animal experiments, using knock-out mice for genes for certain phosphatases, indicate that subsequent stimulation of such animals with LPS, which targets the TLR-4/Md2/CD14 complex, can lead to excessive cytokine production resulting in a cytokine storm and multiple organ failure.
- GWASs have defined polymorphisms in a human phosphatase, which has been associated with dysregulated inflammatory responses and with a range of autoimmune disorders.
- In humans, genetic polymorphisms associated with NOD2 are linked to Crohn's disease, a chronic inflammatory bowel disease (see Chapter 8) and polymorphisms in the tyrosine phosphatase PTPN22 are linked to autoimmune diseases. These polymorphisms appear to dysregulate mechanisms and lead to excessive signalling and inflammation.
- Within the GIT, evidence demonstrates that epithelial cell TLR signalling, triggered by commensals of the gut microflora, can induce anti-inflammatory responses [11]. The basal activity within the host MALT and associated microflora aids homeostasis. Note the interesting contrast of TLR signalling associated with recognition of PAMPs by epithelial cells, compared with immune cells. Reactions of immune cells generally result in the production of proinflammatory cytokines, such as TNF-α

and IL-1 via NF-κB activation, whereas epithelial cell signalling appears to be anti-inflammatory.

- Innate DCs found in MALT (GIT and respiratory tract) are often of an immature phenotype. They can be induced by cytokines (e.g. IL-10) from other innate cells to express suppressive functions. Such DCs, in turn, produce more IL-10 and TGF-β which regulate, control, and limit inflammatory responses in MALT.
- The fundamental process of apoptosis (see below) which ensures the engulfing and disposal of effete cells without exciting inflammation (in contrast to necrosis), is being recognized as more than a passive process. Phagocytes of innate immunity which engulf apoptotic cells have been demonstrated experimentally to develop a suppressive phenotype. When challenged with LPS or other stimuli, rather than elaborating proinflammatory cytokines (e.g. TNF-α), such phagocytes with engulfed apoptotic bodies elaborate suppressive cytokines (e.g. IL-10).
- An alternative pathway of macrophage activation is also now considered an important regulatory mechanism in innate immunity, ensuring that tissue damage initiated by inflammatory responses is, in turn, directed towards resolution and repair [23]. Cytokines linked to activating the alternate macrophage pathway include IL-4 and IL-10. Innate immune cells, such as basophils and tissue mast cells, are now known to be key sources of IL-4 in tissue sites and are activated in sites of inflammation. The broadly suppressive cytokine IL-10 is produced by a wide range of immune and nonimmune cells [44,45].
- Intriguing recent experiments, using animals depleted of subsets of T cells, indicate that such cells play an important role in regulating innate immune responses. T-cell-depleted animals, challenged via PAMP–PRR systems, show markedly excessive production of proinflammatory cytokines. Replacement of the missing T cells significantly dampens the response. Mechanistic data suggests that T cells exert their inhibitory effects via actions against proteins of the inflammasome complex.
- Rare human autoinflammatory diseases (see Chapter 8), which are linked to gain or loss of function mutations, are revealing fundamental mechanisms that are important in the regulation of innate immunity. These diseases are seen as dysregulation of innate immunity.
- Other areas of innate immunity have long illustrated the need for tight regulation within the system. This is evident in the complement system where loss of regulatory mechanisms, such as the loss of the C1 inhibitor protein, leads to severe acute, potentially life-threatening, inflammation. Other complement cell-associated molecules and fluid-phase regulators are well defined and include CD46, CD55, factor H, and factor I. More recently attention has been paid to the possible role of complement activation being linked to regulation of lymphocyte responses. T and B lymphocytes express several receptors for complement components. These have mainly been studied for their augmenting role in a range of adaptive immune responses. However, recent studies of molecules (such as CD55) found on T cells indicate that such molecules may be important in the generation of suppressive Tregs.

- Tregs provide good examples of bidirectional regulation between adaptive and innate immunity [46]. It is known that Tregs can induce marked suppressive phenotypes in innate DCs (see above). DCs in the MALT systems are good inducers of Tregs.

The study of immune regulation of innate immunity and of the bidirectional influence of innate and adaptive responses is an exponentially expanding area. Such studies will undoubtedly yield new understanding and insight into the control of diseases ranging from rare autoinflammatory conditions to common disease such as cancer. Noteworthy links between persistent inflammation and the induction of neoplasia are established (see 'Overview of immunology', above, and Chapter 4). Understanding of these innate immunoregulatory pathways will also undoubtedly inform studies of autoimmunity.

Studies of immune regulation of adaptive immunity have a long and well-documented history. Key mechanisms relate to central and peripheral tolerance for T and B cells, the process of anergy, immune suppression by regulatory T cells, and major cell deletion events in peripheral tissues associated with AICD. These mechanisms are explored in 'Apoptosis and autophagy', below. A fundamental process mediating many of these adaptive immune regulatory mechanisms is apoptosis. Much effort is being directed to modulating apoptosis as a means of controlling and treating a wide range of diseases encountered in medical and surgical practice. Some key features of apoptosis, as it relates to immunology and wider cell biology/physiology in medicine, are outlined below together with comments on autophagy, another physiological process that is becoming recognized as important in immunity.

Apoptosis and autophagy

Apoptosis

The process of apoptosis may be considered as the physiological master controller of cell death. It counterbalances cell proliferation to ensure cellular homeostasis. Apoptosis is a fundamental process in cell biology and development; it takes centre stage where tissues undergo massive periods of remodelling requiring cell proliferation (mitosis) and concomitant cell death. Apoptotic cells are cleared by viable neighbouring cells or by professional phagocytes. The removal of apoptotic cells is thus achieved without exciting inflammation, as occurs in the process of necrosis, and is characterized by cell swelling, membrane disruption with release of intracellular contents, and induction of inflammation.

Apoptotic cells can be characterized by molecular and cellular features that flag them for phagocytosis. The seminal paper published by Curry *et al.* in the early 1970s documented the key cellular/morphological changes of apoptosis. These are summarized in Table 1.9 and are compared with features and functions of necrosis.

In central and peripheral lymphoid tissues, massive numbers of nonselected lymphocytes (potentially deleterious and anti-self reactive) die daily and are removed by apoptosis. In innate immunity the bone marrow generates in the order of a billion neutrophils per day; the lifespan of such cells ranges from hours to a few days. The massive cell death and turnover of such cells, which possess very potent intracellular inflammation-inducing molecules, must be regulated to maintain homeostasis and

Table 1.9 Cardinal features associated with apoptosis and necrosis

Apoptosis	Necrosis
Physiological (can also be pathological)	Pathological
Specific stimuli induce genetic events leading to apoptosis (genetically controlled)	Toxic stimuli
DNA condensation, internucleosomal fragmentation producing a DNA laddering pattern	No condensation or laddering but large random DNA fragments may be detected
Cell membrane remains intact (excludes various dyes) and expresses on the surface phosphatidyl serine molecules (detectable by binding of annexin V)	Loss of membrane integrity
Leads to an anti-inflammatory clearance (passive and active induction of suppressive phagocytes)	Inflammatory clearance
Suppressive phagocytes on stimulation secrete IL-10 and TGF-β	The tissue inflammation favours the production of proinflammatory cytokines (e.g. TNF-α, IL-12)

survival—this is achieved through apoptosis. Apoptosis can be considered as constitutive in the physiology of immune cell development and in developmental biology generally with regard to tissue remodelling.

In certain situations, dysregulation of the process of apoptosis occurs and can manifest in disease. In some areas, such as cancer and autoimmunity, evidence indicates inadequate apoptosis, due in part to genetic susceptibility events that contribute to disease development (see below for apoptosis in autoimmunity). In the area of cancer, the master regulatory proto-oncogene p53 normally detects DNA damage in cells and triggers the process of apoptosis. However, p53 is often noted to be mutated in many cancers, resulting in a failure in apoptosis, a major factor contributing to survival of tumour cells. By contrast, an ever-growing list of diseases and disorders are being defined as associated with the aberrant induction of excessive apoptosis. These diseases range from cardiovascular disorders (strokes and myocardial infarction), acute liver failure, and spinal cord injuries to neurodegenerative diseases and AIDS. In some of these disorders, it is suggested that the excessive apoptosis overcomes the normal cell clearance mechanisms, resulting in degeneration of nonphagocytosed apoptotic cells which release their contents by undergoing secondary necrosis. This, in turn, can induce tissue inflammation. Thus, inflammation is seen as a significant process in all of these diseases.

The *in vivo* effectiveness of phagocyte clearance of apoptotic cells is evident; microscopic examination of tissue sections can rarely demonstrate apoptotic cells. Historically, the description of 'tingible body' macrophages within sections of thymus tissue is an indicator of cells that have engulfed and destroyed apoptosed thymocytes.

It is important to recognize that a whole range of stimuli can induce apoptosis. Figure 1.30 illustrates some well-known inducers of apoptosis. It is evident that some of these stimuli are already exploited in medical practice, particularly in the use of

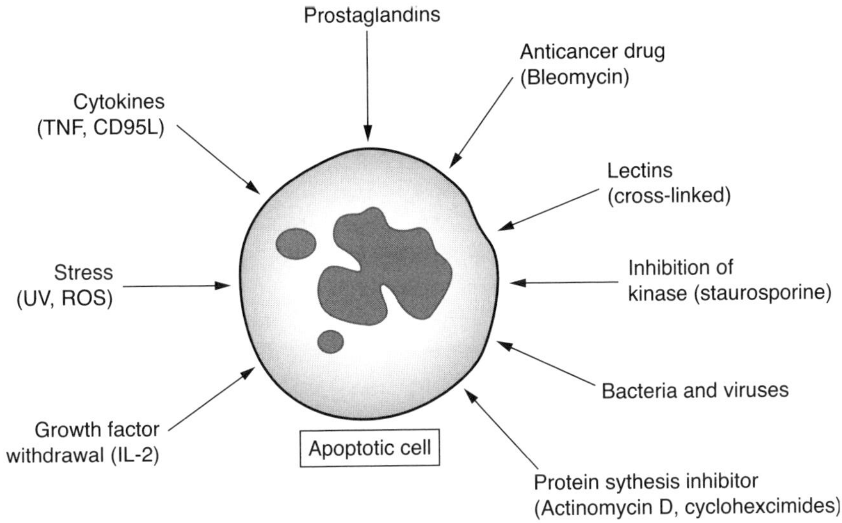

Fig. 1.30 Inducers of apoptosis. Various stimuli which are known to induce apoptosis in target cells are indicated. ROS, reactive oxygen species.

anticancer drugs. Other stimuli give insight into peripheral pathways that exploit apoptosis; cytokines, such as TNF-α, and also the FasL can induce apoptosis. These are pertinent to death-inducing responses in adaptive and innate immunity.

The genetic control of apoptosis is a highly regulated and complex area and beyond the scope of this text. More than 50 genes are known to be involved in apoptosis [47]. However, certain key areas with particular pertinence to immunology can be summarized as follows. There are two predominant pathways that provide signals for apoptosis, the *extrinsic* and *intrinsic* pathways, the latter being associated with mitochondria. Of the many genes linked to apoptosis, there are some whose products favour the induction of apoptosis, e.g. Bax and Bak. The proapoptotic Bax is particularly active in the mitochondrial intrinsic pathway. A well-known antiapoptotic gene and protein is Bcl2. The pro- and antiapoptotic proteins ultimately target the enzyme systems which lead to the expression of apoptosis. These enzymes are proteases of the caspase system: some 10 caspases have been defined in human cell biology. Caspases 8 and 10 are linked to the essential cell cleavage processes which ultimately result in the well-characterized features of apoptosis such as DNA laddering. The caspases act in a cascade activation manner analogous to that seen in the complement system. They exist as proproteins which undergo cleavage and activation, the active compound then cleaving downstream caspase targets. Ultimately, the active caspases lead to cleavage/disruption of cytoplasmic and nuclear proteins.

The extrinsic pathway leading to apoptosis is particularly pertinent in immunology, as it is exploited by cytotoxic cells such as NK cells and CD8$^+$ CTLs in their effector functions (see 'Effector cells and receptors', above). It is also the prominent pathway used for maintenance of peripheral tolerance induced by the mechanism of AICD

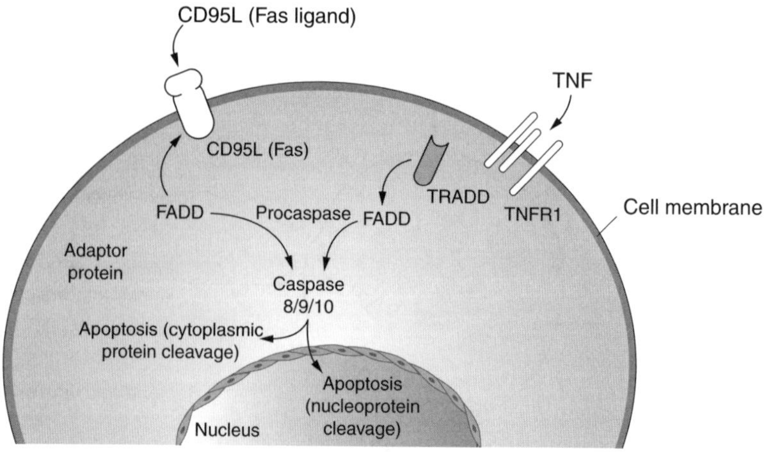

Fig. 1.31 Extrinsic pathway of activation (via death receptors) of the caspases to induce cell apoptosis. Shown are the receptors CD95 (Fas) and TNFR1, which both have cytoplasmic 'death domains'. On binding their respective ligands, their cytoplasmic death domains attract the adaptor proteins FADD and TRADD, which ultimately leads to activation of procaspases that are cleaved to generate terminal caspases, enzymes that cause the apoptotic death of the cell. FADD, Fas-associated death domain; TNFR1, tumour necrosis factor receptor 1; TRADD, TNFR-associated death domain.

(see below). Key molecules within the extrinisic pathway are shown in Figure 1.31. This pathway has associated membrane receptors, referred to as death receptors; particularly well-characterized examples are the Fas (CD95) molecule and the TNF receptor (TNFR). The cytoplasmic portion of these receptors have linkages to adapter proteins, termed Fas-associated death domain (FADD) and TNFR-associated domain (TRADD), respectively. These have other linkages downstream that ultimately generate from procaspases the key molecules, activated caspases 8 and 10, which mediate the apoptotic cleavage events. The death receptor Fas/CD95 and its ligand FasL/CD95L can both be expressed on activated T cells. Engagement of Fas with its ligand triggers the extrinsic apoptotic pathway and is particularly pertinent in the process of AICD. The TNFR family proteins, upon ligand binding, can also trigger proapoptotic pathways (Figure 1.31).

Mutations in apoptosis-associated genes have been linked as causal or contributory factors in some rare but important human diseases. Examples include mutations in *TNFR1* which leads to some forms of familial autoinflammatory diseases (see Chapter 8). Mutations in CD95 or CD95L have been associated with some forms of non-Hodgkin's lymphoma and, importantly, with autoimmune lymphoproliferative syndromes (see 'Autoimmunity: re-establishing homeostatic regulation', below). Perforins are key mediators of lymphocyte cytotoxicity (used by NK cells and CD8^{+} CTLs); genes for perforin have been found to be mutated in some forms of familial haemophagocytic lymphohistiocytosis syndromes. It is also noteworthy that mutations of the proapoptotic gene *BAX* have also been documented in significant numbers of malignant neoplasms with p53 mutations.

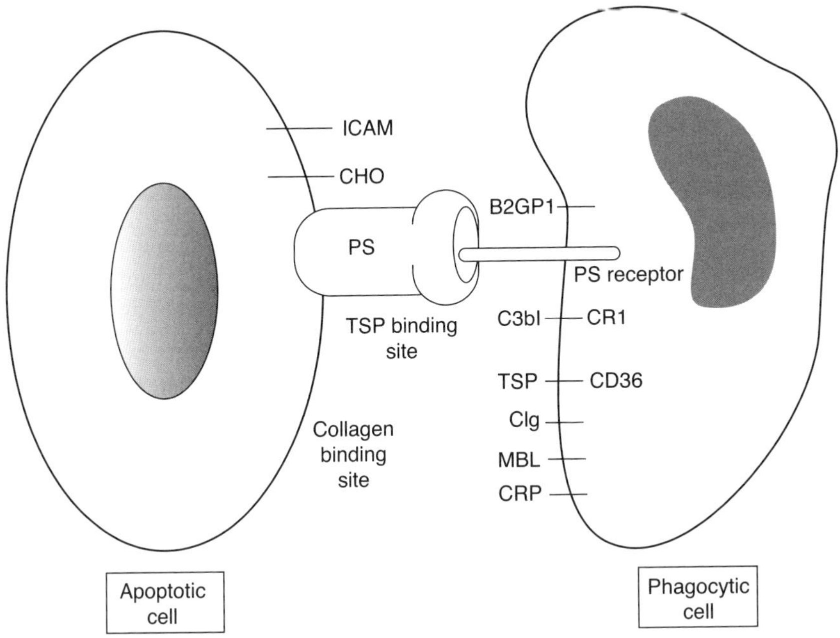

Fig. 1.32 Molecular interactions that occur between apoptotic cells and phagocytes. The pre-eminence of the reacting pairs of molecules in the process is an area of intense study. B2-GP1, β2-glycoprotein1; CHO, modified carbohydrates; CRP, C-reactive protein; ICAM, intercellular cell adhesion molecule; MBL, mannan-binding lectin; PS, phosphatidylserine; TSP, thrombospondin.

Apoptotic cells have a range of membrane-associated molecules (Figure 1.32) which have counter receptor molecules defined on the phagocytic cells. Much research has been carried out in exploring the hierarchy associated with these interactions. Some of the well-known molecules which bind to the surface of apoptotic cells and cross-link with phagocytes include CRP, C1q, MBL and annexin V. The molecule phosphatidylserine, which flips from the intracellular surface of the cell membrane to the extracellular surface early in the process of apoptosis, is exploited in laboratory experiments to demonstrate early apoptosis by the binding of labelled annexin V. This analysis for detecting apoptotic cells can be done by flow cytometric methods (see Chapter 9).

Autophagy

Autophagy is a catabolic process which is important in cell growth, development and homeostasis. It is being recognized as a fundamental process in the regulation of innate and adaptive immune responses [48]. In autophagy, cell cytoplasmic constituents are sequestered into a double-membrane autophagosome and delivered for degradation. This is perceived as a housekeeping process involved in the daily turnover of cell constituents. Autophagy is being linked to aspects of innate and adaptive immunity. For example, it is considered to play a role in the cross-presentation of antigens, whereby, intracellular/cytosolic-processed peptides that would normally be destined for the

HLA class I presentation pathway, can, as autosomes, be delivered for presentation via the HLA class II pathway for recognition by $CD4^+$ T cells. Autophagy in DCs, in particular in plasmacytoid DCs, has been shown to favour high production of type 1 IFNs, important in innate antiviral responses. GWASs have helped to define autophagy genes and their links to disease and disease processes. A strong linkage has been found for a particular autophagy gene, *ATG61*, which has been linked to susceptibility to Crohn's disease. Autophagy has also been generally thought to favour negative regulation of cytokine signalling and inflammation. Thus, loss-of-function mutations may favour excessive inflammation; polymorphisms or mutations in such autophagy genes may favour the emergence of inflammatory conditions as typified by Crohn's disease (see Chapter 8).

Immune tolerance: central and peripheral tolerance

Introduction

The ability of the adaptive immune response to react specifically against vast arrays of antigens/non-self, but not to react against host self cell tissues in a pathological way is the essence of immune tolerance or unresponsiveness to self. T and B cell lymphocyte receptors are generated by massive somatic rearrangement of limited germ-line genes (see 'B cells, receptors, and antibodies', above). This occurs mainly in the central lymphoid organs—the thymus and the bone marrow. The process is stochastic and lymphocytes with receptors against self molecules must, therefore, arise frequently. However, in normal physiology there is little evidence of such self-reactive clones of cells inducing disease. Self molecules (potential antigens) are constantly seen by developing lymphocytes. Accordingly, there must exist powerful and robust mechanisms preventing response to self while simultaneously favouring effective immune responses against non-self (microbial) antigens. These mechanisms of immunological tolerance are induced by exposure of T and B cells to potential self antigens in very particular situations.

Normally, immune competent T and B cells outside the central lymphoid organs, with appropriate stimuli from signals 1–3 (see 'T cells, receptors, and effectors: $CD4^+$ Th1, Th2 and Th17; $CD4^+$ Tregs and $CD8^+$ CTLs', above) respond positively by activation, proliferation, differentiation, and generation of effector and memory cells. The result is a productive immune response to the exciting non-self molecule termed the immunogen. In contrast, in the situation of immunological tolerance, exposure of T and B cells in the central and peripheral lymphoid organs to antigens can result either in cell death (by apoptosis), cell inactivation (anergy), or apparent neutral non-responsiveness (immunological ignorance). This lack of responsiveness is the defining element of tolerance. Self antigens that have the particular property of being able to induce this response are termed *tolerogens* in contrast to the immunogens (microbial antigens). What determines the choice between immune responsiveness and tolerance is, in part, determined by the nature of the specific T and B lymphocytes, as well as the nature of the antigen, and how it is presented to the immune system.

A great deal of experimental evidence, over many decades, has demonstrated that immunological tolerance of self antigens is strongly induced when developing lymphocytes meet antigens in the central lymphoid organs; this is known as *central tolerance*.

When tolerance is noted in the reactions of cells outside the thymus and bone marrow, in peripheral lymphoid tissue, the term *peripheral tolerance* is used.

Central tolerance for T and B lymphocytes

Central tolerance mechanisms have been described for T and B lymphocytes. The processes of central tolerance for T cells is associated with cell death (apoptosis) in the thymus and also by the generation of $CD4^+$ nTregs in that organ, and their subsequent exit to the peripheral lymphoid compartment. The randomly generated TCRs in the thymic lymphocytes can be shown to have specificity for self and non-self antigens. As described in 'Central and peripheral lymphoid organs; lymphocyte recirculation' above, if immature thymocytes strongly react to self antigens bound to HLA, these cells receive negative signals that trigger their apoptotic death in the process called negative selection. Many self antigens are expressed in the thymic environment, including some proteins abundant elsewhere in the body. These latter proteins are produced in the thymus by the action of the *AIRE* gene transcription factor regulator [49]. Negative selection destroys $CD4^+$ and $CD8^+$ T cells that have strong anti-self reactivity. T lymphocytes engaged in immunological ignorance also 'die by neglect' via apoptosis.

Clearly, defective negative regulation (failure of apoptosis) or malfunction of the *AIRE* gene, resulting in the lack of self antigen for negative selection, could lead to unwanted outcomes associated with lack of deletion of potentially self-reactive clones (see 'Autoimmunity: re-establishing homeostatic regulation', below). Positive selection processes operate for wide ranges of $CD4^+$ and $CD8^+$ T cells which survive and exit the thymus to become the naive immunocompetent T cells in the periphery. In the periphery they have the potential for reactivity against antigenic peptides linked to self HLA molecules (see 'T cells, receptors, and effectors: $CD4^+$ Th1, Th2 and Th17; $CD4^+$ Tregs and $CD8^+$ CTLs', above) due to their selection and education in the thymus. The nTregs are also among the $CD4^+$ populations emerging from the thymus. The selection processes within the thymus for generating nTregs are not fully understood, but the cytokines IL-2 and IL-7 appear particularly important for this process.

Central tolerance mechanisms operate in a similar manner in the bone marrow, to delete immature B cells with receptors with strong reactivity against self antigens. These cells undergo apoptosis. Another process also operates for B cells in the bone marrow, whereby, some BCRs with high affinity and strong anti-self reactivity, rather than being destroyed, are modified by a genetic process called *receptor editing*. In this situation, the *RAG* genes responsible for somatic recombination and generation of functional receptors (see 'B cells, receptors, and antibodies', above) are reactivated, particularly for the BCR light chains. Random generation of new light chains occurs, some combined with the existing heavy chains. Some of the productive combinations result in new BCR specificities that have moved away from strong anti-self reactivity. Those B cells that survive exit the bone marrow to function in the peripheral lymphoid tissues. The central tolerance mechanisms, although very efficient, are not absolute. Clones of T and B cells can be found (and isolated) from peripheral lymphoid tissues and shown *in vitro* to have TCRs and BCRs with self antigen reactivity. However, *in vivo* such clones do not normally mediate apparent deleterious autoimmunity (see Chapter 8). Such cells are kept nonreactive by the peripheral tolerance mechanisms.

Peripheral tolerance for T and B lymphocytes

The mature immunocompetent T and B cell clones in the periphery have the opportunity of constantly meeting the widely expressed and persistent self antigens. However, recognition events between such cells and their cognate antigens result not in cell activation, but in functional inactivation. The mechanisms responsible are lack of effective costimulator signals (signals 2 and 3). Normal self tissues containing immature DCs express very low levels of signal-2-inducing molecules such as CD80/CD86, although physiologically they are constantly processing and presenting self molecules to T cells. The lack of adequate signals 2 and 3, including the lack of innate inflammatory signals (e.g. TNF-α and IL-1), leads to lack of adequate TCR signalling downstream from signal 1. It is suggested that the T cells fail to reach an appropriate threshold for activation. Additionally, some studies have shown that anergic T cells constitutively express low but functional levels of CTLA-4$^+$ (the inhibitory receptor of the CD28 family of molecules on CD8$^+$T cells). This receptor on engagement transmits negative inactivating signals helping to maintain the anergic state of the T cells.

B cells with self-reactive specificity in the periphery, when encountering high concentrations of self antigens, can also be shown to become anergic. Mechanistically, this is explained in part by such B cells being unable to receive help from T cells. The T cells with specificity for peptides of the same antigen may also be anergic. TI antigens (e.g. some human polysaccharide antigens and microbial polysaccharides), may trigger self-reactive B cells. These may account for some of the so-called natural antibodies found at low levels, and the IgM class in blood. Such antibodies are believed to play useful physiological roles in cell turnover, contributing to removal of effete cells.

Activation-induced cell death

AICD represents another significant use of the process of apoptosis in immune regulation, this time in peripheral lymphoid tissues. AICD results in the deletion of mature self-reactive T and B lymphocytes. Within the T cell compartments, when self antigens are strongly recognized, experimental data shows that this can result in increased expression of proapoptotic proteins (e.g. Bax and Bak), which trigger cell death via the mitochondrial pathway (see 'Apoptosis', above). Self-reactive T cells in anergy are assumed to exhibit intermediate or weak self recognition. In contrast, when T cells react against non-self (microbial antigens), with appropriate costimulation from DCs (CD80/CD86) or with costimulation from cytokines of innate immune responses, such reacting cells switch on their antiapoptotic genes and proteins such as Bcl2 and survive. In some models of AICD, lymphocyte recognition of self antigens leads to coexpression of death receptors (Fas/CD95). Signalling via these up-regulated receptors, following engagement with FasL, uses the death receptor pathway to activate intracellular caspases and results in apoptosis (see 'Apoptosis', above).

AICD is also seen to be the key process in re-establishing homeostatic levels of lymphocytes in the body following normal immune responses. In some antiviral responses massive expansion of lymphocytes can be demonstrated (at times as much as 10% of blood lymphocytes), which need to be disposed of subsequently. After effector cells control the infection and there is generation of long-lived memory cells, the excess lymphocytes are dealt by AICD using the pathways described.

Another area where apoptosis occurs in the peripheral immune system is within B cell areas, such as secondary follicles and germinal centres. In these areas, there is generation of memory B cells and of cells undergoing hypermutation to generate high-affinity receptors. It can be shown that there is a significant amount of apoptosis within these areas. This is believed to be associated with removal of nonproductive potentially deleterious mutations, as well as with removal of highly self-reactive B cells generated by chance by new point mutations.

Overall, the processes of central and peripheral tolerance are evidently very successful, as evidenced by the survival of the species and maintenance of effective reactivities against non-self antigens without any significant evidence of deleterious anti-self autoimmune reactions. Nevertheless, it is apparent that human autoimmune diseases do occur (see Chapter 8) and must indicate situations where failure of immune tolerance occurs. These maladaptations—linked to the generation of autoimmunity—are explored in the next section.

Autoimmunity

The distinction between autoimmunity and autoimmune disease is explored in Chapter 8. The discussion here is focused on the anti-self reactions of T and B lymphocytes that are deemed to be pathological and indicate failure in some or most of the regulatory mechanisms of tolerance outlined above.

Although autoimmune disorders are heterogeneous (>80 different diseases have been defined) they nevertheless have several common features which relate to aetiology and pathogenesis that can be seen in humans and in experimental models of autoimmunity. There is a genetic susceptibility linked with defective immune responses and, in some cases, documented aberrant responses to environmental agents [50,51]. There is also a very apparent but poorly understood gender (female sex) linkage.

Genetic factors in autoimmunity

For many decades, it has been recognized that patients with autoimmune diseases have a strong family history of autoimmunity and increased association with other disorders such as specific IgA primary antibody deficiency, and some apparent linkage with nonimmunological disorders, such as Down's syndrome (see Chapter 8). Significant correlations were subsequently established in individual patients and on a population basis with the occurrence of increased associations of certain autoimmune diseases with various HLA alleles and haplotypes encoded in the MHC region (see Major histocompatibility complex, above). The pattern of disease inheritance in the vast majority of autoimmune diseases does not follow simple mendelian rules of genetics: they are clearly polygenic disorders. Additionally, twin studies demonstrate that concordance for an autoimmune disease such as type 1 diabetes was of the order of 50% in monozygotic twins. This clearly demonstrates that genetic factors alone are

Table 1.10 HLA association (class I or II) and risk of autoimmune disease

Class I	Class II	Disease	Approximate relative risk (RR)[a]
A29		Birdshot retinopathy	>200
	DR2(DQB1*0602)	Narcolepsy[b]	>100
B27	-	AS	~90
B27	-	Reiter's syndrome	~40
	DR3 DR4 DR3 and 4	Insulin dependent (type 1) diabetes mellitus	~5 ~5 20
	DR4	RA	~5
	DR4	IgA nephropthy	~4
	DR2	Pemphigus vulgaris	24
	DR3 and DR7 (DQ2 and DQ8)	Coeliac disease	~30
	DR3	SLE	~4
	DR3	Graves' disease	~3

AS, ankylosing spondylitis; RA, rheumatoid arthritis; SLE, systemic lupus erythematosus.

[a]The relative risk (RR) is a statement of the chance an individual, with the disease-associated HLA allele, has of developing the disease compared with an individual who lacks that HLA type. The higher the RR the more frequent is that HLA allele represented in the patient population.

[b]In excess of 95% of narcolepsy patients are reported to be HLA-DR2 but subsequent and larger studies, using the related subtype HLA DBQ1 *0602, has resulted in a RR >100.

not sufficient to cause an autoimmune disease (with some rare exceptions of single-gene defects outlined below).

The overall evidence for induction of autoimmunity is of a genetic susceptibility, best exemplified by linkages to HLA alleles, which may be linked in various ways to failure of self-tolerance acting in concert with various environmental triggers, and probably some other random events.

Table 1.10 illustrates examples of human autoimmune diseases with their association with HLA alleles and the concept of relative risk.

It is important to note that these HLA alleles can be found in controls in the normal population, but usually at significantly lower frequency than in the disease cohorts. Some HLA alleles have strong association with a range of different diseases, e.g. HLA-DR2, HLA-DR3. Historically, the associations have been found to be predominantly with alleles of HLA class II D region genes. However, there are some very notable and strong associations with HLA class I alleles. In Table 1.10, note the association of HLA-B27 with AS and HLA-A29 with birdshot retinopathy. With refinements in HLA typing, in particular the development of molecular techniques (see Chapter 9), some earlier documented associations, such as linkage of narcolepsy with HLA-DR2 and coeliac disease with HLA-DR3/DR7 have now been shown to have even stronger linkages with subsets of molecules associated with these loci. Thus, narcolepsy has now an even stronger linkage described as HLA-DQB1*0602.

What does HLA disease association mean in terms of disease aetiology and or pathogenesis? The definition of the functional role of HLA molecules in presenting peptide antigens to T cells clearly led to much effort to link the autoimmune disease associations to that function in various patient groups. Clearly, this approach is limited by the fact that in most autoimmune diseases the important antigen (i.e. self/autoantigen or possibly cross-reacting environmental antigen) is not known. However, studies of a few autoimmune diseases have been particularly enlightening regarding the role of HLA molecules and pathology. One of the best worked out is that of patients with coeliac disease who are known to generate aberrant immune responses to dietary gluten protein complex. Such patients have a strong HLA association with molecularly defined subsets of the HLA-DQ2 and HLA-DQ8 alleles; they also have autoantibodies to isoforms of an enzyme called tissue transglutaminase (tTG; see Chapter 8). The links between coeliac disease patients' presentation of gluten peptides, cross-reactions and binding to tTG, and the results of catalysis contributing to peptide-binding affinity and presentation to relevant T cells have all been well worked out, as expanded on in Chapter 8, 'Coeliac disease'. Mechanistically, the HLA associations, antigen presentation, and induction of autoimmunity appear to be linked and robustly explained. There is no other human autoimmune disease where the linkages to HLA and disease have been so closely worked out to explain disease induction and/or maintenance. The strong association of HLA-B27 with AS has similarly been explored looking at subtypes of B27 and variations in antigen peptide-binding presentation to T cells. Indeed, B27 peptides which cross-react with microbial antigen triggers have been examined in a similar manner to the experimental approaches in coeliac disease. Currently, however, there is no proven mechanistic linkage that can be documented as clearly as that produced in coeliac disease. Caution must also be exercised when it is recognized that established HLA associations may not, in themselves, necessarily reflect the most relevant genes. This is a result of the strong linkage disequilibrium associated with HLA haplotypes and with the extended MHC type (see 'Recognition elements, cells, and receptors in adaptive immunity', above).

With the technological advances in gene sequencing linked to postgenomic technologies and, in particular, the use of whole GWASs (see Chapter 9), more information has been gathered linking sequence variants to autoimmune disease. Concurrently, deep genetic analysis of rare human single-gene defects that have been linked to the expression of autoimmunity, together with analysis of useful animal models using gene knock-out mice and some spontaneous mutations, have given new mechanistic insights into the development of autoimmunity. Some of the findings clearly indicate the importance of failure in mechanisms of immune tolerance.

Table 1.11 shows some of the documented human single-gene defects with the parallel mouse models, and the biologically plausible mechanism in humans and proven mechanisms in the animal models that lead to autoimmunity. The table lists the non-MHC genes that, when defective, have been linked to the development and clinical expression of human autoimmunity. The known functional role of the normal genes is well characterized immunologically. Parallel experiments knocking out the target

Table 1.11 Single-gene defects and associated autoimmunity in humans and mouse models

Human gene	Disease	Mouse model	Mechanism of autoimmunity
AIRE	APECED	Knock-out mice AIRE	Decrease expression of self antigen in the thymus, leading to failure in negative selection
FOXP3	IPEX	Knock-out mice FOXP3; spontaneous mutation	Deficiency of $CD4^{+}$ $CD25^{+}$ Tregs
CD95/CD95L	ALPS	Spontaneous mutations in CD95 or CD95L	Failure of peripheral lymphocyte apoptosis, maintenance of self-reactive clones
Complement (C2, C4)	Lupus-like syndrome	Knock-out mice	Poor clearance of immune complexes, poor clearance of apoptotic cells
FcγRIIb	Lupus-like syndrome	Knock-out mice	Defective inhibitory signals to B cells. Augmentation of mast cell degranulation
IL-2/CD25	Increase in range of autoantibodies–lupus-like syndrome		Deficiency of Tregs
CTLA-4	Associated with Graves' disease and other organ specific autoimmunity	Knock-out mice	Failure of peripheral T cell anergy, reduce threshold of activation of self-reactive T cells
IL-10	Crohn's disease	Knock-out mice	Failure of cytokine IL-10 suppressive action in GIT host/microbe interactions

AIRE, autoimmune regulator; ALPS, autoimmune lymphoproliferative syndrome; APECED, autoimmune polyendocrinopathy candidiasis and ectodermal dysplasia; CD25, low affinity IL-2α receptor; CTLA-4 (CD152), cytotoxic T lymphocyte-associated antigen 4; IPEX, immunodysregulation–polyendocrinopathy/enteropathy X-linked syndrome;

genes in mouse model systems support the autoimmune associations with the natural human mutations. Some long-known mouse spontaneous mutants which show problems with marked lymphoid proliferation and autoimmunity (e.g. lpr–/lpr– mouse) parallel the human disease associated, for example, with mutations in Fas (CD95) or FasL (CD95L)—see above.

These rare single-gene disorders strongly support the need for central and peripheral tolerance mechanisms to prevent autoimmunity. The mechanisms of autoimmunity, associated with these genetic defects, fit in well with the basic and essential immunological reactions described throughout this text. For instance, the key role of the transcription factor $Foxp3^{+}$ in the generation of $CD4^{+}$, $CD25^{+}$ Tregs (lost in immunodysregulation polyendocrinopathy enteropathy X-linked syndrome, IPEX), the key role of CTLA-4, a molecule that engages with costimulators (CD80/86) but results in inhibitory signals for T cell activation [52].

Other interesting and strong associations derived from GWAS analysis include the polymorphisms associated with NOD2 in Crohn's disease (see Chapter 8, 'Crohn's disease and ulcerative colitis') and of a protein, PTPN22, which is linked to several autoimmune diseases including RA. Defective PTPN22 is shown to result in abnormal phosphatase regulation of lymphocyte activation (see 'Innate and adaptive immunity', above). This is believed to contribute to autoimmunity by lack of checks on kinase signalling and a generation of proinflammatory reactions.

The above examples of association of single-gene defects and of susceptibility genes obtained via GWAS are linked mainly to non-MHC genes. However, the importance of the MHC associations have been confirmed; important MHC associations occur with type 1 diabetes and RA—prototypic organ-specific and systemic autoimmune diseases, respectively (Wellcome Trust Consortium, 2007) [53]. The mechanistic role of MHC associations with common autoimmune disease, with a few exceptions (e.g. coeliac disease), still remains unclear.

Hormonal and environmental factors in autoimmunity

Hormonal factors: It is well documented that, after puberty, there is a significantly increased susceptibility to connective tissue autoimmunity in females, compared with males. This could represent the effects of oestrogen and/or permissive alleles on the X chromosome. Current evidence indicates that oestrogen, and many other endocrine hormones, can directly modulate the action of lymphocytes. Thus, receptors for testosterone and for thymic hormones are expressed on T cells, and the functions of such cells are enhanced by receptor occupancy by the appropriate hormone. In contrast, oestrogen has been shown to down-regulate the reactivity of some T cells which, it is speculated, facilitates the expression of autoimmunity in women. Recent data has firmly demonstrated that oestrogen activates the expression of the *AID* gene which is known to drive the mechanisms of antibody diversification (see 'B cells, receptors, and antibodies', above), including probably autoantibodies.

Environmental factors: Drugs that are well documented as inducers of autoimmunity (e.g. penicillamine) may adsorb on to cells and alter the structure of self molecules, so that they become antigenic. Environmental trauma, which leads to the release of sequestered antigens (e.g. in the eye, heart, or urogenital tract), can lead to the induction of autoimmune responses. Interestingly, the autoimmune responses which commonly follow trauma and surgery are transient (see Chapter 8). They illustrate that induction of autoantibodies may not be sufficient in itself for induction of clinical autoimmunity; other 'factors' in the individual's immunogenetic background are required.

The role of microorganisms as triggers for autoimmunity is still a matter for debate. There is not a simple correlation of infection with autoimmunity, but microorganisms, or their products, may induce autoimmunity in individuals with an appropriate immune, genetic, and hormonal background. Microorganisms may share molecular similarity (molecular mimicry) with self molecules of some individuals and, thus, perturb the organism's homeostasis without an appropriate induction of protective immunity.

Research also indicates that various ubiquitous organisms, such as mycobacteria, possess glycoproteins which cross-react strongly with certain cellular HSPs. Immune reactions to such molecules appear to correlate with certain rheumatic autoimmune disorders. It has long been known that some antigens of particular streptococcal serotypes cross-react with heart antigens and, in appropriate individuals, infection with streptococci has resulted in the induction of rheumatic fever. Other microorganisms, such as EBV, can be shown to act as polyclonal activators of B cells, thus, bypassing the need for Th cells. By circumventing the need for T 'help', such organisms could contribute to the overcoming of clonal anergy. Once there is a genetic susceptibility to autoimmunity, as described above, a range of different environmental antigens can operate on that permissive background via various mechanisms of mimicry, epitope spreading, etc.—all culminating in a common presentation of autoimmunity. Indeed, epidemiological associations, clinical observations (including serology), and microbiological studies have linked a whole range of different viruses and some bacteria in the triggering of type 1 diabetes. Similarly, various microbes have been linked to the development of RA, MS, and inflammatory bowel disease. These findings should inform future studies of autoimmunity, whereby these assumed environmental triggers should be considered as important in the early, acute, and likely subclinical phase of induction of autoimmunity. However, once disease is triggered and self-reactive clones are directed to internal self antigens then a chronic autoimmune disorder, with persistent (self) antigenic stimulation, may ensue.

Autoimmunity and epigenomics: Most autoimmune diseases clearly have a genetic predisposition, as evidenced in twin and family studies, by HLA associations, and in GWASs. Additionally, there are clearly interacting environmental factors as described above. The search for gene variants encoded in the DNA sequence has not, so far, yielded enough data to lead to clear biological models for the induction and maintenance of autoimmunity (with a few exceptions, e.g. coeliac disease—see Chapter 8). Most autoimmune diseases are complex genetic disorders, not simple single-gene or mendelian inheritance disorders. New ways of pursuing the aetiology of autoimmunity are being explored by using the science of epigenetics. Analysis of epigenetic modifications (i.e. changes in gene expression caused by mechanisms other than changes in the underlying DNA sequence) is developing rapidly. Epigenetic modifications include methylation of DNA, particularly around cytosine bases, and modifications of the histone proteins which encircle the coiled double helix. Such modifications can regulate genetic functions in their own right. Such regulation by the epigenome has been well demonstrated in plants and in various mouse model systems. The latter have indicated that environmental factors, such as sex hormones, microbial products, and drugs, can modify the epigenome. The epigenome is thus seen as the critical integrator linking the environment to key functions of genes, and hence a determinant of disease predisposition. The probing and cataloguing of the human epigenome is predicted to give new insights into complex diseases such as those linked to autoimmunity, thereby, allowing a better understanding of gene environment interactions in aetiopathology [50,51,54–57]. An international consortium, the Human Epigenome Project, is currently working with state-of-the-art high-throughput sequencers and sophisticated microarray systems (see Chapter 9). This should yield rapid and accurate maps of the epigenomes associated with a wide range of complex human diseases, including those due to autoimmunity.

Another new area of study that may yield deeper insights into autoimmunity is exploration of the role of micro RNAs (miRNAs). The human genome encodes more than 1000 miRNAs. These are recently defined biological regulators, mainly post-transcriptional regulators, that bind to complementary sequences of target mRNA and induce modifications of gene function. miRNAs have been shown to be critical regulators in Th17 cells, which are known to be key effectors in inflammation and autoimmunity [58].

Attempts at targeting or modulating autoimmune disease will need to focus on the following points:

- The specificity of the autoimmune reaction at the level of lymphocyte receptors recognizing the self antigens. In most cases, those self antigens cannot be removed (an exception being discrete organ-specific immunity, e.g. thyroid—see Chapter 8, 'Introduction'). Targeting of the receptors, therefore, is the only practical approach at specific immune therapy. Some other forms of specific immunotherapy are based on the activation of adaptive Tregs by harnessing the process and mechanisms of oral tolerance.
- Studies will need to address ways of interrupting the downstream mediators of the chronic immune/inflammatory reactions, targeting, for instance, costimulatory molecules, chemokines, cytokines, and their receptors. Some significant progress has been made in these immunotherapeutic attempts to modulate autoimmunity (see 'Monoclonals and other biological therapies', above) [54].

In summary, the adaptive immune response is generally useful, protective, and self-regulatory. Nevertheless, in some situations the response can be seen as inappropriately linked to breakdown in regulatory mechanisms and the induction of harmful autoimmunity. Broad, relatively nonspecific immune suppressive regimens (steroids, cytotoxics, etc.) are used in clinical practice to overcome excessive and prolonged autoimmune responses. The ultimate goal of autoimmune suppression is to selectively inhibit the specific self reactive T and B lymphocyte clones, leaving intact other clones and effector mechanisms which are normally useful and protective.

Attempts at suppression have progressed from the use of nonspecific drugs to using cell-specific MABs and other biological constructs. Immune modulation using such approaches is outlined below.

Immune modulation

Autoimmunity: re-establishing homeostatic regulation

The detailed knowledge of immune interactions, along with technological advances in generating MABs (including human antibodies) and other biological therapies, has provided windows of opportunity in modulating autoimmune disease for the benefit of patients (see 'Monoclonals and other biological therapies', above). The 'holy grail' of re-establishing immune regulatory tolerance mechanisms is still being pursued, but is proving difficult in the setting of human disease. Experimental models clearly indicate the possibility of such resetting of tolerance mechanisms, but it is debatable how relevant those models are to the human situation.

Current immune modulatory approaches to human autoimmunity exploit drugs beyond the established areas of broad immunosuppression associated with cytotoxic agents as well as steroids. Calcineurin blockers, such as ciclosporin, tacrolimus, mycophenolate mofetil, and other agents used in transplantation (see Chapter 3), have all been tried in different autoimmune diseases with variable success. Often there is initial success, but with time effectiveness is lost and there are problems associated with toxicity. With long-term use, there is the additional risk of developing immunosuppression-linked neoplasms. Agents such as rapamycin, known to target important signalling pathways (e.g. p13K–AKT–mTOR), are also being used in various clinical trials in autoimmunity [59].

Some considerable success is being achieved in the immunotherapy of autoimmune diseases, using relatively non-antigen-specific modalities: anticytokine and/or anticytokine receptor antibodies, fusion proteins, and antiintegrin antibodies. These approaches have proved particularly useful in treating RA and some other connective tissue diseases, as well as MS and Crohn's disease.

Other experimental/investigational approaches are attempting to target various cell signalling pathways by way of 'selective' antikinases, as well as targeting transcription factors within the STAT family of proteins. These approaches are not without problems: targeting molecules that have many physiological functions beyond immune responses appears daunting. Nevertheless, there are reasons to believe these approaches are worthy of further studies (see 'Innate and adaptive immunity', above).

Immune modulation of human autoimmunity will continue to yield benefits by way of biological entities (or indeed small-molecule agonists) targeting the non-antigen-specific pathways, thus, blocking mediators and/or cell trafficking. Attempts are being pursued to exploit generation of Tregs *in vivo* or expanded *ex vivo* to be reintroduced as a means of controlling undesirable autoimmunity (see 'T cells, receptors, and effectors: $CD4^+$ Th1, Th2 and Th17; $CD4^+$ Tregs and $CD8^+$ CTLs', above). However, these approaches, like most nonspecific approaches, have the attendant risk of infections (see 'Monoclonals and other biological therapies', below) and the possible longer-term development of neoplasia. This makes it necessary and important to continue pursuing possible antigen-specific approaches or means of re-establishing tolerance. Long-term antigen-specific therapy, targeting specific TCRs and BCRs to destroy those clones or to make them anergic, is still a worthy quest in search of that 'holy grail' of immunology.

Neuroimmunology: integration and interactivity

The central and peripheral nervous systems (CNS and PNS) together with the neuroendocrine system, exemplified by the hypothalamic–pituitary–adrenal axis (HPA), are major modulators of the innate and adaptive immune responses [60]. The burgeoning science of neuroimmunology (encompassing studies of the bidirectional interactions between the nervous system and immune system) has, over the past 20 years, revealed detailed interactions involved in the normal development of the host, response to injury, and homeostasis. The physiological and pathological interactions defined are also contributing to new and better understanding of the aetiopathology of certain nervous system diseases and their therapeutic management.

For example, in MS, myelin-specific T cells and B cells secreting antimyelin antibodies are believed to play a dual role in initiating and inducing CNS autoimmunity [61].

Historically, the CNS was considered to be an immune-privileged site, partly due to its lack of a lymphatic system and the existence of the blood–brain barrier (BBB), which normally excludes access of leucocytes and macromolecules. Additionally, classical experiments demonstrated that foreign tissue transplanted directly into the CNS survived for long periods without exciting inflammation or immune rejection.

However, experiments from the 1970s onwards repeatedly demonstrated that systemic infections or induction of systemic inflammatory disease (e.g. using LPS) affected CNS responses. This was subsequently shown to be due to the effects of the systemic cytokines (TNF-α, IL-1, and IL-6) binding to and triggering receptors on cells in the hypothalamus and other areas of the brain. Brain glial cells were further demonstrated to express TLRs and were capable of responding to PAMPs and self DAMPs, via NF-κB activation and induction of proinflammatory mediators. It was rapidly appreciated that neural tissues triggered by systemically derived cytokines accounted for changes such as fever, anorexia, behavioural and mood changes, and somnolence [62].

The CNS itself was also noted to be a source of cytokine production in some neurodegenerative diseases and following some infections of the nervous system. The CNS production of cytokines is due mainly to parenchymal/glial cells and is generally not exhibited by neuronal cells. The induction of innate-driven inflammatory lesions by activated glial cells that follows infections of the CNS is also seen following traumatic brain injury and other insults such as postischaemic stroke (these latter insults leading to the release of DAMPs). Concomitant studies demonstrated that the HPA axis had major effects, quantitative and qualitative, on the immune system. Anatomical studies have also revealed significant innervation of peripheral immune tissues such as spleen and gut-associated lymphoid tissue (GALT) by various cholinergic, catecholaminergic, peptidergic, and other neurons. Currently, the distinction between immune system cytokines and neural tissue transmitters (neuropeptides) is blurred. A neuropeptide, such as vasoactive intestinal peptide (VIP) is now known to be produced by immune cells (e.g. T cells) as well as by neurons. Additionally, immune cells have receptors for VIP and respond to it.

The autonomic nervous system, as exemplified by the vagus nerve, mediates responses which have been shown experimentally in animal model systems and in limited human studies to be a major modulator of the innate immune response. Vagal stimulation leads to the release of neural substances such as acetylcholine which act on receptors in the secondary lymphoid tissues, resulting in major changes in leucocyte migration and in suppression of proinflammatory mediators (TNF-α, IL-1, IL-6) produced during innate immune responses. The vagal nerve also informs the higher CNS centres regarding the presence of systemic inflammatory lesions, to enhance HPA interactions. Recent elegant neurophysiological and immunological experiments in animals have demonstrated an immune–neural inflammatory reflex. Afferent nerves sense mediator and ionic changes associated with peripheral tissue inflammation. These induce action potentials which transmit to the intercalated neurons and result in efferent nerves producing molecules which help to modulate the immune–inflammatory tissue response [62].

These important observations have firmly established that the immune system is not a stand-alone, autonomous entity, detecting and responding to antigen and stressors that perturb homoestasis. Neuroimmunology studies clearly indicate that the nervous system is a major factor in modulating responses of innate immunity and of subsequent downstream adaptive immunity. The nervous system helps to 'set the thermostat' of immune responsiveness—neural circuits directly regulate innate immunity. There is growing evidence that the immune system and its basal reactions can, in turn, influence and modulate brain cell development and plasticity [60].

Neuroimmunology: pathological disturbances

It has long been recognized that if the BBB is disrupted, and there is an excessive innate immune response with glial activation, then the ingress of lymphocytes and induction of adaptive immune reponses in the CNS is facilitated. Recent studies have documented changes in cytokines, chemokines, and their receptors that favour leucocyte migration into the CNS. Such findings are offering potential newer therapies for diseases such as MS by the use of biologicals (MABs) or small-molecule inhibitors (SMIs) of cytokines, receptors, and adhesion molecules that are important in the migration and action of cells responsible for pathological immune neuron-inflammatory responses [63].

Biologically, it is also recognized that controlled use of potential innate immune responses in the CNS may be manipulated to beneficial ends in the early phases of a range of neurodegenerative diseases. Alzheimer's is characterized, in part, by the accumulation of damaging amyloid plaques. Experimental models have revealed that activation of CNS glial cells and perivascular macrophages may counteract the accumulation and formation of such plaques. Similarly, the importance of enhancing and exploiting the adaptive immune system in CNS disease is also demonstrated in models of postischaemic injury associated with stroke in animal model systems. They have unequivocally demonstrated that $CD4^+$ $CD25^+$ $Foxp3^+$ Tregs can modulate (limit) the amount of tissue inflammatory damage associated with stroke. Predictably, such a positive role for Tregs is also demonstrated in animal model systems of MS. In MS, myelin-specific T cells cross the BBB, are reactivated by APCs presenting myelin, triggering the recruitment of macrophages and monocytes inducing demyelination and axonal damage. $CD4^+$ Th1 cells secreting IFN-γ, IL-2 and TNF-α, and $CD8^+$ CTLs play important roles in MS. B cell responses are equally important as a source of antibodies against myelin and axons, as APCs and controlling Treg activity [61].

Psychoneuroimmunology

A fascinating and continually developing area, boosted from the insights into the bidirectional interaction of the nervous and immune system, is to be found in studies of psychoneuroimmunology. 'Mind and body' medicine is striving to reveal the biological basis and consequences of their interactions beyond philosophical and psychological considerations [64]. Observational studies have long demonstrated that activities, such as aerobic exercise, controlled breathing, relaxation therapy, and consumption of fish oils—ω-3, eicosapentaenoic acid (EPA), and docosahexaenoic acid (DHA)—can affect immune–inflammatory diseases and disorder. Recent studies (in human and experimental animals) have shown that these varied activities can all be shown to increase vagus nerve activity with subsequent suppression of proinflammatory cytokines (TNF-α, IL-6) (see Chapter 4 for more details).

In summary, neuroimmunological studies have clearly indicated that the immune and nervous systems are not autonomous entities, but are deeply interactive in a bidirectional manner. Significant further progress will come from interdisciplinary studies, involving immunologists, neuroscientists, behavioural psychologists, and others exploring these bidirectional interactions in diverse situations (e.g. autism, schizophrenia, and other developmental disorders), in neurodegeneration and in neuroinflammatory conditions. Exploitation of neural influences on the immune response may yield new treatment modalities for chronic autoimmune/inflammatory conditions (e.g. RA, SLE), as well as for more acute systemic inflammatory conditions. Mind–body interaction exploiting state-of-the-art functional magnetic resonance imaging (fMRI), positron emission tomography (PET), and molecular imaging, along with immunological studies, should prove enlightening and provide new knowledge and better understanding in this still orphan area of neuroimmunological studies.

Immunopathology and tissue damage, immune deficiency and immunotherapeutics

Immunopathological processes: hypersensitivity (types I–IV) and tissue damage

Mechanisms underlying the hypersensitivity reactions

Humoral and CMI usually are beneficial and protective host defence mechanisms. Nevertheless, situations occur where either one or both reactions can result in more tissue damage than protection. The mechanistic and descriptive cataloguing of such immunopathology is embodied in the term *hypersensitivity*, which was originally crystallized by Gell and Coombs as type I–IV hypersensitivity reactions. Types I, II, and III are mediated mainly by antibodies and type IV by cells of CMI. These reactions can be directed against extrinsic antigens or autoantigens. The unifying feature is that once the specific reactants are triggered they recruit complement, neutrophils, eosinophils, and basophils, which act as the mediators of damage. Although the description of type I–IV hypersensitivity conveniently summarizes the mechanisms of the reactions, the classification does not consider the possible aetiological factors. Outlined below is the classification of type I–IV hypersensitivity reactions, with appropriate clinical examples, followed by a case study of latex allergy—a condition of particular importance to surgeons and other health care workers.

Type I hypersensitivity: Type I hypersensitivity is also referred to as immediate hypersensitivity. Within this grouping can be found disorders (called 'allergic' reactions in common parlance) such as hay fever, asthma, and anaphylaxis associated with reactions to agents such as penicillin and other drugs. Type I reactions are due to IgE antibodies, which are bound in high numbers to the membrane receptors (termed FcεR) of tissue mast cells and blood basophils: see Figure 1.33. In contrast, the amount of IgE in blood is very low, compared with the other isotypes.

Although everyone produces IgE antibodies, it is evident on examination of family histories of 'allergy' sufferers that there is a genetic predisposition for developing type I hypersensitivity. The inheritance and exhibition of the hypersensitivity phenotype is denoted by the term *atopy*, the hypersensitive individual being termed *atopic*. Atopic individuals usually have raised serum IgE levels; they usually have a strong family history of type I allergic reactions and often have multiple IgE antibodies to several different antigens. The basis of their genetic predisposition is far from clear, but in some cases an association with certain HLA phenotypes is documented and appears to relate to the strength of their immune response to allergens. Also, the induction of IgE antibodies is highly dependent on and is controlled by $CD4^+$ Th2 lymphocytes [65].

Recent genetic research, using GWAS and SNP analyses in extended families of patients with type I allergic diseases, have identified a plethora of genes. Associations are documented with receptors and effector cells linked to allergy as well as to IgE at its receptors. Strong associations have been found in several studies linking allergy and asthma risk to the chromosomal region Ch.5q31. Within that region is found a cluster of genes for cytokines linked to allergy, namely IL-4, IL-5, IL-9, and IL-13, that characterize Th2 responses. The genetics of allergy is clearly complex; the findings suggests there is no single allergy gene but a collection of them which may segregate to different individuals in varying ways to contribute to the allergy phenotype. Interestingly, some GWASs have found associations with asthma, such as the *ADAM33* gene, which is not linked to type I IgE responses but rather to the tissue remodelling events of long-standing asthma disease. Clinically, it has long been known that psychological factors (*stressors*) can precipitate or intensify 'allergic' type I reactions. Recent evidence has demonstrated that neuroendocrine-linked reactions can clearly trigger type I reactions in highly sensitized experimental animals, apparently without the presence of the allergen. Genetic studies of patients with atopic dermatitis have shown linkages to genes expressed in cutaneous tissue which have receptors for hormonal ligands, giving biologically plausible neuroimmunological links of stress responses to the allergic phenotype.

From Figure 1.33a it can be seen that when the 'antigen' cross-links (bridges) two IgE molecules on the surface of the mast cell, a stimulatory transmembrane signal is sent, which ultimately activates the mast cell to release its preformed stored mediators and to synthesize further mediators. It is the released products of the tissue mast cells and of blood basophils that lead to the dramatic clinical manifestations of type I reactions. The released mediators are potent stimulators of acute inflammation, and also act on smooth muscle and the blood-vessel endothelium. The release of the preformed mediators accounts for the rapid time course of type I reactions which occur within minutes of exposure to the antigen (also called an allergen).

Current laboratory tests designed to document type I reactions include PRIST for total IgE, and RAST and ELISA-based systems for specific IgE antibodies (see Chapter 9). For suspected type I reactions to anaesthetic agents, such as halothane, suxamethonium, and procainamide as well as to other drugs, the current tests are far from ideal and are of unproven value. Depending on the methods employed for data collection, e.g. population surveys, or anaesthetic, surgical, and post-mortem records, the incidence of such type I reactions to drugs is variously reported (in different surveys) as from approximately 1 in 400 to less than 1 in 10 000!

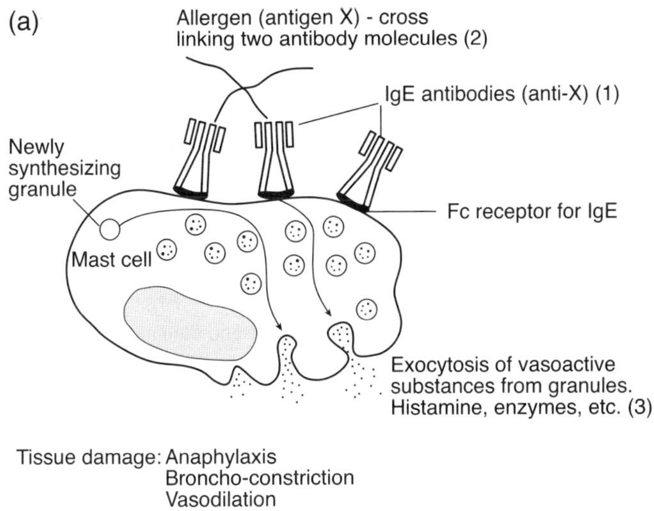

Fig. 1.33a Type I hypersensitivity.

Treatment of type I reactions is based ideally on prophylaxis/prevention rather than just symptomatic control as occurs with antihistamines. Drugs that antagonize various pathways involved in type I reactions have proved extremely useful, together with agents that help to inhibit or modify the damage caused to the target organs. Sodium cromoglicate acts on the mast cell, at various biochemical levels, to inhibit its reaction to the allergen–IgE signal of activation and its consequent release of mediators. β_1- and β_2-adrenergic agonists (isoprenaline, salbutamol) help to relax the bronchial smooth muscle and vascular spasm induced by mast cell mediators. Steroids administered locally and systemically have a broad-based 'anti-inflammatory reaction' against many agents and mediators involved in the type I reaction. Attempts at hyposensitization, by injecting various forms of purified allergens, has to date proved clinically less successful (with a few striking exceptions) than predicted from basic research. Undoubtedly, part of the problem is inadequate purification and definition of the appropriate 'allergens', and lack of knowledge of the best injection protocols with respect to timing and dosage. It is hoped that some of these problems will be overcome in the near future.

Type II hypersensitivity: Type II hypersensitivity involves antibodies directed to and reacting with antigens which are part of a cell membrane. The antigen may be an integral membrane component, or can be of extrinsic origin that becomes adsorbed to the cell (e.g. a drug). The result of this membrane-bound location is that antibodies, mainly of the IgG and IgM class, after reacting with the cell membrane antigen, recruit and activate effectors such as complement or cells with appropriate Fc receptors. The latter then mediate cellular and tissue damage at the site of the bound antibodies (see Figure 1.33b). In some situations, if the antibodies bind to a functional receptor (antigen) on the cell membrane, it may trigger the associated cell function. An important example of this stimulatory damaging type II reaction is that involved in the pathogenesis of

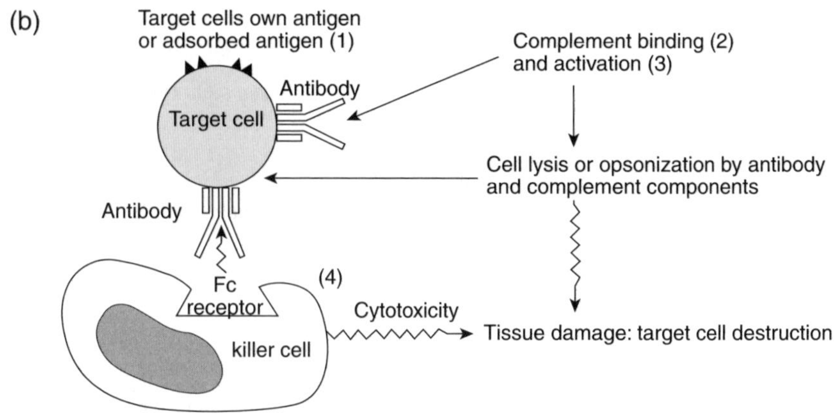

Fig. 1.33b Type II hypersensitivity.

Graves' disease. The IgG autoantibody, termed long-acting thyroid stimulator (LATS) or, more appropriately, thyroid stimulating immunoglobulin (TSI), binds to the thyroid stimulating hormone receptor (TSHR) on the surface of thyroid cells. The resulting enhanced activity of the thyroid cells leads to excessive and continued release of the thyroid hormones and clinical hyperthyroidism. Some authorities have tried to classify 'stimulatory' type II reactions into a separate (but perhaps unnecessary) type V category.

Some well-known examples of type II reactions include reactions against blood cells in mismatched transfusions, autoimmune haemolytic anaemias, drug-induced reactions to blood cells, and haemolytic disease of the newborn. Certain autoimmune diseases have type II reactions as the main imunopathological basis of damage, e.g. myasthenia gravis and Goodpasture's syndrome.

Type III hypersensitivity: Type III hypersensitivity involves preformed antibody interacting with antigen; the resultant *immune complexes* mediate tissue damage when they precipitate in tissue sites. The deposited complexes recruit and activate complement and effector cells which can result in severe tissue damage. Classical examples of type III systemic reactions are embodied by the serum sickness syndromes, and the more localized form of type III by the so-called Arthus reaction (see Figure 1.33c). The reactions triggered by the immune complexes are usually manifested as clinical inflammation, 4–6 hours following exposure to the antigen. Serum sickness was historically associated with treatments such as the administration of passive antisera (e.g. horse Ig to treat patients exposed to tetanus bacilli). Over a period of time (4–10 days) the patient develops high levels of anti-horse immunoglobulin antibodies. These form immune complexes in the systemic circulation with the declining levels of the administered horse proteins, the resultant immune complex-mediated inflammation being manifested as an acute serum sickness syndrome. The patients develop urticaria, arthralgia, and glomerulonephritis, due to the soluble immune complexes precipitating in associated tissue sites. In the Arthus reaction, the preformed antibodies interact with antigens, which are present in high concentration in local sites, e.g. the dermis, or

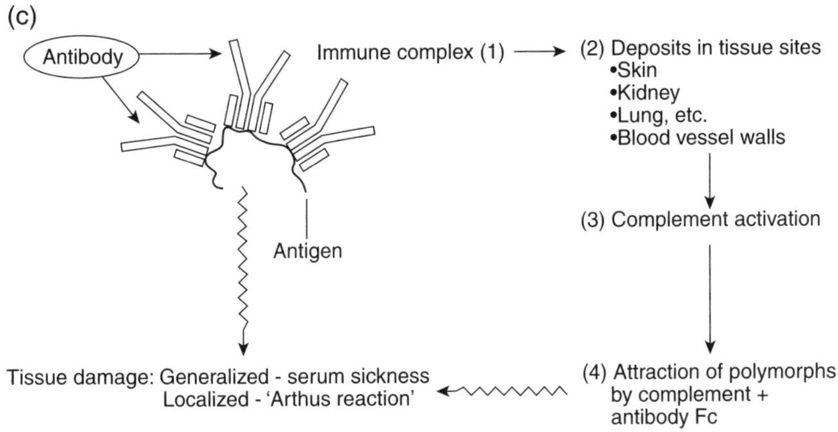

Fig. 1.33c Type III hypersensitivity.

the bronchial tree. The resultant local concentrations of immune complexes induce severe localized immune inflammation. Well-known examples of type III reactions include some forms of immune complex-induced glomerulonephritis and dermatitis, associated with extrinsic antigens (microorganisms) and with autoantigens in autoimmune diseases, such as SLE.

Type IV hypersensitivity: Type IV reactions, which are associated with specific $CD4^+$ T lymphocytes (see Figure 1.33d), are interpreted as excessive tissue-damaging CMI. The clinical description of this is termed delayed-type hypersensitivity (DTH), because of the time taken for maximal clinical expression—2–3 days compared with the minutes to hours for types I, II, and III reactions. The sensitized T lymphocytes recognize

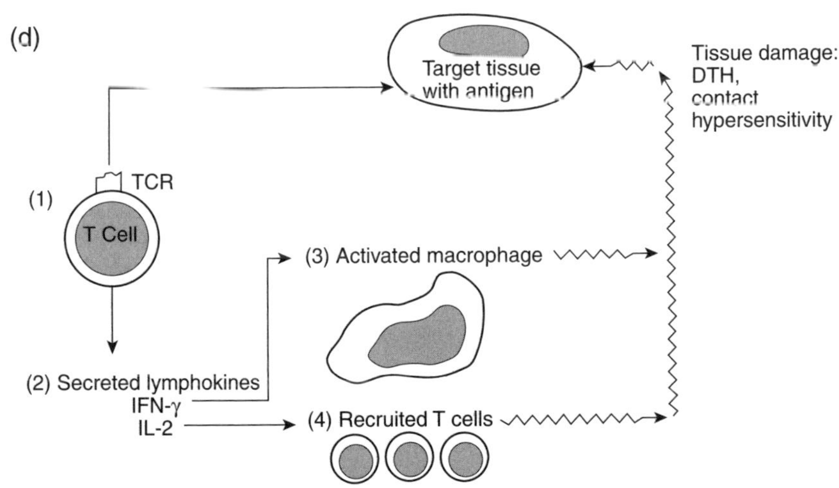

Fig. 1.33d Type IV hypersensitivity.

antigen appropriately and secrete cytokines which attract other T lymphocytes and macrophages to the antigen site. The crucial factors that result in this CMI becoming overtly pathological rather than physiologically protective are not fully elucidated. Undoubtedly, in some situations it is due to the nature of the antigen, which persists because it is biologically nondegradable (e.g. metal ions, resistant intracellular organisms) and, thus, leads to continued and excessive stimulation of CMI. Some well-known DTH type IV reactions include certain viral-induced skin rashes, the iatrogenic Mantoux test, dermatitis associated with 'allergy' to metals and industrial chemicals, and the tuberculoid form of leprosy.

Although the hypersensitivity tissue-damaging reactions can be conveniently described in the type I–IV compartments, such distinctions are less readily discernible *in vivo* and are a gross oversimplification. Thus, the patient manifesting a severe and protracted asthmatic attack triggered by a type I reaction may, with time, concurrently develop elements of type II and III reactions. Similarly, many highly sensitized patients experiencing type IV reactions can, on examination, be shown to have elements of type II hypersensitivity reactions. The clarification of the *in vivo* interactions of the various elements of hypersensitivity reactions will lead to more efficient forms of therapy, particularly combinational treatment, and ultimately prophylaxis.

Case study of latex allergy

An 8-year-old boy with spina bifida, requiring frequent urinary catheterization and several surgical procedures over the years, attended a follow-up clinic. He described to the clinician several episodes of urticaria (with itching and nettle rash type skin lesions). He also noticed an episode of nonitchy facial swelling when blowing up a balloon at a recent school party. The swelling description fitted well with an episode of angioedema. Further clinical questioning indicated other episodes of angioedema associated with eating bananas or avocado pears. The surgeon recognized that he was dealing with a likely case of hypersensitivity/allergic reactions and conferred with his allergist/clinical immunology colleagues. With the history, it was very probable that the boy had an allergy to latex, consequent to his exposure to latex during his surgical management and catheterization episodes. The diagnosis was confirmed by the clinical skin prick test (SPT) conducted by the allergist in the hospital setting with appropriate resuscitation support. The SPT involved administration of latex antigens along with controls and resulted within minutes in the characteristic localized acute inflammatory reaction strongly suggestive of a type I IgE-mediated reaction. The diagnosis was further confirmed by the *in vitro* detection of specific IgE antilatex antibodies. The patient was advised to avoid latex-containing materials. As the potential existed for more severe reactions, he was supplied with and taught how to use a device for self-administering an IM injection of adrenaline, if an extensive acute attack of angioedema or possible anaphylaxis was developing. A great deal of educational material was shared with the patient and his family. He was also supplied with a medical alert bracelet indicating his diagnosis.

Allergy to rubber latex is not uncommon and can be serious. It is a significant problem for health care workers. Many proteins/polypeptides have been isolated from latex, and tests show they vary in their allergenic potency. The talcum powder associated with the use of latex gloves absorbs residual minute amounts of latex proteins remaining after rubber processing. Additionally, other residual proteins remain on the surface of latex materials, e.g. balloons or condoms. Latex sensitization—induction of the primary T and B cell responses resulting in IgE production—occurs after skin or mucosal contact. Abdominal surgical procedures can cause sensitization via peritoneal exposure. The full spectrum of clinical type I hypersensitivity reactions can occur in latex-allergic patients, ranging from localized inflammation to generalized anaphylaxis. Indeed, anaphylaxis has been documented intraoperatively in patients undergoing abdominal surgery. Latex is considered the second most common cause of intraoperative anaphylaxis (after drugs) and should be borne in mind if such reactions occur unexpectedly, and at a time when the patient is unable to communicate their clinical symptoms.

Evidence suggests an increased incidence of type I latex hypersensitivity in atopic individuals. However, latex allergy occurs in many nonatopic individuals. Other clinical syndromes occur with latex, including type IV hypersensitive reactions producing features of contact dermatitis. The type IV reactions which develop 24–72 hours after exposure tend to occur to chemical allergens used in latex processing, rather than to proteins. The sensitization for type IV occurs via a hapten–protein complex, i.e. the chemical–protein complex which is taken up, processed, and presented by skin LCs and other local DCs to T cells in regional lymphoid tissues, ultimately generating strong $CD4^+$ Th1 responses. HLA class II alleles have been linked to the increased risk of producing IgE antibodies to latex.

Interestingly, as shown in the clinical case, it has become apparent that cross-reacting antigens occur between latex proteins and those of several fruits, including banana, papaya, avocado, kiwi, peach, and nectarine.

Latex allergy is increased in individuals who are chronically exposed to latex. Severe type I and type IV reactions in health care workers can jeopardize careers. Additionally, latex products are ubiquitous in the environment. Beyond medical treatments for different aspects of latex allergy, prevention is better than cure. Attempts should be made to minimize exposure to latex within working and home environments. For health care workers, where possible, eliminating powdered latex gloves should be considered. There are less allergenic latex gloves or high-quality nonlatex gloves; although they are expensive, an overall cost–benefit analysis may favour the adoption of nonlatex gloves. Tentative experimental latex desensitization studies have been pursued, but they carry significant risks as anaphylaxis to latex is not uncommon. Some authorities are not supportive of this approach.

Drug allergy

Acute systemic reactions, including anaphylaxis and angioedema due to type I IgE-mediated hypersensitivity, are well documented with muscle relaxants, pencillins (including cephalosporins), and other antibiotics where the allergic cross-reactions appear to be due to structural homologies. Drugs, such as opiates, radiocontrast media, ACE inhibitors, and nonsteroidal anti-inflammatory drugs (NSAIDs), can produce acute syndromes of angioedema or anaphylaxis-like reactions that are considered to be due to non-IgE-mediated mechanisms. Drug allergy represents a common and, at

Box 1.2 Some common drugs and agents associated with adverse reactions (immune type I–IV and nonimmune reactions)

- Pencillin and other antibiotics
- Reactions associated with general anaesthesia and surgery:
  anaesthetic agents
  neuromuscular blockers
  latex (see 'Case study of latex allergy')
  patent blue V*
  aspirin and other NSAIDs
  opiates
  skin disinfectants, chlorhexidine and povidone iodine
  local anaesthetics (rare)
- Radiocontrast media
- ACE inhibitors

* Patent blue V is a synthetic dye used originally for lymphography. It is now more widely used to identify sentinel lymph nodes in staging procedures for breast cancer, melanoma, and cervical cancers. Recent publications have highlighted the dye as a cause of type I IgE-mediated anaphylaxis. This may be uncommon, but clinicians and surgeons should be aware of this possible side-effect.

the same time, a most difficult problem faced by many clinicians. Hypersensitivity reactions to drugs can cause appreciable harm in many patients. Adverse drug reactions can be immune-mediated types I–IV (see Table 1.12 and Box 1.2) but many involve nonimmune mechanisms and in many cases the mechanisms are not well understood.

Diagnosis, investigations, and management of drug allergy, including desensitization, require collaborative working between the specialist clinician/surgeon, allergist, anaesthetist, etc., together with a great deal of patient education. Sound history-taking and examination may be supplemented with tests such as SPT and intradermal (ID) injection of antigens in the investigation of IgE-mediated responses. Blood testing may include measurement of tryptase levels (see 'Mast cells and basophils', above). Tryptase is a specific indicator of mast cell degranulation but does not define the mechanism causing such degranulation. This could be due to type I IgE hypersensitivity or to non-IgE-mediated/direct mast cell degranulation, as caused by some agents used in anaesthesia. Other specialist tests that are used include patch tests for type IV hypersensitivity reactions and, under appropriate supervision, drug provocation tests. Practitioners should read, use, and follow authoritative guidelines to inform their investigation and management of drug allergy. International and national guidelines are available in the UK. Excellent guidelines, appropriately updated, are produced by the British Society for Allergy and Clinical Immunology [66].

Table 1.12 Summary of type I–IV hypersensitivity reactions with key clinical features and investigations used in the evaluation of drug allergies

Reaction	Mechanism	Clinical presentation	Investigations
Type I	IgE-mediated	Urticaria/angioedema Anaphylaxis	SPT, ID skin tests, specific IgE in blood, drug provocation test
Type II	Drug absorbs to host cell surface. IgG/IgM cytotoxicity by complement activation or ADCC	Cytopenias, anaemia, thrombocytopenia	Blood counts Coombs test
Type III	Antibody (IgG/IgM) antigen-antibody immune complexes	Vasculitis, serum sickness, skin rashes, fever	Serology, complement assays, histology, ANCA testing
Type IV	$CD4^+$/$CD8^+$ T cells, Th1 and Th2 cytokines	Contact hypersensitivity, various skin rashes	Patch test

ADCC, antibody-dependent cellular cytoxicity; ANCA, anti-neutrophil cytoplasmic antibody; ID, intradermal; SPT, skin prick test.

Allergy, immunotherapy, and new vaccines

Allergic disease in the developed world has been increasing steadily for more than two decades, and there are indications that the same is now occurring in the developing world. The aetiological causes are, in part, speculative. A central idea is contained in the 'hygiene hypothesis' which suggests that the relatively clean environment found in more economically advanced societies results in lack of exposure in early life to microbes (antigens that would favour and drive Th1 responses). The lack of this Th1 stimulation is considered to lead by default to an immune environment favouring Th2. Th2 mechanisms, in turn, favour the development of allergic reactions to a range of environmental molecules, which result in the emergence of IgE-mediated reactions. Whatever the aetiology, it is clear that allergic diseases (ranging from rhinoconjunctivitis, to some forms of asthma, to anaphylaxis) are associated with many allergens and, therefore, require newer therapeutic modalities beyond those associated with the established use of antihistamines, β-agonists, steroids, and LT inhibitors.

As many of the allergens exciting inflammatory disease in atopic and nonatopic subjects are known, together with details of the sequence of events associated with Th2 immune responses, there is now a resurgence in interest in treating allergic disease with specific immunotherapy. The concept of injecting allergens as a means of specific immunotherapy is not new. Research published in the early part of the 20th century suggested that specific immunotherapy (SI) could be used to treat hay fever. During the latter part of the 20th century, some forms of limited SI, referred to as hyposensitization or desensitization, found wide acceptance in clinical practice. They are targeted to agents such as bee and wasp venom allergens, and pollen antigens associated with severe hay fever. Randomized clinical trials have strongly indicated the efficacy of those targeted therapies. Other specific immunotherapeutic regimens are directed to allergies to animal-associated allergens (cats, dogs, and horses), and also to house dust mite allergens. The general assumption is that SI somehow modulates and resets the immune response to the allergen, moving it away from the Th2 pathway and IgE production. There have been significant problems militating against the wider use of SI in the treatment of severe allergy and asthma:

- The regimens, mainly involving SC injection of allergens/allergen extracts in escalating doses are prolonged, lasting many months, together with maintenance doses over several years.
- The procedure, though simple in principle, carries the risk of inducing severe anaphylaxis and, therefore, needs to be carried out in a safe environment with resuscitation facilities and with the appropriate clinical expertise.
- In many allergic diseases, pure and quality-controlled allergen preparations are not available for systematic use and study.

Studies in asthma, especially in patients with long-standing disease, have tended to be less successful with SI, compared with other allergic diseases such as rhinoconjunctivitis. This is partly explained by long-standing asthma having a pathogenesis beyond that definable by Th2 IgE immune responses. There are also fundamental changes associated with mesenchymal and smooth muscle reactions, leading to potentially irreversible (nonimmune mediated) tissue remodelling.

Over the past 20 years, there has been a much greater understanding of the immunological science of Th2 responses. The definition of chemokines and cytokines involved and the central role of IgE, together with deeper understanding of immnoregulatory pathways associated with Tregs and suppressive cytokines, have all helped to rejuvenate studies of SI. Additionally, by the use of molecular biological and biochemical techniques, a range of pure allergens (including recombinant allergens) is becoming available. One consequence of this knowledge base is seen in the use of specific allergy immunotherapy, using routes beyond SC injection of allergens. Currently, there are regimens using the oral sublingual forms of therapy, e.g. for grass pollen allergies. Allergen vaccines using recombinant and modified allergens are in use (e.g. for pollen allergy) which are resulting in less prolonged immunization schedules. They are being used, for instance, in preseasonal immunization/desensitization schedules for grass and birch pollen and for some other allergens.

Newer findings are helping to explain the efficacy of SI. The repeated use of high doses of SC allergens leads to the secretion of IL-10 by subsets of DCs/APC which then stimulate the production of Tregs which further amplify the production of IL-10 and/or TGF-β. These changes result in the widespread suppression of the Th2 cell cytokines (IL-4, IL-5, IL-9, and IL-13) as well as some Th1 cytokines (IFN-γ and IL-2) which can add to the late inflammatory allergic response. For many years SI has been known to result in decreases in serum IgE antibodies with concomitant increases in IgG4, particularly after prolonged therapy. It is suggested that the IgG4 antibodies compete with IgE for the allergen. Recent data also shows increase in allergen-specific IgG1. Some researchers have suggested that the IgG antibodies may bind via their constant Fc regions to some types of Fc receptors on mast cells and basophils that are known to transduce negative signals (the receptors contain ITIM motifs). These negative signals suppress mast cell degranulation events.

Deeper understanding of the immune mechanisms associated with SI may provide more specific targeting by new vaccines or other immunotherapeutic protocols to overcome severe allergic reactions. For instance, our long-standing knowledge of IgE binding to FcεR1, and that cross-linking of the bound IgE molecule leads to signal transduction and mast cell degranulation, has led to the development of agents that act directly by interrupting that process. A newer therapy interrupting the IgE pathway involves using anti-IgE MABs, such as the prototype agent omalizumab. This antibody, which is administered parentally, antagonizes IgE binding and leads consequentially also to the down-regulation of unoccupied, high-affinity FcεR1 receptors. This therapy, albeit with limited efficacy, is now added to the armamentarium to treat severe forms of rhinoconjunctivitis and some particular groups of asthmatics.

Recent clinical and laboratory studies of patients receiving sublingual immunotherapy have shown strong correlation of efficacy with the emergence of Tregs ($CD4^+$, $CD25^+$, $Foxp3^+$ Tcells). Newer vaccines are being considered which may enhance the appearance of Tregs or which will redirect the immune response to the allergen from Th2 towards Th1. A major focus of research towards newer vaccines for SI is based on the targeting of TLRs. It is known that such innate immune receptors can help to direct the types of downstream adaptive immune responses that are induced. TLR antagonist formulations with allergens are being used to direct responses to the Th1 pathway rather than to the Th2 response. A main focus has been on TLR-9 as a target. DNA plasmid vaccines encoding allergen sequences and injected intradermally or intramuscularly have been shown in animal experiments to generate strong Th1 rather Th2 responses to the allergen. This vaccination protocol, like the existing SC immunotherapeutic approaches, bypasses the epithelial TLRs which may favour Th2 induction (as occurs in the MALT system). The intracellularly located TLR-9 stimulation may favour endosomal pathways for antigen presentation via the HLA class II pathway and, thus, to $CD4^+$ Th1 cells. Other TLR antagonists with novel adjuvants, such as MPL (see 'Central and peripheral lymphoid organs; lymphocyte recirculation', above), are also being explored.

Primary (congenital) and secondary (acquired) immune deficiencies (including HIV/AIDS)

Innate and adaptive immune systems

Clinical immunodeficiency diseases have been described associated with defects in many key molecules and cells of innate and adaptive immunity. The manifestation of such diseases are predictable problems associated primarily with infections—serious, persistent, unusual, or recurrent (SPUR). There is also noted to be increased incidence of certain cancers. These observations clearly reinforce the *raison d'être* of the immune system in defence against infections and development of some cancers. Immune deficiencies are commonly considered as primary, often with clearly defined genetic, biochemical, or metabolic lesions. Many patients present soon after birth (hence the term 'congenital immune deficiency' is often used). Primary immune deficiencies are rare to relatively rare. Acquired immune deficiencies, sometimes called secondary immune deficiencies, are much more common and immune defects can be demonstrated to be caused by clear nonimmune aetiological agents or other nonimmune diseases. Causes of secondary/acquired immune deficiency range from viruses (e.g. HIV, EBV, CMV) in immune suppressed patients to secondary immune deficiency associated with malignancy, with medical therapies, or consequent on surgical procedures, e.g. post-splenectomy (see Chapter 7).

SPUR infections dominate the clinical presentation of immune deficiencies. Other features may, however, raise suspicion of such diseases, including patients presenting with chronic diarrhoea without obvious faecal isolates and with the exclusion of inflammatory bowel disease. In childhood immune deficiency, there may be unexplained failure to thrive (children significantly below the physiological growth milestones/centiles for age). Atypical skin rashes may characterize certain prime immune deficiencies. Deep-seated chronic bacterial infections/abscesses and disorders such as osteomyelitis may indicate defects in phagocytic cells. Interestingly, some primary antibody deficiency syndromes are associated with features of clinical autoimmunity. The family history is important in the diagnosis of primary immune deficiencies, as many of the disorders have an autosomal recessive inheritance. However, a few are autosomal dominant—e.g. major forms of complement C1 inhibitor deficiency associated with hereditary angioedema. Other disorders are X-linked, including some forms of primary antibody deficiency (e.g. Bruton's hypogammaglobulinaemia, with no B cells in blood and very low levels or absence of all serum Igs). The commonest form of SCID, which occurs in 1 in 50 000 to 1 in 70 000 births, presents because of severe defects in T and B lymphocyte numbers and in their functions. The commonest form of SCID is X-linked, as is the commonest form of genetic defect in phagocytes of patients with chronic granulomatous disease (CGD); there is also an autosomal recessive form of CGD. Some prime immunodeficiency syndromes have specific clinical features which can alert clinicians to the diagnosis, e.g. the occurrence of ataxia telangiectasia (AT) in young children. Individuals with AT tend to have defects in antibody production and, over time, also in T cell numbers and functions. Partial albinism is noted in patients with rare defects involving their NK cells (Chediak–Higashi syndrome). Presentation of neonatal tetany (due to maldeveloped parathyroid glands and hypocalcaemia) is noted in patients with the Di George syndrome due to lack of or limited development of the thymus and, thus, of peripheral T cell development. These patients are now clustered into a syndrome, referred to as the 22q11 deletion syndrome, referring to the precise location of the genetic lesion on the long arm of chromosome 22 which leads to the defective pharyngeal pouch developmental anomaly responsible for the thymic defects.

Primary immune deficiencies, as indicated above, are relatively rare but clinical awareness of their occurrence and a high index of suspicion is needed by all clinicians to avoid missing these diagnoses. Many patients with immune deficiencies have significant morbidity, namely endstage organ damage (e.g. bronchiectasis) and mortality because of missed diagnoses. Our advances in knowledge in immunology, together with therapies such as bone marrow transplantation, and replacement of missing antibodies by IV or SC Ig therapy, can transform significantly the quality of life of patients with primary immune deficiencies. Emerging uses of newer recombinant DNA-derived products and tentative steps with clinical gene therapy hold out further specific strategies for effectively treating patients with these disorders. Clinicians suspecting immune deficiency should contact their clinical immunology colleagues early to work collaboratively in establishing the diagnosis. Following careful clinical history-taking and examination, with the formulation of possible differential diagnoses, some simple initial tests may prove helpful. Full blood count and differential (many infants with SCID will have a marked lymphopenia), global tests for T and B cell numbers, and typing of lymphoid subsets are now commonly available, as are global tests for phagocyte enumeration and function. Measurements of serum Ig levels and of specific antibodies are also readily available. Measurement of complement components quantitatively, and a measure of their global function (e.g. by lysis of antibody-coated cells), are also readily available assays.

Some well-characterized primary immune deficiencies of the innate and adaptive immune systems are outlined in Tables 1.13 and 1.14. These experiments of nature have yielded extremely informative data at the scientific level, confirming the basis of immune responses and their interactions. A review of these clinical immune deficiencies and their associated pathology confirms many of the scientific ideas, experimental and hypothetical, that have been discussed throughout this chapter.

Primary immune deficiencies of adaptive immunity, though relatively rare, have been studied in great depth by national and international consortia. Systematically, the documented defects can be shown to lead to blocks in the maturation and/or function of different elements of T and B lymphocytes and their products. Defects causing blocks in the early common pathways of T and B cell development usually present as severe disorders (SCIDs). The precise molecular definitions of lesions in clinical immune deficiencies of adaptive immunity have strongly underpinned our precise understanding of lymphocyte maturation, activation, and functioning.

Acquired (secondary) immune deficiencies

In clinical practice in the developed world, the most frequent cause of acquired immune deficiency is that secondary to cancer *per se* or to the consequences of cancer therapies (see Chapters 4 and 7). Other forms of clinical therapy, e.g. immunosuppressive therapy in autoimmune disease, including the newer biologicals (anticytokines/cytokine receptor MABs), can result in deficiencies in elements of innate and adaptive immunity, and an increased risk of infections (or of particular infections). Indeed, in some situations over time, there may be increased incidence of certain neoplasms. Worldwide, protein–calorie malnutrition, with or without widespread infections (e.g. TB, HIV, malaria and other parasites) is responsible for the greatest number of people presenting with acquired/secondary immune deficiencies (see Chapter 6). The remainder of this section will focus on the ongoing threat and problems associated with AIDS due to HIV infection.

HIV, AIDS, and the surgeon

Aetiopathology

The AIDS pandemic was first recognized in 1981 when a group of men presented with rare opportunistic infections and tumours which were indicative of an underlying cellular immune deficiency, but without any obvious cause for such a deficiency.

Table 1.13 Primary immune deficiencies of the innate immune system

Functional deficiencies	Clinical diseases and presentations; pathophysiological lesions	Lesions and mechanisms
Early complement (C1q, C2 or C4), MBL	Immune complex disease, SLE-like syndromes, serum sickness	Mutations in genes (C1q, C2, C4), additional null alleles (in MHC), MBL—possibly infection with bacteria Failure in activation of complement system which is needed to clear immune complexes and destroy or opsonise microbes
Mid complement (C3)	Very severe infections (especially bacterial)	Mutation in C3 gene (often lethal)
Factors B and H; properdin	Problems with infections	Gene mutations
Late complement (C5–C9)	Recurrent/severe infection (especially with Gram-negative bacteria), meningitis	Mutations in separate genes C5–C9
Phagocytes (polymorphs and macrophages)	Acute and chronic inflammatory lesions, CGDs, deep abscesses	X-linked CGD (mutation), autosomal CGD—mutations in genes for phagocyte intracellular enzyme (oxidases) components
Polymorphs and monocytes	Leucocyte adhesion deficiency (LAD,1 and 2)–recurrent 'abscesses' with limited signs of inflammation; repeated surgical drainage	LAD1 mutation in beta2 integrin gene (CD18/CD11). LAD2 mutations in genes for protein linkage sites for components of selectins (E and P); poor extravastion of phagocytes to site of tissue infection
Regulatory protein C1 esterase inhibition (C1.INH)	Recurrent angioedema (hereditary angioedema) Acute abdomen presentation Upper respiratory tract swelling Angioedema with intubation, with dental operations	80% of cases are mutations in C1.INH gene (lack of protein in blood); 15% have protein in blood but it is nonfunctional Acquired cases of INH deficiency secondary to lymphoid neoplasia and autoimmunity
Cytokines/signalling (IL-I2 or IFN-γ) or their receptors	Problems with infection (especially various mycobacteria, salmonella intracellular microbes); SPUR	Mutations in genes for cytokines or their receptors
NK cells	Severe viral (especially HSVs) infections which are recurrent	Some cytoskelatal intracellular defects (various, not well defined at present) Defects in numbers and/or functions
TLRs IRAK4 Signalling molecules IKKB	Recurrent infections with selected bacteria and viruses	Gene mutations for IRAK4 and IKK8 TLR polymorphisms, increase susceptibility to some infections

CGD, chronic granulomatous disease; HSV, herpes simplex virus; IRAK4, interleukin1 receptor-associated kinase 4; IKKB: Iκ/κB (natural inhibitor of NF-κB transcription factor); INH, inhibitor (gene); MBL, mannose-binding lectin; SLE, systemic lupus erythematosus; SPUR, serious, persistent, unusual, or recurrent infection; TLR, Toll-like receptor.

Table 1.14 Primary immune deficiencies in adaptive immunity

Diseases	Mechanisms	Laboratory findings/ correlates
Defects in lymphocyte maturation		
X-linked SCID	Mutation in the gene for the common γ chain of the IL-2R which are used by ILs	Very low T cells, B cells low or normal, reduced serum Ig levels
Autosomal SCID	Mutation in genes for enzymes involved in lymphocyte maturation; some forms of RAG1 and RAG2 mutations Enzyme defects (e.g. ADA and PNP) and lymphocytes are unable to clear toxic metabolites	Decreases in T and B cell numbers in blood, reduced serum Ig levels Progressive decrease in T and B cells, reduced serum Igs
Chromosome 22q11 syndrome (including Di George)	Abnormal developmental biology (3rd and 4th pharyngeal pouches) leading to thymic absence/or hypoplasia	Absence or very low T cell numbers, diminished T cell function, B cells normal, decreased serum IgG
B cells X-linked agammaglobulinaemia (Bruton's disease)	Mutation in Brutons tyrosine kinase (signalling) gene Failure of B cell maturation	No or very low numbers of B cells in blood, very low or absent serum Ig
Selective IgA deficiency, (commonest primary antibody deficiency); incidence 1 in 600 of the population	Ig-α chain deletion on chromosome 14	Absence of IgA in blood
Defects in lymphocyte activation and function		
X-linked hyper-IgM syndrome	Failure of B cell heavy chain class switching due to mutation in gene for CD40L on activated I cells	Raised serum IgM, very low IgA and IgG; poor response to immunization
Autosomal recessive hyper-IgM mutations in the AID gene	Limited somatic hypermutation and CSR	Raised serum IgM, very low IgA and IgG; poor response to immunization
CVID; relatively common incidence (1 in 10 000–40 000) and presents at all ages	Varied mechanisms: cytokine genes/ receptor mutation defects; costimulatory defects	Low serum IgG and IgA, poor antibody function; poor response to immunization
MHC class II and class I deficiencies	Lack of expression of HLA class II and I antigens: Poor antigen presentation to $CD4^+$ and $CD8^+$ T cells; poor thymic development, especially of $CD8^+$ T cells in MHC class I deficiency	Defective CMI, defective antibody responses

CMI, cell-mediated immunity; CSR, class switch recombination; CVID, common variable immune deficiency; SCID, severe combined immunodeficiency.

That clinical definition of the syndrome was followed in 1983 by the discovery of the retrovirus, now called human immunodeficiency virus (HIV), which is known to be the central agent in the aetiopathology of AIDS. Retroviruses contain the unique enzyme reverse transcriptase (RT) which allows them to copy their RNA into proviral DNA, reversing the normal flow of genetic events. The delineation of the prototype HIV-1 has been followed by the isolation of another member of the *Lentivirus* group, HIV-2, which is also capable of causing AIDS, albeit significantly less than HIV-1. Distantly related retroviruses, simian immunodeficiency virus (SIV), have also been isolated from several monkey species. Recent molecular genetic and evolutionary biology research, using field isolates of viruses, has indicated that HIV-1 infection has occurred by trans-species transmission from chimpanzees to humans, probably some time in the past 100 years.

Figure 1.34 shows the overall organizational structure of HIV, together with some of the detectable antibodies to viral proteins (antigens) found in infected people. Figure 1.35 shows some of the clinical manifestations of AIDS. In developed countries, most AIDS patients originally presented with opportunistic infections, especially prominent being *Pneumocystis jiroveci* pneumonitis (>60% of cases) and Kaposi's sarcoma (KS). Other infections with pathogenic and opportunistic bacteria, viruses, protozoa, and fungi also cause severe diseases in such patients. Apart from KS, patients with AIDS have an increased incidence of certain other cancers (e.g. lymphomas).

AIDS patients in other parts of the world (e.g. sub-Saharan Africa), with a differing spectrum of environmental microflora, have differing patterns of clinical presentation. In parts of Africa, AIDS patients often present with severe malabsorption and a

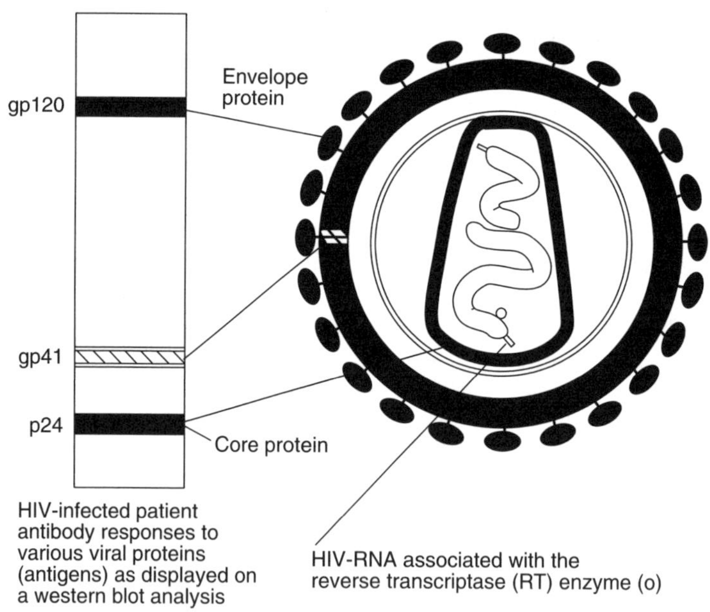

Fig. 1.34 Organization of the HIV-1 retrovirus.

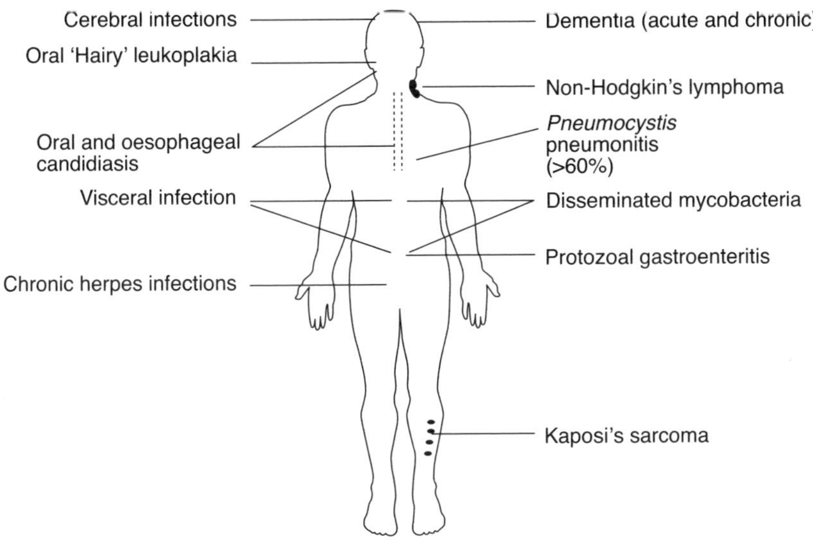

Fig. 1.35 AIDS—some clinical associations/manifestations. The agents associated with AIDS pathology: this involves opportunistic infections (protozoal, fungal, bacterial, and viral) together with well-known pathogens. Neuropathological disorders are well recognized without concomitant infections. Associated tumours are being increasingly recognized, beyond the well-documented Kaposi's sarcoma.

wasting syndrome (called 'slim disease') together with disseminated infections, such as TB. Comorbidity with TB and with protozoal infections makes for a lethal cocktail of diseases in those regions.

Epidemiology and transmission of HIV infection and treatment strategies

AIDS represents only the endstage manifestation of infection, which may take many years to develop following initial infection with HIV. It was commonly estimated that for every documented case of AIDS there may be 20–30 times as many HIV-infected persons. However, with worldwide coordination on HIV surveillance and epidemiology, led by the United Nations AIDS agency (UNAIDS) and the World Health Organization (WHO) working closely with national governments, there is now robust data on the state of the pandemic.

The UNAIDs/WHO 2008 report on the global AIDS epidemic [67] documented in excess of 33 million people living with HIV worldwide and more than 25 million deaths caused by AIDS since the 1980s. Currently, the data indicate that two-thirds of people living with HIV and three-quarters of those dying from AIDS are in sub-Saharan Africa. Globally, the HIV epidemic appears to be levelling off but there are still unacceptably high levels of new AIDS cases and the infection continues to spread worldwide.

HIV-infected individuals may be asymptomatic or present with a spectrum of clinical manifestations, including those associated with AIDS. Various attempts have been made to classify and stage the spectrum of HIV infection. Figure 1.36 shows some of

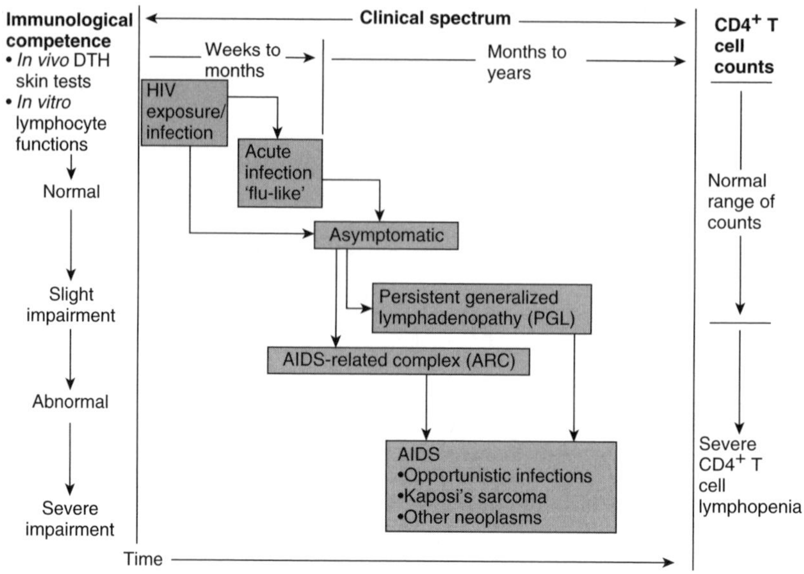

Fig. 1.36 Progression of HIV infection to AIDS. Correlates of clinical spectrum, immunological competence, and $CD4^+$ T cell counts with time.

the recognized features/stages of HIV infection, correlated with time and measureable immunological indices.

Early epidemiological studies (mid–late 1980s) clearly documented the means of spread of the infection which are:

- Sexual intercourse—anal and vaginal
- Needle route—intravenous drug abuse, 'needlestick' injuries, and injections
- Mother-to-child (vertical transmission) route—*in utero,* perinatal, breast milk
- Tissues and organs for transplantation—blood/blood products (e.g. factor VIII), kidneys, skin, bone marrow, etc.

Recognition of the means of viral transmission accordingly indicated some of the means of prevention. At present, transmission by tissues and organs for transplantation is essentially abolished by robust screening, including highly sensitive and specific serological and molecular testing for HIV. Needlestick injuries need to be avoided; however, when they do occur in a defined risk scenario the evidence is that rapid postexposure treatment of the wound and administration of appropriate antiviral drugs can reduce the risk of infection. Additionally, mother-to-child transmission has been markedly reduced by education (avoidance of breast-feeding as appropriate) and by treating pregnant women with antiretroviral drugs. Greater penetrance of such procedures is needed in parts of the developing world; currently 90% of children (<15 years) living with HIV have acquired it from maternal transmission. It is axiomatic that prevention is better than cure, but today, with this particular viral infection, prevention of transmission is still the only cure. Recent (2006–9) strategies aimed at production of novel anti-HIV vaccines or use of vaginal microbicidal gels have not proved efficacious in large-scale clinical and field trials. Recent, as yet unpublished, reports at the 2010 International AIDS Conference have suggested (based on several small studies) that use of vaginal gels containing specific anti-HIV antivirals may provide up to 50% protection from infection. Current policies, national and worldwide, are directed to prevention by way of education and social behaviour strategies—to overcome public ignorance, to teach safe sex, and to change behaviour. There is also substantial ongoing funding for biomedical research, aimed at developing additional suitable pharmaceuticals, newer vaccines, and other treatment modalities to combat HIV infection [68]. Outstanding scientific advances in molecular and cell biology have led to a better understanding of the nature of the virus and its interaction with the host immune system. This knowledge has highlighted the major difficulties which are present and will be encountered in trying to find an effective therapy or vaccine for HIV. It has also, however, revealed possible weaknesses in the viral 'armour' which may be breachable.

Immunology of HIV/AIDS

The pathology and clinical features of HIV/AIDS can be understood in terms of the immunology of HIV–host interaction. The virus targets the CD4$^+$ cells, especially the Th lymphocytes, the central cells of the immune response. The HIV gp120 outer coat molecule targets/uses the CD4 molecule on the T cell as its main receptor along with the chemokine receptors CXCR4 or CCR5 as coreceptors to bind to and enter the cell. Most HIV isolates are CCR5 binders (drugs such as maraviroc have been developed to specifically block that binding). The initial binding of HIV to the CD4 molecule is the major prerequisite for infection. Following fusion of HIV to the T cell membrane a series of events ensues. Having entered the host cell, the retrovirus uses its RT-directed and newly synthesized proviral DNA form to integrate into the host genomic DNA under the control of a viral integrase enzyme. It then uses the cell's hijacked genetic apparatus to make new viruses. Production of new virus is particularly favoured if lymphocytes become activated by responding to antigens/microbes and to cytokine signals—events likely to be more frequent in immunodeficient people. Viral production can be monitored in blood and other tissues by sensitive molecular techniques and assays using the PCR. In fact, the measurement of viral load (viral copy numbers) by PCR is now in common usage, along with CD4$^+$ T cell counts, in monitoring patients' response to antiretroviral drug treatment and for prognosis. Current evidence suggests that serial measurements of absolute CD4$^+$ T cell counts remain the best single prognostic marker. Without significant cell activation the incorporated provirus remains dormant in the cell. This state is not sensitive to current antiviral drugs and thus there exists an efficient reservoir site for the virus. Hence, HIV incorporates itself into the CD4$^+$ T cell, and into any other cell which expresses the CD4 receptor molecule. Macrophages, monocytes, LCs of skin, and other APCs in mucosal and other sites express CD4 along with some cells of the CNS, such as glial cells. Each of these cell types has been demonstrated to be a site of harbouring, incorporation, and expression of HIV. Importantly, APCs at the sites of HIV entry in the genitals and GIT express on their surface membranes, along with CD4, a chemokine receptor CCR5 which acts as a coreceptor for the virus. When HIV breaches the epithelial linings of these sites it readily infects these DCs and other APCs inadvertently, thus facilitating HIV spread to secondary lymphoid organs and to T cells and other APCs in those tissues.

Over a period of time, infected $CD4^+$ T cells, macrophages, and other APCs malfunction and/or are destroyed by a series of incompletely defined mechanisms. The latter include direct viral toxic (cytopathic) effects, and the probable induction of indirect destructive 'autoimmune reactions'—autoantibodies and autoreactive cytotoxic cells have been demonstrated in HIV subjects. Additionally, increased apoptosis of activated infected and noninfected cells has been reported. Over months to years, a decline in $CD4^+$ T cells can be measured and, in fact, it remains currently the most important prognostic monitor of progression of HIV infection towards AIDS. Tissue analysis reveals marked destruction of the anatomy of secondary lymphoid tissues. Many factors involved in the progression of HIV infection to AIDS are still not fully understood. However, as $CD4^+$ T cells are known to be central *regulator* and *effector* cells in the immune response and are responsible for mediating CMI, which protect against intracellular infections and the development of tumours, their loss leads to predictable outcomes. Accordingly, many of the tumours and opportunistic infections seen in HIV/AIDS can be attributed to loss or functional impairment of the critical $CD4^+$ cells. Other associations of HIV infection, such as dementia and neuropathies, are not so readily explained and can be encountered in patients with normal numbers and functional $CD4^+$ T cells. The genesis of AIDS-associated KS is linked to a causative human herpesvirus (HHV8) and may additionally involve stimulation of the target endothelial cells by deregulated cytokine growth factor(s).

Serum antibodies in HIV/AIDS

The serum antibodies detected in HIV-infected people are believed, in the main, to be nonprotective with regard to the natural history and progression to AIDS. Current evidence indicates that, without therapeutic intervention, most HIV-infected individuals will have progressive disease, probably over many years. The laboratory tests designed to detect antibodies (e.g. anti-gp120, anti-gp41, and anti-p24) have been extremely useful for documenting HIV status, for screening blood and organ donors, and for epidemiological studies. The antibody test also indicates that following exposure to the virus, there is a period of several weeks (referred to as the 'window period') during which the individual is probably infectious (HIV can be cultured from infected lymphocytes and p24 antigen can be found in blood) before antibody is detectable. Thus, among the many social, legal, economic, and medical arguments concerning the advantages and disadvantages of antibody screening for HIV status, it must be clearly understood that the antibody tests, though exceedingly useful, are unreliable in the early stages of infection. Currently, molecular assays such as PCR for viral nucleic acid and sensitive newer-generation viral antigen assays are the most useful tests in the early phase of testing, following an assumed or known exposure to HIV infection.

HIV/AIDS and surgical practice

Surgeons realize that there is a growing number of people in the community infected by HIV, some of whom will undoubtedly become patients under their care. Some people who require surgical treatment or invasive investigations will be known to have HIV infection or AIDS. Others will present as patients with a normal spectrum of surgical problems, unrelated to their HIV status. Thus, the question must be asked as to whether surgeons are at high occupational risk and, if so, what can be done to mitigate such risk. Blood and blood products are a major source of transmission of the virus, and are of course constantly in the working arena of surgeons. Surveys show surgeons inflicting self-injury with needles or knives in the course of their duties in up to 10% of all surgical procedures; glove puncture occurs in up to one-quarter to one-third of operations. Although the risk of virus transmission appears potentially high, the number of recorded cases of surgeons or other health care personnel becoming infected with HIV is very low. Perhaps this might change for the worse if current practices continue and HIV infection in the community continues to increase. What, then, should surgeons do? What special precautions or measures should be taken? The following comments (Box 1.3) are the personal opinions by the author, some of which are supported by current national guidelines. Readers should refer to international and UK Department of Health guidelines.

Box 1.3 Suggested precautions against HIV infection

- *Known AIDS/HIV-infected patient*: Adopt similar precautions to those recommended for patients who are positive for hepatitis B virus antigen. Some surgical units in the USA, with a significant community of HIV-positive individuals, assume all patients carry the virus. That may well represent extreme caution, but it should remind all those in medical/paramedical practice to treat blood with the necessary caution. In the UK, it is standard practice to adopt 'universal precautions', i.e. consider everyone as a risk.
- *High-risk groups*: If the patient is known to indulge in 'risky' practices (sex with prostitutes/promiscuous sex, homosexual practices, drug abuse/addiction), either currently or previously, then surgery should be performed assuming that the patient maybe infected with HIV. To require compulsory HIV testing of the patient prior to surgery involves many legal and ethical dilemmas. However, with appropriate supportive discussion and counselling patients may consent to HIV testing. Even if a patient in such a high-risk group was found on testing to be HIV antibody negative, that could never be taken as an absolute guarantee of not being infected with the virus and therefore not infectious (see 'window period', in 'Serum antibodies in HIV/AIDS', above).
- *Donors*: Donors of all organs and semen should be screened for the presence of HIV antibody in blood and, more importantly, potential donors should be made aware of high-risk groups. If they fall into any of the known risk categories they, like blood donors, should desist from donation.
- *Contaminated sources*: HIV has been isolated from plasma, leucocytes, semen, cervical secretions, breast milk, tears, saliva, urine, and cerebrospinal fluid. There is considerable doubt that infection is transmitted from the latter four fluids. If body fluids (from known HIV-positive patients) are spilled on skin, eyes, or other mucus membranes, these should be washed immediately with copious amounts of fluid.

Box 1.3 Suggested precautions against HIV infection *(continued)*

- *Penetrating wounds*: Needlestick or scalpel wounds should be encouraged to bleed, and I would advocate washing with 70% ethanol/isopropyl alcohol or phenolics (which are known to kill the virus). Even in the light of the very few seroconversions documented for needlestick injuries with known HIV-positive blood, the consensus now is that postexposure antiretroviral drug prophylaxis should be used. Institutional guidelines for this are in existence.
- *Reporting*: Any health care worker who sustains needlestick or splash exposure to bodily fluids (especially blood) should report the incident so that a risk assessment can be made and drug prophylaxis offered if necessary.

Guidelines concerning the spillage of HIV-infected blood, decontamination of equipment, and protocols for the control of infection, are clearly documented nationally and internationally.

Antiviral therapy

Several effective antiviral drugs are in general use, based on the detailed understanding of the HIV life cycle. They target key enzymes utilized in viral invasion, integration, replication, and assembly in host cells. The earliest drugs were the nucleoside analogue RT inhibitors typified by zidovudine (AZT). Their blocking of the RT enzyme that is essential for production of the intracellular provirus was extremely effective. However, over time, because of the high mutation rate of HIV, drug resistance rapidly emerged. Additional drugs were soon developed, including other RT inhibitors and drugs targeting other key viral enzyme systems, including a range of protease inhibitors, which interrupt early viral uncoating before the action of RT. Other drugs interfere with downstream viral assembly from preprotein precursors in the cytoplasm, resulting in structurally damaged and noninfectious particles. It was apparent that combinations of different types of antivirals, rather than monotherapy, made the emergence of resistant HIV much less likely. The most effective therapy over the past decade is referred to as highly active antiretroviral therapy (HAART), which is based on a combination of three or more drugs. HAART can be shown to markedly suppress viral copy numbers in blood and lead, at least initially, to increases in blood $CD4^+$ T cell counts. Clearly, these powerful drugs can and do have significant side effects and patient compliance is important to achieve and maintain maximum viral suppression for as long as possible. Current evidence suggest that viral reservoirs—integrated non-replicating HIV provirus in the host cellular DNA—are not affected by drug therapy. HAART is therefore not a cure. It is hoped that long-term suppression of the virus may give the host immune system the opportunity to combat the virus more effectively, especially if other treatment modalities become available (e.g. a vaccine, chemokine or receptor antagonists). These are statements of conjecture and hope, but they are stimulating intense ongoing research into anti-HIV therapy.

A developing principle is the idea of widespread (worldwide) testing and antiviral drug treatment as a means for prevention of HIV transmission [69]. It is known that early drug treatment of pregnant women is very effective in preventing viral transmission to the child. WHO suggests that such a strategy could result in the near elimination of HIV within 50 years. Randomized trials are ongoing in several countries assessing whether such a strategy can lead to durable prevention of transmission in targeted groups. This approach is not without concerns, including the possible emergence of drug-resistant strains of the virus; nevertheless this 'seek, test, and treat' strategy is progressing and its results will be eagerly awaited.

Whatever antiviral therapies eventually prove most beneficial globally, for the individual they will need to be introduced early in the course of infection, before the virus causes irreversible damage to the immune system.

Vaccines for HIV

The holy grail of prophylatic or therapeutic vaccines for HIV in this early part of the 21st century has still to be achieved and appears to be as far away as it was 20 years ago. Even now, with our deep understanding of the molecular and cellular aspects of HIV and its interaction with host cells, together with advances in recombinant DNA technology (enabling the construction of novel HIV DNA vector vaccines known to generate experimentally good anti-HIV T cell responses) the caution remains and disappointments occur. In 2003, two large vaccine trials proved inefficacious; in 2007, one of the most studied and promising vaccines failed in a large international collaborative clinical trial. Much pessimism descended on the vaccination strategies. A glimmer of hope appeared in late 2009 when it was announced that an international anti-HIV vaccine trial in Thailand had cut the risk of becoming infected with HIV by some 30%. The study was hailed as a historic milestone. Subsequent publication of the trial data and expert discussions of the data suggest, at best, cautious optimism. The level of significance of the findings, based on the powering of the study, suggests it could be a chance finding or that the benefits of the vaccine were marginal. Preventive vaccine studies are continuing.

Some authorities have suggested the need to go back to vaccine studies aimed at generating broadly neutralizing anti-HIV antibodies—a task which in the recent past has proved to be largely unsuccessful. The complexity of HIV interactions in the host and over time is far from fully understood. To generate a successful vaccine may need new, holistic systems biology and medicine approaches to model, predict, and garner new insights into the virus–host interactions *in vivo*. Indeed, such a systems study in 2008/9 analysed sequences in HIV isolates from thousands of patients correlated with their HLA alleles known to facilitate strong anti-HIV immune responses. The striking finding from the study indicated that HIV is rapidly evolving to evade human immune responses (escape mutants). Vaccines will be needed that can keep pace with such dramatic viral evolution. Such vaccines may need to harness simultaneously elements of innate immunity along with both significant humoral antibody immunity and CMI against HIV [68].

Monoclonals and other biological therapies (including immunoglobulin replacement)

Monoclonal antibodies

A quiet revolution has occurred in medical therapeutics over the past 15 years, with MABs delivering on their promise from the mid 1970s of making valuable contributions to the management of patients with a wide range of diseases. Therapeutic antibodies, along with other biologicals such as recombinant cytokines, soluble receptor constructs, and fusion proteins (recombinant molecules comprising a ligand or receptor molecule linked to the constant region of Ig, usually IgG Fc region) are the main agents in clinical use. These are now widely used in cancer immunotherapy and the treatment of a range of immune and inflammatory disorders, including RA and other inflammatory or immune diseases, in transplantation, and in IgE-mediated allergy and asthma.

From Kohler and Milstein's publication in 1975 of their seminal work on generating mouse MABs it was hoped that such reagents, with their fine specificity for target antigens and their perceived potential low toxicity (compared with cytotoxic drugs, immunosuppressive agents, etc.), would substantially change the treatment of a range of diseases and disorders. This hope was not fully realized for nearly 20 years (with a few exceptions, e.g. use of anti-T cell MABs in transplantation). The disappointments were a consequence of several factors when mouse MABs were used in humans. Their limited efficacy related to the fact that the mouse Fc region was unable to efficiently recruit *in vivo* human effector systems. Therefore, the benefits of complement activation and the recruitment of cellular effectors by binding to and signalling via Fc receptors of cells such as NK cells and phagocytes could not be exploited. Additionally, mouse MABs, being themselves foreign non-self molecules, were seen as foreign by the recipient's human immune system, which made an appropriate human anti-mouse antibody (HAMA) response. The HAMA response neutralizes and antagonizes subsequent use of therapeutic mouse MABs by forming immune complexes, leading to rapid removal of the agents. In the case of antitumour therapy there are other problems relating to the targeting of the important TAAs, as well as the poor penetration of MABs into tumour tissues.

Notwithstanding these problems, the outstanding success in the late 1990s of anti-TNF MAB therapy in RA, resulting in a paradigm shift in the successful management of that hitherto very destructive inflammatory joint disease, maintained interest in the clinical use of therapeutic MABs. The advancement in recombinant DNA technology, which paralleled the discovery and development of MABs, provided new molecular engineering tools to overcome some of the drawbacks of the mouse MABs. In the 1980s, via the use of DNA technology, researchers were able to retain the CDR specificities of mouse MABs by grafting them as whole mouse V regions into a scaffold of human Ig constant regions, thus, producing a so-called *chimeric* antibody. This theoretically should be much less foreign and antigenic when used to treat humans, since large parts of the foreign mouse protein have been removed. Clinical experience with chimeric therapeutic MABs still demonstrated some (albeit more limited) HAMA responses to the mouse V regions. Further DNA recombinant work resulted in the removal of even more mouse antigens by the generation of partially humanized MABs where only the CDRs from the V region are grafted onto the human Ig scaffold. Currently, advanced cellular and molecular biological techniques are allowing the generation of fully human MABs *de novo* in the laboratory (e.g. using the Greg Winter technology) or as human MABs generated from isolated blood lymphocytes (antibody-secreting B cells) which have predefined specificities. At present, all forms

Box 1.4 Nomenclature of monoclonal antibodies

The nomenclature is varied but there is some agreed systematic usage of the names (Table 1.15). Notation appearing before the letters -mab indicates the origin and type of monoclonal; thus, chimeric (human/mouse) antibodies are designated -ximabs (e.g. rituximab); partially humanized (CDR grafted on antibodies) are termed -zumabs (e.g. bevacizumab—Avastin); fully human antibodies are noted as -umabs (adalimumab—anti-TNF monoclonal). The term -momab indicates the fully mouse monoclonal, a limited number of which are still licensed for therapy (muromomab CD3, the original OKT3 MAB used to treat allograft rejection).

of monoclonals are being used therapeutically in a wide range of diseases. Their nomenclature is described in Box 1.4.

In the field of therapeutic antibodies for cancer, apart from humanizing constructs to reduce antigenicity and to engage effector functions, additional strategies have used the specific antibody to focus delivery of cellular toxins or radio-isotopes to the tumour site by the linkage of these moieties (usually chemically) to the antibody molecule.

Licensed therapeutic MABs have proved their value in well-controlled randomized clinical trials. Some are used off licence where many trials have shown significant efficacy: for example, the use of rituximab in Wegener's vasculitis and in some patients with primary Sjögren's syndrome. As with all therapeutic modalites, side effects are documented ranging from general side effects (e.g. chills, fever, headaches, tiredness, occasional urticaria), to rare but severe adverse drug reactions. Because many of the MABs used to treat RA and other immune-inflammatory diseases target key molecules such as TNF-α it was predictable that side effects would emerge. Various bacterial and viral infections have been documented arising as a consequence of anti-TNF-α therapy, including in particular TB. This is not surprising, as experimental data exist indicating the important role of TNF-α in the formation of granulomas that contain mycobacteria *in vivo*. There are guidelines regarding the prevention and management of TB in patients considered for or undergoing anti-TNF-α therapies. Bacterial infection of the upper and (rarely lower) respiratory tract and of the urogenital tract, and less commonly the GIT, have also been documented. Clearly, a risk–benefit analysis is important in considering MAB therapies. On balance, benefits far outweigh side effects, many of which are usually manageable. Another concern with using immune-modulating or suppressive monoclonals, in the longer term, is the risk of developing cancers. The longest experience of the use of therapeutic MABs is in patients with RA. Surveillance has suggested a slight increase in incidence of some skin cancers and of some non-Hodgkin's lymphomas. This indicates the need for continuous and close monitoring of patients receiving therapeutic MABs. The overall safety data on the use of these reagents and of the constructs (such as fusion proteins) in relation to infection are encouraging. The possibility of problems with neoplasia over time requires more vigilance, and more data. This area is complex, as the natural history of some of the

Table 1.15 Selection of therapeutic MABs licensed and in clinical practice with their major target diseases

Generic name	Proprietary/other name	Molecule targeted	Licensed indication
Infliximab	Remicade	TNF-α	RA, AS, CD, ulcerative colitis, severe PP
Trastuzumab	Herceptin	Epidermal growth factor receptor (c-erb B2: HER2/neu)	Breast cancer, over expressing HER2/neu
Rituximab	Rituxan	CD20	RA, B cell non-Hodgkin's lymphoma
Natalizumab	Tysalori	Integrins: block binding of VLA4 toVCAM1; α4/B7 to MADCAM1	CD, relapsing MS
Muromomab/ CD3	OKT3	CD3 (pan T cells)	Allograft rejection
Omalizumab	Xolair	IgE	Moderate to severe IgE-mediated (Type 1) diseases (specified)
Bevacizumab	Avastin	VEGF	Metastatic/advanced cancers, colorectal and non-small cell lung cancers
Adalimumab	Humira	TNF-α	RA, juvenile RA, AS, CD, PP
Basiliximab	Simulect	CD25 low affinity IL-2 receptor (α chain)	Prevention of acute organ rejection
Tocilizumab	Actemra	IL-6 receptor	RA, juvenile RA
Alemtumzab	Campath (1H)	CD52: cell surface molecule on various leucocytes, especially T and B cells and monocytes	B cell chronic lymphocytic leukaemia
Ustekinumab	Stelara	Anti-IL-12/IL-23	Moderate to severe PP

AS, ankylosing spondylitis; CD, Crohn's disease; MS, muscular sclerosis; PP, plaque psoriasis; RA, rheumatoid arthritis; VEGF, vascular endothelial growth factor.

diseases being treated has an inherent increased incidence of neoplasia. Some rarer side effects of specific therapeutic MABs are documented. These include the development of potentially lethal progressive multifocal leucoencephalopathy (PML) in MS patients treated with the anti-integrin MAB natalizumab. This MAB was withdrawn from usage for a time. However, the perceived benefits in MS patients appear to significantly outweigh this very rare risk of PML and this has resulted in the re-approval of natalizumab by the US Food and Drug Adminstration (FDA) and its reintroduction in clinical practice.

Fusion proteins

The use of fusion proteins in clinical practice is currently much more limited than that of MABs. They exploit the specificity of receptors or counter-ligands with the additional benefit of the fused Fc region of human Ig (usually IgG). The benefits include prolongation of the half-life of the therapeutic molecule receptor or ligand and, additionally, the engagement of the effector functions associated with the Fc region, as described above. Current constructs include etanercept, which is a TNF receptor–IgG1Fc fusion protein, targeting TNF-α in the treatment areas similar to those for the therapeutic anti-TNF-α MABs. Another important molecule is abatacept which is a construct of CTLA-4–human IgGFc. CTLA-4 is a member of the CD28 family of proteins found on responding/activated T cells which acts as a negative regulator of T cell activation when it interacts with its ligands CD80/CD86, found on APCs and on other cell types. This fusion protein switches off T cell reactivity. It is used in the treatment of RA and juvenile RA. A rationally designed construct called belatacept targets CD86 more than CD80 and has shown potent immunosuppression of acute renal transplant rejection. Its approval by the FDA in 2010 for that use adds to the clinician's armenturium of powerful immunosuppressants beyond the calcineurin inhibitors (see Chapter 3). T cell costimulation blockers, with more targeted inhibition of the immune response, should avoid the nephrotoxicity and increased cardiovascular risks associated with ciclosporin and other anticalcineurin agents. However, they will need close monitoring for other possible complications such as post-transplant lymphoproliferative disease and PML, as noted above for some of the other therapeutic MABs.

Soluble receptor constructs

Some soluble receptor constucts have been introduced into clinical practice. One of the best known is anakinra, a recombinant nonglycosylated form of the human IL-1Ra. It combats the proinflammatory action of IL-1 (and indirectly linked downstream inflammatory promoting cytokines such as IL-6). It is used in moderate to severe RA, as is the newer IL-6Ra MAB, tocilizumab. Anakinra is also used (off licence) in some autoinflammatory diseases, where IL-1 is believed to be a significant pathogenic cytokine. Another receptor construct, rilonacept (a complex fusion protein (that binds and neutralises IL-1)) is licensed for use in the same clinical indications as anakinra, as well as for the treatment of some forms of named autoinflammatory diseases (cryopyrin-associated periodic syndrome, Muckle–Wells syndrome) and for chronic infantile neurological cutaneous articular syndrome (see Chapter 8).

Recombinant cytokines

Some recombinant cytokines have been used for many years as licensed therapeutics in well-defined diseases—a range of tumours and viral infections. IFN-α 2A and 2B are used to treat selected groups of leukaemias, lymphomas, and chronic hepatitis B and C. Recombinant IFN-β 1a and 1b are used in the treatment of relapsing MS.

IFN-γ has been used as an adjunct in supportive therapy of severe CGD. The cytokine is known to stimulate cells of innate and adaptive immunity; the hope was that it would help to overcome some of the poor antimicrobial responses seen in patients with CGD. Results have been very variable with regards to efficacy.

The potential for synergistic therapeutic use of MABs, fusion proteins, and inhibitors of signal transduction (anti-tyrosine kinases, anti-STATs) are being explored in carefully designed studies in diseases ranging from cancer to autoimmunity.

Polyclonal immunoglobulin replacement therapy

Polyclonal IVIg or SCIg replacement therapy has for several decades been an efficacious treatment for patients with primary antibody deficiency. It has (in conjunction with antimicrobial drugs) substantially transformed the lives of those patients with regard to morbidity and mortality associated with infections. The advent of home therapy with IVIg or SCIg has also significantly enhanced the patient's quality of life and sense of self with their participation in the control of their disease. If antibody-deficient patients are diagnosed early, replacement Ig has been shown to reduce the rate, severity, and frequency of acute and chronic bacterial infections. The avoidance of recurrent infections prevents permanent structural damage to organs such as the lungs (e.g. bronchiectasis). Some short- and long-term complications are associated with antibody deficiency syndromes including increased incidence of certain autoimmune disorders, in particular cell cytopenias and inflammatory and granulomatous lesions in the GIT and lungs. There is also occurrence of some forms of noninfectious arthritis, as well as some associated with infectious agents. Over time, however, there is an increased incidence of antibody-deficient patients developing non-Hodgkin's lymphoma (NHL). Ig replacement therapy appears to protect against most of these complications, with the exception of the development of NHL. These observations and other evidence suggest that replacement Ig therapy gives protection beyond simply supplying antimicrobial antibody activity.

Replacement Ig is believed (on the basis of limited evidence) to have additional immunomodulatory properties, and this has led to its much wider use in medical and surgical practice. The literature highlights anti-inflammatory and immunoregulatory mechanisms. These include neutralization of superantigens, blockade of FcR interactions, modulation of cytokines, anti-complement system activities, and modulation of the production of Tregs. Each of the cited mechanisms has had some supportive experimental data. Not surprisingly, Ig replacement therapy has been tried in a wide range of conditions with immune and inflammatory pathogenesis or perceived dysregulation. Beyond primary antibody immune deficiency, internationally and nationally licensed indications for the use of some Ig preparations include the treatment of severe idiopathic thrombocytopenic purpura, Guillain–Barré syndrome, CMV-induced pneumonitis post-transplantation, and Kawasaki's disease. Early Ig therapy has been shown to protect against the development of coronary artery aneurysms in patients with Kawasaki's disease if treatment is instituted soon after disease onset. Some Ig preparations are licensed for use in defined cases of chronic lymphocytic leukaemia with associated antibody deficiency.

Various literature reviews have indicated more than 100 other different (off-label) uses of Ig therapy in medicine. These range from severe sepsis in the critically ill patient (see Chapter 5), autoimmune diseases including MS (see Chapter 8), *C. difficile* gut infections, chronic inflammatory polyneuropathies, bullous skin diseases, severe intractable asthma, transplantation for graft versus host disease, and in some situations treatment of highly sensitized patients in preparation for receiving a transplant (see Chapter 3). There is, in addition, a wide range of other secondary (acquired) immune deficiencies where Ig therapy has been tried. International expert panels have reviewed many of these uses and the studies that purport to support them. Consensus guidelines have been promulgated ranking the perceived benefits of Ig replacement in these myriad diseases. This is important for several reasons: perceived efficacy, safety, supply (shortage of Igs), and also economic cost–benefit considerations. Igs for therapeutic use are obtained from sourced pooled human blood plasma, using fractionation and purification methods that also involve anti-infectious agent protocols. As with all human-derived products there is some, albeit at times unquantifiable, risk regarding acquiring infections. IVIg replacement in antibody-deficient patients has, in past decades, been shown to have transmitted viral infection—e.g. hepatitis C with significant morbidity and limited mortality. Steps are now in place which should ensure against this recurrence; nevertheless the risks are still inherent in such human products. Concerns in the past decade have been raised about possible transmission of new variant Creutzfeldt–Jakob disease (nvCJD) by Ig preparations. It is sensible, therefore, that Ig therapy should be used where there is clear benefit that is significantly above any perceived risks and beyond that attainable with other treatment modalities. Additionally, and mainly because of the safety concerns, sourcing of human plasma has become more rigorous and restricted, with consequent falling supplies. This again reinforces the need for prioritizing the beneficial uses of this therapy, a treatment which is also costly.

References and further reading

1. Janeway CA. The immune system evolved to discriminate infectious non-self from non-infectious self. *Immunol Today* 1992; **1**: 11–16.
2. Janeway CA, Medzhitov R. Innate immune recognition: *Annu Rev Immunol* 2002; **20**: 197–216.
3. Human genome special issue. *Science* 2001; **291**: 1145–1434.
4. Initial sequencing and analysis of the human genome. *Nature* 2001; 409; 813–958.
5. Melum E, Franke A, Karlsen TH. Genome-wide association studies–a summary for the clinical gastroenterologist. *World J Gastroenterol* 2009; **15**: 5377–5396.
6. Zak DE, Aderem A. Systems biology of innate immunity. *Immunological Rev* 2008; **227**: 264–282.
7. Hunter CA, Kastelein R. New paradigms in inflammation. *Immunol Rev* 2008; **226**: 6–9.
8. Martinon F, Mayor A, Tschopp J. The inflammasomes: guardians of the body. *Annu Rev Immunol* 2009; **27**: 229–265.
9. Arend WP, Palmer G, Gabay C. IL-1, IL-18 and IL-33 families of cytokines: *Immunol Rev* 2008; **223**: 20–38.
10. Bianchi ME, Manfredi AA. High-mobility group box 1 (HMGB1) protein at the crossroads between innate and adaptive immunity. *Immunol Rev* 2007; **220**: 35–46.
11. Ben-Neriah Y, Schmidt-Supprian M. Epithelial NFκB maintains host gut microflora homeostasis. *Nat Immunol* 2007; **8**: 479–481.
12. Joffre O, Nolte MA, Spörri R, Reis e Sousa C. Inflammatory signals in dendritic cell activation and the induction of adaptive Immunity. *Immunol Rev* 2008; **227**: 234–247.

13. Ley K, Laudanna C, Cybulsky MI, Nourshargh S. Getting to the site of inflammation: the leukocyte adhesion cascade updated. *Nat Rev Immunol* 2007; **7**: 678–689.
14. Katz JB, Muller AJ and Prendergast GC. Indoleamine 2,3-dioxygenase in T cell tolerance and tumoral immune escape. *Immunol Rev* 2008; **222**: 206–221.
15. Lanier LL, Sun JC. Do the terms innate and adaptive immunity create conceptual barriers? *Nat Rev Immunol* 2009; **9**: 302–303.
16. Sun JC, Beilke JN, Lanier LL. Adaptive immune features of natural killer cells. *Nature* 2009; **457**: 557–561.
17. Kohler G, Milstein C. Continuous cultures of fused cells secreting antibody of predefined specificity. *Nature* 1975; **256**: 495–497.
18. Veillette A. Organization of immunoreceptor signalling by adaptors. *Immunol Rev* 2009; **232**: 5–6.
19. Guimond M, Veenstra RG, Grindler DJ, *et al.* IL-7 signalling in dendritic cells regulates the homeostatic proliferation and niche size of CD4+ T cells. *Nat Immunol* 2009; **10**: 149–157.
20. Ghoreschi K, Laurence A, O'Shea JJ. Selective and therapeutic inhibition of kinases: to be or not to be? *Nat Immunol* 2009; **10**: 356–360.
21. Woodland DL, Kohlmeier JE. Migration, maintenance and recall of memory T cells in peripheral tissues. *Nat Rev Immunol* 2009; **9**: 153–161.
22. Pittet M, Mempel TR. Regulation of T cell migration and effector functions: insights from in vivo imaging studies. *Immunol Rev* 2008; **221**: 107–129.
23. Varin A, Gordon S. Alternative activation of macrophages: immune functions and cellular biology. *Immunobiology* 2009; **214**: 630–647.
24. Horton R, Wilming L, Rand V *et al.* Gene map of the extended human MHC. *Nat Rev Genet* 2004; **12**: 889–899.
25. Ford ML and Larsen CP. Translating co-stimulation blockade to the clinic: lessons learned from three pathways. *Immunol Rev* 2009; **229**: 294–306.
26. Mosmann TR, Cherwinski H, Bond MW, Giedlin MA, Coffman RL. Two types of murine helper T cells clone: 1. definition according to profiles of lymphokine activities and secreted proteins. *J Immunol*1986; **136**: 2348–2357.
27. Mosmann TR and Coffman RL. TH1 and TH2 cells: different patterns of lymphokine secretion lead to different functional properties. *Annu Rev Immunol* 1989; **7**: 145–173.
28. Trifari S, Kaplan CD, Tran EH, Crellin NK, Spits H. Identification of a human helper T cell population that has abundant production of IL-22 and is distinct from TH17, TH1 and TH2 cells. *Nat Immunol* 2009; **10**: 884–871.
29. Bluestone JA, Mackay CR, O'Shea JJ, Stockinger B. The functional plasticity of T cell subsets. *Nat Rev Immunol* 2009; **11**: 811–816.
30. Izcue A, Coombes JL, Powrie F. Regulatory lymphocytes and intestinal inflammation. *Annu Rev Immunol* 2009; **27**: 313–338.
31. Ware CF. APRIL and BAFF connect autoimmunity and cancer. *J Exp Med* 2000; **192**: F35–38.
32. Wrammert J, Smith K, Miller J *et al.* Rapid cloning of high-affinity human monoclonal antibodies against influenza virus. *Nature* 2008; **453**: 667–672.
33. Bedoui S, Whitney PG, Waithman J *et al.* Cross presentation of viral and self antigens by skin-derived CD103+ dendritic cells. *Nat Immunol* 2009; **10**: 488–495.
34. Gebhardt T, Wakim LM, Eidsmo L, Reading PC, Heath WR, Carbone FR. Memory T cells in nonlymphoid tissue that provide enhanced local immunity during infection with herpes simplex virus. *Nat Immunol* 2009; **10**: 524–530.

35. Nolting J, Daniel C, Reuter S *et al.* Retinoic acid can enhance conversion of naive into regulatory T cells independently of secreted cytokines. *J Exp. Med* 2010; **206**: 2131–2139.
36. Zheng J, Liu Y, Lau YL, Tu W. CD40 activated B cells are more potent than immature dendritic cells to induce and expand CD4+ regulatory T cells. *Cell Mol Immunol* 2010; **7**: 44–50.
37. Review: immune responses to commensal and environmental microbes. *Nat Immunol* 2007; **8**: 1173–1178.
38. Morretta A, Locatelli F, Moretta L. Human NK cells: from HLA class I specific killer Ig-like receptors to the therapy of acute leukaemia. *Immunol Rev* 2008; **224**: 58–69.
39. Cerundolo V, Silk JD, Masri SH, Salio M. Harnessing invariant NK T cells in vaccination strategies. *Nat Rev Immunol* 2009; **9**: 28–38.
40. Fujii S, Shimizu K, Hemmi H, Steinman RM. Innate Vα14$^+$ natural killer T cells mature dendritic cells, leading to strong adaptive immunity. *Immunol Rev* 2007; **220**: 183–198.
41. Bischoff SC. Physiological and pathophysiological functions of intestinal mast cells. *Semin Immunopathol* 2009; **31**: 185–205.
42. Liew FY, Pitman NI, McInnes IB. Disease associated functions of IL-33: the new kid in the IL-1 family. *Nat Rev Immunol* 2010; **10**: 103–110.
43. Gibson DG, Glass JI, Lartigue C *et al.* Creation of a bacterial cell controlled by a chemically synthesized genome. *Science* 2010; **329**: 52–56.
44. Saraiva M, O'Garra A. The regulation of IL-10 production by immune cells. *Nat Rev Immunol* 2010; **3**: 170–181.
45. Glocker EO, Kotlarz D, Boztug K *et al.* Inflammatory bowel disease and mutations affecting the IL-10 receptor. *N Engl J Med* 2009; **361**: 2033–2045.
46. Vignali DA, Collison LW, Workman CJ (2008). How regulatory T cells work. *Nat Rev Immunol*; **8**, 523–532.
47. Elmore S. Apoptosis: a review of programmed cell death. *Toxicol Pathol* 2007; **35**: 495–516.
48. Virgin HW, Levine B. Autophagy genes in immunity. *Nat Immunol* 2009; **10**: 461–470.
49. Rizzi M, Ferrera F, Filaci G, Indiveri F. Disruption of immunological tolerance: role of AIRE gene in autoimmunity. *Autoimmun Rev* 2006; **15**: 145–147.
50. Krieg AM, Vollmer J. Toll-like receptors 7, 8 and 9: Linking innate immunity to autoimmunity. *Immunol Rev* 2007; **220**: 251–269
51. Rioux JD, Abbas AK. Paths to understanding the genetic basis of autoimmune disease: *Nature* 2005; **435**: 584–589.
52. Fife BT, Bluestone JA. Control of peripheral T cell tolerance and autoimmunity via CTLA-4 and PD-1 pathways. *Immunol Rev* 2008; **228**: 166–182.
53. Wellcome Trust Case Control Consortium. Genome-wide association study of 14,000 cases of seven common diseases and 3,000 shared controls. *Nature* 2007; **447**: 661–678.
54. Feldmann M, Steinman L. Design of effective immunotherapy for human autoimmunity. *Nature* 2005; **435**: 612–620.
55. Kanzler H, Barrat FJ, Hessel EM, Coffman RL. Therapeutic targeting of innate immunity with Toll-like receptor agonists and antagonists. *Nat Med* 2007; **13**: 552–559.
56. Webster KE, Walters S, Kohler RE *et al.* In vivo expansion of T reg cells with IL 2 mAb complexes. Induction of resistance to EAE and long term acceptance of islet allografts without immunosuppression. *J Exp Med* 2010; **206**: 751–760.
57. Maul RW, Gearhart PJ. Women, autoimmunity and cancer: a dangerous liaison between oestrogen and activation-induced deaminase? *J Exp Med* 2010; **206**: 11–13.

58. Wei B, Pei G. microRNAs: critical regulators in Th17 cells and players in diseases. *Cell Mol Immunol* 2010; **7**: 175–181.
59. Thomson AW, Turnquist HR, Raimondi G. Immunoregulatory functions of mTOR inhibition. *Nat Rev Immunol* 2009; **9**: 324–337.
60. Focus on neuroimmunology. *Nat Rev Immunol* 2009; 9 (special issue).
61. Goverman J. Autoimmune T cell responses in the central nervous system. *Nat Rev Immunol* 2009; **9**: 393–407.
62. Tracey KJ. Reflex control of immunity. *Nat Rev Immuno* 2009; **9**: 418–428.
63. Popovich PG, Longbrake EE. Can the immune system be harnessed to repair the CNS? *Nat Rev Neurosci* 2008; **9**: 481–493.
64. Editorial. The emergence of a new science of the mind: immunology benefits the mind. *Mol Psychiatry* 2010; **15**: 337–338.
65. Shakib F, Ghaemmaghami AM, Sewell HF .The molecular basis of allergenicity. *Trends Immunol* 2008; **12**: 633–642.
66. Mirakian R, Ewan PW, Durham SR *et al.* BSACI guidelines for the management of drug allergy. *Clin Exp Allergy* 2008; **39**: 43–61.
67. UNAIDS. *Report on the global AIDS epidemic, 2008.* http://www.unaids.org/en/KnowledgeCentre/HIVData/GlobalReport/2008/2008_Global_report.asp
68. McMichael AJ, Borrow P, Tomaras GD, Goonetilleke N, Haynes BF. The immune response during acute HIV-1 infection: clues for vaccine development. *Nat Rev Immunol* 2010; **10**: 11–23.
69. Hayden E.C. Seek, test and treat slows HIV. *Nature* 2010; **463**: 1006.

Journals

- Current Opinion in Immunology
- Nature Immunology
- Annual Review of Immunology
- Trends in Immunology
- Immunological Reviews
- Journal of Experimental Medicine
- Nature Reviews in Immunology

Online resources

Henry Stewart Talks: the Biomedical& Life Sciences Collection. http://hstalks.com/main/index_category.php?id=252

Video on kinetics of DC–lymphocyte interactions. http://authors.library.caltech.edu/10084/4/NOBblo08video1.avi

Textbooks

Todd I, Spickett G. *Lecture notes: Immunology* (6th edn). John Wiley & Sons, Chichester, 2010.

Murphy KM, Travers P, Walport M. *Janeway's immunobiology* (7th edn). Garland Science/Taylor & Francis, New York, 2007.

Chapter 2

Trauma and tissue injury

John C. Eun, Ernest E. Moore, Winston P. Choi, James H. Wood, Christopher Silliman, and Anirban Banerjee

Key summary points

- MOF is the leading contributor to post-trauma hospital mortality and ICU resource utilization.
- MOF is the result of a hyperactive innate immune system and a suppressed adaptive immune system.
- Gut ischaemia/reperfusion injury is critical for the development of trauma/haemorrhagic shock-induced ALI and mesenteric lymph is the link between the two.
- ALI and subsequent MOF is associated with a 'two-hit' model of events where the first insult recruits and 'primes' inflammatory mediators (such as neutrophils) and the second insult activates these proinflammatory mediators to cause end-organ damage.
- Various signalling molecules are elevated after trauma/haemorrhagic shock such as TNF-α, IL-1β, IL-6, IL-8.
- The coagulation system is a delicate balance between procoagulant factors and the fibrinolytic system and a change in one direction or the other can shift the balance from homeostasis to systemic clotting or coagulopathy.
- The inflammatory response to injury in children appears to be fundamentally distinct from that seen in adults and is probably due to the innate immune system being in a state of flux in children.
- Various therapies have been attempted to augment the body's response to injury by either decreasing inflammation, enhancing the immune system, or modulating the gut via selective nutrition.

Host defences and the metabolic response to injury

Trauma background

According to the Centers for Disease Control and Prevention, 'unintentional injury' was the leading cause of death in the USA for individuals aged 1–44 years in 2006, and was the fifth leading cause of death overall. Adding deaths from homicide and suicide to unintentional injury, 'trauma' then becomes the third leading cause of death, preceded only by heart disease and cancer [1]. Up to 50% of trauma deaths can occur at the scene (from injuries to the heart, great vessels, or brainstem), but in cities with well-integrated trauma systems the patient hospital mortality for trauma can be low: 3% or less [2]. As surgical techniques and critical care have improved, we are now able to keep patients alive with injuries that would have been uniformly fatal 25 years ago. With progress, however, come new challenges. We are now able to artificially prolong life with the use of mechanical ventilators, pressor agents, and renal support, all in the hope of enabling surgical intervention, critical care therapy, or the natural healing process to work. Because of this extension of life, we are now encountering patients with multiple organ failure (MOF) who consume a very large percentage of our health care resources.

Trauma and multiple organ failure

MOF was first identified in 1975, and Ben Eiseman coined the term in 1977 from his experiences with 42 patients in Denver, Colorado [3]. This group of trauma surgeons found that patients who had failure of two or more vital systems had a 69% mortality rate [3]. Over the past 20 years several scoring systems have been proposed [4–6]. The Denver MOF score is one of the most commonly used and is based on the evaluation of four organ systems (respiratory, renal, hepatic, and cardiac), assigning each organ system a score of 0–3 depending on the level of dysfunction. MOF is defined as a score greater than 3, 48 hours after significant trauma. It is the net result of a dysfunctional immune response to injury, characterized by a hyperactive innate immune system and a suppressed adaptive immune system. Acute lung injury (ALI) is the first clinical manifestation of organ failure, followed by renal and hepatic dysfunction. ALI and subsequent MOF remain the leading cause of mortality after the first 24 hours of injury and represent a substantial health care expenditure [5]. Thus, knowledge of MOF pathophysiology and its mediators are essential to the surgeon who is managing the critically ill patient following trauma.

Mechanical tissue disruption and cellular damage trigger a cascade of proinflammatory reactions, namely the systemic inflammatory response syndrome (SIRS). SIRS is defined as having two or more of the following [6]:

- Body temperature greater than 38° C or less than 36° C.
- Heart rate greater than 90 beats per minute.
- Respiratory rate greater than 20 breaths per minute or $PaCO_2$ less than 32 mmHg.
- White blood cell (WBC) count greater than 12.0×10^9/L or less than 4.0×10^9/L, or the presence of more than 10% immature neutrophils.

SIRS primes the innate immune system in such a way that a secondary insult during this vulnerable window provokes an uncontrolled inflammatory response, culminating in early (day 3 postinjury or before) MOF [7,8]. Shock and simultaneous tissue injury initiate events resulting in a depressed adaptive immune response and a resultant compensatory anti-inflammatory response syndrome (CARS). This system is the body's attempt at modulating SIRS but, ironically, it renders the patient at risk for overwhelming infectious complications resulting in late MOF [9] (Figure 2.1).

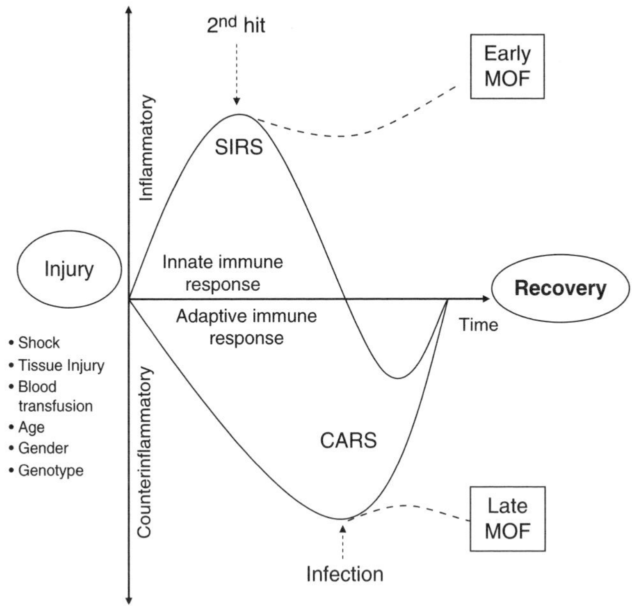

Fig. 2.1 The conceptual framework of multiple organ failure (MOF). CARS, compensatory anti-inflammatory response syndrome; SIRS, systemic inflammatory response syndrome.

The mechanism of trauma-induced immune system priming is currently an active area of research, but it is clear that the neutrophil is critical to this early response and can be used as a surrogate marker for proinflammatory activation of the innate immune system [10,11]. The role of the neutrophil in ALI and subsequent MOF is a well-studied pathophysiological process and is characterized by a two-hit model of events. The first hit (such as trauma) causes the release of soluble inflammatory mediators that can attract circulating neutrophils which are then sequestered in capillary beds such as those found within the lung. The neutrophil is also 'primed' to release potent cytotoxic factors upon activation. Patients at risk for MOF have a remarkably consistent pattern of postinjury neutrophil priming; beginning within 2 hours of injury, peaking at 6–12 hours, and finally resolving by 24 hours if there are no further insults [12,13]. A second hit (such as sepsis or hypotension) within this priming window then has the potential to activate these primed WBCs. The latter then transmigrate to the interstitial space where an amplified cytotoxic response occurs as the result of a substantial release of proteolytic enzymes and reactive oxygen species (ROSs) into the local environment causing indiscriminate tissue damage leading to ALI, and ultimately MOF [8,14].

Haemorrhagic shock has been consistently identified as a major risk factor for postinjury MOF [4], and the gut has been invoked as the mechanistic link between shock and MOF [15,16]. The gastrointestinal (GI) mucosa provides a remarkably effective barrier to the potentially toxic contents of the GI tract, but this barrier is exquisitely vulnerable to postinjury shock. This vulnerability stems from the body's prioritization over mesenteric needs. In response to haemorrhagic shock blood flow is diverted from the gut to more vital organ systems such as the brain, heart, and kidneys. The intestinal villus, the primary site of GI absorption, is uniquely precarious because its blood supply is derived from a single arterial vessel that arborizes at the villus tip into a network of surface capillaries emptying into a single venule. Following haemorrhagic shock, there is selective vasoconstriction of the intestinal inflow arterioles, mediated predominantly via the renin–angiotensin system [17]. Despite restoration of central haemodynamics, there is persistent vasoconstriction at all levels of the intestinal microvasculature due to the net effect of multiple agents such as vasopressin, endothelin, and the reduction of nitric oxide, as well as other circulating vasoactive substances [18,19].

The proinflammatory response stimulated by mesenteric ischaemia/reperfusion is complex, and the processes whereby local gut events translate into distant organ injury remain unclear. We do know that tissue ischaemia, and subsequent oxidant stress with reperfusion [20,21] activates families of protein kinases, such as mitogen-activated protein kinase, that converge on transcription factors, e.g. nuclear factor kappa light-chain-enhancer of activated B cell (NF-κB), CCAAT/enhancer-binding protein beta (C/EBPβ), and activator protein 1 (AP-1), that regulate the expression of inflammatory genes [21,23]. The resultant proinflammatory gene products include the cytokines tumour necrosis factor-alpha (TNF-α), interleukin-1 beta (IL-1β), and IL-6; the chemokine IL-8; intracellular adhesion molecules (ICAM-1); and enzymes such as inducible nitric oxide synthase and phospholipase A_2 (PLA_2); as well as an increase in anti-inflammatory cytokines such as IL-10 and protective enzymes such as haemeoxygenase-1 and cyclooxygenase-2 (COX-2) [24,25].

Multiple organ failure and mesenteric lymph

Initially, the role of the gut in MOF was linked with the concept of bacterial translocation via the portal circulation after circulatory shock. Subsequently, bacteria or endotoxin have not been found in the portal circulation of critically injured patients at risk for MOF [26]. In 1998, Magnotti *et al.* reported the important observation that ligation of the mesenteric duct in rodents, prior to the induction of haemorrhagic shock, prevented ALI [27]. This finding, coupled with subsequent rodent studies, have confirmed that postshock mesenteric lymph (PSML) can have profound systemic inflammatory effects compromising the integrity of distant organs [28,29]. Moreover, the central role of PSML in the pathogenesis of organ dysfunction has been confirmed in swine and nonhuman primates [30,31]. The identification of the toxic factors in PSML, however, remains a challenge. Mesenteric lymph represents a delta, which acts as a collecting basin for the diverse by-products from the gut. In the most basic sense, lymph can be separated into two fractions: an insoluble (lipid) fraction, and a soluble (protein) fraction.

We have had a long-term interest in the lipid mediators as the mechanistic link between splanchnic ischaemia and remote organ injury, and have shown that the nonpolar lipid portion of PSML has the ability to prime neutrophils *ex vivo* [32]. PLA_2 is a well-described proximal enzyme in the generation of proinflammatory lipids invoked in the pathogenesis of a number of hyperinflammatory processes [33]. We have found in human studies that mesenteric ischaemia/reperfusion activates gut PLA_2

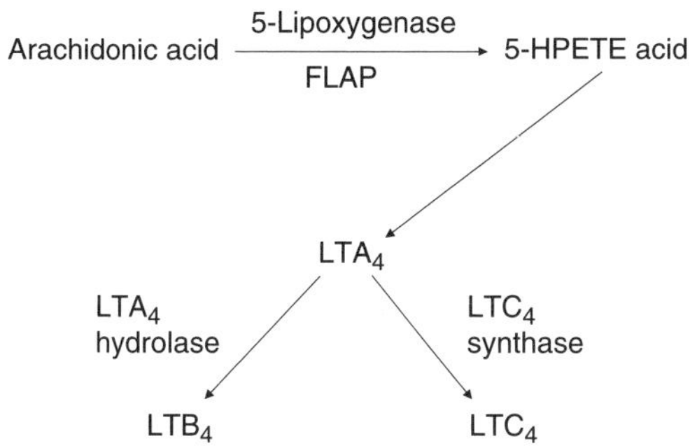

Fig. 2.2 The 5-lipooxygenase (5-LOX) pathway. FLAP, 5-lipoxygenase activating protein; 5-HPETE, 5-hydroxyperoxyeicosatetraenoic (acid); LTs, leukotrienes.

[34]. Also, in rodent experiments a PLA_2 inhibitor prevented haemorrhagic shock-induced ALI [35]. Thus, there is compelling evidence to support the postulate that the predominant proinflammatory lipid in PSML is PLA_2 or its metabolic products. PLA_2 hydrolyses fatty acids from the sn-2 position of a phospholipid backbone. One of the potential fatty acids released from PLA_2 activity is arachidonic acid (ARA). ARA, released by PLA_2, is subsequently modified by COXs and lipooxygenases (LOXs) to generate bioactive eicosanoids. COX-1 is constitutively expressed throughout the gastrointestinal tract and has been suggested to maintain mucosal integrity, while COX-2 is typically activated in response to inflammation [24,29,36]. LOXs, on the other hand, are not constitutively active, but when they are induced the resulting leukotrienes (LTs) are predominately proinflammatory. The LOX system in humans consists of three primary pathways: 5-LOX, 12-LOX, and 15-LOX [37,38]. LTs are metabolites of ARA and are generated by the action of 5-LOX and its coenzyme 5-LOX activating protein (FLAP) to 5-hydroxyperoxyeicosatetraenoic (5-HPETE) acid which is further acted upon by 5-LOX/FLAP to produce the intermediate LTA_4. LTA_4 is a highly unstable epoxide which is enzymatically hydrolysed by LTA_4 hydrolase into LTB_4 or conjugated with reduced glutathione by the action of LTC_4 synthase to produce LTC_4 [39]. Regulation of the biosynthesis of LTs is controlled at several levels, including the amount of ARA available, the presence of the 5-LOX pathway enzymes, the activation state of these enzymes which are modified via protein kinase phosphorylation, and the presence of oxidants and nitric oxide that can further alter enzyme activity [39,40] (Figure 2.2) LTB_4 is one of the most effective chemotactic agents for neutrophils, monocytes, and macrophages [40,41]. LTB_4 stimulates neutrophil chemotaxis, increases their adherence to endothelial cells, stimulates the release and generation of ROSs, and can increase 5-LOX activation in neutrophils to produce more LTB_4 [42,43]. Elevated levels of LTB_4 have also been seen in several inflammatory diseases such as psoriasis, inflammatory bowel disease, and acute respiratory distress syndrome (ARDS) [43,44]. LTC_4 is a potent constrictor of arterioles that increases permeability of the postcapillary venules resulting in capillary leak and oedema formation [40,41].

5-LOX is expressed predominantly in cells of myeloid origin (e.g. neutrophils, monocytes, macrophages). FLAP is a membrane-associated protein that is also essential for LT production via its interaction with 5-LOX, but the precise role/mechanism of action of this protein remains unclear [45,46]. LTA_4 hydrolase is expressed widely in cells including neutrophils, red blood cells (RBCs), endothelial cells, and epithelial cells, and is seen in high levels in the small intestine and the lung [47,48]. LTC_4 synthase is expressed primarily in cells of myeloid origin but is also present in platelets which do not contain 5-LOX [49,50]. Platelets, however, can import LTA_4 through a process termed transcellular metabolism [51]. LTA_4 is produced by a cell that has 5-LOX (such as the neutrophil) and the newly synthesized LTA_4 is transferred to the platelet via unknown mechanisms to produce LTC_4 [51]. The actions of LTB_4 are mediated via at least two distinct G-protein-coupled receptors, referred to as BLT_1 and BLT_2 [52,53]. BLT_2 is expressed ubiquitously but with low affinity, while BLT_1 is expressed primarily on leucocytes and with high affinity. LTB_4 is inactivated by metabolic conversion into a number of products. Various isoforms of the P450 enzyme serve to metabolize LTB_4, including cytochrome P450 (CYP4F) in human neutrophils [54]. The liver serves as the principle site for LTB_4 clearance from the systemic circulation where hepatic CYP4F2 metabolizes LTB_4 to its ω-hydroxylated metabolite 20-hydroxy-leukotriene B_4 (20-OH-LTB_4) which is subsequently carboxylated to 20-carboxy-LTB_4 (20-COOH-LTB_4) [54]. The cysteinyl LTs (LTC_4 and its subsequent products LTD_4, and LTE_4) also bind to G-protein-coupled receptors, $CysLT_1$ and $CysLT_2$. $CysLT_1$ is predominantly responsible for mediating bronchospasm and airway oedema. There is extensive research data and clinical corroboration invoking cysteinyl LTs in the pathogenesis of asthma as well as in atherosclerosis [50]. There is also evidence suggesting a critical role for LTB_4 in the pathogenesis of ALI following both remote ischaemia and local insults [55,56].

It is known that lipids require protein carriers, and that unique carriers exist to target certain lipids. There is also evidence for crosstalk between cytokines and LTs in promoting inflammation [41]. Thus, perhaps changes in the protein fraction of PSML may also play a role in the development of haemorrhagic shock-induced ALI and subsequent MOF. Leak *et al.* have shown that the proteome of mesenteric lymph is quantitatively and qualitatively different from that found in plasma under normal conditions, and that certain proteins seem to be unique to mesenteric lymph [57]. More recent proteomic data investigating the difference between pre- and postshock lymph have shown a decrease in several protease inhibitors such as α_2-macroglobulin, α_1-inhibitor 3, and an increase in lipid carriers such as major urinary protein, apoprotein A-I, and apoprotein A-IV [58]. This decrease in protease activity can result in the uncontrolled action of known neutrophil-associated proteases, such as elastase, to indiscriminately attack the capillary bed of the lung and lead to ALI and finally MOF [58].

MOF can be the end product of an overactive immune system that damages the host it was designed to protect. This maladaptive immune response can be triggered by haemorrhagic shock-induced gut ischaemia/reperfusion injury, which activates PLA_2 and other enzymes to send bioactive mediators to the lung via mesenteric lymph. Not only do neutrophils carry proinflammatory lipids that cause leucocyte recruitment, adhesion, and priming, but also the lipids are depleted of protective factors present in normal lymph. The net result is a state of proinflammation that can ultimately lead to end-organ injury.

Host defences and the critical care setting

Background

The intensive care unit (ICU) was originally developed as a multidisciplinary approach to patients experiencing acute, life-threatening single organ failure as the result of severe illness, trauma, or surgery. Fifty years ago, MOF was unheard of, as it was impossible to keep patients alive long enough for sequential organ dysfunction to develop [59]. With the advances in trauma and acute care surgery, MOF has become the driving force of focused investigation, particularly in the areas of organ failure after trauma [3,60]. Progress in the treatment of the acutely ill surgical patient, in both the operating theatre and the ICU, have yielded significant improvements in patient outcomes, despite a progressively rising risk of MOF [5]. Even so, MOF continues to be the leading contributor to postinjury mortality in hospital and to the utilization of ICU resources [61,62].

Although a great diversity of severe illnesses may incite a common pattern of progressive organ failure, the unifying feature of its pathology is a dysregulated balance between pro- and anti-inflammatory mediators of the innate and adaptive immune systems [59,63]. Ischaemia–reperfusion injury, hypovolaemic shock, burns, extensive soft-tissue injury, and other perturbations result in a progressive increase in systemic derangement along the spectrum of the SIRS [62,64]. MOF is the most severe manifestation of that pathology, responsible for 50–60% of all trauma-related deaths occurring more than 48 hours after injury [5,61,65].

Epidemiology

Factors which place individual patients at risk for prolonged ICU stays are multiple and complex. They involve patterns of pre-existing conditions overlaid on the specifics of antecedent trauma, and the methods by which they are treated [59]. In order to better define the epidemiology of MOF, we carried out a literature review and retrospective study of our ICU patient database to identify and establish pertinent standard definitions [66,67], and then established a prospective postinjury MOF database [63,68]. Over a 4-year period, 457 surgical ICU patients were analysed for host factors, tissue injury indexes, and clinical indicators of shock in an effort to stratify MOF susceptible patients from those less at risk. Injury severity score (ISS), number of transfused RBCs, base deficit, and lactate levels were all significantly associated with the development of MOF. In addition, MOF has a greater incidence and mortality following blunt trauma versus penetrating trauma, with an odds ratio of 1.7 and a mortality rate of 13% versus 3% [7,69,70].

In general, patients who experience postinjury MOF have long stays in ICU (mean 19 days) and a mortality rate of between 27% and 100%, depending on the number of organs involved [63,65,71,72]. Additionally, there appears to be a bimodal pattern of MOF, whereby high-risk patients may be stratified into ‘early’ versus ‘late’ presenters [63]. In a prospectively evaluated cohort of 457 high-risk trauma patients, we demonstrated that of the 70 (15%) patients who developed MOF, 27 (39%) presented early (by admission day 3), and 43 (61%) presented late (after day 3, peak at day 7) [63]. The risk factors for early and late MOF were identified by multiple logistic regression analysis and showed slightly different patterns. Independent risk factors for early

MOF included an ISS of 25 or more, emergency department systolic blood pressure of less than 90 mmHg, early blood transfusion of more than 6 units, and a lactate level of 2.5 mmol/L or greater 13–24 hours after admission. In contrast, risk factors for late MOF included age greater than 55 years, early blood transfusion of more than 6 units, early base deficit of greater than 8 meq/L, and a lactate level of 2.5 mmol/L or greater 13–24 hours after admission [68].

Patterns such as these have been corroborated by other investigators [70,71,72]. These findings underline the complexity of trauma and resuscitation physiology, whereby, the initial insult either promotes severe SIRS (one hit), or primes for an immediate secondary insult (two hits) resulting in early MOF. Alternatively, simultaneous compensatory anti-inflammatory mechanisms promote a relatively immunocompromised state, allowing severe secondary infections to occur, hence late MOF [63] (Figure 2.1).

Multiple longitudinal epidemiological studies of MOF have clarified the changing characteristics of the trauma population, as well as the incidence of organ failure therein. In a 12-year prospective study at a level I trauma centre in Denver, with an overall MOF incidence of 25%, Ciesla *et al.* reported a progressive decrease in adjusted MOF incidence and MOF-related mortality, despite a patient population with increasing ISSs and age [5]. Of the patients who developed MOF, there was a significant decrease in disease severity and duration, although the overall mortality rate remained constant [5]. These improvements were attributed to advances in trauma surgery and ICU treatment protocols, particularly the implementation of a conservative blood transfusion strategy [5].

In a 25-year retrospective study of organ failure after blunt trauma in patients with an ISS greater than 15, Nast-Kolb *et al.* reported an unchanged incidence of MOF, despite steadily increasing patient ages [73]. Overall mortality, however, decreased significantly from 28.7% to 13.9% ($p<0.001$) [73]. Mortality due to organ failure specifically, decreased from 18% to 4.1% ($p<0.001$), while the age of patients dying from organ failure increased from 44 ± 3 years to 63 ± 6 years ($p=0.04$) [73].

These and other studies have shown that trauma-related organ dysfunction remains a persistent problem; however, our ability to treat its sequelae has improved considerably. Although there remains much controversy over whether or not the incidence of MOF itself is decreasing, MOF-related deaths are certainly decreasing. Advances over the last several decades have allowed stepwise optimization in the resuscitation and critical care management of the most challenging injured patients. Improvements such as goal-directed resuscitation, lung-protective ventilator settings, intensive glucose control, immune enhanced and early enteral nutrition, damage control surgery, and the judicious use of blood products have all contributed to decreases in mortality and prevention of secondary injury [5,61,73].

Inflammatory mediators

Severe injury elicits a whole body response which sets into motion both the proinflammatory and anti-inflammatory aspects of the immune system. MOF is the manifestation of a widespread, dysfunctional immune response which occurs via several distinct routes. Massive or multiple sequential insults at the time of injury may elicit severe SIRS and subsequent early MOF [65,68]. A less severe physiological response to injury may prime the cells of the innate immune system such that a secondary, otherwise innocuous, inflammatory stimulus results in overt hyperinflammation and end-organ damage [7,59,61]. Examples of relevant second hits include delayed haemorrhage, blood transfusions, hypoxaemic events, and skeletal fracture fixation. These features have been described by many as the one-hit and two-hit processes, respectively. Late MOF, on the other hand, is a pathophysiologically distinct entity in which the generation of a CARS produces a state of delayed immunosuppression, several days after the inciting trauma [74,75]. The result is a depressed adaptive immune system which predisposes to infection and an increased risk of late MOF (Figure 2.1).

Both SIRS and CARS have been postulated to act simultaneously, even in the early phase after injury. The actual response at specific time points after injury is defined by the relative levels of each mechanism as they pertain to the innate (SIRS) and adaptive (CARS) immune systems [76]. In other words, if there is no second hit during the vulnerable windows either early or late in the postinjury course, MOF is not likely to occur.

Signalling molecules

Inflammatory and anti-inflammatory mediators, as well as the phenotype of associated leucocytes, have been widely used to characterize the systemic responses to trauma. Patients who develop MOF have higher levels of proinflammatory cytokines in their circulation. The role of TNF-α and IL-1β in the pathophysiology of sepsis and MOF has been well established [77]. Evidence has been compiled from three major sources of data: (1) circulating levels of cytokines in animals and patients correlate with outcome; (2) injection of inflammatory agents into humans and animals elicits a similar response; and (3) blockade of those cytokines decreases the organ failure and mortality that occurs with sepsis [78]. Unlike septic shock, however, the role these cytokines play in trauma and haemorrhagic shock is less clear.

Both TNF-α and IL-1β are present in the bronchoalveolar lavage fluid (BALF) of patients at risk for ARDS and with established ARDS, thus reflecting a possible pathophysiological role in ALI [79,80]. The highest concentrations of TNF-α and IL-1β occur in the BALF of patients with sustained ARDS, and the ratios of BALF to serum cytokine concentrations suggest a pulmonary origin [80,81]. On the other hand, data regarding TNF-α and IL-1β as plasma markers of inflammation after trauma have not demonstrated such convincing correlations.

IL-6 has been shown to be consistently elevated in both animal models of haemorrhagic shock, as well as in humans experiencing trauma or undergoing major surgery [78]. Unlike TNF-α, plasma IL-6 levels are not significantly elevated until 2 hours posthaemorrhage, and the levels remain elevated up to 24 hours after the induction of haemorrhage [82]. Elevations in IL-6 levels in patients have been shown to correspond with the windows of organ failure susceptibility [83]. IL-6 also correlates with the degree of injury [76,84], and high levels are predictive of subsequent organ failure and mortality [85,86].

In post-trauma patients with established ARDS, levels of the chemotactic chemokine IL-8 in BALF correlate with the levels of neutrophil infiltration, but not necessarily with the severity of lung injury, or the subsequent clinical course [80,87,88]. IL-8 levels are also elevated systemically in conjunction with IL-6, promoting a generalized proinflammatory state.

The cytokine response after injury is not restricted to those cytokines which specifically recruit and activate leucocytes, and is accompanied by a compensatory anti-inflammatory milieu. Elevated levels of anti-inflammatory immunosuppressive mediators such as IL-4, IL-10, prostaglandin(PG)-E2, and transforming growth factor-beta (TGF-β) are all found after trauma with a similar dynamic profile to their proinflammatory counterparts [74]. Although these mediators are likely to have a profound effect on the crosstalk of involved leucocytes, their precise roles are not well established [74].

There is mounting evidence that patients who experience MOF differ markedly in terms of their cytokine expression profile from those who do not. In addition to early predictors of MOF, as described previously, cytokine expression also follows a consistent temporal relationship with the time of injury that stratifies patients by risk [83,89]. Jastrow *et al.* demonstrated that trauma patients who had MOF exhibited substantially increased levels of both proinflammatory and anti-inflammatory signalling molecules, when compared with trauma patients who did not have MOF [89]. Serum levels of chemokine ligand 10 (IP-10), macrophage inflammatory protein 1 beta (MIP-1β), IL-10, IL-6, IL-receptor agonist (IL-1Ra), and eotaxin were each identified as independent predictors of MOF [89]. In a separate study, Maier *et al.* demonstrated that late MOF patients exhibited higher serum levels of soluble TNF-α receptors p55 and p75 than all other subgroups. The initial values (<24 hours from injury) of these receptors were also predictive of late MOF development [90].

Haemorrhagic shock and resuscitation, as the prototype of trauma-related immune priming, results in the entry into the circulation of multiple active mediators, including proinflammatory lipids and proteins, in addition to the aforementioned cytokines and chemokines. Diverse substances such as platelet-activating factor (PAF), LTB_4, C5a, substance P, TNF, IL-8, granulocyte–macrophage colony-stimulating factor (GM-CSF), interferon (INF), and lipopolysaccharide (LPS) may all act as neutrophil priming agents [7,61]. Investigation into the mechanisms of shock-mediated priming have identified postischaemic gut PLA_2 activation as an important early event [41]. Mesenteric lymph is the conduit for proinflammatory lipids generated in the reperfused splanchnic bed [7].

Pattern recognition receptors

The innate immune system neutralizes a broad diversity of extracellular microorganisms via the Toll-like receptors (TLRs). These pattern recognition receptors (PRRs) have recently been associated with ischaemia and reperfusion-mediated proinflammatory states relevant to trauma [91]. Ligands for the TLRs were first described as the well-known pathogen-associated molecular patterns (PAMPs). They include substances such as peptidoglycan (TLR1, TLR2, TLR6), CpG DNA motifs (TLR9), viral RNA (TLR3, TLR7, TLR8), and LPS (TLR4) [92,93]. Endogenous antigens released by cells after trauma may also activate immune cells via these same primordial PRRs.

TLR activation, for example, is integral to the pathogenesis of several noninfectious conditions including ischaemia [90], atherosclerosis [94], osteoporosis [95], and obesity [96]. The concept of cellular crosstalk via damage-associated molecular patterns (DAMPs) during inflammation or tissue injury describes the process by which sterile tissue disruption initiates or propagates noninfectious inflammatory states [91,97,98].

TLR4, in particular, has been shown to mediate the inflammatory response in experimental models of shock. Prince *et al.* demonstrated that mice deficient in TLR4 were protected from liver injury after haemorrhagic shock and resuscitation (HS/R) as evident by decreased levels of circulating proinflammatory cytokines, and decreased NF-κB activation [99]. In the lung, it was demonstrated that TLR4 signalling was necessary for lung injury induced by haemorrhagic shock, as seen by decreased lung TNF-α levels, protein leak, and accumulation of neutrophils in TLR4-deficient mice [100]. Thus, during ischaemic insult, the release of DAMPs may represent the link between oxidative stress and inflammation.

Several putative danger signals have been studied as potential mediators of immune activation after oxidative stress. Heat shock proteins (HSPs) exhibit increased circulating levels after cardiac and hepatic ischaemia and reperfusion injury [101,102]. They have been shown to mediate inflammatory responses in a variety of ischaemia and reperfusion models [103,104]. As endogenous chaperone and antigen presentation molecules, HSPs may function to deliver PAMPs to their respective TLRs, as highly purified HSPs do not function as TLR agonists alone [105].

The calcium-regulating protein S100 is a DAMP which is released after TLR4 receptor signalling. Its levels have been shown to be up-regulated in murine cardiac tissue exposed to LPS, with overexpression leading to decreases in calcium influx and cardiac ejection fraction [106]. The S100B isoform has also been shown to mediate infarct size and neurological deficits in cerebral ischaemia [107].

High-mobility group box 1 (HMGB1) protein is another DAMP which has received particular attention because of its involvement in many important infectious and noninfectious inflammatory processes [91]. After identification of its role as a late mediator in sepsis, HMGB1's additional properties as a DAMP were discovered through its release by necrotic cells, and its subsequent activation of inflammatory and tissue repair processes [108,109]. Serum levels of HMGB1 are also increased in models of ischaemia and reperfusion and haemorrhagic shock [91]. In an animal model of haemorrhagic shock, it was demonstrated that neutralizing antibodies to HMGB1 not only decreased systemic levels of IL-6 and IL-10, but also reduced gut permeability, bacterial translocation, and improved overall survival [110]. Although the putative cellular receptors for HMGB1 are still controversial, they are likely to include TLR2, TLR4, and the immunoglobulin superfamily member RAGE (receptor for advanced glycation end-products) [111–113].

Cellular immunity

Neutrophils are widely recognized to be the primary mediators of end-organ damage. Once primed, neutrophils enter into the vascular circulation, resulting in prominent neutrophilia 3 hours after injury [7,62,114]. Up-regulated adhesion molecules, including L-selectin and CD18, enable them to roll along the endothelium and marginate out of the circulation [114,115]. In patients who experience MOF, this event is then associated with a subsequent neutropenia by 6–12 hours, indicating a massive infiltration of primed neutrophils into peripheral organs [115]. End-organ damage then ensues via neutrophil activation and degranulation, releasing various cytotoxic elements including nitric oxide, ROSs, and proteolytic enzymes [7]. There is also an associated release of cytokines and chemokines from activated neutrophils including IL-6, IL-8, and TNF-α. In patients who do not experience MOF, there is no subsequent neutropenia, and priming resolves over the next 36 hours without end-organ damage [9].

The endothelium is also a very active participant in the inflammatory process. Neutrophil-mediated infiltration and tissue damage requires the up-regulation of adhesion molecules on both neutrophils and the microvascular endothelium. Endothelial adhesion molecules include the selectins (E-selectin, P-selectin), and molecules that belong to the immunoglobulin superfamily ICAM-1, vascular cell adhesion molecule-1 (VCAM-1). These cell surface components allow for rolling contact and tight adhesion, respectively. Increased expression of ICAM-1 on endothelial cells has been shown to be sufficient for neutrophil-mediated cytotoxicity [78,116]. This is a common pathway for microvascular and tissue injury.

In patients with haemorrhagic or septic shock, a second hit by proinflammatory cytokines or LPS induces an endothelial up-regulation of cell surface adhesion molecules, release of PAF, and potentiation of end-organ dysfunction [117–119]. Multiple studies of haemorrhagic shock in rat models have shown significant leucostasis in lung and liver, measured by the myeloperoxidase assay and intravital fluorescence microscopy [120,121]. Once tight adhesion between the endothelium and neutrophils occurs, the adherent leucocytes are able to transmigrate through the intercellular junctions and direct their movement via a chemotactic gradient into the tissue microenvironment. When excessive adhesion occurs, the cytotoxic arsenal of primed and activated neutrophils induce damage on host endothelial and parenchymal cells.

Conclusion

MOF remains the leading cause of mortality in patients surviving the initial resuscitation period after trauma and haemorrhagic shock. Advances in the ability of the acute care surgeon to treat severely injured patients have improved mortality when adjusted for age, ISS, and blood transfusion. However, the incidence of MOF in surgical ICUs continues unabated, consuming enormous amounts of health care resources.

Immunological priming via release of factors from reperfused splanchnic beds results in a bimodal window of susceptibility to subsequent end-organ damage. A second hit during this time period promotes widespread dysregulated inflammation, with neutrophils as the primary mediators of end-organ injury. Although elevations in cytokine and chemokine levels have been strongly associated with MOF prognosis and mortality, their pathophysiological relevance has yet to be completely elucidated. Newly described signalling molecules such as the DAMPs highlight the ever increasing complexity in the cellular mechanisms of ischaemia and reperfusion injury. These and other events which occur early in the post-traumatic treatment phase are likely to be responsible for the subsequent ICU length of stay and outcome. Thus, intense investigation continues in the search for immunomodulating agents which may prevent initial priming events, and maintain the homeostasis of the immune system throughout the recovery period.

Trauma and coagulation

Haemostasis and fibrinolysis

Haemostasis is the arrest of blood flow from or within a blood vessel and involves (1) the interaction of the vessel and the supporting structure, (2) the circulating platelets and their interactions with the disrupted vessel, (3) the formation of fibrin, (4) the regulation of clot extension, and (5) the repair of the injury following the cessation of bleeding [122]. When damage occurs to a blood vessel, the endothelial barrier is disrupted exposing collagen and tissue factor (TF). Platelets are recruited to the site of injury and a haemostatic plug is created, mediated by von Willebrand factor (vWF) and fibrinogen, which acts to temporarily slow down bleeding as well as providing a surface for further enzymatic reactions [122]. Concurrently, the coagulation system is triggered via TF activation of factor VII, producing thrombin. Thrombin activates platelets leading to the exposure of a site for clotting factor assembly on the platelets themselves. This allows for increased thrombin production, resulting in the establishment of an insoluble fibrin assembly with cross-linking by factor XIII [122]. This haemostatic plug is anchored by clot retraction and regulated by several 'anticoagulant' proteins such as antithrombin III, thrombomodulin, and the protein C and S systems, which inactivate the thrombin accelerator factors Va and VIIIa. In summary, coagulation is kept in check by three main routes: (1) inhibition of the initiation complex by TF pathway inhibitor (TFPI), (2) reduced thrombin generation by activation of the protein C pathway, and (3) direct inhibition of activated coagulation proteases by antithrombin III [123]. Over time, the clot is lysed by plasmin through activation of the fibrinolytic system.

Fibrinolysis is the clearing of excess fibrin from the circulation and is vital for anchoring the haemostatic plug, as well as limiting coagulation to the site of injury [122]. The deposition of fibrin activates tissue plasminogen activator (tPA) from the adjacent endothelium, which attaches to the fibrin strands converting circulating plasminogen to plasmin. Plasmin then acts to dissolve the fibrin clot. Localization of this process is due to immediate inactivation of any free plasmin by α_2-antiplasmin or α_2-macroglobulin and inhibition of tPA by plasminogen activator inhibitor-1 (PAI-1), which circulates in the plasma or is released by endothelial cells and platelets. Plasmin can also be inhibited by PAI-2 released from neutrophils [122]. Systemic fibrinolysis occurs when fibrinolytic proteases or plasminogen activators circulate and damage the clotting proteins and/or the haemostatic plugs, resulting in clinical bleeding; importantly, systemic fibrinolysis also impairs fibrin formation and inhibits platelet function [122]. In short, the coagulation system is a delicate interplay between factors that are circulating in the plasma or generated by the disruption of tissue. A change in one or other direction can move the balance from homeostasis to systemic clotting or coagulopathy.

Acute coagulopathy of trauma

Acute coagulopathy of trauma occurs in 25–30% of patients upon presentation to the emergency department, and its recognition and management varies widely [124]. Many surgical treatment approaches rely on traditional approaches and surgical dogma rather than on evidence-based medicine [124]. Diagnosis is based on a variety of variables, including estimated blood loss, temperature, pH, platelet counts, prothromin time (PT)/international normalized ratio (INR), partial thromboplastin time (aPTT), and overall clinical assessment [124]. Only 40% of trauma centres employ massive transfusion protocols; however, it is not known if they are activated immediately or only when the number of units transfused is excessive [124]. Most centres do not use specific triggers for the transfusion of fresh frozen plasma (FFP) or packed RBCs (PRBCs) and only a few have employed FFP:PRBC ratios [124]. Hypothermia and acidosis appear to be addressed more uniformly; thus, the approach to the injured patients with significant bleeding and an acute coagulopathy varies widely [124]. Awareness is crucial for these patients because coagulopathy is the fuel that continuously supports bleeding, and its presence can make the difference between responders and nonresponders in injured patients with significant haemorrhage [124]. Moreover, acute coagulopathy of trauma has remained the most prevalent and compelling reason for damage control, using a staged laparotomy which has become standard practice for all severely injured patients [125,126].

Massive transfusion is defined as more than 10 units of PRBCs in 24 hours, with special attention to those patients requiring greater than 10 units of PRBCs in the first 12 hours because of their predisposition to develop MOF. Both trauma and massive transfusion have inherent coagulation deficits, which are diverse, and it is important to understand both the background and influence of traumatic injury on homeostasis, which has led to the development of newer resuscitation strategies. The coagulopathy of massive transfusion has long been considered dilutional, and haemodilution of coagulation factors begins with the drawing of interstitial and cellular fluids into the plasma followed by resuscitation with crystalloid and PRBCs [125,127,128]. Although haemodilution remains a major cause of the acute coagulopathy of trauma, numerous studies suggest that there is no significant correlation between total blood transfused and the severity of the haemostatic defect; rather, the consumption of coagulation factors and platelets appears paramount [125,129,130]. The rubric of haemodilution requires a focus on the platelet count, and data from injured, massively transfused patients who received early platelet transfusions displayed a survival advantage, which supported this hypothesis [129,131]. Despite this intuitively reasonable explanation, in injured patients prophylactic platelet transfusions did not result in increased platelet counts over those that did not receive them. For injured patients who required massive transfusion, the majority did not experience platelet counts less than 100 000/mm^3 until 18 units of PRBCs were administered [132,133]. Additionally, in this patient group only 43% of the variations in platelet counts could be ascribed to the amount of blood transfused [132]. Taken together, these studies suggested that factors other than simple dilution affect the platelet count [132,133]. Furthermore, previous mathematical modelling of dilutional thrombocytopenia did not reflect the measured platelet counts in these severely injured patients [134]. Importantly, given the fact that the bleeding time, the best test for platelet function, has little clinical utility in massively transfused trauma patients, it appears logical to consider that coagulopathy in trauma patients results from a combined deficit of platelets and fibrinogen; therefore, focusing on platelets or specific clotting factors alone may lead to improper conclusions [125]. Moreover, when one takes into account the constitutional effects of hypothermia, acidosis, shock, and injury severity, a much more complicated coagulopathy may be present [125].

Shock appears to be a primary mediator of early coagulopathy after injury. There is a proportional relationship between the severity of tissue hypoperfusion and the degree of coagulopathy upon admission (via PT/aPTT) for patients with a base deficit of 6 or greater [135,136]. Although shock is intimately associated with acidaemia, which impairs protease activity, decreases the activity of coagulation factor complexes, and increases the degradation of fibrinogen, shock itself induces a coagulopathy that persists despite the return to normal pH by the instillation of parenteral buffers [137–139]. Such a coagulopathy may be secondary to widespread endothelial damage or stimulation inducing protein C activation, as determined by increased thrombomodulin activity and thrombin formation resulting in fibrinolysis [140,141]. This evidence is indirect but does offer activated protein C (APrC)-induced PAI-1 consumption or reduced activation of thrombin-activatable fibrinolysis inhibitor (TAFI) as explanations for the observed systemic hyperfibrinolysis.

Hypothermia (<35° C) slows the activity of the coagulation cascade, both intrinsic and extrinsic, through decreases in enzymatic activity, reduction of the synthesis of coagulation factors, increased fibrinolysis, and decreased platelet function [142,143]. Platelets are probably most affected due to the reduced effect of vWF traction on the GpIb/IX platelet receptor complex that mediates signalling essential for progress from simple platelet adhesion to activation [137,142,143]. Mild hypothermia is quite common, and significant reduction in enzymatic protease activity does not occur until core temperatures fall below 34° C, with increasing mortality seen at core temperatures less than 32° C [137,139,144]. However, at core temperatures commonly seen in injured patients (33–36° C) isolated hypothermia may not effect coagulation [137].

Coagulation and the immune system

Coagulation and immunity are intimately linked in the response to severe injury. Proteases are crucial in plasma-based coagulation and proteases may serve as signalling molecules via activation of specific protease-activated receptors (PARs) [145,146]. PARs are unique G-protein-coupled receptors activated by protease cleavage of their extracellular N-terminal domain leading to G-protein-mediated signalling [145]. Thrombin can activate PAR1, PAR3, and PAR4. TF:FVIIa and TF:FXa complexes can activate PAR1 and PAR2, respectively, and retention of APrC to the endothelial cell surface induces PAR1 activation [147,148]. PARs are expressed in the vascular endothelium and are responsible for changes in vascular tone and permeability such that PAR1 activation elicits ALI via increases in permeability of alveolar epithelium and pulmonary vascular endothelium [148–150]. PAR activation is required for platelet activation, but there are significant differences between animal models and humans [148].

PAR activation by thrombin or other proteases increases P-selectin expression, induces vWF release, and causes the synthesis and release of chemokines [151]. Low levels of PAR1 activity by APrC may mediate a very different response from thrombin [148]. In trauma, TF-based activation of PARs modulates inflammatory responses and appears to impact on MOF. Patients with postinjury ARDS had high levels of TF, which was not counterbalanced by TFPI, indicating that systemic production of TF and its interactions with other inflammatory mediators may play a role in postinjury ALI [152,153]. Moreover, PAR activation induced a proinflammatory response as shown by synthesis and/or release of IL-8, MCP-1, ICAM-1, and P-selectin [123]. Likewise, thrombin activates human microvascular endothelial cells (HMVECs) *in vitro*, resulting in neutrophil adherence through the production of proinflammatory membrane lipids including PAF, which was abrogated by $sPLA_2$ antagonists [154]. Importantly, the coagulation system is not the only source for proteases with the ability to induce signalling. Neutrophils can also release proteases from their granules that cause activation of PAR4 (via cathepsin G) and PAR2 (via proteinase 3), and activation of mast cells released tryptase which can also activate PAR1 [154,155].

ALI is a product of diffuse endothelial injury and increased capillary permeability [156]. The coagulation system is a major participant in ALI, and activation of coagulation both mediates ALI and is a consequence of it [156]. Sepsis and ALI represent a shift towards a procoagulant state, as demonstrated by marked increases in fibrinopeptide A, FVII, and D-dimer as well as decrease in fibrinolysis activity as seen in BALF fluid [156,157]. Extravascular fibrin deposition is also a hallmark of ALI/ARDS with increases in TF and the TF:FVIIa and TF:TXa complexes [158]. Additionally, TNF-α and IL-6 display procoagulant activity without affecting fibrinolysis by increasing the synthesis and release of TF [158]. Increased pulmonary coagulation in combination with decreased fibrinolysis results in ongoing pulmonary injury, which is counteracted by APrC through alterations in thrombin-induced permeability by binding the endothelial protein C receptor (EPCR) and increasing endothelial barrier protection [156,159]. Furthermore, the lowest protein C levels in patients with ALI correlated with the greatest mortality, and protein administration diminished the increases in IL-8 and ICAM-1 [160]. The many anti-inflammatory properties of APrC have been documented both *in vitro* and *in vivo*; however, clinical trials have not demonstrated its ability to attenuate ALI [161, 162].

ALI induced by sepsis and other causes is different from trauma-induced ALI [163], as shown by the following:

- Clinical—Trauma patients are young and less likely to have comorbidities, such as AIDS, diabetes, immunosuppression, renal failure, and significantly lower APACHE II scores.
- Blood pressure—Trauma patients have higher mean arterial blood pressures, lower incidence of vasopressor administration, and higher urine output.
- Respiratory support—Trauma patients have a lower mean (ventilated) respiratory rate, higher PaO_2/FiO_2 and higher peak plateau and end-expiratory pressures, although injured patients have higher incidences of pneumothorax, subcutaneous emphysema, and tube thoracostomy.

- Laboratory findings—Trauma patients have a significantly lower haematocrit, platelet count, leucocyte count, serum creatinine and albumin but higher levels of bicarbonate.
- Biomarkers—Trauma patients have significantly lower baseline biomarkers including decreased ICAM-2, surfactant protein-D (SP-D), vWF, PAI-1, IL-8, and sTNFR-1.

In summary, patients with ALI as the result of injury have less endothelial and epithelial injury than nontrauma patients, resulting in the observed decreases in ALI-induced mortality for the trauma patient. Thus, further studies are required to elucidate the aetiology of trauma-induced ALI which may be related to injury severity, shock, and transfusions of plasma and stored blood components, which directly affect haemostasis and innate immunity of the host.

Transfusion-related acute lung injury

Transfusion-related ALI (TRALI) is the most common serious complication of blood transfusions worldwide with a reported incidence of 1/1333–1/5000 per unit transfused in North America, and associated with a mortality rate of 5–35%. Critically ill patients are more susceptible to TRALI, with a prevalence of 8–11% [164,165]. TRALI occurs within 6 hours of transfusion, with the majority of patients developing clinical features within 2 hours of transfusion. TRALI is defined as ALI with an acute onset, hypoxaemia with a PaO_2/FiO_2 less than 300 mmHg, radiographic evidence of bilateral pulmonary oedema despite normal cardiac function (pulmonary artery occlusion pressure ≤18 mmHg), in patients who received blood transfusions within 6 hours of developing symptoms [166]. All blood products have been associated with TRALI, but those that contain plasma, such as FFP, and whole blood-derived platelet concentrates (WB-PLTs) are the most common perpetrators [166].

The neutrophil and its interaction with the vascular endothelium is a key mediator in the development of TRALI. After trauma or infection, soluble proinflammatory mediators are released into the circulation that cause the activation of the vascular endothelium and, thus, the increase in adhesion molecules (selectins). As the neutrophils travel through the pulmonary vasculature, they are slowed in the pulmonary capillaries by the interaction between L-selectin on the neutrophil and P- and E-selectins on the endothelial cell [166,167]. Within the lung, chemokines such as IL-8 cause a change in adhesion molecule expression whereby the L-selectins are shed and replaced by β_2-integrins on the neutrophil, which adhere to ICAM-1 on the endothelial cell, thereby, sequestering neutrophils in the lung. Along with activation of the endothelium, the neutrophils becomes 'primed' and experience changes that not only increase adherence to endothelial cells but also stimulate the antibacterial mechanisms for an enhanced respiratory burst [166,167]. These primed hyperactive neutrophils sequestered in the lung can then be activated to release their antibacterial products to cause endothelial cell damage, and subsequent ALI [166–168].

There are currently three hypotheses for the pathogenesis of TRALI:

- Antibody-mediated TRALI—The infusion of donor antibodies specific for human leucocyte antigen (HLA) class I and their reaction with these on neutrophils and endothelium of the recipient.

- Antibody-mediated TRALI—The infusion of donor antibodies specific for HLA class II antigens expressed by the immune and vascular endothelial cells of the recipient.
- The two-event model of TRALI—The initial insult leading to hospital admission is the first event that causes priming of the neutrophils and activation of the endothelial cells, and transfusion itself is the second event—either from donor-derived antileucocyte antibodies or biological response modifiers (BRMs) in the transfused product itself [166]. This postulate of initial neutrophil priming and subsequent activation is analogous to the two-hit model of trauma-associated MOF, described previously.

The incidence of TRALI does not seem to be affected by the leucocyte reduction of transfusion products, but there appears to be evidence that increased age of the blood products carries an increased risk, as do blood products from multiparous female donors [164]. It appears that the only effective method for the treatment and/or decrease in TRALI is education and prevention of the overuse of blood products, especially in the critically ill patient [164].

TRALI is the end result of an inflammatory response triggered or activated by an injury and subsequent blood transfusion. Although the exact cause is unknown, what is known is that TRALI is the result of a hyperactive immune system, which leads to end-organ dysfunction manifested by lung injury. TRALI is dependent on the activation of pulmonary vascular endothelial cells and the priming of neutrophils triggered by an initial proinflammatory insult, followed by a blood transfusion that provides additional proinflammatory stimuli to cause lung injury. TRALI has a high mortality, and the judicious use of blood products is critical to preventing this hospital-associated disease entity.

Host defences and the metabolic response to injury in children

Background

Surgeons have long believed that children are unlikely to develop MOF in the setting of major trauma, but so far only one study has specifically investigated rates of MOF in injured children [169]. In a retrospective review of 579 children (age <16 years) with ISSs greater than 15, it was found that the incidence of MOF in severely injured children who survived greater than 24 hours was only 1%. There were no adult patients for direct comparison in this study, but a subsequent analysis of 1244 comparably injured adult patients (age >16 years, ISS>15) followed prospectively over a 12-year period at the same institution revealed an incidence of MOF of 25% [5]. These findings are consistent with other reports (range 13–26%) [170,171]. The findings of these two studies strongly support the conclusion that MOF occurs at a significantly lower rate in traumatically injured children than in adults.

Furthermore, children tend to develop MOF in a different temporal pattern from adults. In contrast to adults, progressive, sequential organ failure beginning at least 48 hours after injury is the exception in children [172]. In the small number of children who developed postinjury MOF, in the study by Calkins *et al.* all did so within the first week of admission [169]. Other studies, which included noninjured, critically ill children with sepsis or bone marrow transplantation, found that MOF tends to occur early in the course of paediatric ICU admissions and in an overwhelming, organ-simultaneous manner [173,174].

These findings suggest that the inflammatory response to injury in children may be fundamentally different from that of adults. However, the mechanisms by which the less mature immune system may confer a cumulative protective effect in injured children remains unclear.

Development of the immune system

Several aspects of the neonatal immune system may increase susceptibility to infection and decrease susceptibility to diseases of hyperinflammation [175–177]. These include down-regulation of complement, phagocytic activity, and macrophage function, as well as an anti-inflammatory cytokine predisposition [178–180].

At birth, the immune system begins to change from a state of 'foetal lethargy,' in which a strong T helper 2 (Th2) anti-inflammatory predisposition presumably protects the infant from allogeneic immune responses to maternal antigens *in utero* [180]. The Th2 predominance is maintained in the neonatal period by an intrinsic bias of costimulatory cells (monocytes and antigen-presenting cells) against Th1 immune responses [181–183]. For example, stimulation of mononuclear cells from cord blood (serving as a surrogate for foetal blood) by agonists of TLRs 1–7 results in 1–3 log less production of proinflammatory TNF-α, than equivalent stimulation of adult peripheral blood mononuclear cells (PBMCs) [183]. Furthermore, TLR4 stimulation in cord blood and neonatal blood produces an anti-inflammatory-biased pattern of cytokine production, with increased IL-10 (anti-inflammatory) and decreased IL-12 (proinflammatory) production, as compared with adults [181].

This paradigm has now been called into question by Halonen *et al.*, who report a 2–10-fold decrease in production of both Th1 and Th2 cytokines by foetal and infant-derived mononuclear cells, with no significant Th2 cytokine bias, when compared with adults [184]. These findings suggest that Th1/Th2 balance in the foetus and newborn infant is more complex than previously thought, but corroborate the notion of an immune system in a state of flux.

Several studies have demonstrated phenotypical and functional changes in immune cells throughout childhood, and the cumulative evidence of these data suggest that paediatric immunity maintains the Th2, anti-inflammatory predisposition. This has been demonstrated in studies using monocytes, PBMCs, $CD4^+$ T cells, and peritoneal macrophages [185–189].

There is a well-correlated relationship between age and cytokine production by circulating cells of the immune system for most cytokines and chemokines. For example, there appears to be a direct proportional relationship between age and monocyte production of IFN-γ, TNF-α, IL-2, IL-12, whereas IL-10 production showed no age pattern [186]. Others have also reported age-related increases in IL-12 production by PBMCs [187].

In contrast to circulating immune cells, resident tissue macrophages in children appear to have a more prominent cytokine response to stimulation than those from adults [189,190]. However, these macrophages maintain a strong anti-inflammatory balance with the IL-10 to TNF-α ratio being consistently greater in macrophages from children compared with adults.

The duration of these changes during childhood is unclear. Maximal levels of IL-10 and IL-12 production by PBMCs do not appear to reach adult levels during the first decade of life, but there may be a reversal of the IL-10 to IL-12 ratio from high to low by age 5 [187]. Furthermore, although not directly related to postinjury inflammation, $CD4^+$ T cell production of IFN-γ in response to staphylococcal toxin appears to reach adult levels around age 10 [188]. These data suggest that the immune system persists in a state of transition, at least into the second decade, with some responses and cytokines approaching adult levels more quickly than others.

Injury-induced inflammation in children

The implications of a maturing immune system for the response to injury are not immediately evident. Furthermore, it is uncertain how differences of immunity observed *in vitro* translate into clinical outcomes, where the response to injury involves the coordination of several complex biological systems.

There are no clinical laboratory data on cytokine levels in paediatric trauma. However, data from patients with burns may offer insight into the cytokine responses likely to occur after traumatic injury. Finnerty *et al.* examined the circulating levels of 22 cytokines in 25 adults and 24 children who sustained and survived burns of >20% total body surface area [191]. Cytokines were measured at multiple time points, ranging from 0 to 66 days, and only two cytokines, GM-CSF and IL-6, were different at more than two time points. This suggests that age-related outcome discrepancies in burned patients may not be attributed to significant differences in circulating levels of cytokines. It is not known whether this is also true for trauma-induced inflammation. However, this study suggests that future research should focus on nuances of paediatric immunity, such as the CARS mechanisms which could account for the differences of postinjury inflammation not explained by circulating cytokine levels.

Using a rat model, researchers have validated an age-related proclivity for haemorrhagic shock-induced ALI and SIRS, and they demonstrated that systemic and end-organ manifestations of uncontrolled inflammation are regulated at the nuclear level by changes in expression and function of peroxisome proliferator-activated receptor-N (PPAR-N) [192]. PPAR-N is down-regulated in the lung tissue of older rats, and major haemorrhage causes an additional, age-dependent, down-regulation of PPAR-N expression and activity, which is proportional to the severity of ALI.

In addition to suggesting mechanistic explanations for age-dependent ALI, the findings of this study reinforce the importance of paediatric-specific interventions for SIRS and MOF. Zingarelli *et al.* found that administration of a PPAR-N ligand attenuated inflammation in the lungs of young rats, but failed to confer a protective effect in mature rats [192]. They suggested that exogenous activation of PPAR-N may be an effective therapeutic strategy for the prevention of ALI in young injured patients.

There is great interest in immunomodulatory therapy in adults subjected to trauma [193] (discussed in the next section), but the findings published by Zingarelli *et al.* [192] suggest that caution is required when applying such therapy to paediatric patients, as the intended effects may be achieved only in the appropriately aged population.

Therapeutic modulation of host defences

The critically ill trauma patient has a dysfunctional immune system where the innate immune system is overactive and the adaptive immune system is underactive. These immune aberrations are triggered by cellular injury causing the release of a variety of immune-modulating signals that can lead to end-organ dysfunction and ultimately MOF. Thus, treatment of the trauma patient may take several forms, each trying to deal with a specific problem. One way to organize the variety of potential therapies is by their target goal: (1) decreasing inflammation, (2) enhancement of the immune system, and (3) gut modulation.

Decreasing inflammation

Hyperosmolar therapy

Earlier work with hypertonic saline (HTS) resuscitation in trauma patients suggested some clinical benefit [194]. However, more recent clinical trials have been discontinued because mortality was not significantly improved over standard resuscitation [195,196]. On the other hand, these trials have proven the inherent safety of HTS treatment. An apparent weakness in the use of HTS resuscitation (typically 4 mL/kg of 7.5% NaCl) is the short duration of elevated plasma osmolarity. In pigs, plasma sodium levels peak at 180 mM (which correlated to 380 mOsm) and plateaus at 150 mM (320 mOsm) for less than 1 hour [197]. As expected, osmolar changes in humans also appear to be temporary [196,198]. From *in vitro* experiments, however, it would appear that at least 180 mM of sodium (380 mOsm) is required to produce a beneficial effect [197–200].

Evidence suggests that the benefit of HTS on ALI and ARDS stems from the anti-inflammatory effects of HTS itself [196,201,202]. HTS has been shown to decrease alveolar macrophage activation and neutrophil recruitment into the lungs [199,203–205]. In the neutrophil, it has been shown that HTS decreases inflammatory receptor internalization and depresses the activation of the mitogen-activated protein (MAP) kinase pathway [206]. In cell culture experiments with pulmonary epithelial cells, HTS inhibited NF-κB, which has been associated with clinical ARDS. Furthermore, blocking NF-κB has been associated with decreased neutrophil infiltration and cytokine production [207–210].

Instead of using systemic HTS therapy, several studies have looked at targeted, inhaled HTS which has been shown to be beneficial in the treatment of cystic fibrosis and bronchiectasis [211,212]. While the mechanism of action of inhaled HTS remains to be elucidated, a likely explanation is the anti-inflammatory role HTS plays in immunomodulation [213]. Thus, the role of targeted hyperosmolar therapy may prove to be beneficial in the future.

Recent work in our laboratory has shown the potential benefit of inhaled HTS in a murine trauma/haemorrhagic shock (T/HS) model. In these experiments, rats underwent haemorrhagic shock (30 for 45 minutes with a base deficit of at least 20) and were

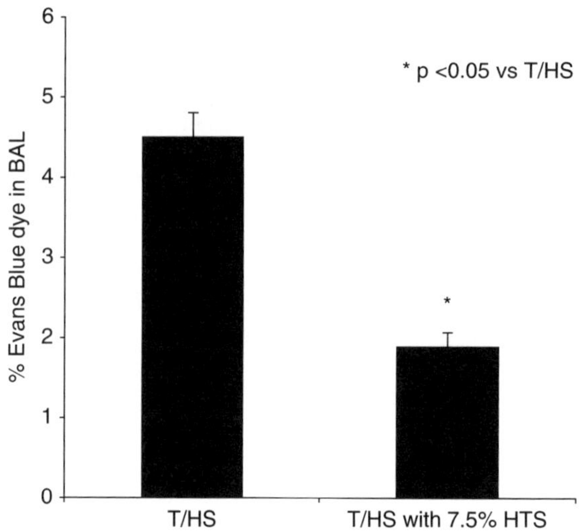

Fig. 2.3 The administration of 7.5% hypertonic saline (HTS) reduced the level of lung injury seen in animals who underwent trauma/haemorrhagic shock (T/HS).

then resuscitated with a combination of normal saline and shed blood [214]. At the end of a 3 hour resuscitation period, the animals were injected with Evans Blue dye, and BAL was then performed. Various experiments have shown that the level of Evans Blue dye in the BALF correlated with the severity of lung injury [215]. In this set of experiments, administration of inhaled HTS (7.5% HTS) during the resuscitation period managed to significantly attenuate lung injury in animals that underwent T/HS (Figure 2.3).

While further work needs to be done with inhaled HTS to determine optimal timing and dose, the initial data are encouraging for translation into future human studies.

Steroids

The development of ALI, ARDS, and MOF is the end result of a hyperactive immune system where the body's own defences against foreign antigens act indiscriminately and, ultimately, damage the host. In the case of ALI and ARDS, the circulating neutrophils are recruited into the capillaries of the lungs by proinflammatory mediators such as IL-6 and IL-8 [216]. Corticosteroids are anti-inflammatory drugs used in the treatment of a wide variety of inflammatory diseases [217–219]. These drugs act by both up-regulating anti-inflammatory molecules and reducing proinflammatory molecules synthesized by the cell [218]. Moreover, steroids inhibit PLA_2 activity via the activation of annexin I (formerly known as lipocortin-I). Although it may seem logical that reducing the inflammatory state seen after traumatic injury would reduce the rate of MOF seen, clinical data do not support this idea. In a randomized controlled trial involving 180 patients with ARDS, there was an increase in 60-day and 180-day mortality in patients who received methylprednisone versus placebo. These results suggest that global inhibition of the inflammatory response with steroid administration is too broad-based a treatment for the severely injured patient [193]. However, the optimal dosage and duration of steroids has yet to be determined and low-dose steroid treatment may still prove to be a beneficial form of therapy.

Enhancement of the immune system

Interferon-γ

Traumatic injury has been shown to reduce the capacity of circulating monocytes to react to an inflammatory stimulus. Trauma also decreases the level of IL-2 and INF-γ released from antigen-presenting cells [193,220]. Furthermore, trauma decreases the expression of HLA-DR on the monocyte which is critical to T-cell-mediated adaptive immunity [193,220]. Various clinical trials have shown an increase in infection and related mortality in trauma patients who had decreased expression of the HLA-DR antigen on circulating monocytes [193,220–222]. INF-γ is a potent activator of monocytes and can increase the expression of HLA-DR in the trauma patient [193,223]. Several clinical trials looking at the role of administering INF-γ to trauma patients have shown an increase in the expression of the HLA-DR antigen, a decreased incidence in ventilator-associated pneumonia, and a decrease in infection-related death and overall deaths [224–226]. Thus, the therapeutic administration of INF-γ appears to be feasible, but further work needs to be done to determine the optimum dose, route of administration, and timing of the INF-γ.

Human recombinant granulocyte colony-stimulating factor (rh-G-CSF)

G-CSF stimulates haematopoiesis and is used to augment the innate immune system in neutropenic patients [227]. G-CSF also blunts the response of monocytes to various proinflammatory stimulants such as TNF-α, IL-1β, and IL-12 [228]. It appears that G-CSF not only enhances aspects of the body's innate immune defences, but can also attenuate the proinflammatory milieu seen in the trauma patient. In a double-blind randomized controlled trial looking at the administration of rh-G-CSF versus placebo [228], there was an increase in circulating anti-inflammatory mediators (IL-1ra, sTNFR-2) following surgery and a decrease in trauma-induced acute phase response (as measured by a decrease in C-reactive protein) [228]. Schneider *et al.* concluded in the above study that the administration of G-CSF can conserve the 'innate immune system . . . under [the] most stressful conditions such as major surgery, thus, preventing life-threatening clinical scenarios such as second-hit multiple organ failure.' Further trials need to be performed to determine optimal dose and timing [228].

Oestrogen

It is known that in animal models of sepsis and haemorrhagic shock, females have better outcomes than their male counterparts [229,230]. It appears that this gender advantage exists in humans as well [229,231]. In a study looking at over 4000 trauma patients, hormonally active females had lower serum lactate levels, and received less blood than their ISS-matched male counterparts, suggesting a better physiological response to trauma [231]. This gender advantage possibly stems from the protective activity of oestrogen [119,232].

Oestrogen acts via the α- and β-oestradiol receptors which are located throughout the body, although the overall distribution of the oestrogen receptor in trauma-susceptible organs has yet to be fully established [229, 233]. Oestrogen has several anti-inflammatory effects throughout the body. It has been shown to inhibit IL-1 and IL-6 in vascular smooth muscle cells, and the administration of oestrogen in rat models has shown decreased lung neutrophil sequestration, as well as a decrease in TNF-α, IL-β, and IL-6 compared with placebo [234]. Thus, the potential benefit of oestrogen therapy in the trauma patient appears to be promising. The increased risk of thrombosis, however, or the lack of consensus regarding the mechanism of action of oestrogen, have prevented any clinical trials looking at the role of oestrogens as a treatment. More work needs to be done to further elucidate the role of this important sex hormone in trauma and inflammation.

Gut modulation

Immunonutrition

Immunonutrition is the ability of nutrients (macro and micro) to augment or influence the immune system [193, 235] (see Chapter 6). The nutrients involved in immunonutrition are those that have been shown in various animal models to improve immune function, attenuate inflammation, augment gut barrier function, or have enhanced antioxidant effects [235]. Various nutritional supplements have been shown to be beneficial to the trauma patient. Also, early enteral nutrition has been shown to be associated with decreased infection rates, shorter hospital stay, and improved survival [193,235,236]. L-Glutamine has been shown to enhance the immune system by increasing blood lymphocyte counts and also has several clinical advantages such as decreased infectious complications, decreased length of hospital stay, and reduction in mortality [193,235,237]. ω-3 Fatty acids have been shown to be anti-inflammatory and to be beneficial in patients with ARDS [193,235,238]. Treatment with ω-3 fatty acids was associated with an improved arterial oxygenation, decreased time on the ventilator, and shorter ICU stay. Other nutrients that have been shown to show some benefits in the critically ill patient are L-arginine, *N*-acetylcysteine, antioxidant vitamins (e.g. vitamin E), and trace elements (e.g. zinc, copper, selenium) [193,235]. It appears that extrinsic factors delivered though the gut can modulate the immune response in ways that improve survival in the critically ill patient through either anti-inflammatory properties or the ability to enhance the immune system to prevent MOF.

Summary and conclusions

Trauma and haemorrhagic shock induce a multitude of changes that can alter the homeostatic balance in the human host defences. This aberration in homeostasis can manifest as derangements in the coagulation system, injury to specific organ systems such as the lung, or failure of multiple critical organ systems. MOF remains the leading cause of mortality in patients surviving the initial resuscitation period after trauma and haemorrhagic shock. Advances in the management of the critically ill patient have improved mortality; however, the incidence of MOF in surgical ICUs continues to consume substantial amounts of health care resources. MOF is the result of a maladaptive immune response that is triggered by a two-hit model of events that lead to priming, recruitment, and the eventual activation of neutrophils to release cytotoxic mediators. PSML is the mechanistic link between gut ischaemia and reperfusion injury, ALI, and eventual MOF. PSML not only carries proinflammatory lipids, but the protective factors present in normal lymph are depleted. The net result is a state of proinflammation that can ultimately lead to end-organ injury. This proinflammatory state can be detected by elevations in various cytokine and chemokine levels which have been strongly associated with MOF prognosis and mortality, as well as signalling molecules such as the DAMPs. Treatment of the critically ill patient can be targeted towards the derangements of these factors, focusing on decreasing inflammation or enhancing the immune system itself. Continued research on the aetiology of MOF, and its associated factors, is needed to decrease the high cost of trauma-related injury and resultant complications.

References

1. Centers for Disease Control and Prevention. *Ten leading causes of death and injury (charts)*. http://www.cdc.gov/injury/wisquars/LeadingCauses.html; accessed 18 January 2010.
2. Shackford SR, Hollingworth-Fridlund P, Cooper GF *et al.* The effect of regionalization upon the quality of trauma care as assessed by concurrent audit before and after institution of a trauma system: a preliminary report. *J Trauma* 1986; **26**: 812–820.
3. Eiseman B, Beart R, Norton L. Multiple organ failure. *Surg Gynecol Obstet* 1977; **144**: 323–326.
4. Sauaia A, Moore EE, Johnson JL *et al.* Validation of postinjury multiple organ failure scores. *Shock* 2009; **31**: 438–447.
5. Ciesla DJ, Moore EE, Johnson JL *et al.* A 12-year prospective study of postinjury multiple organ failure: has anything changed? *Arch Surg* 2005; **140**: 432–8; discussion 438–40.
6. Bone RC, Balk RA, Cerra FB *et al.* Definitions for sepsis and organ failure and guidelines for the use of innovative therapies in sepsis. The ACCP/SCCM Consensus Conference Committee. American College of Chest Physicians/Society of Critical Care Medicine. *Chest* 1992; **101**: 1644–1655.
7. Moore EE, Moore FA, Harken AH *et al.* The two-event construct of postinjury multiple organ failure. *Shock* 2005; **24 Suppl 1**, 71–74.
8. Moore FA, Moore EE. Evolving concepts in the pathogenesis of postinjury multiple organ failure. *Surg Clin North Am* 1995; **75**: 257–277.
9. Murphy TJ, Paterson HM, Mannick JA *et al.* Injury, sepsis, and the regulation of Toll-like receptor responses. *J Leukoc Biol* 2004; **75**: 400–407.
10. Anderson BO, Moore EE, Moore FA *et al.* Hypovolemic shock promotes neutrophil sequestration in lungs by a xanthine oxidase-related mechanism. *J Appl Physiol* 1991; **71**: 1862–1865.
11. Botha AJ, Moore FA, Moore EE *et al.* Postinjury neutrophil priming and activation states: therapeutic challenges. *Shock* 1995; **3**: 157–166.
12. Biffl WL EE Moore, G Zallen *et al.* Neutrophils are primed for cytotoxicity and resist apoptosis in injured patients at risk for multiple organ failure. *Surgery* 1999; **126**: 198–202.
13. Zallen, G, Moore EE, Johnson JL *et al.* Circulating postinjury neutrophils are primed for the release of proinflammatory cytokines. *J Trauma* 1999; **46**: 42–48.

14. Partrick DA, Moore FA, Moore EE *et al.* Neutrophil priming and activation in the pathogenesis of postinjury multiple organ failure. *New Horiz* 1996; **4**: 194–210.
15. Hassoun HT, Kone BC, Mercer DW *et al.* Post-injury multiple organ failure: the role of the gut. *Shock* 2001; **15**: 1–10.
16. Clark JA, Coopersmith CM. Intestinal crosstalk: a new paradigm for understanding the gut as the 'motor' of critical illness. *Shock* 2007; **28**: 384–393.
17. Redfors S, Hallback DA, Haglund U *et al.* Blood flow distribution, villous tissue osmolality and fluid and electrolyte transport in the cat small intestine during regional hypotension. *Acta Physiol Scand* 1984; **121**: 193–209.
18. Moore EE, Moore FA, Francoise RJ *et al.* The postischemic gut serves as a priming bed for circulating neutrophils that provoke multiple organ failure. *J Trauma* 1994; **37**: 881–887.
19. Reilly, PM Wilkins, KB Fuh, KC *et al.* The mesenteric hemodynamic response to circulatory shock: an overview. *Shock* 2001; **15**: 329–343.
20. Ichikawa H, Wolf RE, Aw TY *et al.* Exogenous xanthine promotes neutrophil adherence to cultured endothelial cells. *Am J Physiol* 1997; **273**: G342–347.
21. Poggetti RS, Moore FA, Moore EE *et al.* Simultaneous liver and lung injury following gut ischemia is mediated by xanthine oxidase. *J Trauma* 1992; **32**: 723–7; discussion 727–8.
22. Wulczyn FG, Krappmann D , Scheidereit C. The NF-kappa B/Rel and I kappa B gene families: mediators of immune response and inflammation. *J Mol Med* 1996; **74**(12), 749–769.
23. Yeh KY, M Yeh, J Glass *et al.* Rapid activation of NF-kappa B and AP-1 and target gene expression in postischemic rat intestine. *Gastroenterology* 2000; **118**: 525–534.
24. Blikslager AT Roberts MC, Rhoads JM *et al.* Prostaglandins I2 and E2 have a synergistic role in rescuing epithelial barrier function in porcine ileum. *J Clin Invest* 1997; **100**: 1928–1933.
25. Ryter SW, Alam J, Choi AM. Heme oxygenase-1/carbon monoxide: from basic science to therapeutic applications. *Physiol Rev* 2006; **86**: 583–650.
26. Moore FA, Moore EE, Poggetti R *et al.* Gut bacterial translocation via the portal vein: a clinical perspective with major torso trauma. *J Trauma* 1991; **31**: 629–36; discussion 636–8.
27. Magnotti LJ, Upperman JS, Xu DZ *et al.* Gut-derived mesenteric lymph but not portal blood increases endothelial cell permeability and promotes lung injury after hemorrhagic shock. *Ann Surg* 1998; **228**: 518–527.
28. Adams CA, Jr, Hauser CJ, Adams JM *et al.* Trauma-hemorrhage-induced neutrophil priming is prevented by mesenteric lymph duct ligation. *Shock* 2002; **18**: 513–517.
29. Gonzalez RJ, Moore EE, Ciesla DJ *et al.* Mesenteric lymph is responsible for post-hemorrhagic shock systemic neutrophil priming. *J Trauma* 2001; **51**: 1069–1072.
30. Sarin EL, Moore EE, Moore JB *et al.* Systemic neutrophil priming by lipid mediators in post-shock mesenteric lymph exists across species. *J Trauma* 2004; **57**: 950–954.
31. Deitch EA, Feketeova E, Adams JM *et al.* Lymph from a primate baboon trauma hemorrhagic shock model activates human neutrophils. *Shock* 2006; **25**: 460–463.
32. Gonzalez RJ, Moore EE, Ciesla DJ *et al.* Phospholipase A(2)—derived neutral lipids from posthemorrhagic shock mesenteric lymph prime the neutrophil oxidative burst. *Surgery* 2001; **130**: 198–203.
33. Murakami, M, Kudo I. Phospholipase A2. *J Biochem* 2002; **131**: 285–292.

34. Partrick DA, Moore EE, Silliman CC *et al.* Secretory phospholipase A2 activity correlates with postinjury multiple organ failure. *Crit Care Med* 2001; **29**: 989–993.
35. Koike, K, Moore EE, Moore FA *et al.* Gut phospholipase A2 mediates neutrophil priming and lung injury after mesenteric ischemia-reperfusion. *Am J Physiol* 1995; **268**, G397–403.
36. Mifflin RC, Saada JI, Di Mari JF *et al.* Regulation of COX-2 expression in human intestinal myofibroblasts: mechanisms of IL-1-mediated induction. *Am J Physiol Cell Physiol* 2002; **282**: C824–834.
37. Haeggstrom JZ, Wetterholm A. Enzymes and receptors in the leukotriene cascade. *Cell Mol Life Sci* 2002; **59**: 742–753.
38. Soberman RJ, Christmas P. The organization and consequences of eicosanoid signaling. *J Clin Invest* 2003; **111**: 1107–1113.
39. Murphy RC, Gijon MA. Biosynthesis and metabolism of leukotrienes. *Biochem J* 2007; **405**: 379–395.
40. Peters-Golden M, Henderson WR Jr. Leukotrienes. *N Engl J Med* 2007; **357**: 1841–1854.
41. Radmark O, Samuelsson B. Regulation of 5-lipoxygenase enzyme activity. *Biochem Biophys Res Commun* 2005; **338**: 102–110.
42. Crooks SW, Stockley RA. Leukotriene B4. *Int J Biochem Cell Biol* 1998; **30**: 173–178.
43. Tager AM, Luster AD. BLT1 and BLT2: the leukotriene B(4) receptors. *Prostaglandins Leukot Essent Fatty Acids* 2003; **69**: 123–134.
44. Sala A, Zarini S, Bolla M. Leukotrienes: lipid bioeffectors of inflammatory reactions. *Biochemistry (Moscow)* 1998; **63**: 84–92.
45. Dixon RA, Diehl RE, Opas E *et al.* Requirement of a 5-lipoxygenase-activating protein for leukotriene synthesis. *Nature* 1990; **343**: 282–284.
46. Woods JW, Evans JF, Ethier D *et al.* 5-lipoxygenase and 5-lipoxygenase-activating protein are localized in the nuclear envelope of activated human leukocytes. *J Exp Med* 1993; **178**: 1935–1946.
47. Haeggstrom JZ. Leukotriene A4 hydrolase/aminopeptidase, the gatekeeper of chemotactic leukotriene B4 biosynthesis. *J Biol Chem* 2004; **279**: 50639–50642.
48. Tholander F, Kull F, Ohlson E *et al.* Leukotriene A4 hydrolase, insights into the molecular evolution by homology modeling and mutational analysis of enzyme from *Saccharomyces cerevisiae*. *J Biol Chem* 2005; **280**: 33477–33486.
49. Scoggan KA, Jakobsson PJ, Ford-Hutchinson AW. Production of leukotriene C4 in different human tissues is attributable to distinct membrane bound biosynthetic enzymes. *J Biol Chem* 1997; **272**: 10182–10187.
50. Tornhamre S, Sjolinder M, Lindberg A *et al.* Demonstration of leukotriene-C4 synthase in platelets and species distribution of the enzyme activity. *Eur J Biochem* 1998; **251**: 227–235.
51. Maclouf JA, Murphy RC. Transcellular metabolism of neutrophil-derived leukotriene A4 by human platelets. A potential cellular source of leukotriene C4. *J Biol Chem* 1988; **263**: 174–181.
52. Serhan CN, Prescott SM. The scent of a phagocyte: Advances on leukotriene b(4) receptors. *J Exp Med* 2000; **192**: F5–8.
53. Yokomizo T, Masuda K, Kato K *et al.* Leukotriene B4 receptor. Cloning and intracellular signaling. *Am J Respir Crit Care Med* 2000; **161**: S51–55.
54. Jin R, Koop DR, Raucy JL *et al.* Role of human CYP4F2 in hepatic catabolism of the proinflammatory agent leukotriene B4. *Arch Biochem Biophys* 1998; **359**: 89–98.

55. Byrum RS, Goulet JL, Snouwaert JN *et al.* Determination of the contribution of cysteinyl leukotrienes and leukotriene B4 in acute inflammatory responses using 5-lipoxygenase- and leukotriene A4 hydrolase-deficient mice. *J Immunol* 1999; **163**: 6810–6819.
56. Caironi P, Ichinose F, Liu R *et al.* 5-Lipoxygenase deficiency prevents respiratory failure during ventilator-induced lung injury. *Am J Respir Crit Care Med* 2005; **172**: 334–343.
57. Leak LV, Liotta LA, Krutzsch H *et al.* Proteomic analysis of lymph. *Proteomics* 2004; **4**: 753–765.
58. Peltz ED, Moore EE, Zurawel AA *et al.* Proteome and system ontology of hemorrhagic shock: exploring early constitutive changes in postshock mesenteric lymph. *Surgery* 2009; **146**: 347–357.
59. Bone RC. Immunologic dissonance: a continuing evolution in our understanding of the systemic inflammatory response syndrome (SIRS) and the multiple organ dysfunction syndrome (MODS). *Ann Intern Med* 1996; **125**: 680–687.
60. Eiseman B, Sloan R, Hansbrough J *et al.* Multiple organ failure: clinical and experimental. *Am Surg* 1980; **46**: 14–19.
61. Dewar D, Moore FA, Moore EE *et al.* Postinjury multiple organ failure. *Injury* 2009; **40**: 912–918.
62. Baue AE, Durham R, Faist E. Systemic inflammatory response syndrome (SIRS), multiple organ dysfunction syndrome (MODS), multiple organ failure (MOF): are we winning the battle? *Shock* 1998; **10**: 79–89.
63. Moore FA, Sauaia A, Moore EE *et al.* Postinjury multiple organ failure: a bimodal phenomenon. *J Trauma* 1996; **40**: 501–10; discussion 510–2.
64. Talmor M, Hydo L, Barie PS. Relationship of systemic inflammatory response syndrome to organ dysfunction, length of stay, and mortality in critical surgical illness: effect of intensive care unit resuscitation. *Arch Surg* 1999; **134**: 81–87.
65. Sauaia A, Moore FA, Moore EE *et al.* Epidemiology of trauma deaths: a reassessment. *J Trauma* 1995; **38**: 185–193.
66. Hassoun HT, Weisbrodt NW, Mercer DW *et al.* Inducible nitric oxide synthase mediates gut ischemia/reperfusion-induced ileus only after severe insults. *J Surg Res* 2001; **97**: 150–154.
67. Hernandez LA, Grisham MB, Twohig B *et al.* Role of neutrophils in ischemia-reperfusion-induced microvascular injury. *Am J Physiol* 1987; **253**: H699–703.
68. Sauaia A, Moore FA, Moore EE *et al.* Early predictors of postinjury multiple organ failure. *Arch Surg* 1994; **129**: 39–45.
69. Walker L, Eiseman B. The changing pattern of post-traumatic respiratory distress syndrome. *Ann Surg* 1975; **181**: 693–697.
70. Mannick JA, Rodrick ML, Lederer JA. The immunologic response to injury. *J Am Coll Surg* 2001; **193**: 237–244.
71. Faist E, Baue AE, Dittmer H *et al.* Multiple organ failure in polytrauma patients. *J Trauma* 1983; **23**: 775–787.
72. Fry DE, Pearlstein L, Fulton RL *et al.* Multiple system organ failure. The role of uncontrolled infection. *Arch Surg* 1980; **115**: 136–140.
73. Waydhas C, Nast-Kolb D, Jochum M *et al.* Inflammatory mediators, infection, sepsis, and multiple organ failure after severe trauma. *Arch Surg* 1992; **127**: 460–467.
74. Nast-Kolb D, Aufmkolk M, Rucholtz S *et al.* Multiple organ failure still a major cause of morbidity but not mortality in blunt multiple trauma. *J Trauma* 2001; **51**: 835–41; discussion 841–2.

75. Flohe S, Flohe SB, Schade FU *et al.* Immune response of severely injured patients—influence of surgical intervention and therapeutic impact. *Langenbecks Arch Surg* 2007; **392**: 639–648.
76. Gebhard F, Pfetsch H, Steinbach G *et al.* Is interleukin 6 an early marker of injury severity following major trauma in humans? *Arch Surg* 2000; **135**: 291–295.
77. Dinarello CA. Cytokines as mediators in the pathogenesis of septic shock. *Curr Top Microbiol Immunol* 1996; **216**, 133–165.
78. Yao YM, Redl H, Bahrami S *et al.* The inflammatory basis of trauma/shock-associated multiple organ failure. *Inflamm Res* 1998; **47**: 201–210.
79. Park WY, Goodman RB, Steinberg KP *et al.* Cytokine balance in the lungs of patients with acute respiratory distress syndrome. *Am J Respir Crit Care Med* 2001; **164**: 1896–1903.
80. Goodman RB, Strieter RM, Martin DP *et al.* Inflammatory cytokines in patients with persistence of the acute respiratory distress syndrome. *Am J Respir Crit Care Med* 1996; **154**: 602–611.
81. Bhatia M, Moochhala S. Role of inflammatory mediators in the pathophysiology of acute respiratory distress syndrome. *J Pathol* 2004; **202**: 145–156.
82. Ertel W, Morrison MH, Ayala A *et al.* Chloroquine attenuates hemorrhagic shock-induced suppression of Kupffer cell antigen presentation and major histocompatibility complex class II antigen expression through blockade of tumor necrosis factor and prostaglandin release. *Blood* 1991; **78**: 1781–1788.
83. Maier B, Lefering R, Lehnert M *et al.* Early versus late onset of multiple organ failure is associated with differing patterns of plasma cytokine biomarker expression and outcome after severe trauma. *Shock* 2007; **28**: 668–674.
84. Giannoudis PV, Smith MR, Evans RT *et al.* Serum CRP and IL-6 levels after trauma. Not predictive of septic complications in 31 patients. *Acta Orthop Scand* 1998; **69**: 184–188.
85. Nast-Kolb D, Waydhas C, Gippner-Steppert C *et al.* Indicators of the posttraumatic inflammatory response correlate with organ failure in patients with multiple injuries. *J Trauma* 1997; **42**: 446–54; discussion 454–5.
86. Pape HC, Remmers D, Grotz M *et al.* Levels of antibodies to endotoxin and cytokine release in patients with severe trauma: does posttraumatic dysergy contribute to organ failure? *J Trauma* 1999; **46**: 907–913.
87. Meduri GU, Headley S, Kohler G *et al.* Persistent elevation of inflammatory cytokines predicts a poor outcome in ARDS. Plasma IL-1 beta and IL-6 levels are consistent and efficient predictors of outcome over time. *Chest* 1995; **107**: 1062–1073.
88. Wiedermann FJ, Mayr AJ, Kaneider NC *et al.* Alveolar granulocyte colony-stimulating factor and alpha-chemokines in relation to serum levels, pulmonary neutrophilia, and severity of lung injury in ARDS. *Chest* 2004; **125**: 212–219.
89. Jastrow KM 3rd, Gonzalez EA, McGuire MF *et al.* Early cytokine production risk stratifies trauma patients for multiple organ failure. *J Am Coll Surg* 2009; **209**: 320–331.
90. Zhai Y, Shen XD, O'Connell R *et al.* Cutting edge: TLR4 activation mediates liver ischemia/reperfusion inflammatory response via IFN regulatory factor 3-dependent MyD88 independent pathway. *J Immunol* 2004; **173**: 7115–7119.
91. Gill R, Tsung A, Billiar T. Linking oxidative stress to inflammation: Toll-like receptors. *Free Radic Biol Med* 2010; **48**: 1121–1132.
92. was 93. Poltorak A, He X, Smirnova I *et al.* Defective LPS signaling in C3H/HeJ and C57BL/10ScCr mice: mutations in Tlr4 gene. *Science* 1998; **282**: 2085–2088.

93. Kawai T, Akira S. Toll-like receptor downstream signaling. *Arthritis Res Ther* 2005; **7**: 12–19.
94. Kiechl S, Lorenz E, Reindl M *et al.* Toll-like receptor 4 polymorphisms and atherogenesis. *N Engl J Med* 2002; **347**: 185–192.
95. Johnson GB, Riggs BL, Platt JL. A genetic basis for the 'Adonis' phenotype of low adiposity and strong bones. *FASEB J* 2004; **18**: 1282–1284.
96. Tang AH, Brunn GJ, Cascalho M *et al.* Pivotal advance: endogenous pathway to SIRS, sepsis, and related conditions. *J Leukoc Biol* 2007; **82**: 282–285.
97. Gallucci, S., M Lolkema and P Matzinger. Natural adjuvants: endogenous activators of dendritic cells. *Nat Med* 1999; **5**: 1249–1255.
98. Ohashi K, Burkart V, Flohe S *et al.* Cutting edge: heat shock protein 60 is a putative endogenous ligand of the toll-like receptor-4 complex. *J Immunol* 2000; **164**: 558–561.
99. Prince JM, Levy RM, Yang R *et al.* Toll-like receptor-4 signaling mediates hepatic injury and systemic inflammation in hemorrhagic shock. *J Am Coll Surg* 2006; **202**: 407–417.
100. Barsness KA, Arcaroli J, Harken AH *et al.* Hemorrhage-induced acute lung injury is TLR-4 dependent. *Am J Physiol Regul Integr Comp Physiol* 2004; **287**: R592–599.
101. Dybdahl B, Wahba A, Lien E *et al.* Inflammatory response after open heart surgery: release of heat-shock protein 70 and signaling through toll-like receptor-4. *Circulation* 2002; **105**: 685–690.
102. Kimura F, Itoh H, Ambiru S *et al.* Circulating heat-shock protein 70 is associated with postoperative infection and organ dysfunction after liver resection. *Am J Surg* 2004; **187**: 777–784.
103. Kim BS, Lim SW, Li C *et al.* Ischemia-reperfusion injury activates innate immunity in rat kidneys. *Transplantation* 2005; **79**: 1370–1377.
104. Chen LW, Chang WJ, Chen PH *et al.* TLR ligand decreases mesenteric ischemia and reperfusion injury-induced gut damage through TNF-alpha signaling. *Shock* 2008; **30**: 563–570.
105. Tsan MF, Gao B. Heat shock proteins and immune system. *J Leukoc Biol* 2009; **85**: 905–910.
106. Boyd JH, Kan B, Roberts H *et al.* S100A8 and S100A9 mediate endotoxin-induced cardiomyocyte dysfunction via the receptor for advanced glycation end products. *Circ Res* 2008; **102**: 1239–1246.
107. Mori T, Tan J, Arendash GW *et al.* Overexpression of human S100B exacerbates brain damage and periinfarct gliosis after permanent focal ischemia. *Stroke* 2008; **39**: 2114–2121.
108. Wang H, Bloom O, Zhang M *et al.* HMG-1 as a late mediator of endotoxin lethality in mice. *Science* 1999; **285**: 248–251.
109. Scaffidi P, Misteli T, Bianchi ME. Release of chromatin protein HMGB1 by necrotic cells triggers inflammation. *Nature* 2002; **418**: 191–195.
110. Yang R, Harada T, Mollen KP *et al.* Anti-HMGB1 neutralizing antibody ameliorates gut barrier dysfunction and improves survival after hemorrhagic shock. *Mol Med* 2006; **12**: 105–114.
111. Park JS, Gamboni-Robertson F, He Q *et al.* High mobility group box 1 protein interacts with multiple Toll-like receptors. *Am J Physiol Cell Physiol* 2006; **290**: C917–924.
112. Hori O, Brett J, Slattery T *et al.* The receptor for advanced glycation end products (RAGE) is a cellular binding site for amphoterin. Mediation of neurite outgrowth and co-expression of rage and amphoterin in the developing nervous system. *J Biol Chem* 1995; **270**: 25752–25761.

113. Tian J, Avalos AM, Mao SY *et al.* Toll-like receptor 9-dependent activation by DNA-containing immune complexes is mediated by HMGB1 and RAGE. *Nat Immunol* 2007; **8**: 487–496.

114. Ciesla DJ, Moore EE, Johnson JL *et al.* The role of the lung in postinjury multiple organ failure. *Surgery* 2005; **138**: 749–57; discussion 757–8.

115. Botha AJ, Moore FA, Moore EE *et al.* Early neutrophil sequestration after injury: a pathogenic mechanism for multiple organ failure. *J Trauma* 1995; **39**: 411–417.

116. Barnett CC, Moore EE, Moore FA *et al.* Intercellular adhesion molecule-1 promotes neutrophil-mediated cytotoxicity. *Surgery* 1995; **118**: 171–5; discussion 176.

117. Redl H, Dinges HP, Buurman WA *et al.* Expression of endothelial leukocyte adhesion molecule-1 in septic but not traumatic/hypovolemic shock in the baboon. *Am J Pathol* 1991; **139**: 461–466.

118. Pober JS, Cotran RS. Cytokines and endothelial cell biology. *Physiol Rev* 1990; **70**: 427–451.

119. Gedeit RG Tumor necrosis factor-induced E-selectin expression on vascular endothelial cells. *Crit Care Med* 1996; **24**: 1543–1546.

120. Yao YM, Bahrami S, Leichtfried G *et al.* Significance of NO in hemorrhage-induced hemodynamic alterations, organ injury, and mortality in rats. *Am J Physiol* 1996; **270**: H1616–1623.

121. Marzi I, Bauer C, Hower R *et al.* Leukocyte-endothelial cell interactions in the liver after hemorrhagic shock in the rat. *Circ Shock* 1993; **40**: 105–114.

122. Hathaway WE, Hathaway HS, Belhasen LP Coagulation Factors in Newborn Animals. *J Lab Clin Med* 1964; **63**: 784–790.

123. Shrivastava S, McVey JH, Dorling A. The interface between coagulation and immunity. *Am J Transplant* 2007; **7**: 499–506.

124. Hoyt DB, Dutton RP, Hauser CJ *et al.* Management of coagulopathy in the patients with multiple injuries: results from an international survey of clinical practice. *J Trauma* 2008; **65**: 755–64; discussion 764–5.

125. Hardy JF, De Moerloose P, Samama M. Massive transfusion and coagulopathy: pathophysiology and implications for clinical management. *Can J Anaesth* 2004; **51**: 293–310.

126. Kashuk JL, Moore EE, Johnson JL *et al.* Postinjury life threatening coagulopathy: is 1:1 fresh frozen plasma: packed red blood cells the answer? *J Trauma* 2008; **65**: 261–70; discussion 270–1.

127. Boldt J New light on intravascular volume replacement regimens: what did we learn from the past three years? *Anesth Analg* 2003; **97**: 1595–1604.

128. Brazil EV, Coats TJ. Sonoclot coagulation analysis of in-vitro haemodilution with resuscitation solutions. *J R Soc Med* 2000; **93**: 507–510.

129. Cosgriff N, Moore EE, Sauaia A *et al.* Predicting life-threatening coagulopathy in the massively transfused trauma patient: hypothermia and acidoses revisited. *J Trauma* 1997; **42**: 857–861; discussion 861–2.

130. Hardy JF, Moerloose P de, Samama CM. The coagulopathy of massive transfusion. *Vox Sang* 2005; **89**: 123–127.

131. Cinat ME, Wallace WC, Nastanski F *et al.* Improved survival following massive transfusion in patients who have undergone trauma. *Arch Surg* 1999; **134**: 964–8; discussion 968–70.

132. Counts RB, Haisch C, Simon TL *et al.* Hemostasis in massively transfused trauma patients. *Ann Surg* 1979; **190**: 91–99.
133. Reed RL 2nd, Ciavarella D, Heimbach DM *et al.* Prophylactic platelet administration during massive transfusion. A prospective, randomized, double-blind clinical study. *Ann Surg* 1986; **203**: 40–48.
134. Miller RD, Robbins TO, Tong MJ *et al.* Coagulation defects associated with massive blood transfusions. *Ann Surg* 1971; **174**: 794–801.
135. Brohi K, Cohen MJ, Ganter MT *et al.* Acute traumatic coagulopathy: initiated by hypoperfusion: modulated through the protein C pathway? *Ann Surg* 2007; **245**: 812–818.
136. Niles SE, McLaughlin DF, Perkins JG *et al.* Increased mortality associated with the early coagulopathy of trauma in combat casualties. *J Trauma* 2008; **64**: 1459–63; discussion 1463–5.
137. Hess JR, Brohi K, Dutton RP *et al.* The coagulopathy of trauma: a review of mechanisms. *J Trauma* 2008; **65**: 748–754.
138. Martini WZ, Dubick MA, Wade CE *et al.* Evaluation of tris-hydroxymethylaminomethane on reversing coagulation abnormalities caused by acidosis in pigs. *Crit Care Med* 2007; **35**: 1568–1574.
139. Meng ZH, Wolberg AS, Monroe DM 3rd *et al.* The effect of temperature and pH on the activity of factor VIIa: implications for the efficacy of high-dose factor VIIa in hypothermic and acidotic patients. *J Trauma* 2003; **55**: 886–891.
140. Bajzar L, Jain N, Wang P *et al.* Thrombin activatable fibrinolysis inhibitor: not just an inhibitor of fibrinolysis. *Crit Care Med* 2004; **32**(5 Suppl): S320–324.
141. Harke H, Rahman S. Haemostatic disorders in massive transfusion. *Bibl Haematol* 1980; **46**: 179–188.
142. Kermode JC, Zheng Q, Milner EP. Marked temperature dependence of the platelet calcium signal induced by human von Willebrand factor. *Blood* 1999; **94**: 199–207.
143. Valeri CR, Feingold H, Cassidy G *et al.* Hypothermia-induced reversible platelet dysfunction. *Ann Surg* 1987; **205**: 175–181.
144. Wolberg AS, Meng ZH, Monroe DM 3rd *et al.* A systematic evaluation of the effect of temperature on coagulation enzyme activity and platelet function. *J Trauma* 2004; **56**: 1221–1228.
145. Cirino G, Vergnolle N. Proteinase-activated receptors (PARs): crossroads between innate immunity and coagulation. *Curr Opin Pharmacol* 2006; **6**: 428–434.
146. Vu TK, Hung DT, Wheaton VI *et al.* Molecular cloning of a functional thrombin receptor reveals a novel proteolytic mechanism of receptor activation. *Cell* 1991; **64**: 1057–1068.
147. Camerer E, Huang W, Coughlin SR. Tissue factor- and factor X-dependent activation of protease-activated receptor 2 by factor VIIa. *Proc Natl Acad Sci U S A* 2000; **97**: 5255–5260.
148. Coughlin SR. Protease-activated receptors in hemostasis, thrombosis and vascular biology. *J Thromb Haemost* 2005; **3**: 1800–1814.
149. Chambers RC, Laurent GJ. Coagulation cascade proteases and tissue fibrosis. *Biochem Soc Trans* 2002; **30**: 194–200.
150. Howell DC, Johns RH, Lasky JA *et al.* Absence of proteinase-activated receptor-1 signaling affords protection from bleomycin-induced lung inflammation and fibrosis. *Am J Pathol* 2005; **166**: 1353–1365.

151. Johnson K, Choi Y, DeGroot E *et al.* Potential mechanisms for a proinflammatory vascular cytokine response to coagulation activation. *J Immunol* 1998; **160**: 5130–5135.
152. Gando S Tissue factor in trauma and organ dysfunction. *Semin Thromb Hemost* 2006; **32**: 48–53.
153. Gando S, Nanzaki S, Morimoto Y *et al.* Systemic activation of tissue-factor dependent coagulation pathway in evolving acute respiratory distress syndrome in patients with trauma and sepsis. *J Trauma* 1999; **47**: 719–723.
154. Rastogi P, McHowat J. Inhibition of calcium-independent phospholipase A2 prevents inflammatory mediator production in pulmonary microvascular endothelium. *Respir Physiol Neurobiol* 2009; **165**: 167–174.
155. Sambrano GR, Huang W, Faruqi T *et al.* Cathepsin G activates protease-activated receptor-4 in human platelets. *J Biol Chem* 2000; **275**: 6819–6823.
156. Finigan JH The coagulation system and pulmonary endothelial function in acute lung injury. *Microvasc Res* 2009; **77**: 35–38.
157. Idell S, Koenig KB Fair DS *et al.* Serial abnormalities of fibrin turnover in evolving adult respiratory distress syndrome. *Am J Physiol* 1991; **261**: L240–248.
158. Nieuwenhuizen L, de Groot PG, Grutters JC *et al.* A review of pulmonary coagulopathy in acute lung injury, acute respiratory distress syndrome and pneumonia. *Eur J Haematol* 2009; **82**: 413–425.
159. Finigan JH, Dudek SM, Singleton PA *et al.* Activated protein C mediates novel lung endothelial barrier enhancement: role of sphingosine 1-phosphate receptor transactivation. *J Biol Chem* 2005; **280**: 17286–17293.
160. McClintock D, Zhuo H, Wickersham N *et al.* Biomarkers of inflammation, coagulation and fibrinolysis predict mortality in acute lung injury. *Crit Care* 2008; **12**: R41.
161. Ware LB, Fang X, Matthay MA. Protein C and thrombomodulin in human acute lung injury. *Am J Physiol Lung Cell Mol Physiol* 2003; **285**: L514–521.
162. Ware LB, Camerer E, Welty-Wolf K *et al.* Bench to bedside: targeting coagulation and fibrinolysis in acute lung injury. *Am J Physiol Lung Cell Mol Physiol* 2006; **291**: L307–311.
163. Calfee CS, Eisner MD, Ware LB *et al.* Trauma-associated lung injury differs clinically and biologically from acute lung injury due to other clinical disorders. *Crit Care Med* 2007; **35**: 2243–2250.
164. Benson AB, Moss M, Silliman CC. Transfusion-related acute lung injury (TRALI): a clinical review with emphasis on the critically ill. *Br J Haematol* 2009; **147**: 431–443.
165. Gajic O, Rana R, Winters JL *et al.* Transfusion-related acute lung injury in the critically ill: prospective nested case-control study. *Am J Respir Crit Care Med* 2007; **176**: 886–891.
166. Silliman CC, Fung YL, Ball JB *et al.* Transfusion-related acute lung injury (TRALI): current concepts and misconceptions. *Blood Rev* 2009; **23**: 245–255.
167. Silliman CC The two-event model of transfusion-related acute lung injury. *Crit Care Med* 2006; **34**(5 Suppl): S124–131.
168. Silliman CC, Kelher M. The role of endothelial activation in the pathogenesis of transfusion-related acute lung injury. *Transfusion* 2005; **45**(2 Suppl): 109S–116S.
169. Calkins CM Bensard DD Moore EE *et al.* The injured child is resistant to multiple organ failure: a different inflammatory response? *J Trauma* 2002; **53**: 1058–1063.
170. Crump JM, Duncan DA, Wears R. Analysis of multiple organ system failure in trauma and nontrauma patients. *Am Surg* 1988; **54**: 702–708.

171. Sauaia A, Moore FA, Moore EE *et al.* Multiple organ failure can be predicted as early as 12 hours after injury. *J Trauma* 1998; **45**: 291–301; discussion 301–3.
172. Proulx F, Joyal JS, Mariscalco MM *et al.* The pediatric multiple organ dysfunction syndrome. *Pediatr Crit Care Med* 2009; **10**: 12–22.
173. Wilkinson JD, Pollack MM, Ruttimann UE *et al.* Outcome of pediatric patients with multiple organ system failure. *Crit Care Med* 1986; **14**: 271–274.
174. Tantalean JA, Leon RJ, Santos AA *et al.* Multiple organ dysfunction syndrome in children. *Pediatr Crit Care Med* 2003; **4**: 181–185.
175. Johnston RB Jr, Altenburger KM, Atkinson AW Jr *et al.* Complement in the newborn infant. *Pediatrics* 1979; **64**(5 Pt 2 Suppl): 781–786.
176. Johnston RB Jr. Function and cell biology of neutrophils and mononuclear phagocytes in the newborn infant. *Vaccine* 1998; **16**: 1363–1368.
177. Calkins CM, Bensard DD, Partrick DA *et al.* Altered neutrophil function in the neonate protects against sepsis-induced lung injury. *J Pediatr Surg* 2002; **37**: 1042–7; discussion 1042–7.
178. Chelvarajan RL, Collins SM, Doubinskaia IE *et al.* Defective macrophage function in neonates and its impact on unresponsiveness of neonates to polysaccharide antigens. *J Leukoc Biol* 2004; **75**: 982–994.
179. Marodi L, Kaposzta R, Campbell DE *et al.* Candidacidal mechanisms in the human neonate. Impaired IFN-gamma activation of macrophages in newborn infants. *J Immunol* 1994; **153**: 5643–5649.
180. Johnston RA, Theman TA, Lu FL *et al.* Diet-induced obesity causes innate airway hyperresponsiveness to methacholine and enhances ozone-induced pulmonary inflammation. *J Appl Physiol* 2008; **104**: 1727–1735.
181. Belderbos ME, van Bleek GM, Levy O *et al.* Skewed pattern of Toll-like receptor 4-mediated cytokine production in human neonatal blood: low LPS-induced IL-12p70 and high IL-10 persist throughout the first month of life. *Clin Immunol* 2009; **133**: 228–237.
182. Langrish CL, Buddle JC, Thrasher AJ *et al.* Neonatal dendritic cells are intrinsically biased against Th-1 immune responses. *Clin Exp Immunol* 2002; **128**: 118–123.
183. Levy O, Zarember KA, Roy RM *et al.* Selective impairment of TLR-mediated innate immunity in human newborns: neonatal blood plasma reduces monocyte TNF-alpha induction by bacterial lipopeptides, lipopolysaccharide, and imiquimod, but preserves the response to R-848. *J Immunol* 2004; **173**: 4627–4634.
184. Halonen M, Lohman IC, Stern DA *et al.* Th1/Th2 patterns and balance in cytokine production in the parents and infants of a large birth cohort. *J Immunol* 2009; **182**: 3285–3293.
185. Smart JM, Kemp AS. Ontogeny of T-helper 1 and T-helper 2 cytokine production in childhood. *Pediatr Allergy Immunol* 2001; **12**: 181–187.
186. Hartel C, Adam N, Strunk T *et al.* Cytokine responses correlate differentially with age in infancy and early childhood. *Clin Exp Immunol* 2005; **142**: 446–453.
187. Upham JW, Lee PT, Holt BJ *et al.* Development of interleukin-12-producing capacity throughout childhood. *Infect Immun* 2002; **70**: 6583–6588.
188. Hanna-Wakim R, Yasukawa LL, Sung P *et al.* Age-related increase in the frequency of CD4(+) T cells that produce interferon-gamma in response to staphylococcal enterotoxin B during childhood. *J Infect Dis* 2009; **200**: 1921–1927.
189. Barsness KA, Bensard DD, Partrick DA *et al.* Endotoxin induces an exaggerated interleukin-10 response in peritoneal macrophages of children compared with adults. *J Pediatr Surg* 2004; **39**: 912–5; discussion 912–5.

190. Barsness KA, Bensard DD, Partrick DA *et al.* IL-1beta induces an exaggerated pro- and anti-inflammatory response in peritoneal macrophages of children compared with adults. *Pediatr Surg Int* 2004; **20**: 238–242.
191. Finnerty CC, Jeschke MG, Herndon DN *et al.* Temporal cytokine profiles in severely burned patients: a comparison of adults and children. *Mol Med* 2008; **14**: 553–560.
192. Zingarelli B, Hake PW, O'Connor M *et al.* Lung injury after hemorrhage is age dependent: role of peroxisome proliferator-activated receptor gamma. *Crit Care Med* 2009; **37**: 1978–1987.
193. Stahel PF, Smith WR, Moore EE. Role of biological modifiers regulating the immune response after trauma *Injury* 2007; **38**: 1409–1422.
194. Mattox KL, Maningas PA, Moore EE *et al.* Prehospital hypertonic saline/dextran infusion for post-traumatic hypotension. The U.S.A. Multicenter Trial. *Ann Surg* 1991; **213**: 482–491.
195. Bulger EM, Jurkovich GJ, Nathens AB *et al.* Hypertonic resuscitation of hypovolemic shock after blunt trauma: a randomized controlled trial. *Arch Surg* 2008; **143**: 139–148; discussion 149.
196. Rizoli SB, Rhind SG, Shek PN *et al.* The immunomodulatory effects of hypertonic saline resuscitation in patients sustaining traumatic hemorrhagic shock: a randomized, controlled, double-blinded trial. *Ann Surg* 2006; **243**: 47–57.
197. Ciesla DJ, Moore EE, Zallen G *et al.* Hypertonic saline attenuation of polymorphonuclear neutrophil cytotoxicity: timing is everything. *J Trauma* 2000; **48**: 388–395.
198. Angle N, Cabello-Passini R, Hoyt DB *et al.* Hypertonic saline infusion: can it regulate human neutrophil function? *Shock* 2000; **14**: 503–508.
199. Ciesla DJ, Moore EE, Biffl WL *et al.* Hypertonic saline attenuation of the neutrophil cytotoxic response is reversed upon restoration of normotonicity and reestablished by repeated hypertonic challenge. *Surgery* 2001; **129**: 567–575.
200. Ochi, H., J Masuda and M.A. Gimbrone. Hyperosmotic stimuli inhibit VCAM-1 expression in cultured endothelial cells via effects on interferon regulatory factor-1 expression and activity. *Eur J Immunol* 2002; **32**: 1821–1831.
201. Cuschieri J, Gourlay D, Garcia I *et al.* Hypertonic preconditioning inhibits macrophage responsiveness to endotoxin. *J Immunol* 2002; **168**: 1389–1396.
202. Junger WG, Coimbra R, Liu FC *et al.* Hypertonic saline resuscitation: a tool to modulate immune function in trauma patients? *Shock* 1997; **8**: 235–241.
203. Staudenmayer KL, Maier RV, Jelacic S *et al.* Hypertonic saline modulates innate immunity in a model of systemic inflammation. *Shock* 2005; **23**: 459–463.
204. Angle N, Hoyt DB, Coimbra R *et al.* Hypertonic saline resuscitation diminishes lung injury by suppressing neutrophil activation after hemorrhagic shock. *Shock* 1998; **9**: 164–170.
205. Powers KA, J Woo RG Khadaroo *et al.* Hypertonic resuscitation of hemorrhagic shock upregulates the anti-inflammatory response by alveolar macrophages. *Surgery* 2003; **134**: 312–318.
206. Eckels PC, Banerjee A, Moore EE *et al.* Amantadine inhibits platelet-activating factor induced clathrin-mediated endocytosis in human neutrophils. *Am J Physiol Cell Physiol* 2009; **297**: C886–897.
207. Nydam TL EE Moore RC McIntyre, Jr. *et al.* Hypertonic saline attenuates TNF-alpha-induced NF-kappaB activation in pulmonary epithelial cells. *Shock* 2009; **31**: 466–472.
208. Schwartz MD, Moore EE, Moore FA *et al.* Nuclear factor-kappa B is activated in alveolar macrophages from patients with acute respiratory distress syndrome. *Crit Care Med* 1996; **24**: 1285–1292.

209. Shenkar R, Schwartz MD Terada LS *et al.* Hemorrhage activates NF-kappa B in murine lung mononuclear cells in vivo. *Am J Physiol* 1996; **270**: L729–735.
210. Blackwell TS, Christman JW. The role of nuclear factor-kappa B in cytokine gene regulation. *Am J Respir Cell Mol Biol* 1997; **17**: 3–9.
211. Wills P, Greenstone M. Inhaled hyperosmolar agents for bronchiectasis. *Cochrane Database Syst Rev* 2006; **2**: CD002996.
212. Kuzik BA, Al-Qadhi SA, Kent S *et al.* Nebulized hypertonic saline in the treatment of viral bronchiolitis in infants. *J Pediatr* 2007; **151**: 266–270.
213. Guggino WB Cystic fibrosis and the salt controversy. *Cell* 1999; **96**: 607–610.
214. Masuno T, Moore EE, Cheng AM *et al.* Prehospital hemoglobin-based oxygen carrier resuscitation attenuates postinjury acute lung injury. *Surgery* 2005; **138**: 335–341.
215. Kelher MR, Masuno T, Moore EE *et al.* Plasma from stored packed red blood cells and MHC class I antibodies causes acute lung injury in a 2-event in vivo rat model. *Blood* 2009; **113**: 2079–2087.
216. Weiss SJ Tissue destruction by neutrophils. *N Engl J Med* 1989; **320**: 365–376.
217. Thongprasom, K and K Dhanuthai. Steriods in the treatment of lichen planus: a review. *J Oral Sci* 2008; **50**: 377–385.
218. Mullol J, Obando A, Pujols L *et al.* Corticosteroid treatment in chronic rhinosinusitis: the possibilities and the limits. *Immunol Allergy Clin North Am* 2009; **29**: 657–668.
219. Krishnan JA, Davis SQ, Naureckas ET *et al.* An umbrella review: corticosteroid therapy for adults with acute asthma. *Am J Med* 2009; **122**: 977–991.
220. Schinkel C The role of IFN-gamma in surgical patients. *J Interferon Cytokine Res* 2003; **23**: 341–349.
221. Hershman MJ, Cheadle WG, Wellhausen SR *et al.* Monocyte HLA-DR antigen expression characterizes clinical outcome in the trauma patient. *Br J Surg* 1990; **77**: 204–207.
222. Cheadle WG, Hershman MJ, Wellhausen SR *et al.* HLA-DR antigen expression on peripheral blood monocytes correlates with surgical infection. *Am J Surg* 1991; **161**: 639–645.
223. Livingston DH, Malangoni MA. Interferon-gamma restores immune competence after hemorrhagic shock. *J Surg Res* 1988; **45**: 37–43.
224. Polk HC Jr, Cheadle WG, Livingston DH *et al.* A randomized prospective clinical trial to determine the efficacy of interferon-gamma in severely injured patients. *Am J Surg* 1992; **163**: 191–196.
225. Nakos G Malamou-Mitsi VD, Lachana A *et al.* Immunoparalysis in patients with severe trauma and the effect of inhaled interferon-gamma. *Crit Care Med* 2002; **30**: 1488–1494.
226. Dries DJ, Jurkovich GJ, Maier RV *et al.* Effect of interferon gamma on infection-related death in patients with severe injuries. A randomized, double-blind, placebo-controlled trial. *Arch Surg* 1994; **129**: 1031–41; discussion 1042.
227. Crawford J, Glaspy JA, Stoller RG *et al.* Final results of a placebo-controlled study of filgrastim in small-cell lung cancer: exploration of risk factors for febrile neutropenia. *Support Cancer Ther* 2005; **3**: 36–46.
228. Schneider C, von Aulock S, Zedler S *et al.* Perioperative recombinant human granulocyte colony-stimulating factor (Filgrastim) treatment prevents immunoinflammatory dysfunction associated with major surgery. *Ann Surg* 2004; **239**: 75–81.
229. Bullard MK, Bir N, Kwan R *et al.* Women rule. *Surgery* 2010; **147**: 134–137.

230. Angele MK, Schwacha MG, Ayala A *et al.* Effect of gender and sex hormones on immune responses following shock. *Shock* 2000; **14**: 81–90.
231. Deitch EA, Livingston DH, Lavery RF *et al.* Hormonally active women tolerate shock-trauma better than do men: a prospective study of over 4000 trauma patients. *Ann Surg* 2007; **246**: 447–53; discussion 453–5.
232. Yu HP, Chaudry IH. The role of estrogen and receptor agonists in maintaining organ function after trauma-hemorrhage. *Shock* 2009; **31**: 227–237.
233. Choudhry MA, Chaudry IH. 17beta-Estradiol: a novel hormone for improving immune and cardiovascular responses following trauma-hemorrhage. *J Leukoc Biol* 2008; **83**: 518–522.
234. Gatson JW, Maass DL, Simpkins JW *et al.* Estrogen treatment following severe burn injury reduces brain inflammation and apoptotic signaling. *J Neuroinflammation* 2009; **6**: 30.
235. Calder PC Immunonutrition in surgical and critically ill patients. *Br J Nutr* 2007; **98** Suppl 1, S133–139.
236. Heyland DK, Novak F, Drover JW *et al.* Should immunonutrition become routine in critically ill patients? A systematic review of the evidence. *JAMA* 2001; **286**: 944–953.
237. Murray SM, Pindoria S. Nutrition support for bone marrow transplant patients. *Cochrane Database Syst Rev* 2008; **4**: CD002920.
238. Gadek JE, DeMichele SJ, Karlstad MD *et al.* Effect of enteral feeding with eicosapentaenoic acid, gamma-linolenic acid, and antioxidants in patients with acute respiratory distress syndrome. Enteral Nutrition in ARDS Study Group. *Crit Care Med* 1999; **27**: 1409–1420.

Chapter 3

Transplantation immunology

Eleanor M. Bolton and J. Andrew Bradley

Key summary points

- The immune response to a transplant involves both innate immunity and the adaptive (or acquired) immune response. The basis of the latter response is the ability to recognize certain proteins as foreign or non-self.
- Allograft rejection is dependent upon recipient T lymphocytes responding to highly polymorphic class I and class II cell surface molecules encoded by the MHC genes (the HLA system in humans), and may be avoided by matching donor and recipient MHC (HLA) molecules.
- The expression of HLA molecules on tissues and organs acts as both a stimulus and a target for an immunological rejection response. HLA class I (-A, -B, -C) molecules are expressed by most nucleated cells; HLA class II (-DR, -DP, -DQ) are expressed on DCs, B cells, and macrophages/monocytes.
- HLA matching (ABO blood groups, six-antigen class I and II typing) is important in selection of suitable donors; a priority for kidney and bone marrow transplants, but less so for heart and liver transplants, and not established for small bowel and pancreatic transplants. Serological cross-match is done (donor lymphocytes and recipient serum) to detect circulating anti-HLA antibodies—likelihood of hyperacute rejection.
- Incompatibility between the donor graft and recipient for antigens encoded by genes of MHC is the most important cause of rapid graft rejection. Long-term (20 year post-transplant) graft survival correlates with level of HLA mismatch.
- The innate immune response is induced by stressed and damaged cell interactions with PRRs on neutrophils, monocytes, and DCs and releases ROSs and cytokines (e.g. TNF-α). Donor-derived DCs are activated within the transplant and migrate to local lymph nodes in recipient and activate the adaptive immune response.
- T cells recognize donor MHC molecules either *directly*, as intact molecules on the cell surface of donor APCs and transplanted tissues, or *indirectly* as processed donor MHC peptides complexed with self MHC on recipient APCs. Indirect recognition is tenfold lower than direct recognition. Direct recognition plays a

major role in acute rejection; indirect recognition is responsible for chronic rejection.

- Costimulatory molecules (CD80, CD86) on APCs are necessary for T cell activation, through interaction with CD28 molecules on T cells. Expression of CTLA-4 on T lymphocytes down-regulates activation.
- $CD4^+$ T cells coordinate the rejection response through secretion of cytokines (IFN-γ, TNF-α, IL-2, IL-4, IL-5), mediate delayed-type hypersensitivity, CTL (perforin, granzyme B) activation, and production of alloantibody (ADCC, complement and coagulation cascades and autoantibodies).
- Rejection (acute and chronic) is mediated by cellular and/or humoral mechanisms. Cellular infiltrate consists of $CD4^+$ T and $CD8^+$ T lymphocytes destroying parenchymal structures; alloantibodies and complement (C4d) damage vascular endothelium. Chronic rejection is the major cause of graft loss; characteristic features include thickened interlobular arteries—intimal oedema, lipid-laden macrophages, smooth muscle proliferation, disruption of elastic lamina.
- Rejection may be controlled by treatment with immunosuppressive drugs (azathioprine, steroids, ciclosporin, and MABs) and induction of specific tolerance. Choice of agent is dependent on phase of rejection—induction, maintenance.
- Infections are not infrequent and most common in the early phase of transplantation; opportunistic infections include viruses (CMV, HHV, EBV), toxoplasmosis, TB, and fungal infections.
- Malignancy is a long-term risk in transplantation (4.3-fold increase); SCC is the commonest cancer (50%) seen, with 30-fold increase in the incidence of PTLD (3% of transplant recipients).
- Desensitization protocols (plasmapheresis, IVIg) are being used to overcome ABO and HLA incompatibility; achieving an optimal reduction of antibody titres in recipient is problematic.
- Tolerance is dependent on $CD4^+$ $CD25^+$ $FOXP3^+$ Tregs through direct cell contact or secretion of suppressive IL-10 and TGF-β. MABs blocking APC costimulatory molecules and induction of mixed chimaerism are being explored.

Background

Introduction and historical perspective

Tissue transplantation is the preferred, and often life-saving, treatment pathway for a range of clinical conditions including endstage renal, liver, heart, and lung failure, and certain causes of blindness. Until the mid-20th century, transplantation was no more than an interesting surgical experiment since attempts at tissue transplantation inevitably ended in failure. The idea that certain terminal illnesses could be treated by transplantation was vindicated when the first successful kidney transplant was performed in 1954 between identical twins, by Joseph Murray and colleagues in Boston.

Routine renal transplantation today owes its position as an established form of treatment to three major developments:

- Skin transplantation studies carried out by Peter Medawar in the 1940s and 1950s, on patients with burns and in experimental rabbits, demonstrated unequivocally the immunological basis of graft rejection. Importantly, Medawar also found that, experimentally at least, induction of neonatal tolerance could reliably result in long-term transplant survival.
- The use of vascular anastomosis techniques, originally developed by Jaboulay and Carrel in the early 1900s.
- The discovery in 1959, by Schwarz and Damashek, of the immunosuppressive action of 6-mercaptopurine; further developed by Roy Calne who used azathioprine, a derivative of 6-mercaptopurine, to prevent kidney graft rejection in experimental dogs.

These important developments offered not only an explanation for graft failure but also hope for future successful transplantation with the use of immunosuppression to overcome the rejection response.

The basis of an immune response is the ability to recognize certain proteins as foreign, or non-self. This applies as much to the 20th-century medical advance of tissue transplantation as it does to the threat of dangerous pathogens, including bacteria and viruses.

Terminology

A number of technical terms are used that describe the origin of a transplant and imply its likely outcome (Table 3.1). Although the original reports published by Murray and colleagues referred to 'homotransplants' or homografts, meaning a graft of a replacement tissue from another individual (as opposed to self), this term did not distinguish between a transplant from an unrelated donor and from a genetically identical donor, and is not used today. More commonly used, especially with reference to experimental studies, are the terms *allograft* and *syngeneic graft*, meaning a replacement graft from, respectively, a genetically nonidentical donor and an identical donor. Implicit is the acknowledgement that without immunosuppression, an allograft will elicit a strong immune response that will destroy the graft, while a syngeneic graft will be regarded as 'self' tissue by the immune system and will be permanently accepted. The term *autograft* refers to tissue, such as a skin graft, transplanted from the same individual, while a *xenograft* is tissue transplanted from one species to another (an experimental procedure).

Tissues and histocompatibility

Introduction

All nucleated cells of the body express molecules within the cell membrane that signify the identity of the individual, called major histocompatibility complex (MHC) molecules, whose function is to present small fragments of endogenous and exogenous

Table 3.1 Terms used in transplantation immunology

Term	Explanation
Allograft	Tissue or organ transplant between genetically dissimilar individuals
Syngeneic graft	Transplant between genetically identical individuals
Autograft	Transplantation of tissue or organs from the same individual
Xenograft	Transplantation of tissues or organs from one species to another
MHC	Major histocompatibility complex: the conserved gene region encoding highly polymorphic class I and class II cell surface molecules that present antigenic peptides to T lymphocytes
HLA complex	Human leucocyte antigen complex: synonym for the human MHC, located on chromosome 6
H-2 complex	Histocompatibility-2: synonym for the mouse MHC, located on chromosome 17
RT1 complex	Synonym for the rat MHC, located on chromosome 20
MLR	Mixed lymphocyte reaction: a laboratory test demonstrating alloreactivity, where mononuclear leucocytes from two genetically distinct individuals are cultured together for several days, and each population of leucocytes is stimulated by the other to proliferate. In a one-way MLR, one of the leucocyte populations is prevented from proliferating, by irradiation or mitomycin treatment, prior to coculture

proteins (peptides) to T lymphocytes which establish whether the peptide–MHC complex (pMHC) represents a 'self' or a 'non-self' complex and potentially threatening antigen, thereby, eliciting an immune response. In humans, the MHC is termed the human leucocyte antigen (HLA) system (Table 3.1).

A wide range of tissues, including cellular transplants, organ transplants and, more recently, composite tissue grafts (arm, face), are transplanted in current clinical practice. The expression of HLA molecules on these tissues and organs act as both a stimulus and a target for an immunological rejection response. Different transplants require different approaches to managing the immunological considerations of tissue matching to minimize rejection, and immunosuppression. Some transplants, such as corneas, bone grafts, or heart valves, are either transplanted to a relatively immunologically privileged site where rejection is uncommon (cornea), or they are treated and preserved prior to transplantation to reduce their immunogenicity and minimize the risk of rejection.

Among cellular transplants, blood transfusion is the commonest procedure and ABO blood group antigen matching ensures a safe and successful transfusion. Red blood cells (RBCs) express very low levels of HLA molecules; instead, they express protein–carbohydrate molecules called H antigens that have three allelic forms, such that the terminal carbohydrate chain is of the A antigen form, the B antigen form, or the unchanged H antigen, designated O. Every individual possesses naturally occurring IgM antibodies against their nonexpressed A or B antigens that develop during infancy in response to bacteria colonizing the gastrointestinal tract, which express cross-reactive antigens; blood group AB individuals have no antibodies to blood group antigens. ABO matching is a requirement not only for blood transfusion but also for composite tissue and organ transplantation, although there is now an effective plasmapheresis procedure for absorbing out circulating anti-A or anti-B antibodies. It is not necessary to match for rhesus (Rh) blood group antigens because Rh antigens are expressed only on erythrocytes. Rh-negative individuals can develop anti-Rh antibodies following blood transfusion or pregnancy, and any effect of circulating anti-Rh antibodies is likely to be short-lived and limited in extent.

Bone marrow transplantation involves the transfer of precursor cells of the immune system or stem cells, and is undertaken to restore defective immunity. However, bone marrow also includes mature immune cells that not only express high levels of HLA molecules, but also are able to mount a potentially lethal rejection response against the genetically distinct patient—called a 'graft-versus-host' (GVH) reaction. Bone marrow transplantation is consequently performed only in very well-matched patients such as close relatives. Strategies such as T cell depletion and $CD34^+$ stem cell selection are routinely employed to minimize the risk of GVH disease.

Transplantation of tissues and organs is usually from donors who are genetically nonidentical and is therefore likely to trigger rejection. Hence there is a need for tissue matching and immunosuppression strategies to maximize graft survival that vary according to the tissues transplanted. Skin grafting, for practical reasons, is almost always an autograft, involving transplantation of healthy skin from another part of the patient's body; skin xenografting (using a sterile medical product) may be used as a temporary graft to protect against infection prior to a skin autograft.

Among organ transplants, kidney transplantation has the longest and most successful history stemming partly from the important invention of the kidney dialysis machine by Willem Kolff in 1944,. The complexity, diversity and inheritance of MHC and HLA molecules were established by Snell, Benacerraf and Dausset, among others [1–3], and their importance in allograft rejection was clearly illustrated by Medawar's studies. Subsequently, the practical considerations of tissue matching for kidney transplantation became possible when artificial dialysis bought sufficient time for the patient to enable a well-matched donor to be identified. Since the 1960s, HLA matching has remained a priority in selection of a suitable donor kidney for transplantation.

For other types of organ transplantation (heart and liver), HLA matching is not a priority since other nonimmunological considerations take precedence, such as the length of time an organ remains viable when removed from a deceased donor, and the size match of the available organ with respect to the recipient. The importance of tissue matching for transplantation of small bowel and pancreas or pancreatic islet is not established. Retrospective comparisons of degree of tissue matching with graft outcome continue to provide useful information.

Both liver and small bowel have large numbers of mature lymphocytes and their contribution to transplant outcome is much debated. There is experimental evidence, however, that as well as potentially contributing to organ rejection and GVH disease, such 'passenger leucocytes' may also contribute to graft survival. Clinical studies suggest that combined organ transplants may be preferable to multiple organs from different donors transplanted sequentially over a longer period of time. This appears to be the case for liver and small bowel, or kidney and pancreas organ transplants.

Immunological considerations in organ transplantation

The importance of antigenically different cell surface histocompatibility molecules in graft rejection was first proposed by Gorer, Snell and colleagues in the early 1950s, although it had long been recognized that variability in the rejection response to transplanted tissues was genetically controlled [4]. Early studies on transplanted tumours in Japanese waltzing mice had demonstrated the influence of approximately a dozen dominant genes that are now known to encode some of the MHC antigens. Incompatibility between the graft donor and recipient for antigens encoded by genes of the MHC is the most important cause of rapid graft rejection. Minor histocompatibility (mH) antigens, such as the male-specific H-Y antigen, are encoded by genes outside the MHC and are not expressed as intact cell surface molecules, but rather as peptides; incompatibility in this region may also cause graft rejection, but usually with a markedly delayed time course.

During the early trials of clinical renal transplantation, attempts were made to match donor and recipient in order to reduce the risk of graft rejection. Serological methods were developed from 1958 onwards by the pioneer, Jean Dausset, to type the MHC gene products expressed on peripheral blood leucocytes. The existence of another class of MHC antigens became apparent when it was found (initially in mice and later in humans) that cells from individuals that were identical on the basis of serological typing responded strongly to each other when tested in the mixed lymphocyte reaction (MLR) *in vitro*. This second class of MHC antigens has a more limited cellular distribution and constitutes class II MHC antigens; the serologically defined molecules are class I MHC antigens.

The HLA system

The HLA system of cell surface molecules is encoded within the MHC, a large group of around 200 genes on chromosome 6 in humans (Figure 3.1). It includes 3 highly polymorphic class I α-chain genes which combine with the β_2-microglobulin (β2M) chain to form the classical class I molecules HLA-A, HLA-B, and HLA-C, as well as three pairs of polymorphic class II α- and β-chain genes that combine to form the HLA-DR, -DP, and -DQ class II molecules. Other relatively nonpolymorphic class II genes encode a series of proteins involved in antigen processing and presentation, including *LMP* genes encoding proteasome components, the TAP1, TAP2, and tapasin molecules involved in class I–peptide assembly, and the DM and DO molecules that perform a similar peptide-loading function in the class II complex. In addition to these loci, class III genes encode various serum proteins of the immune system, including components of the complement system.

The cellular distribution of HLA molecules is determined largely by their function. Peptides presented by class I HLA molecules are derived from cytosolic proteins, such as viral pathogens and their gene products. Thus, HLA class I molecules are expressed constitutively by most nucleated cells of the body (since they are susceptible

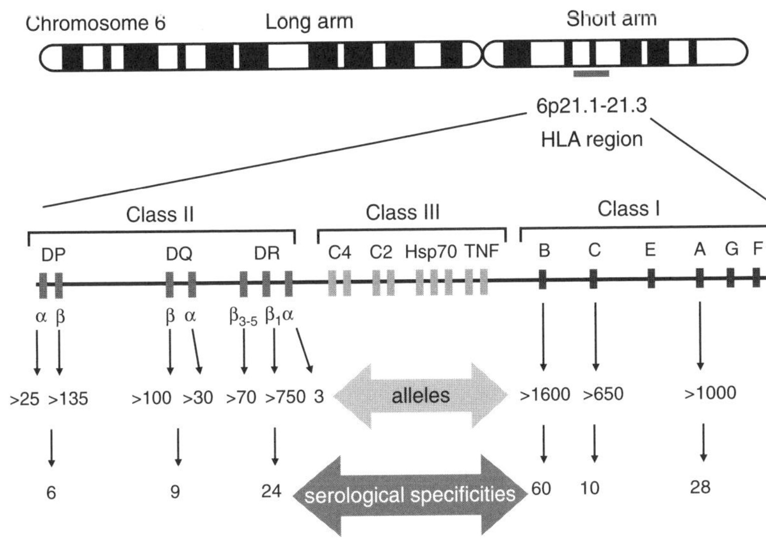

Fig. 3.1 The human leucocyte antigen (HLA) gene complex. The HLA class I and class II membrane molecules, together with soluble inflammatory proteins (class III), are encoded by a set of genes located on the short arm of chromosome 6. A total of 3296 HLA-A, -B and–C α-chain alleles encode 2520 proteins, of which 98 are recognized as distinct class I molecules by specific antibodies. Similarly, 1222 α- and β-chain alleles encode 931 class II molecules of which 39 are recognized by specific antibodies. HSP70, heat shock protein 70; TNF, tumour necrosis factor.

to viral attack) and, in particularly high density, by cells of the immune system. Increased expression may be induced by an inflammatory milieu characteristic of an active immune response. Peptides presented by class II molecules are generated by breakdown of endosomal proteins; class II expression is thus much less widespread and largely restricted to cells that have the capability to process and present exogenous soluble and particulate antigen. Cells with these characteristics include B lymphocytes, dendritic cells (DCs), macrophages, and monocytes; class II molecules may be induced, in inflammatory conditions, on certain types of epithelial and endothelial cells (ECs). Class II expression on activated human T lymphocytes may be induced or may result from membrane sharing with, for example, DCs.

The HLA system is the most polymorphic gene system in the entire human genome and mostly results from gene duplication. Each individual expresses only a relatively small number of HLA alleles: one allele each of HLA-A, -B and -C classical class I molecules from each parent together with one allele each of the three principal class II molecules (HLA-DR, -DP, -DQ) from each parent, with little or no crossover between the chromosomes supplying these alleles (Figure 3.2). The number of permutations of particular peptide-binding sites covered by these few alleles means that most potentially dangerous antigens may be presented and recognized by T cell receptors (TCRs). Throughout the human population, there is a survival advantage to this extensive polymorphism since it is unlikely that a member of the population will

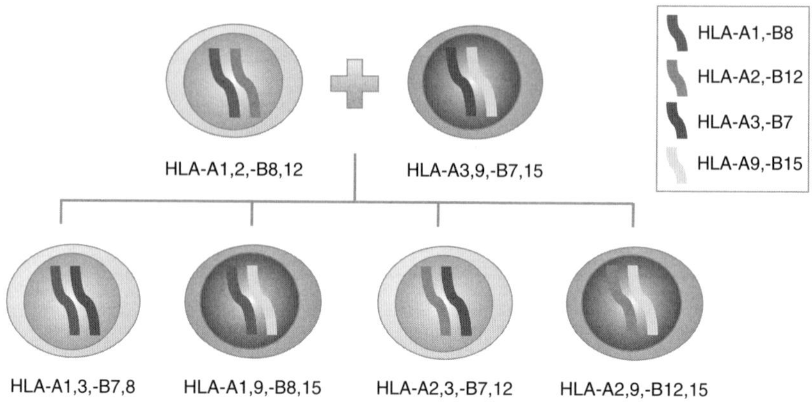

Fig. 3.2 Mendelian inheritance of codominantly expressed HLA types. An individual inherits one copy (haplotype) of the full complement of MHC genes from each parent, and expresses them codominantly. Chromosomal crossover within the MHC is rare. There is a 25% chance that an individual will have a two-haplotype match with a sibling, a 25% chance of a two-haplotype mismatch, and a 50% chance of a one-haplotype match. HLA, human leucocyte antigen; MHC, major histocompatibility complex (see also colour plate section).

encounter a particular antigen to which it is unable to respond. For transplantation, however, this is a disadvantage because it makes the chance of finding a well-matched donor more difficult, although within ethnic groups certain combinations of alleles are represented with a higher than random frequency (termed 'linkage disequilibrium') that indicates they have a particular evolutionary advantage.

According to the latest data available from the IMGT/HLA database (http://www.ebi.ac.uk/imgt/hla/stats.html), a total of 3296 HLA-A, -B, and -C α-chain alleles have been identified and these are expressed as 2520 distinct proteins. For class II loci, there are 1222 α- and β-chain alleles expressed as 931 distinct class II molecules. Among class I genes, the HLA-B locus is the most polymorphic, and for class II it is HLA-DR, with the class II β-chain genes being the more polymorphic and the DR α-chain being notably nonpolymorphic (three alleles, two proteins). These molecules are expressed at the cell surface and are accessible to T and B cells. In a transplant setting they are potentially antigenic, but additionally, since they are expressed to some degree on foetal tissues and in blood, any potential transplant recipient who has been pregnant or who has had a blood transfusion may have already developed immunological memory and circulating antibodies to non-self HLA molecules and will, thus, be 'sensitized' against certain HLA molecules. In practical terms, this has hitherto been managed by performing (1) a tissue type, to determine the HLA genotype of donors and recipients prior to kidney transplantation, in order to select the closest HLA match, and (2) a cross-match test, between the selected donor–recipient pair, to exclude the presence of existing circulating alloantibodies against donor cells that would result in rapid or hyperacute graft rejection.

HLA matching

The primary consideration when selecting a suitable donor for organ and tissue transplantation is to ensure compatibility for ABO blood group antigens, since all individuals have pre-existing circulating IgM antibodies against the ABO blood types that they do not possess. Thus, a blood group A recipient may receive a transplant from a blood group A or O donor, a group B patient may be transplanted from a group B or O donor, a group AB patient may receive tissue from a donor of any ABO group, and a group O patient may receive a transplant only from another group O donor.

HLA matching is a secondary, but important, issue [5]. An individual's complement of class I and class II HLA molecules is inherited from each parent in mendelian fashion and expressed codominantly as a haplotype, and usually an individual shares one identical haplotype with each parent because chromosomal crossover within the MHC is a very rare event (Figure 3.2).

In practice, three of the HLA loci are usually typed and matched for in kidney transplantation: HLA-A, HLA-B, and HLA-DR. In the absence of a suitably matched relative who is able to donate a kidney, there is a reasonable chance, over a period of time (months to years) on a recipient waiting list, that a kidney from a well-matched deceased donor will become available. For bone marrow transplantation, where matching requirements are more stringent to avoid both rejection of the stem cells and GVH disease, it is common to HLA-match for 10 antigens: HLA-A, -B, -C, -DR, and -DQ. Deceased donor kidney transplantation is the most common organ transplantation procedure and has provided the most information on benefits of HLA matching, association between degree of matching and transplant outcome, pathology of rejection, and effects of immunosuppression.

HLA matching is always performed in deceased donor kidney transplantation and there has been a continuous trend of improved tissue typing and matching methods, correlating with improved kidney transplant outcome. In recent years, however, acute transplant rejection has been usually well controlled by immunosuppression so that the added beneficial effect of tissue matching has become much less important. There is currently a debate about whether tissue matching should continue to be performed in the absence of evidence that it improves graft survival. The strongest argument in favour of continuing to match for HLA is that when a transplanted kidney eventually fails, the patient is likely to have become immunologically sensitized to the mismatched HLA alleles and the pool of potential donors for a subsequent transplant, therefore, is much reduced.

Tissue typing

The role of the tissue typing laboratory in kidney transplantation is: (1) to determine the HLA type of the patient and of potential donors in order to advise on the best match; (2) to perform a cross-match test to exclude the presence of existing circulating antibodies against HLA alleles expressed by donor lymphocytes; and (3) to identify the HLA specificity of circulating antibodies when patients are found to be sensitized in order to pre-emptively exclude unsuitable donor HLA types [5,6]. The ideal scenario is to achieve a six-antigen match between donor and recipient—that is, identity at the

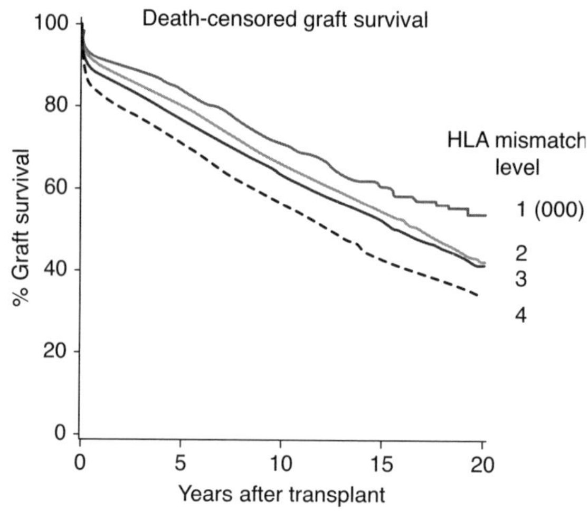

Fig. 3.3 Effect of HLA mismatch on survival of deceased donor kidney transplants. Data from NHSBT deceased donor renal transplant database. Kaplan–Meier plot of 20-year, death-censored kidney graft survival according to level of HLA mismatch (mm) between donor and recipient where level 1 represents zero HLA mm; level 2 = 0 HLA-DR and 0/1 HLA-B mm; level 3 = 0 DR + 2 B mm, or 1 DR + 0/1 B mm; and level 4 = 1 DR + 2 B mm, or 2 DR mm, demonstrating the beneficial effect of HLA matching. HLA, human leucocyte antigen.

HLA-A, -B, and -DR locus antigens. Although there exist thousands of distinct HLA proteins, the number of antigenically identifiable HLA epitopes (that are capable of eliciting an immune response) recognized by conventional antibody-based (serological) typing methods is in the low hundreds (Figure 3.1). Serological tissue typing methods use a panel of antibodies that identify distinct cell surface class I HLA antigens on T lymphocytes and class II molecules on B lymphocytes. More commonly now, molecular techniques are used for tissue typing which depend on the polymerase chain reaction (PCR) to identify specific nucleotide sequences within HLA genes in DNA prepared from peripheral blood. These methods provide a tissue type for each individual, for example HLA-A1, A2; B8, B7; DR3, DR15, where each allele is codominantly expressed and the individual is likely, partly because of linkage disequilibrium, to have inherited the separate haplotypes HLA-A1 B8 DR3 and HLA-A2 B7 DR15 from either parent (Figure 3.2). It is not uncommon for an individual to have a 'null' allele at one or more loci because the parents were identical for those particular loci. Thus, an individual's HLA type may be HLA-A2, A3; B7; DR15 because they inherited the two similar haplotypes: HLA-A2 B7 DR15 and HLA-A3 B7 DR15.

Large national transplant databases clearly show that, in spite of improving immunosuppression, the higher the number of HLA antigen matches, the better the outcome following kidney transplantation (Figure 3.3).

Having selected a suitable donor–recipient match on the basis of six-antigen HLA typing, a serological cross-match test is undertaken prior to transplantation by incubating the patient's serum with donor lymphocytes. Lymphocytes are prepared from a sample of donor lymphoid tissue or peripheral blood by mixing with magnetic microbeads coated with antibodies against B and T lymphocytes. The resultant bead–lymphocyte complexes are then isolated with a magnet; the beads are small enough that they do not interfere with the cross-match. The donor T and B lymphocytes are then incubated with current and previous samples of patient serum in microtitre plates, in the presence of rabbit complement together with an indicator dye that is excluded from live cells. Donor lymphocyte cytotoxicity indicates the presence of circulating anti-HLA antibodies and this usually rules out that particular transplant because of the high likelihood of hyperacute rejection of the kidney occurring within hours of the operation. The specificity of antibodies in the patient's serum is then determined, using single antigen bead technology, to identify all the HLA alleles against which the patient is sensitized [7]. This involves incubating patient's serum with a panel of fluorescent latex beads, each coated with molecules of a single purified HLA allele (Luminex technology). The panel of beads covers the spectrum of HLA types and bound serum is detected using a fluorescently-labelled secondary detection antibody. The reaction is read by flow cytometry where the combination of fluorescent signals provides a unique light scatter pattern for each HLA specificity.

Immunology of transplant rejection

Introduction

In spite of stringent tests to maximize tissue matching and minimize sensitization, the natural response of the body following transplantation is to identify a change to the status quo and to respond appropriately. The immune response that aims to eliminate the transplant consists of the innate immune system and the adaptive immune system, which are triggered in different ways and differ in speed and specificity of the pathophysiological responses elicited (see Chapter 1).

Contribution of innate immunity

The innate immune system, on its own, is not sufficient to cause allograft rejection; numerous experimental studies have clearly shown an absolute requirement for adaptive immunity. The innate response contributes to adaptive immunity through a system of molecules, highly conserved between species, for distinguishing between self and non-self. Certain simple and repeating pathogen-associated molecular patterns (PAMPs) in many microorganisms (e.g. on bacterial cell walls) are recognized by pattern recognition receptors (PRRs) such as the Toll-like receptors (TLRs) expressed by macrophages, neutrophils, natural killer (NK) cells, and DCs (Figure 3.4). DCs activated by TLR recognition are then able to function as antigen processing and presentation cells, thus initiating the adaptive immune response. Certain TLRs, such as TLR4, are also known to bind molecules associated with cell damage through recognition elements termed damage-associated molecular patterns (DAMPs) expressed on heat shock proteins (HSPs) and other chaperones that are induced by cellular stress, and whose purpose is to scavenge harmful molecules such as reactive oxygen species (ROSs) that can induce cell apoptosis.

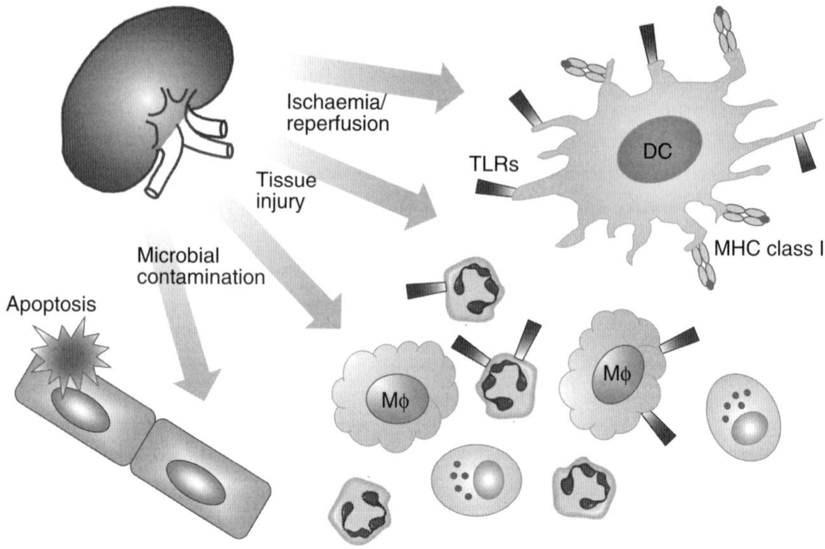

Fig. 3.4 Activation of the innate immune response following transplantation. TLRs expressed on DCs, neutrophils, NK cells, and macrophages (Mϕ) engage with a range of molecules released during transplantation-associated ischaemia/reperfusion injury and donor tissue injury, as well as with PAMPs expressed by microbial contaminants. ROS induced by ischaemia/reperfusion injury cause EC activation and apoptosis, while TLR signalling induces a nonspecific inflammatory response, and activates DCs that are then able to engage the adaptive immune (rejection) response. DC, dendritic cell; MHC, major histocompatibility complex; PAMP, pathogen-associated molecular pattern; ROS, reactive oxygen species; TLR, Toll-like receptor.

Innate immunity is highly effective as a first line of defence for combating infection and cell damage, and its armoury includes signalling pathways that induce gene transcription and production of inflammatory cytokines, chemokines and adhesion molecules. For example, release of tumour necrosis factor-alpha (TNF-α) results in vascular EC activation which permits leucocyte transmigration into tissues. Inflammation also results in locally enhanced vascular permeability so that increased drainage of extracellular fluid into the lymphoid system transports free antigens from the site of infection or cellular damage to the draining lymph nodes.

There is accumulating evidence from rodent studies of transplantation that tissue damage in the donor organ contributes to the adaptive immune response through activation of the innate response [8,9] (Figure 3.4). Nevertheless, triggering of the adaptive immune response remains dependent on highly regulated and specific interactions between peptide-specific T cells and antigen-presenting cells (APC), as evidenced by numerous animal studies showing that T cells are essential for graft rejection.

A number of apparently nonimmune considerations in transplantation are now recognized to contribute to the innate response via the release of ROSs, such as the status of deceased organ donors (age, physiological stability), treatment with inotropes, and periods of organ ischaemia followed by reperfusion, as well as recipient factors including hypertension, hyperlipidaemia, viral infection, and immunosuppressive drug toxicity [10]. There is future scope, therefore, for investigating the potential benefits of including agents to inhibit the innate response in the immunosuppressive treatment regimens of transplant patients, such as antioxidants and agents to block TLR signalling.

Allorecognition: direct and indirect pathways

While the innate response clearly contributes to the adaptive immune response, it is unclear whether the adaptive immune system can function in the absence of innate immunity. It is likely that the innate immune system functions as part of the complex arrangements of checks and balances that are essential for regulating adaptive immunity in order to avoid the tissue-destructive and, at times, life-threatening effects of inappropriate adaptive immune responses, as occurs in autoimmune disease, allergies, and anaphylaxis. Perhaps the critical contribution of the innate immune response in transplantation is to activate donor-derived DCs residing within the transplanted organ, providing them with the stimulus to migrate to local lymph nodes in the recipient where they interface with and activate the adaptive immune system.

The initial step in the immune response to a transplant is recognition that the transplanted tissue is non-self and represents a threat equivalent to that of an exogenous protein or pathogen. Transplant rejection results from triggering of the immune response that has evolved over time to manage infection and to protect against further reinfection. It is helpful, therefore, to consider rejection mechanisms in terms of current knowledge of the conventional immune response. During infection and cell damage, DCs become activated in response to innate immune recognition of PAMPs and DAMPs by TLRs. DCs are able to take up infectious agents and cell debris by receptor-mediated endocytosis, or by macropinocytosis. Antigenic material is then processed intracellularly and presented in the form of small peptides (12–20 amino acids in length) embedded in the peptide-binding cleft of membrane-bound MHC class II molecules. Virally infected DCs present newly synthesized viral peptides (9–11 amino acids), in the cleft of MHC class I molecules. Thus activated, these APCs begin to mature, up-regulating the expression of MHC class II proteins and expressing costimulatory molecules (CD80, CD86), adhesion molecules (CD40), and chemokine receptors (CCR7), and migrate through the lymphatic system to the local draining lymph nodes where their interaction with responding lymphocytes is further regulated. Macrophages and B lymphocytes also function as APCs, macrophages principally by engulfing particulate matter, while B cells bind soluble antigens via their surface immunoglobulin receptors. Migration and interaction with naive T and B cells is mediated by chemokines and their specific receptors. For example, DCs that have been licensed by TLR signalling to express the chemokine receptor CCR7 are then able to interact with the chemokine CCL21 present in a concentration gradient in lymphoid tissue to facilitate the correct location of the DC within the lymph node for effective interaction with naive T cells (see Chapter 1).

In a transplant situation, the newly transplanted allograft induces an immune response because the class I and class II MHC molecules expressed (to a varying extent by every cell of the transplant) differ, depending on the degree of mismatch from that

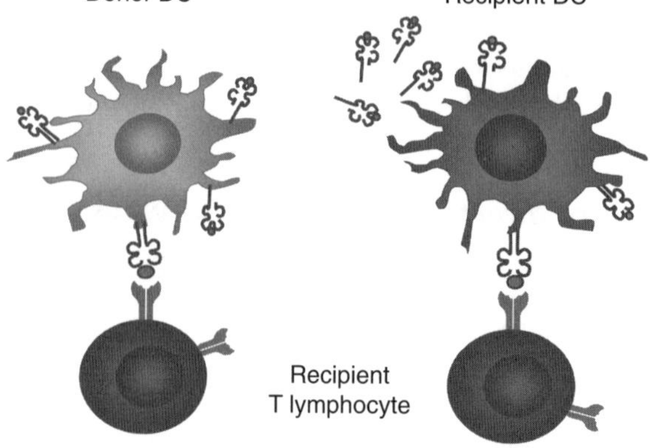

Fig. 3.5 Two pathways of allorecognition. In direct allorecognition, recipient T lymphocytes recognize (by cross-reactivity) and respond to intact, non-self class I and class II HLA molecules expressed on donor-derived APCs. In indirect allorecognition, recipient CD4$^+$ T lymphocytes recognize and respond to donor HLA molecules that have been taken up and processed by recipient APCs, and presented as peptide fragments in the peptide binding cleft of recipient HLA class II molecules (recognition by MHC restriction). APC, antigen-presenting cell; DC, dendritic cell; HLA, human leucocyte antigen (see also colour plate section).

of the patient. As soon as a blood supply to the transplanted organ is re-established, recipient APCs enter the organ encountering cell material shed from the transplant, become activated, and migrate to the recipient's draining lymph nodes. The graft itself also contains many donor-derived DCs, which may become activated as a result of cell injury incurred during the transplant procedure and migrate to the recipient's draining lymph nodes. At the same time, the transplant sheds soluble MHC molecules that become a target for processing and presentation by B cells. Transplantation is unique in that both donor and recipient DCs may function as APCs giving rise to two distinct pathways of allorecognition [11] (Figure 3.5).

The *indirect pathway* of antigen presentation and allorecognition is analogous to the pathway whereby T cells become activated in response to pathogens, or following immunization. Recipient APCs (DCs and B cells) internalize donor material, such as cell membrane fragments and soluble MHC molecules, into endocytic vesicles which move through the cell towards the Golgi apparatus. They become increasingly acidic, thereby activating protease enzymes that break down the vesicle contents into peptides. Fusion of late endosomes with lysosomes completes the degradation process and peptides are then loaded on to newly synthesized MHC class II molecules for transport to the cell surface where they integrate into the cell membrane to present peptides to nearby CD4$^+$ T cells. CD4$^+$ TCRs engage with the class II MHC–peptide complex and are able to recognize the peptides as representative of either normal self-proteins (e.g. enzyme fragments) or of foreign proteins. In the former case the T cell disengages and separates from the DC. However, the peptide may be derived from mismatched donor

HLA molecules and is recognized as foreign, resulting in prolonged contact between the $CD4^+$ T cell and the APC. This latter cell contact effectively initiates T cell activation and instigates a rejection response. This pathway also results in presentation of peptides derived from m(minor)HC antigens.

The *direct pathway* of allorecognition is dependent upon donor DCs, present within the transplanted tissue, migrating to the local lymph nodes to interact with $CD4^+$ and $CD8^+$ T lymphocytes. DCs express a high density of both class I and class II MHC molecules and, in contradiction to the laws of MHC restriction, recipient $CD4^+$ T cells respond directly to donor class II MHC–peptide complexes while recipient $CD8^+$ T cells respond directly to donor class I MHC–peptide complexes on the cell membrane of donor DCs. From laboratory experiments in which lymphocytes of HLA-mismatched individuals are cultured together, it has long been recognized that this results in surprisingly high levels of T cell proliferation. This was unexpected, because Zinkernagel and Doherty showed clearly in 1974 that T cells responding (by proliferating) to viral peptides do so only if the viral peptides are presented by cells expressing the same MHC as responding cells; if viral peptides were presented by third-party cells the responders would not proliferate, implying lack of recognition [12]. This fundamental pattern of recognition was termed MHC restriction, for which Zinkernagel and Doherty were awarded the Nobel prize in 1996. It is now apparent that T cell proliferation is initiated by close molecular interaction between a specific TCR and its ligand, which is the complex comprising peptide and MHC α-helices forming the peptide-binding cleft. The ability of T cells to proliferate in response to non-self MHC can be explained by cross-reactivity: a TCR that has higher affinity for the peptide than for the MHC α-helices of the MHC–peptide complex will be able to engage with a similar but different MHC molecule presenting the same peptide, while a TCR with higher affinity for the MHC portion than for the peptide will be able to engage with an identical MHC molecule presenting a different peptide. The former condition represents the case in *direct allorecognition* where the peptides are often derived from tissue components common to all individuals of the species. Direct TCR engagement with the combined 'self' peptide–foreign MHC complex induces T cell activation (see Chapter 1).

In vitro experiments have demonstrated that the frequency of T cells responding to donor MHC that is processed and presented as peptides by recipient DCs (indirect recognition) is at least tenfold lower than the frequency of T cells responding to foreign MHC expressed on donor DCs (direct recognition) [13]. The likely explanation for this disparity is that the great majority of T cells are nonresponsive to, or tolerant of, self peptides presented by self MHC, and most recipient APCs sampling the cell environment will be presenting self peptides with only a small proportion of class II molecules presenting foreign (donor MHC) peptides and, thereby, initiating T cell proliferation. In contrast, when T cells encounter donor DCs, because they already recognize endogenous peptides they can respond by cross-reaction to most of the MHC molecules presenting self peptides on donor DCs (Figure 3.6). Since the self-peptide–MHC complex is highly similar but not identical, T cells will become activated instead of becoming anergic, resulting in higher levels of T cell proliferation. Thus, when the blood circulation through the transplanted tissue is re-established,

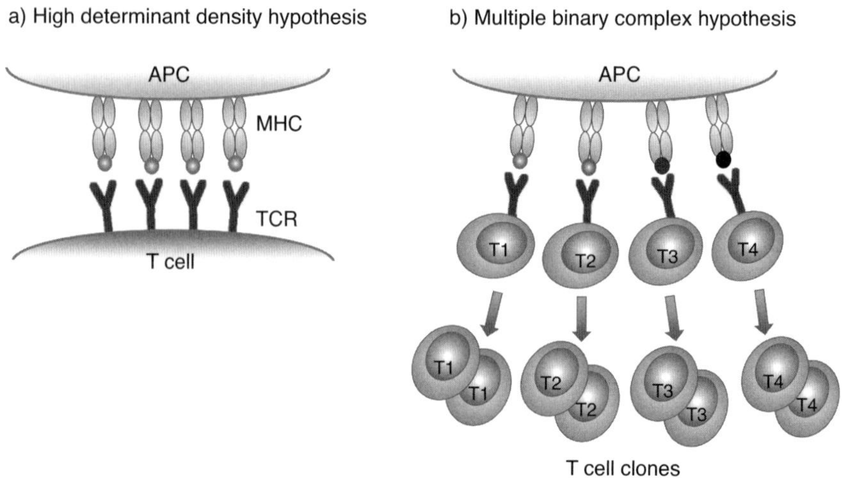

Fig. 3.6 High frequency of alloreactive T cells. Two theories have been proposed to account for the high frequency of recipient T cells responding directly to donor MHC [13]. (a) The *high determinant density* hypothesis proposes T cells preferentially recognizing the MHC part of the MHC–peptide complex encounter alloantigen (donor MHC) that is expressed at high frequency on donor APCs, so many T cells can respond to individual APCs. (b) The *multiple binary complex* hypothesis proposes that T cells that preferentially recognize the peptide part of the MHC–peptide complex are able to respond by cross-reaction to many donor MHC–peptide complexes presenting different endogenous peptides. APC, antigen-presenting cell; MHC, major histocompatibility complex.

migration of donor DCs from the graft to the local lymphoid tissue is a very effective mechanism for initiating immunity against the graft.

The relative contribution of direct and indirect pathways of allorecognition to the graft rejection response is unknown, but it is likely that the direct pathways plays a major role in acute rejection when donor DCs migrate from the graft immediately after transplantation, to be replaced subsequently by recipient DCs. Donor DCs probably do not persist for more than a few days after transplantation, since they themselves will become a target of the graft rejection response. In contrast, recipient DCs are able to continually sample, process, and present donor MHC molecules and it is thought that indirect recognition is responsible for chronic allograft rejection.

A third pathway of (semi-direct) allorecognition has been proposed that is based on a well-recognized biological process of contact-dependent membrane sharing between DCs and other cell types [11]. *In vitro* studies have demonstrated that cocultured allogeneic DCs exchange and express each other's MHC molecules; it is possible that they acquire membrane fragments from contact with apoptotic cells. The physiological purpose of membrane sharing is not known, but in a transplantation setting it may enhance recipient T cell activation by combining direct and indirect antigen presentation on the same cell.

Initiation and amplification of the alloimmune response

A rejection response is initiated, as with responses to conventional antigens, when naive T cells with specificity for a particular peptide–MHC complex encounter their ligand on an APC. Trafficking DCs that have acquired antigens migrate to the local lymph node where this encounter is facilitated through expression of adhesion molecules, chemokines, and chemokine receptors on immune cells and on the stroma of the lymphoid tissue. Naive T lymphocytes circulating in the blood enter the lymph node via the afferent lymphatic vessels where, though expression of the adhesion molecule L-selectin, they pass into high endothelial venules and thence, through expression of the chemokine receptor CCR7, into the T cell zones in the lymph node paracortex where stromal cells produce the chemokine ligand CCL21. T cells then encounter and interact with DCs. When an antigen-specific interaction occurs, further molecular interactions extend the contact time between the T cell and DC to enable full T cell activation. Naive T cells that fail to make prolonged contact pass through to the cortical sinus and the collecting system of the medullary sinuses, through their expression of a receptor for the signalling lipid molecule sphingosine-1-phosphate, leaving the lymph node to return to the circulation via the efferent lymphatics.

T lymphocytes that encounter specific antigen in the lymph node, whether expressed by DCs, B cells, or macrophages, remain there for 3–4 days where they are fully activated through costimulatory molecules to undergo clonal expansion.

T cell activation requires that the initial specific interaction (signal 1) between the TCR and the peptide–MHC complex, together with docking of the CD4 or CD8 molecules with the class II or class I MHC molecules on the APC, respectively, is followed by the second, costimulatory signal which involves interaction between the B7 molecules on the APC (CD80 and CD86) with the CD28 molecules on the T lymphocyte. This second signal is rapidly followed by lymphocyte expression of cytotoxic lymphocyte antigen-4 (CTLA-4) which is thought to regulate T cell activation by engaging with B7 in preference to CD28, either to limit the proliferative response or to induce anergy instead of activation. A number of costimulatory molecules have been identified (PD-1, ICOS) that contribute to either full lymphocyte activation, anergy, apoptosis, or termination of T cell activation; their relative contribution is not fully understood.

Costimulation through CD28 signals the T cell to enter the G_1 phase of the cell cycle to achieve clonal expansion and at the same time causes induction of the nuclear factor of activated T cells (NFATs) family of DNA-binding factors that activate transcription of the interleukin-2 (IL-2) gene. The cytokine IL-2 may be regarded as signal 3 of lymphocyte activation since it is necessary for the differentiation of activated lymphocytes into functional effector cells [12] (see Chapter 1).

Following transplantation, the recipient immune response is initiated directly by graft DCs migrating to regional lymphoid tissue where they engage with T cells via cross-reactive MHC-restricted recognition. At the same time, indirect T cell activation occurs when recipient DCs enter the graft, encounter alloantigens, and migrate to the lymph nodes to present them as peptides to recipient T cells. Responding T cells then differentiate into effector cells to mediate allograft rejection. In the absence of immunosuppressive therapy, the endpoint of this rejection response is destruction of the foreign tissue within the graft, and failure of the transplant to function and survive. As this is achieved, the immune response is down-regulated and only memory T and B cells persist, ready to respond rapidly if the graft-specific MHC antigens are re-encountered.

In addition to the recipient antigraft rejection response, donor lymphocytes that are transplanted as 'passenger leucocytes' within the graft may themselves engage in T cell activation following recognition of recipient tissues as foreign. This initiates GVH disease, which can cause significant problems following allogeneic bone marrow transplantation. This may also occur after organ transplantation, especially of liver and small bowel which carry particularly large numbers of donor lymphocytes. The primary targets of the GVH reaction are the skin, gastrointestinal tract, liver, and lungs of the recipient.

Effector mechanisms: cellular and humoral responses

T cell activation and differentiation is sustained over a prolonged period by a continuum of direct and indirect presentation, together with production of a range of cytokines that mediate T cell differentiation [13].

The $CD4^+$ T cell is of central importance in allograft rejection and essentially orchestrates the various effector responses (Figure 3.7) [14–16]. It secretes IL-2 that acts in an autocrine (and paracrine) manner to initiate up-regulation of the inducible chain of the IL-2 receptor. Activated naive $CD4^+$ T cells thus differentiate into T helper (Th) cells that can secrete a range of cytokines—e.g. IL-2, IL-4, IL-5, and interferon-gamma (IFN-γ)—to coordinate the three principal mechanisms of graft rejection: cytotoxic T cell (CTL) responses, antibody-mediated responses, and delayed-type hypersensitivity (DTH) responses.

Graft antigen-specific $CD8^+$ CTLs are induced following direct recognition of donor MHC class I antigens, most likely expressed on donor DCs migrating to recipient lymphoid tissue. $CD8^+$ T cells receive help from IL-2 secreted by $CD4^+$ Th cells and differentiate into cytotoxic effector cells that engage, via the TCR and $CD8^+$ molecules, with donor class I molecules expressed on most cells of the transplanted organ. Help is probably delivered most effectively by noncognate interaction in a three-cell cluster consisting of a $CD8^+$ T cell recognizing donor class I MHC on the donor APC and a direct pathway with recipient $CD4^+$ T cells recognizing donor class II MHC. There are additional possible scenarios, whereby $CD8^+$ T cells receive help in a noncognate fashion by way of three- and four-cell clusters involving donor and/or recipient APCs [17]. Cell damage occurs through the formation of an immune synapse with the target cell that facilitates passage of perforins and granzymes from the granules of CTLs into the target cell, resulting in cell death by apoptosis.

B lymphocytes, whose surface immunoglobulin receptors engage with donor MHC target antigens, receive help for differentiation into plasma cells because of their ability to process and present antigen. Thus, self-restricted, indirect pathway $CD4^+$ T cells

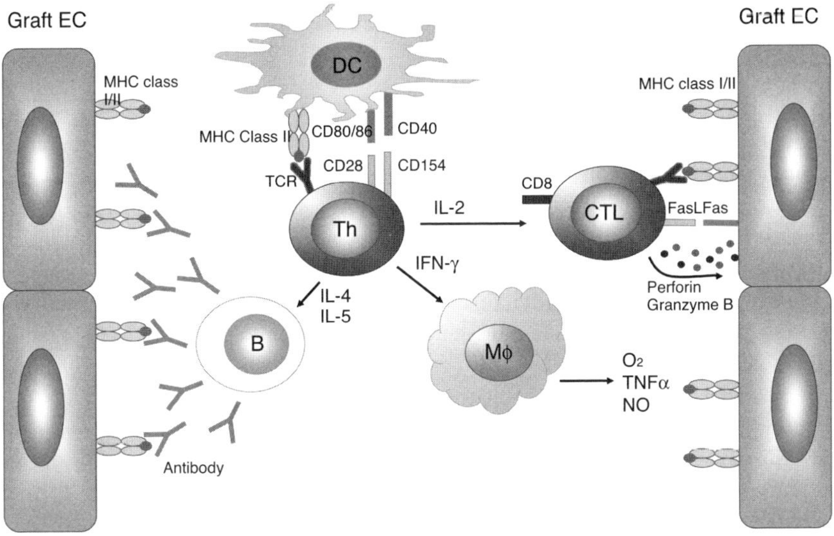

Fig. 3.7 Mechanisms of allograft rejection. The CD4$^+$ Th cell is a key player in the adaptive immune response to a transplant. CD4$^+$ T cells engage with activated APCs and are themselves activated, resulting in cytokine production that is necessary for maturation of B lymphocytes and production of graft-specific alloantibodies, generation of donor-specific CTLs that lyse target cells via release of perforins and granzymes inducing apoptosis, and initiation of a nonspecific inflammatory response or DTH reaction, whereby macrophages, NK cells, and granulocytes release mediators that enhance the rejection response and cause EC activation and apoptosis. CTL, cytotoxic T lymphocyte; DC, dendritic cell; EC, endothelial cell; FasL, Fas ligand; MHC, major histocompatibility complex; Mϕ, macrophage; TCR, T cell receptor.

recognizing processed donor MHC peptides through MHC class II molecules on B cells provide help in a cognate fashion to the B cells. The latter are then able to mature and differentiate into plasma cells that secrete specific alloantibodies against the transplant. The primary target of the alloantibody response is the layer of ECs lining the donor organ vasculature (Figure 3.7). Antibody-induced cell damage is mediated by a range of mechanisms including activation of both the classical complement and coagulation cascades, and also possibly by antibody-dependent cell-mediated cytotoxicity (ADCC). In ADCC Fc receptors on NK cells and macrophages recognize tissue-bound antibody and mediate damage via perforins and granzymes, as well as by release of various small molecules such as ROSs and nitric oxide (NO) [18]. ADCC has long been demonstrated in *in vitro* responses by NK cells and activated macrophages against target cells coated with antibody, but there is contradictory evidence regarding its role in contributing to graft rejection. In addition, alloantibody binding to graft endothelium induces characteristic changes in the ECs themselves that may result in alterations in cell surface expression of integrins and adhesion molecules, and secretion of cytokines [19,20]. These changes contribute to EC activation, leucocyte recruitment, and cell proliferation associated with graft damage. In certain circumstances, the persistent presence of low-level alloantibodies may have a protective effect on the graft through EC accommodation, a term implying that ECs become resistant to caspase-dependent apoptosis.

The DTH response is initiated by alloantigen-specific $CD4^+$ T cells that secrete proinflammatory cytokines, including IFN-γ and TNF-α, which help to recruit and activate non-antigen-specific cells such as monocytes and macrophages. These cells secrete additional cytokines and mediate leucocyte chemotaxis, and the resulting local inflammation, oedema, and cellular infiltrate, characteristic of allograft rejection, contribute to tissue damage. On its own, however, the DTH pathway is not an efficient process: experimental studies in transgenic mice bearing only a monoclonal population of donor MHC-specific $CD4^+$ T cells have shown that skin allografts are rejected but in a much delayed manner [21].

In addition to alloantigen-specific responses, mechanical damage during transplantation may result in presentation of tissue peptides that initiate an autoimmune response; autoantibodies are increasingly being recognized as contributing to graft rejection [22].

Privileged sites, immunoisolation

Certain anatomical sites are relatively protected from the immune system. One such site is the testis, where immunological privilege ensures that, during puberty, exposure to the immune system by a range of new and potentially antigenic proteins does not have detrimental effects on developing germ cells. Similarly, the developing foetus, which expresses both maternal MHC antigens and foreign, paternal MHC antigens, is protected from the mother's immune system [23]. The eye is also relatively protected from the immune system. The brain is an immunologically privileged site and is protected from circulating lymphocytes and proteins, including antibodies, by the blood–brain barrier. This latter is a physical barrier, but in other cases immune protection is provided by secretion or expression of anti-inflammatory proteins such as Fas ligand (FasL), transforming growth factor-beta (TGF-β), or indoleamine 2,3-dioxygenase (IDO), while protection in the eye is provided by a poor blood and lymph supply and absence of APCs. A combination of anergy and immunological ignorance normally maintains the lack of T cell responses to the privileged tissues, but in some cases, such as the eye and the testis, some of the antigens are novel and hitherto not exposed to the immune system. Following trauma, the novel antigens may become exposed, resulting in the development of an autoimmune response that causes significant and long-term tissue damage and, in the case of pregnancy, loss of the foetus.

As a privileged site, the eye usually, but not always, accepts corneal transplants. For the most part, the transplants are successful without the need for tissue matching or systemic immunosuppression. It is also a useful site for experimental transplantation, for studying mechanisms of tolerance, suppression, and immune avoidance. Interestingly, it has been shown that an allograft transplanted to such a site is not only not rejected but also induces a state of systemic and specific tolerance. A subsequent challenge by cells from the same donor to the skin of the recipient failed to induce a

DTH reaction, but there was a normal response to a third-party challenge [24]. It should be noted, however, that corneal graft rejection is not an infrequent event in the long term [25].

Research into privileged sites has prompted investigation of other approaches for avoiding contact with the recipient's immune system, such as encapsulation of the transplanted material within a biocompatible polymer material. This methodology has been used experimentally, with some success, for pancreatic islets, mesenchymal stem cells, and embryonic stem cell-derived neurons [26].

Clinical patterns of rejection

Introduction

Transplant rejection is diagnosed by a combination of criteria, and transplant biopsies reveal distinct pathological lesions that are characteristic of the mechanisms causing tissue damage. These are described below.

Hyperacute rejection

Hyperacute rejection is the most rapid and aggressive form of transplant rejection and it is mediated by pre-existing circulating antibodies against the graft. A well-known example is the anti-ABO antibodies responsible for the transfusion reaction when patients receive an ABO-mismatched blood transfusion. Similar, naturally occurring antibodies exist in humans and primates. These react against the galactose α1–3 galactosyl-4-*N*-acetylglucosamine (α-Gal) epitope, which is a widespread cell surface epitope in other mammalian species. The anti-ABO antibodies are capable of causing hyperacute rejection of ABO-mismatched organ transplants and the latter pose a major hurdle for the use of animal tissues for transplantation. Damage is caused to the transplant when these antibodies bind to their target antigens on ECs in the graft and activate the complement and coagulation cascades. This results in extensive thrombosis in the graft vasculature, interstitial haemorrhage, and irreversible tissue injury, all of which are initiated within minutes of re-establishing the blood supply to the transplant.

Hyperacute rejection can also be triggered by anti-HLA antibodies in patients sensitized by a previous transplant, blood transfusions, or pregnancies. The pre-transplant cytotoxic cross-match test is routinely performed by the tissue typing laboratory prior to renal transplantation, to detect circulating antibodies in the recipient's serum against HLA molecules on the donor's lymphocytes. Donor lymphocyte cytotoxicity is usually a contraindication to renal transplantation; as a consequence, hyperacute rejection is now rare. All types of organs are prone to hyperacute rejection but the kidney is particularly susceptible. Because preservation times are short for heart and liver transplantation, a pretransplant cross-match test is not routine practice. Interestingly, liver transplantation may be performed in the presence of known anti-HLA antibodies with relatively little likelihood of graft rejection because of the great resilience and regenerative capacity of the liver.

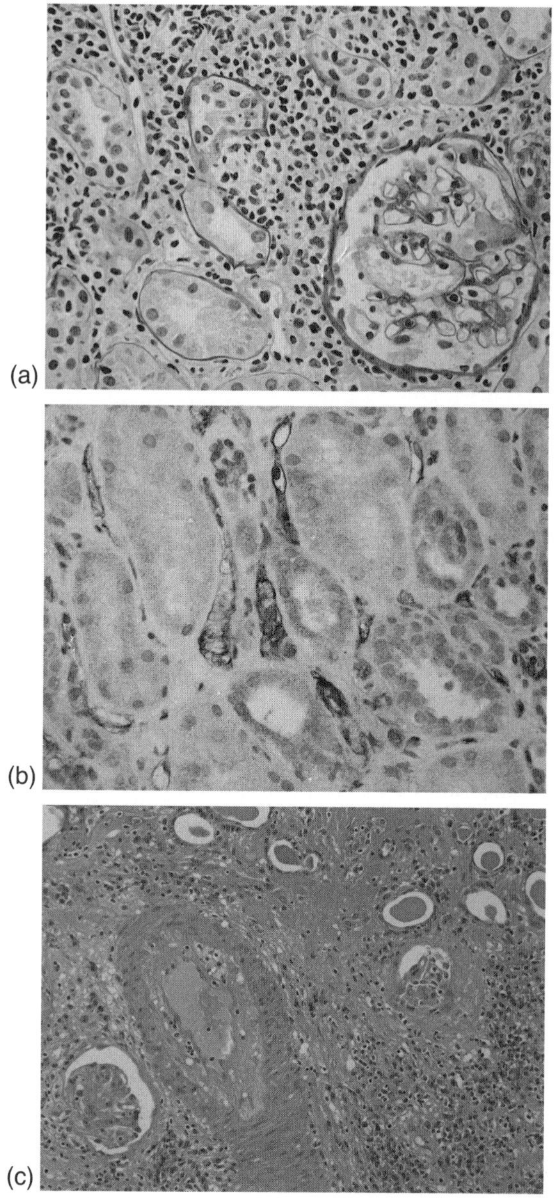

Fig. 3.8 Pathology of renal allograft rejection: (a) Inflammatory infiltrate characteristic of acute cellular rejection. The tubules are separated by an interstitial infiltrate of lymphocytes, and lymphocytes have infiltrated the tubular epithelium (tubulitis). PAS ×400. (b) C4d deposition in a renal transplant with acute humoral rejection. C4d is demonstrated circumferentially in peritubular capillaries using immunohistochemistry (brown staining). ×400. (c) Characteristic appearance of graft vasculopathy in a renal transplant with chronic rejection. The wall of the interlobular artery is thickened by fibrosis and an infiltrate of lymphocytes and macrophages. There is associated atrophy of tubules and glomeruli. H&E ×200. Images kindly supplied by Dr Meryl Griffiths, Consultant Pathologist, Addenbrooke's Hospital, Cambridge (see also colour plate section).

Acute cellular and humoral rejection

Acute rejection is the result of the immune system recognizing new, foreign antigens and involves both humoral and cellular components. It is most likely to happen within the first few weeks after transplantation but may be triggered at a much later stage, most likely by infection or reduction of immunosuppression. Continuous advances in immunosuppressive therapy have resulted in a steady decrease in the incidence of acute rejection following transplantation. Fewer than 20% of recipients of first renal transplants now experience acute rejection during the first year after transplantation.

Clinical diagnosis of acute rejection usually makes a distinction, on the basis of graft pathology, between acute cellular rejection and acute humoral rejection, and this may influence the type of rescue therapy, although sometimes both components contribute to rejection. Features characteristic of cellular rejection include an inflammatory infiltrate, consisting largely of mononuclear leucocytes that initially have a focal perivascular distribution, where the targets are graft ECs. This becomes denser and more diffuse and involves graft parenchymal cells (Figure 3.8a). The early infiltrate comprises mostly $CD4^+$ T and $CD8^+$ T lymphocytes, some of which are activated and proliferating, and this is followed by the appearance of activated macrophages, plasma cells, neutrophils and eosinophils. The diffuse infiltrate is accompanied by destruction of the tissue parenchyma and a degree of oedema. Graft blood vessels are also a target of the inflammatory response and endotheliitis is characterized by leucocyte adherence to vessel endothelium, together with infiltration underneath the endothelium and separation and oedema of the endothelial layer.

Humoral rejection involves formation of alloantibodies that bind primarily to the vascular endothelium, resulting in complement fixation and deposition of complement components, particularly C4d, on the walls of the vasculature (Figure 3.8b). There is also graft oedema and haemorrhage together with accumulation of neutrophils. Fibrinoid necrosis of smaller vessels is characteristically found in renal allograft rejection. The prevalence and contribution of antibody-mediated graft damage in acute rejection is probably underestimated.

Acute rejection is typically associated with release of inflammatory cytokines and both up-regulation and novel induction of MHC class I and II expression, all of which serve to amplify the rejection response.

Chronic rejection

Since fewer grafts now fail as a result of acute rejection, chronic rejection has become the major cause of graft loss. It has benefited little from recent advances in immunosuppression. Chronic rejection usually develops slowly and insidiously over months and years, and is characterized by a progressive decline in graft function. Its primary cause is most likely due to an antigraft immune response, as supported by the fact that development of chronic rejection is strongly associated with previous episodes of acute rejection, and also with the degree of HLA mismatch. Other risk factors for chronic rejection include ischaemia/reperfusion injury, immunosuppressive drug toxicity, hyperlipidaemia, and infection, all of which invoke innate immune responses. Diagnosis is confirmed by biopsy appearance, the most characteristic features being changes to small arteries in clusters throughout the organ. Features include a thickened intima caused by oedema and infiltration, frequently with foamy, lipid-filled macrophages; there may be fibrin deposition in the lumen (Figure 3.8c). Smooth muscle cell proliferation in the medial layer is a classic hallmark of chronic rejection; it may progress to partial or complete obliteration of the vessel lumen, and the elastic lamina may become disrupted, or may demonstrate proliferation. These features strongly resemble those of atherosclerosis, except that in chronic graft vasculopathy the lesions develop in a concentric fashion. Elsewhere in the graft, the parenchyma shows only sparse leucocyte infiltration but there may be patches of necrosis, interstitial fibrosis, and loss of parenchymal structures.

The contribution of antibodies to chronic rejection is supported by a number of studies demonstrating presence of circulating anti-HLA antibodies against both class I and class II MHC proteins at the time of diagnosis, and complement deposition in graft vessels [27]. There is also increasing evidence that autoantibodies directed against structural components (vimentin, cardiac myosin) may develop in the course of chronic rejection and may have a functional role, especially where the protein is also expressed as a component of extracellular matrix [28].

Immunosuppressive therapy

Introduction

The earliest experimental use of immunosuppressive agents in transplantation demonstrated that acute rejection could be prevented and provided a justification for clinical renal transplantation between genetically nonidentical individuals. Azathioprine and steroids were the standard form of immunosuppressive treatment following renal transplantation for 20 years until the next breakthrough in the late 1970s. Ciclosporin, alongside azathioprine and steroids, then became the treatment of choice for the next 20 years, and permitted the successful introduction of heart and liver transplantation programmes. Since the 1990s, a number of new agents have been licensed for use in patients and successfully introduced into clinical transplantation. Currently, there is no longer a uniform approach to antirejection therapy and, to some extent, treatment is tailored to individual needs since it is unrealistic to expect a single form of intervention in the rejection response to be fully effective in all cases [29–31].

The immunosuppressive agents described in the following section are grouped according to their mode of action (Table 3.2).

Calcineurin blockers: ciclosporin and tacrolimus

Ciclosporin (cyclosporin A) and tacrolimus (FK506, Prograf) are calcineurin inhibitors that bind to immunophilins within the lymphocyte.

Ciclosporin is a lipid-soluble cyclic peptide metabolite, secreted by the fungus *Tolyplocadium inflatum*, that binds to cytoplasmic cyclophilins. The ciclosporin/cyclophilin complex blocks the protein phosphatase, calcineurin, whose function is to activate the transcription factor NF-AT by dephosphorylating it. NF-AT is thus unable to translocate to the nucleus where it would normally initiate transcription of a number of genes, especially IL-2, pivotal in Th cell activation and clonal expansion.

Table 3.2 Immunosuppressive agents used to control rejection

Category	Agent
Calcineurin inhibitors	Ciclosporin (cyclosporin A)
	Tacrolimus (FK 506)
Nucleotide synthesis inhibitors	Azathioprine
	Mycophenolate mofetil
	Leflunomide
Target of rapamycin (mTOR) inhibitors	Sirolimus
	Everolimus
Corticosteroids	Prednisolone
Depleting anti-T/B cell MABs	ATG (antithymocyte globulin)
	Anti-CD3 (orthoclone OKT3)
	Anti-CD52 (campath-1H)
	Anti-CD20 (Rituximab)
Blocking MABs, fusion proteins	Anti-CD25 (daclizumab, basiliximab)
	CTLA-4-Ig (belatacept)

The current formulation of the drug (Neoral) is a microemulsion that has improved absorption and bioavailability over that of the original formulation (Sandimmun). Its efficacy is dependent on careful monitoring of its blood trough levels. One of the potential side effects of ciclosporin is that it enhances production of TGF-β which promotes renal fibrosis. Nephrotoxicity, hypertension, and dyslipidaemia are the major side effects of ciclosporin but others include diabetes, neurotoxicity, and cosmetic changes (gingival hyperplasia and hirsutism).

Tacrolimus is structurally unrelated to ciclosporin and is an antibiotic isolated from *Streptomyces tsukubaensis*. It was approved for use in 1994 and became a direct alternative to ciclosporin. It is more potent than ciclosporin and functions similarly by binding to immunophilins (FK binding proteins or FKBP). As with ciclosporin, it inhibits calcineurin activity to prevent dephosphorylation of NF-AT, thus, blocking T cell activation and proliferation. Tacrolimus is well absorbed and its use is associated with a reduced number of acute rejection episodes in comparison with ciclosporin, although overall short-term results for patient and graft survival are similar [32]. It has similar side effects to ciclosporin, including nephrotoxicity. Hypertension, dyslipidaemia, and cosmetic changes are less frequent but diabetes and neurotoxicity are more common.

Antiproliferative agents: azathioprine and mycophenolate mofetil

The antiproliferative agents azathioprine and mycophenolate both inhibit lymphocyte proliferation by limiting the availability of purines that, as nucleotide bases, are critical components of DNA and RNA. Both are prodrugs that are converted to active agents by metabolic processes in the liver, and both are well absorbed. Lymphocytes are a particular target of these agents since, during an immune response, they are a rapidly proliferating and protein-producing cell population. Other rapidly proliferating cell types, such as bone marrow and gut ECs, are similarly affected.

Azathioprine was first used as an immunosuppressive agent in clinical transplantation by Roy Calne who had demonstrated the efficacy of its more toxic predecessor, 6-mercaptopurine, in experimental renal transplantation. Together with steroids, it formed the mainstay of clinical antirejection therapy until the introduction of ciclosporin. Its major side effect is bone marrow suppression and this limits the safe dose range, so that it is now more commonly used as adjunctive therapy to calcineurin inhibitors, where the combination of agents is effective at lower individual doses. Other side effects are typical of antiproliferative agents and include gastrointestinal symptoms.

Mycophenolate (and its prodrug form, mycophenolate mofetil) is a more recently used antiproliferative agent that was approved for use in organ transplantation in 2000 [33]. It was originally isolated from the fungus *Penicillium stoloniferum;* its use and side effects are very similar to azathioprine. Its bone marrow suppressive effects are somewhat less, but diarrhoea is a significant side effect, attributed in part to its inactive metabolite, mycophenolate glucuronidase, being reabsorbed in the gut. Like azathioprine, mycophenolate is commonly used with calcineurin inhibitors or sometimes with calcineurin-sparing agents such as sirolimus.

Corticosteroids

Corticosteroids have a wide range of immunosuppressive activity; oral prednisolone and intravenous methylprednisolone are the two main formulations used in transplantation, and both are readily absorbed. Corticosteroids are commonly used for inflammatory and autoimmune conditions because of their broad effects, which include decreasing vascular permeability and inhibiting histamine release, decreasing leucocyte infiltration through inhibition of adherence to endothelium, and inhibition of IL-1 and IL-6 production, thus leading to an overall reduction in production of cytokines and chemokines, and expression of adhesion molecules (see Chapter 7). The numerous side effects are well known and include impaired wound healing, and cosmetic effects such as thinning of the skin, acne, fluid retention, and fat redistribution. Long-term use is also associated with increased susceptibility to serious infections, hypertension, hyperlipidaemia, hyperglycaemia, and osteoporosis, among other effects.

mTOR inhibitors: sirolimus and everolimus

Sirolimus (rapamycin, Rapamune) and its derivative, everolimus, are macrolides isolated from the soil bacterium *Streptomyces hygroscopicus*. Sirolimus has a similar structure to tacrolimus and also binds to the FKBP12 immunophilin. However, it does not inhibit calcineurin; instead, the complex binds to the mTOR Complex1, thereby, inhibiting the mTOR (mammalian target of rapamycin) pathway [34]. mTOR regulates gene translation and protein synthesis, and the effect of sirolimus is to inhibit IL-2 production and lymphocyte activation. It is well absorbed, has low bioavailability and a long half-life, and produces less renal toxicity than ciclosporin. It may be used in conjunction with mycophenolate or with ciclosporin but, in the latter case, each drug increases the blood levels of the other, and this needs to be managed carefully. Because its side effects include thrombocytopenia and impaired wound healing, its use is often delayed until several weeks after transplantation.

Biological agents: anti-CD3, anti-CD25, anti-CD20

A number of polyclonal and monoclonal antibodies (MABs) directed against molecules expressed on lymphocyte cell surfaces are approved for therapeutic use in transplantation, based on the rationale that removal or lysis of the target cell will diminish the immune response against an allograft [35]. Polyclonal antibodies were raised initially in goats, rabbits, and horses by immunizing them with separated mature or thymus-derived lymphocytes to yield antilymphocyte serum and antithymocyte serum, respectively—known collectively as antithymocyte globulin (ATG). ATG is purified from the gammaglobulin fraction of the pooled immune serum by absorbing out cross-reactivity with other cellular proteins, and it comprises a mixture of antibodies targeting B and T lymphocytes, NK cells, and macrophages. ATG is administered intravenously, daily for several days, and is used for induction therapy and to treat severe rejection or steroid-resistant rejection. It has unpleasant side effects, mostly related to release of inflammatory cytokines resulting from partial lymphocyte activation through cross-linking of cell surface molecules. Its use has consequently diminished in the presence of recent antiproliferative agents and more focused MABs.

Most MABs were raised in rats or mice against specific human leucocyte expressed proteins and have been modified, or 'humanized', so that they do not induce an antispecies response in patients. They have minimal cross-reactivity or batch variability, and their effective dose is therefore more predictable. The first MAB to be licensed for clinical treatment was OKT3, approved for use in patients in 1986 and directed against the CD3 part of the TCR expressed on mature T lymphocytes. Anti-CD3 rapidly causes partial T cell activation followed by apoptosis and disappearance from the circulation and is effective in transplantation and in autoimmune diseases. It has been used as an alternative to ATG for induction therapy and for treating acute rejection. This antibody is not available in a humanized form (although preclinical trials are in progress) and administration is associated with side effects due to cytokine release as well as diminishing efficacy due to antispecies responses. It is used infrequently now and alternative, humanized MABs are preferred in most instances.

Two anti-CD25 MABs, basiliximab and daclizumab, are commonly used for induction therapy following transplantation and are humanized MABs directed against the α-chain of the high affinity IL-2R expressed on activated lymphocytes. One of the earliest events in a normal immune response to specific antigen is production of IL-2 following engagement of the TCR. IL-2 binds to the $\alpha\beta$-subunit of the IL-2R that, in turn, recruits the γ-subunit to form a very stable complex involved in intracellular signalling via the phosphatidylinositol 3 (PI3) kinase, mitogen-activated protein, (MAP) kinase, and Janus kinase-signal transducer and activator (JAK/STAT) pathways.

This amplifies T cell proliferation through increased IL-2R expression and IL-2 production. Anti-CD25 effectively blocks the formation of this stable complex by binding preferentially to the α-chain, thereby inhibiting T cell proliferation. It is used in induction therapy and has minimal side effects but is relatively ineffective for treating acute rejection.

A number of more recently developed MABs are in use for transplantation but there is, as yet, a lack of consensus regarding optimal treatment regimens. Anti-CD52, or Campath-1H, marketed as alemtuzumab, is a MAB directed against the CD52 molecule expressed on thymocytes, T and B lymphocytes (but not plasma cells), and neutrophils. The antibody is highly effective in destroying human lymphocytes, which are depleted from the circulation for several weeks. It was initially used in patients with lymphoma and leukaemia and has since been used in renal and liver transplant patients. It also appears to have some efficacy in treating patients with multiple sclerosis [36].

Rituximab is a humanized anti-CD20 MAB that targets the CD20 molecule expressed on developing and mature B lymphocytes but not on plasma cells. It was approved initially for treatment of B cell lymphomas and has been used subsequently in transplant patients and in the treatment of rheumatoid arthritis [37] (see Chapter 8). B cells are rapidly eliminated from the circulation, most likely by complement-mediated cell lysis, and B cell numbers remain low for several months after treatment. There is some evidence that B cells are less effectively depleted from certain microenvironments such as the marginal zone of secondary lymphoid tissues. When B cells do reappear, they are more likely to be of a naive rather than the memory phenotype. As with other antibody treatments, side effects appear to be associated with cytokine release and are more severe when the B cell number is greatest, so that subsequent treatments have reduced side effects.

A number of antibodies and fusion proteins that interfere with, for example, $CD4^+$ T cell function, or costimulatory molecule signalling, are being assessed in clinical trials in transplant patients, or are being developed for future assessment. Of particular interest are those that have been shown experimentally to promote transplantation tolerance, such as those that target the CD154 and CTLA-4 signalling pathways. The BENEFIT clinical trial, for example, is currently assessing the efficacy of belatacept (a CTLA-4 formulation where the molecule is complexed with a human IgG1 immunoglobulin Fc fragment) as a replacement for ciclosporin in renal transplant patients [38].

As well as antibodies, several other agents are under investigation for their efficacy in preventing rejection, treating acute rejection, or promoting tolerance [39]. Some of these are newer formulations of existing drugs and some are novel agents, and they include fingolimod (FTY720), leflunomide, and deoxyspergualin. Fingolimod disrupts signalling via sphingosine 1-phosphate, which results in lymphocytes being sequestered in lymphoid tissue instead of migrating to sites of inflammation. Its further clinical development for transplantation has, however, been discontinued because of concerns that it causes ocular disorders and transient bradycardia. Leflunomide is an antimetabolite that inhibits proliferation by limiting pyrimidine synthesis, while deoxyspergualin belongs to the group of calcineurin-blocking agents that inhibit IL-2 production. Another promising approach is the use of bortezomib for treating refractory antibody-mediated rejection [40,41]. This is a tripeptide molecule that inhibits proteasome function through binding to its catalytic site. It is effective against antibody-secreting plasma cells and was originally developed for treating patients with multiple myeloma.

Induction and maintenance immunosuppression; treatment of acute rejection

The choice of immunosuppressive agent depends on the phase of activation of the immune response against the transplanted organ. During the *induction phase*, immediately prior to transplantation as well as peri- and postoperatively, the aim of immunosuppression is to minimize the response of the immune system against the challenge of the transplanted organ. At this stage, a number of different agents may be used. The induction phase is followed by the *maintenance phase*, which lasts for the life of the transplanted organ. The challenge here is to achieve a balance of adequate immunosuppression while allowing sufficient reserve to deal effectively with infection and any malignancy that may arise. It is also necessary to monitor possible side effects of maintenance therapy that may result in gradual attrition of graft function, as well as additional comorbidities that may require an alteration in drug administration. During the induction phase, a patient may be treated with a course of anti-CD25 MAB to eliminate activated T lymphocytes, together with a relatively high dose of a calcineurin inhibitor. During the maintenance phase, this dose is reduced to prevent toxicity but the patient will receive additional immunosuppression, such as azathioprine together with prednisolone. Acute rejection episodes are generally treated with a short course of relatively high-dose steroids, sometimes combined with ATG. Chronic rejection is difficult to manage but may respond to simply raising the level of immunosuppression. However, most immunosuppressive agents in current clinical use have little efficacy in treating chronic rejection and the emphasis, therefore, is on preventing chronic rejection by careful monitoring of drug levels, lymphocyte counts and graft function.

Complications of nonspecific immunosuppression

Introduction

The aim of immunosuppression is to prevent graft rejection by suppressing the immune response, but in the absence of strategies that target only the donor-specific response the unwanted outcome is that patients have increased susceptibility to infection and malignancy.

Infection

Infections occurring after transplantation are most common during the first few months, when levels of immunosuppression are at their highest, and may be life-threatening in patients who are already critically ill prior to transplantation [42,43]. Perioperative infections arising from the surgical procedures are frequently bacterial, and prophylaxis with broad-spectrum antibiotics is employed. Opportunistic infections occur during the first few months following transplantation and may be transmitted within the graft itself; viral reactivation commonly occurs when the graft is implanted in the suppressed seronegative recipient. Cytomegalovirus (CMV) is a particularly problematic viral infection and may require reduction in immunosuppression in addition to antiviral therapy; some immunity to the virus is attained. Other important opportunistic infections include Epstein–Barr virus (EBV), human herpesvirus (HHV) 8, toxoplasmosis, *Pneumocystis jirovecii*, and tuberculosis (TB), as well as a range of fungal infections including candidiasis and aspergillosis. Antimicrobial therapy is therefore routinely given during the first few months after transplantation. A particular problem in immunosuppressed transplant recipients with fever and malaise is distinguishing between graft rejection and opportunistic infection. Clearly, it is extremely important to rule out infection before administering additional immunosuppression, if acute rejection is suspected.

Malignancy

The risk of malignancy developing following transplantation is high, particularly in the long-term, as a result of continued immunosuppression. A recent European study revealed that renal transplant patients had a 4.3-fold increased rate overall of developing cancer, of any type, and that the risk of cancer increased with length of time following transplantation and with the patient's age [44]. Particular types of cancer may be associated with certain forms of immunosuppression; for example, the link between treatment with ALG and OKT3 and the development of post-transplant lymphoproliferative disease (PTLD). In general, cancers associated with renal transplantation are not the common cancers in the general population, whose rates were not significantly raised, but tend to be nonmelanoma skin cancers, kidney cancers (which may be related to the original renal disease), and cancers believed to be induced by viruses (e.g. lymphomas, cervical carcinoma).

Squamous cell carcinoma (SSC) is the most common cancer following transplantation, and accounts for more than 50% of all cancers. PTLD develops in up to 3% of transplant patients and its rate of occurrence is 30-fold higher than in the general population [45,46]. When the malignancy is believed to be of viral origin, treatment requires reduction of immunosuppression to encourage re-establishment of viral immunity. As with infection, there is a fine balance between rejection and susceptibility to malignancy resulting from over-immunosuppression (see Chapter 4).

Cardiovascular disease and diabetes

Current immunosuppressive regimens, although highly effective at improving short-term transplant patient survival and reducing acute rejection, are themselves associated with significant morbidity and mortality due to their side effects. Patients with renal disease on long-term renal dialysis and cardiac transplant patients are likely to have established vascular disease and this is worsened after transplantation by the effects of several immunosuppressive agents. Corticosteroids and calcineurin blockers are implicated in increased blood pressure and weight gain, while sirolimus and everolimus contribute to hypercholesterolaemia; tacrolimus is associated with new-onset diabetes [47]. Transplant patients are consequently advised on lifestyle (diet, smoking, and exercise) and are commonly treated with antihypertensive and lipid-lowering agents.

Desensitization

As discussed above, patients with renal failure awaiting transplantation may be excluded from receiving a particular organ because they have an incompatible blood group, or because they have circulating IgG antibodies against donor HLA types. Because of the chronic shortage of donor organs, access to the donor pool is being widened through the use of increasingly marginal donors (older donors, longer ischaemia times, non-heart-beating donors). A particularly successful additional source of donors in renal transplantation involves live donation, where the patient has a relative, spouse, or partner who is willing to donate a kidney, and for sensitized patients (with anti-HLA antibodies) this bypasses what might be a lengthy wait on the list for a deceased donor organ. However, it is frequently the case that the willing donor has an incompatible blood group, particularly for group O recipients, or HLA type, and one strategy that is increasingly used to facilitate live donation is patient desensitization. This approach is designed to remove anti-ABO blood group and anti-HLA circulating antibodies from patients awaiting transplantation [48].

Desensitization protocols have been introduced over many years. During the late 1980s studies were published that demonstrated successful ABO-incompatible renal transplantation in patients who were treated with plasmapheresis and immunoabsorption prior to transplantation to reduce the level of circulating anti-ABO antibodies. This was followed by a splenectomy carried out at the time of transplantation, and immunosuppressive induction therapy that included the use of ALG. Although a significant number of transplants were lost through acute rejection, these studies prompted further research. Prior to these studies, repeated plasmapheresis had been used to rescue kidneys transplanted across ABO barriers in error, but this was largely unsuccessful. With improved desensitization protocols it is now generally accepted that splenectomy is unnecessary, and most patients are treated before and after transplantation either with multiple high-dose intravenous immunoglobulin (IVIg) infusions or with several courses of plasmapheresis and immunoabsorption together with low-dose IVIg. In some cases, anti-CD20 therapy is also used to deplete circulating B lymphocytes.

IVIg is a formulation of IgG fractionated from pooled plasma from thousands of donors. Its mode of action is unclear, since it consists of a random pool of antibodies circulating in normal healthy individuals. It is possible that it functions through induction of anti-idiotype antibodies, opsonization, binding to inhibitory Fc receptors, blocking T cell activation, cytokine activity, and complement fixation. Desensitization prior to transplantation involves multiple episodes of plasmapheresis together with analysis of antibody titres until the titre level is acceptably low (Figure 3.9). A particular problem with achieving a 'safe' titre (typically 1/16) is the variability of techniques and reagents for measuring these antibody titres; some modern techniques, such as Luminex single antigen bead technology, are especially sensitive but not consistently so for a range of different HLA specificities. This has resulted in some patients being

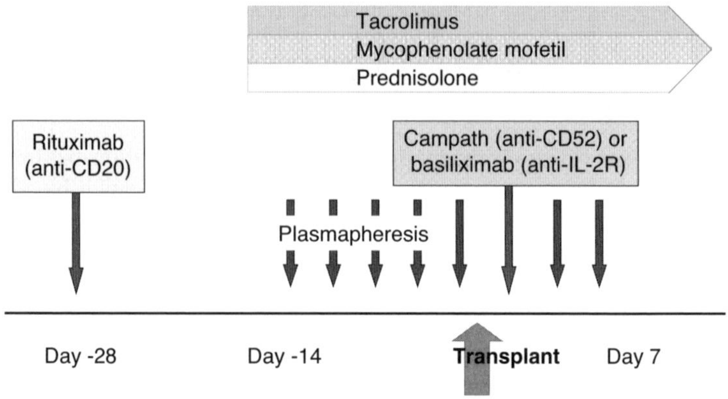

Fig. 3.9 Desensitization protocol for ABO-i/HLAi living donor transplantation. The aim of desensitization protocols is to reduce the level of circulating anti-ABO or anti-HLA antibodies to a safe titre prior to transplantation and to prevent continuing and novel antibody production following transplantation. A typical protocol may involve treatment with rituximab to reduce the pool of B lymphocytes that might mature into plasma cells, together with multiple rounds of plasmapheresis to remove existing circulating antibodies. Patients receive immunosuppressive therapy to minimize continued antibody production, together with standard induction therapy at the time of transplantation, and additional episodes of plasmapheresis, with maintenance immunosuppression following transplantation. ABOi, blood group; HLAi, human leucocyte antigen; IL-2R, interleukin-2 receptor.

unnecessarily desensitized because of anti-HLA antibodies that may be barely detectable using an alternative technique.

There is a concern that transplantation outcomes in desensitized patients are worse than in nonsensitized patients and that more stringent efforts to find a better match with a live donor would be beneficial. One approach that is increasingly being adopted is that of 'paired donation' where a donor and recipient pair who are ABO and/or HLA incompatible exchange with another similar pair where the second donor provides a better matched kidney for the first recipient, and vice versa [48,49]. This arrangement can be extended to include more incompatible pairs, termed domino-paired donations.

Future prospects

Introduction

Transplantation is clearly an effective treatment for endstage organ failure, and improvements in immunosuppression have ensured that few grafts are lost through acute rejection. However, there has been little improvement in long-term kidney graft survival over the past 15 years, and chronic allograft rejection continues to be the main cause of graft failure more than 1 year after transplantation. Certain immunosuppressive agents that effectively prevent acute rejection may themselves contribute to chronic graft damage, and the requirement for long-term immunosuppression increases the risk of infections, malignancy, and cardiovascular damage. Moreover, transplant waiting lists continue to expand more quickly than organ donation rates, leading to ever-increasing numbers of patients who are unable to receive a transplant. These two problems are driving significant research efforts into strategies for inducing immunological tolerance and alternative sources of tissue for transplantation. Immunological tolerance to the graft would obviate the need for immunosuppression and was first demonstrated in experimental studies more than five decades ago. However, it remains an elusive goal in clinical transplantation. Alternative sources of organs include xenotransplantation and regenerative medicine.

Transplant tolerance

Immunological tolerance was first observed independently by Owens in 1945, who identified shared blood groups in twin cattle [50], and by Billingham and Medawar in 1952 who performed skin grafts between twin cattle in an attempt to demonstrate that twins were either monozygotic or dizygotic [51]. To their surprise, skin grafts between either monozygotic (identical) or dizygotic (nonidentical) twins were not rejected. They concluded that the dizygotic twins shared a blood supply *in utero* and had become 'desensitized' or immunologically tolerant to each other through exchange of tissue antigens via the circulation while the immune system was developing. Medawar went on to demonstrate that injection of allogeneic cells into newborn mice resulted in allospecific tolerance such that the mice subsequently tolerated a skin graft from the same inbred strain as the cell donor but rejected a third-party graft [52] (see Chapter 1).

Evidence that organ transplantation tolerance is achievable derives from two groups of transplant patients. One group, principally liver transplant recipients, consists of patients who have decided to stop taking immunosuppression and, unusually, have not rejected their transplant. Current research aims to be able to identify, on the basis of biological markers and *in vitro* assays, those patients most likely to be or to become tolerant in order to gradually wean them off immunosuppression [53]. The second group is a small number of patients who had a bone marrow transplant to treat a haematological malignancy, and subsequently received a renal transplant from the bone marrow donor [54]. The degree of tolerance in this group is being explored in current clinical trials.

A wide range of experimental protocols have been reported to consistently result in transplant tolerance, largely in rodent models [55]. The likely mechanisms for tolerance induction fall into three broad categories—deletion, suppression, and anergy. Clonal deletion implies that all alloreactive cells have undergone apoptosis either centrally in the thymus, as for neonatal tolerance induction or injection of allogeneic cells into the adult thymus, or peripherally where circulating immune cells have been deleted through bone marrow chimaerism and mixed haematopoietic chimaerism. Suppression is achieved either through the presence of suppressor or regulatory cells, or through a suppressive environment. T regulatory cells (Tregs) are known to maintain a state of immunological unresponsiveness in normal individuals but, in certain strains of mice, if Tregs are removed by treatment with MABs against $CD4^+$ $CD25^+$ T cells, the mice develop autoimmune disease (see Chapter 8). Similarly, in transplanted mice, allograft rejection may be prevented by infusion of $CD4^+$ $CD25^+$ Tregs that achieve their effect, in part, through secretion of tolerogenic cytokines such as IL-10 [56]. Alternatively, allograft tolerance may be achieved experimentally by gene therapy or antibody treatment to alter the balance of local and circulating cytokines in favour of those that maintain tolerance, including enhancing the levels of IL-10 and TGF-β (see Chapter 1).

Anergy, or unresponsiveness, may result in transplant tolerance when T cell activation is initiated by TCR engagement with MHC–peptides on APCs but costimulatory signals are prevented by using MABs or proteins that block CD28 and CD154 signalling. This results in apoptosis of the incompletely activated T cells and favours generation of Tregs.

Although modern immunosuppressive induction protocols and drug combinations have enabled an overall reduction in drug treatment for maintenance therapy, tolerance remains an elusive goal for most transplant patients. There is significant interest in the development of new agents that may be combined in an attempt to achieve tolerance since it would have such a profound effect not only for patients with transplanted organs but also for those patients with autoimmune diseases. The use of MABs targeting the costimulatory molecules CD28 and CD154 has looked particularly promising in preclinical trials. Such outcomes should, however, be regarded with caution. A recent UK trial in six healthy human volunteers of a new formulation of anti-CD28 ended disastrously when all six rapidly developed life-threatening inflammatory reactions to the treatment.

On a more optimistic note, the use of nonmyeloablative preconditioning together with donor haematopoietic stem cell or bone marrow transplantation to generate mixed chimaerism is a particularly promising approach for inducing tolerance to a subsequent organ transplant from the stem cell or bone marrow donor. Since the initial trial in 1998 in patients with a haematological malignancy, success has now been achieved in a number of patients whose nonmyeloablative treatment involved cytotoxic agents and antibodies to deplete alloreactive T cells, with or without thymic irradiation. Following stem cell or bone marrow transplantation from HLA-matched or, in some cases, mismatched donors, development of mixed chimaerism was a prerequisite to subsequent renal transplantation from the same donor. Mixed chimaerism was indicated by the presence of both donor and recipient immune cells in the circulation that were cotolerant following thymic selection of T cell precursors. Most kidney transplants are surviving with good renal function and no immunosuppression several years on, although in some cases chimaerism has not persisted. It remains possible that these patients have microchimaerism, where the number of remaining donor cells is below the detectable level.

The mixed chimaerism approach lends itself to the development of regenerative medicine which, despite much publicity, is in its early stages. There are, as yet, no confirmed strategies for inducing human stem cells to proliferate and develop into multicellular organized tissues suitable for replacing or repairing diseased and damaged adult tissues. When this is eventually achieved, using unrelated and HLA-mismatched stem cells, there will be no need for immunosuppression since the stem cells may be simultaneously differentiated into haematopoietic cells for inducing chimaerism. Alternatively, a new development in the stem cell field will enable the generation of HLA-identical replacement tissues from the patient's own adult cells that have been 'reprogrammed' or induced to become pluripotent stem cells.

Xenotransplantation

The possibility of animal tissues being used for human transplantation has been actively researched for decades but has not, as yet, developed into a therapeutic option [57]. Certain groups of species possess naturally circulating antibodies against other groups of species, which cause hyperacute rejection in the minutes following transplantation, in much the same way as for ABO-incompatible transplants. The primary target is expressed on vascular ECs and hyperacute rejection results from antibody binding and activation of the complement and coagulation cascades. The target antigens resemble the human ABO blood group antigens and α-Gal is the target in pig tissues for inducing xenoantibodies in humans. Some progress in surmounting this obstacle has been made on the basis that certain complement regulatory proteins, including CD55 or decay accelerating factor and membrane cofactor protein (CD46), are species-specific. Thus, genetically modified pig kidneys that express one or more human complement regulatory proteins may be transplanted into nonhuman primates without causing hyperacute rejection. Nevertheless, the additional challenges of antibody-mediated and cellular rejection must still be overcome, apart from the risk of transmitting lethal pig viruses.

Summary and conclusions

The cellular and molecular basis of acute allograft rejection is now well understood and modern immunosuppressive therapy is sufficiently effective that only a few transplanted organs fail because of acute rejection. However, the side effects of the nonspecific immunosuppressive agents used are considerable and there is a need for the development of novel biomarkers that predict the likely strength of the graft rejection response so that the overall level of immunosuppression given to a patient can be tailored to the needs of the individual.

In contrast to acute rejection, our understanding of the pathophysiology of chronic rejection is more limited and available immunosuppressive agents are less effective at preventing it. A better understanding of the molecular basis of chronic rejection is required and may reveal novel and more effective therapeutic targets. Clinically applicable strategies for inducing donor-specific tolerance to an allograft would be the ideal solution to overcoming chronic rejection but these remain elusive. A more immediate prospect is the identification of biomarkers that accurately identify the small number of patients who have spontaneously developed a degree of transplant tolerance so that their immunosuppressive therapy can be reduced or even stopped altogether. The most challenging problem for solid organ transplantation remains the severe shortage of available donor organs. Xenotransplantation offers a potential solution but the barriers, both immunological and nonimmunological, remain formidable and, in the short to medium term, efforts should be directed towards increasing the longevity of the organs and tissues available through a better understanding of transplant immunobiology.

References

1. Snell GD. Methods for the study of histocompatibility genes. *J Genetics* 1948; **49**: 87–108.
2. Benacerraf B, McDevitt HO. Histocompatibility-linked immune response genes. *Science* 1972; **175**: 273–279.
3. Dausset J, Degos L, Fellous M, Legrand L. Formal genetics of the HL-A region. *Genetics* 1975; **79**: 251–262.
4. Gorer PA, Lyman S, Snell GD. Studies on the genetic and antigenic basis of tumour transplantation. Linkage between a histocompatibility gene and 'fused' in mice. *Proc R Soc Lond (Biol)* 1948; **135**: 499–505.
5. Fuggle SV, Taylor CJ. Histocompatibility in renal transplantation. In Morris PJ, Knechtle SJ (eds) *Kidney transplantation: principles and practice*. Saunders Elsevier, Philadelphia, 2008; pp. 140–57.
6. Taylor CJ, Kosmoliaptsis V, Summers DM, Bradley JA. Back to the future: application of contemporary technology to long-standing questions about the clinical relevance of human leukocyte antigen-specific alloantibodies in renal transplantation. *Hum Immunol* 2009; **70**: 563–568.
7. Fuggle SV, Martin S. Tools for human leukocyte antigen antibody detection and their application to transplanting sensitized patients. *Transplantation* 2008; **86**: 384–390.
8. LaRosa DF, Rahman AH, Turka LA. The innate immune system in allograft rejection and tolerance. *J Immunol.* 2007; **178**: 7503–7509.
9. Kim IK, Bedi DS, Denecke C, Ge X, Tullius SG. Impact of innate and adaptive immunity on rejection and tolerance. *Transplantation* 2008; **86**: 889–894.
10. Land WG. Innate immunity-mediated allograft rejection and strategies to prevent it. *Transplantation Proceedings* 2007; **39**: 667–672.
11. Afzali B, Lombardi G, Lechler RI. Pathways of major histocompatibility complex allorecognition. *Curr Opin Organ Transplant* 2008; **13**: 438–444.
12. Zinkernagel RM, Doherty PC. Restriction of in vitro T cell-mediated cytotoxicity in lymphocytic choriomeningitis within a syngeneic or semiallogeneic system. *Nature* 1974; **248**: 701–702.
13. Lechler RI, Lombardi G, Batchelor JR, Reinsmoen N, Bach FH. The molecular basis of alloreactivity. *Immunol Today* 1990; **11**: 83–88.
14. Arakelov A, Lakkis FG. The alloimmune response and effector mechanisms of allograft rejection. *Semin Nephrol* 2000; **20**: 95–102.
15. Alegre ML, Florquin S, Goldman M. Cellular mechanisms underlying acute graft rejection: time for reassessment. *Curr Opin Immunol* 2007; **19**: 563–568.
16. Valujskikh A, Baldwin WM, Fairchild RL. Recent progress and new perspectives in studying T-cell responses to allografts. *Am J Transplant* 2010; **10**: 1117–1125.
17. Bolton EM, Bradley JA, Pettigrew GJ. Indirect allorecognition: not simple but effective. *Transplantation* 2008; **85**: 667–669.
18. Wasowska BA. Mechanisms involved in antibody- and complement-mediated allograft rejection. *Immunol Res* 2010; **47**: 25–44.
19. Zhang X, Reed EF. Effect of antibodies on endothelium. *Am J Transplant* 2009; **9**: 2459–2465.
20. Al-Lamki RS, Bradley JR, Pober JS. Endothelial cells in allograft rejection. *Transplantation* 2008; **86**: 1340–1348.

21. Valujskikh A, Matesic D, Gilliam A, Anthony D, Haqqi TM, Heeger PS. T cells reactive to a single immunodominant self-restricted allopeptide induce skin graft rejection in mice. *J Clin Invest* 1998; **101**: 1398–1407.
22. Jurcevic S, Ainsworth ME, Pomerance A et al. Antivimentin antibodies are an independent predictor of transplant-associated coronary artery disease after cardiac transplantation. *Transplantation* 2001; **71**: 886–892.
23. Koch CA, Platt JL. T cell recognition and immunity in the fetus and mother. *Cell Immunol* 2007; **248**: 12–17.
24. Hori J, Niederkorn JY. Immunogenicity and immune privilege of corneal allografts. *Chem Immunol Allergy* 2007; **92**: 290.
25. Williams KA, Coster DJ. The immunobiology of corneal transplantation. *Transplantation.* 2007; **84**: 806–813.
26. Beck J, Angus R, Madsen B, Britt D, Vernon B, Nguyen KT. Islet encapsulation: strategies to enhance islet cell functions. *Tissue Eng* 2007; **13**: 589–599.
27. Colvin RB. Pathology of chronic humoral rejection. *Contrib Nephrol* 2009; **162**: 75–86.
28. Dragun D. Humoral responses directed against non-human leukocyte antigens in solid-organ transplantation. *Transplantation* 2008; **86**: 1019–1025.
29. Torpey N, Bradley JA, Fung JJ. Immunosuppressive therapy in solid organ transplantation. In Zbar AP, Guillou P, Bland KI, Syrigos KN (eds): *Immunology for surgeons.* Springer, New York 2002; pp. 127–54.
30. Taylor AL, Watson CJ, Bradley JA. Immunosuppressive agents in solid organ transplantation: Mechanisms of action and therapeutic efficacy. *Crit Rev Oncol Hematol* 2005; **56**: 23–46.
31. Kahan BD. Individuality: the barrier to optimal immunosuppression. *Nat Rev Immunol.* 2003; **3**: 831–838.
32. Margreiter R. Efficacy and safety of tacrolimus compared with ciclosporin microemulsion in renal transplantation: a randomised multicentre study. *Lancet* 2002; **359**: 741–746.
33. Kahan BD. Mycophenolate mofetil. In Morris PJ, Knechtle SJ (eds): *Kidney transplantation: principles and practice.* Saunders Elsevier, Philadelphia, 2008; pp. 277–92.
34. Watson CJE, Bradley JA. mTOR inhibitors: Sirolimus and everolimus. In Morris PJ, Knechtle SJ (eds): *Kidney transplantation: principles and practice.* Saunders Elsevier, 2008; pp. 293–308.
35. Kirk AD. Antibodies and fusion proteins. In Morris PJ, Knechtle SJ (eds): *Kidney Transplantation: principles and practice.* Saunders Elsevier 2008; pp. 309–32.
36. Watson CJ, Bradley JA, Friend PJ et al. Alemtuzumab (CAMPATH 1H) induction therapy in cadaveric kidney transplantation—efficacy and safety at five years. *Am J Transplant* 2005; **5**: 1347–1353.
37. Pescovitz MD. Rituximab, an anti-CD20 monoclonal antibody: history and mechanism of action. *Am J Transplant* 2006; **6**: 859–866.
38. Vincenti F, Charpentier B, Vanrenterghem Y et al. A phase III study of belatacept-based immunosuppression regimens versus cyclosporine in renal transplant recipients (BENEFIT study). *Am J Transplant* 2010; **10**: 535–546.
39. Vincenti F, Kirk AD. What's next in the pipeline. *Am J Transplant* 2008; **8**: 1972–1981.
40. Walsh RC, Everly JJ, Brailey P et al. Proteasome inhibitor-based primary therapy for antibody-mediated renal allograft rejection. *Transplantation* 2010; **89**: 277–284.

41. Everly JJ, Walsh RC, Alloway RR, Woodle ES. Proteasome inhibition for antibody-mediated rejection. *Curr Opin Organ Transplant* 2009; **14**: 662–666.
42. Marty FM, Rubin RH. The prevention of infection post-transplant: the role of prophylaxis, preemptive and empiric therapy. *Transpl Int* 2006; **19**: 2–11.
43. Special Issue: AST Infectious Diseases Guidelines 2nd Edition. Eds: *Am J Transplantation* 2009; **9**(Suppl 4): S1–S281.
44. Wimmer CD, Rentsch M, Crispin A et al. The janus face of immunosuppression–*de novo* malignancy after renal transplantation: the experience of the Transplantation Center in Munich. *Kidney Int* 2007; **71**: 1271–1278.
45. Ulrich C, Kanitakis J, Stockfleth E, Euvrard S. Skin cancer in organ transplant recipients—where do we stand today? *Am J Transplant* 2008; **8**: 2192–2198.
46. Taylor AL, Marcus R, Bradley JA. Post-transplant lymphoproliferative disorders (PTLD) after solid organ transplantation. *Crit Rev Oncol Hematol* 2005; **56**: 155–167.
47. Knight SR, Morris PJ. Steroid avoidance or withdrawal after renal transplantation increases the risk of acute rejection but decreases cardiovascular risk. A meta-analysis. *Transplantation* 2010; **89**: 1–14.
48. Montgomery RA. Renal transplantation across HLA and ABO antibody barriers: integrating paired donation into desensitization protocols. *Am J Transplant* 2010; **10**: 449–557.
49. Johnson RJ, Allen JE, Fuggle SV, Bradley JA, Rudge C; Kidney Advisory Group, UK Transplant NHSBT. Early experience of paired living kidney donation in the United Kingdom. *Transplantation.* 2008; **86**: 1672–1677.
50. Owen RD. Immunogenetic consequences of vascular anastomoses between bovine twins. *Science* 1945; **102**: 400–401.
51. Billingham RE, Lampkin GH, Medawar PB, Williams HLL. Tolerance to homografts, twin diagnosis, and the freemartin condition in cattle. *Heredity* 1952; **6**: 201–212.
52. Billingham RE, Brent L, Medawar PB. `Actively acquired tolerance' of foreign cells. *Nature* 1953; **172**: 603–606.
53. Martínez-Llordella M, Lozano JJ, Puig-Pey I et al. Using transcriptional profiling to develop a diagnostic test of operational tolerance in liver transplant recipients. *J Clin Invest* 2008; **118**: 2845–2857.
54. Kawai T, Cosimi AB, Spitzer TR, et al. HLA-mismatched renal transplantation without maintenance immunosuppression. *N Engl J Med* 2008; **358**: 353–361.
55. Kingsley CI, Nadig SN, Wood KJ. Transplantation tolerance: lessons from experimental rodent models. *Transpl Int* 2007; **20**: 828–841.
56. Hara M, Kingsley CI, Niimi M et al. IL-10 is required for regulatory T cells to mediate tolerance to alloantigens in vivo. *J Immunol* 2001; **166**: 3789–3796.
57. Yang YG, Sykes M. Xenotransplantation: current status and a perspective on the future. *Nat Rev Immunol* 2007; **7**: 519–531.

Chapter 4

Cancer and the immune response

Mark Aloysius, Leslie Walker, and Oleg Eremin

Key summary points

- Innate and adaptive immunity play key roles in surveillance against mutated and/or malignant cell clones, resulting in the destruction and inhibition of tumour cell proliferation, albeit this may not always be adequate to prevent the establishment and progressive growth of the cancer.
- 'Danger' signals (e.g. HSPs) released from malignant cells (necrotic, hypoxic, stressed) stimulate PRRs on DCs and macrophages within the tumour microenvironment, inducing activation of innate immunity with release of proinflammatory cytokines (e.g. IL-2, IL-6, IL-12, IFN-γ), producing the crucial signal 3 for optimizing the adaptive immune response and production of an effective antitumour CTL response. Provides an explanation for spontaneous tumour regression following infections, noncurative surgery, and radiotherapy.
- Mouse models lacking specific components of innate immunity (NK cells, MHC expressing DCs, IFN-γ) and adaptive immunity (T, B lymphocytes) have an increased incidence of spontaneous solid cancers (lung, colon, breast) and lymphomas.
- Chronic inflammation (autoimmune or infection-induced) is associated with an increased incidence of spontaneous tumours in mice. Mice deficient in IFN-γ and GM-CSF develop chronic inflammatory lesions; treatment with antibiotics can prevent or delay the onset of tumours in certain mouse models.
- Experimental carcinogenesis (MCA, DMBA, TPA, UV light) in immunodeficient mice has demonstrated the key role played by both adaptive immunity (αβ T cells) and innate immunity (γδ T, NK, and NK T cells) in preventing tumour inductions and in tumour rejections. Lack of functional IL-12 increased but lack of IL-23 inhibited tumour growth (also, in human tumours), possibly through reduced production of IL-17.
- Human tumours are infiltrated, to a variable degree by TILs. The presence of TILs (intratumoural, not peritumoural) in a variety of solid cancers (colon, melanoma) has been shown to be an independent beneficial prognostic factor. Prominent NK cell tumour infiltrate has been documented with colorectal, gastric, and lung cancers. Tregs ($CD4^+$ $CD25^+$ $Foxp3^+$) infiltrate most solid cancers

and inhibit NK cell cytotoxity, generation of $CD8^+$ CTLs and function of DCs (*in situ*) by secretion of TGF-β, IL-10, and CTLA-4.

- Most solid tumours (in humans and animals) show a prominent infiltrate by TIMs. They secrete a range of growth promoting factors (e.g. PGs), stimulatory (IL-1, TNF-α, IFN- γ) and inhibitory (TGF-β, IL-10) cytokines, chemokines (CCL22) which attract Tregs, and show defective release of anticancer cytolytic/cytostatic molecules and free radicals.
- Immunocompromised patients (primary or secondary) have an increased risk (3–100-fold increase) of developing malignancies—lymphomas, skin cancers, solid tumours. Paraneoplastic syndromes are due to cross-reactivity between an anticancer immune response and neurological self antigens; they often antedate onset of overt malignancy.
- Tumour cells escape antitumour regulation by: downgrading expression of tumour cell MHC class I antigens; generation of a chronic inflammatory infiltrate via mast cells secretory granules, and humoral B cell responses; production of VEGF and TNF-α; reduced expression of vascular endothelial adhesion molecules; secretion of various growth promoting PGs by TIMs; inhibition of optimal $CD8^+$ CTLs through inadequate activation of DCs and generation of key signals (2 and 3) by $CD4^+$ $CD25^+$ $Foxp3^+$ Tregs and MDSCs; secretion of IL-10 and TGF-β; switching off of DC activity by CTLA-4 signalling, and; tumour cell killing of immune cells by FasL.
- There is a good correlation between the presence of TAMs and clinical outcome in many solid cancers in humans. In tumours, macrophages switch from M1 to M2 phenotype and promotion of tumour growth. TAMs compete with DCs for antigen presentation. TIM chemotaxis is regulated by CSF-1, GM-CSF, VEGF, and CCL24. TAMs secrete TGF-β, and switch off host defences. TGF-β expression is up-regulated in human cancers; produced by both tumour cells and immune cells. Inhibits cells of both innate and adaptive immunity. Promotes tumour cell proliferation, mobility, and invasion, and plays a key role in angiogenesis and metastasis formation.
- Malignant cells can express a range of tumour-specific and/or TAAs and proteins: products of mutated oncogenes, pan tumour survivin and hTERT, oncogenic viral proteins, oncofetal (CEA, AFP) antigens, chromosomal translocations, deletions, and mutations (erB-B2, p53).
- Generation of an effective anticancer CMI is dependent on various factors: Optimal activation of *in situ* DCs (signals 1–3) expressing tumour peptides (8–10 amino acids), linked to class I and II antigens and interacting with $CD8^+$ αβ T and $CD4^+$ T cells, respectively, and generating CTLs; optimal NK cell activity and tumour cell lysis (granzyme/perforin); involvement of IFN-γ secreting NK T cells and IL-17 secreting γδ T cells, interacting with CD1d and CD1c lipid tumour-associated molecules, respectively; overcoming the inhibitory activity of $CD4^+$ $CD25^+$ $Foxp3^+$ Tregs and MDSCs.

- Humoral immunity (IgM antibodies) is well documented in cancer, can induce ADCC (through NK cells). DCs readily take up opsonized TAAs, enhancing $CD4^+$ and $CD8^+$ T cell responses through cross-presentation (DC Fcγ); complement proteins enhance immune surveillance in cancer.
- Metastasis formation is a complex biological process. TAMs play a key role in inducing tumour cells to invade and intravasate through release of various proteases and MMPS. Hypoxia is a strong signal for accumulation of TAMs, production of cytokines and growth factors (GM-CSF, TGF-β, VEGF, PDGF, FGF) and the active stimulation of angiogenesis; pericytes play a key role. Macrophages and other leucocytes prepare the niches for metastasis. Vascular, endothelial and tumour cells express CXCR4 and are attracted to these metastatic niches by *in situ* TAMs secreting CXCL12.
- Differential Th1/Th2 cytokine secretion profiles in tumour microenvironment, associated with enhancement/reduction in chronic inflammation, have an impact on cancer development. Tumour angiogenesis is inhibited by IFN-γ (Th1), while IL-6 and IL-10 (Th2) stimulate angiogenesis. IL-13 inhibits CMI and stimulates cancer cell growth. IL-23 promotes chronic inflammation, inhibits CTL responses, and enhances tumourigenesis.
- Chemotherapy inhibits host defences, usually temporarily; but augments aspects of both CMI and humoral immunity. Various drugs both inhibit host defences (neutrophils, antibody production, NK cell activity, usually temporarily) and augment aspects of humoral immunity (via enhanced TAA presentation) and CMI (NK cells, ADCC, suppression of Tregs).
- Radiotherapy induces lymphopenia (T and B cells), affecting especially $CD4^+$ Th cells, $CD4^+$ $CD25^+$ Tregs and naive T cells; extent is dependent on volume of blood/body irradiated. Local irradiation of tumours can reduce distant metastases (abscopal effect).
- Immunotherapy in cancer is an emerging therapeutic strategy: Adoptive cellular transfer (e.g. TILs in melanoma and renal cell carcinoma); MABs against tumour cell growth factors (HER2/neu in breast cancer, EGFR in colon cancer); malignant T and B cell clones (lymphomas, leukaemia); VEGF (lung, breast, colon); active immunotherapy: vaccination with TAA peptide/protein-pulsed DCs and adjuvants, recombinant viral vectors, DNA and RNA, tumour cell extracts.
- Cachexia occurs to a variable degree in patients with cancer; associated with weight loss (depending on tumour type and tumour cell mass), often with anorexia; exacerbated by cancer treatments. IL-1 and TNF-α affect brain regulatory areas for food intake; IL-6 levels in blood correlate with degree of cachexia. MIC-1 implicated in anorexia and weight loss. Leptin contributes to loss of body fat and energy expenditure. Treatment of cachexia is being evaluated through blocking mechanisms thought to induce cachexia and improving appetite.

- Diagnosis and treatment of cancer are associated with high levels of psychosocial and psychiatric morbidity. The CNS and PNS can modulate host defences via HPA, SMA, and neural innervation of lymphoid tissues. Chronic stressors are associated with suppressed immune function; depression has a negative relationship on survival. Psychosocial interventions can influence aspects of immunity— mitogen responses, NK and LAK cell activities, Th1 (IFN-γ) and Th2 (IL-4) profiles—and improve coping and quality of life; no evidence that immunological changes produced by psychosocial interventions prolong survival.

Introduction

Cancer is an abnormal growth of tissue arising from uncontrolled and uncoordinated proliferation of cells and stroma, resulting in disruption of local tissue architecture, infiltration of adjacent structures, and invasion of lymphatic and vascular channels. If progressive and unchecked, it leads to dissemination of malignant cells, establishment of distant foci of metastatic disease, and the eventual death of the host.

Approximately one in three of the population in industrialized Western societies will develop cancer, and one in four people die from a malignancy (>150 000 people per year in the UK). There is an increasing incidence of cancer worldwide due to various factors—ageing population, diet, environmental pollution, and others (many unknown).

There is evidence to suggest that the immune system plays a crucial role in preventing the establishment of malignant disease and progressive tumour growth. This is thought to occur via several key mechanisms:

- The immune system can protect the host against virus-induced tumours by eliminating or suppressing viral infections.
- By prompt elimination of pathogens and rapid resolution of the pathogen-induced inflammatory process, which is favourable for carcinogenesis, the immune system removes the environmental milieu for malignant transformation and survival of malignantly transformed cells.
- The immune system can specifically identify and eliminate mutated or malignant cells by their recognition of various tumour-associated antigens (TAAs) or molecules induced by cellular stress, such as heat shock proteins (HSPs), generated at the site of malignant transformation.

This last process is referred to as *tumour immune surveillance*, whereby the immune system (innate and adaptive) identifies cancerous and/or transformed precancerous cells and eliminates them before they become established and lead to progressive and uncontrolled tumour growth. The concept that the immune system, which plays a crucial role in protecting the host from microbial pathogens, may also play an important role in recognizing and destroying tumour cells was first suggested over a century ago, and has recently been critically reviewed and re-evaluated [1]. Despite antitumour immune surveillance, tumours do develop and progress in the presence of a functioning immune system; this is explained by the concepts of *tumour escape* and *immunoediting* [1]. This is a more modern explanation for the role of the immune system in preventing or otherwise the initiation and subsequent tumour development and progression of the malignant process.

Immune surveillance and host responses in cancer

The 'danger' hypothesis

Several theories have been proposed to explain the remarkable ability of the immune system to discriminate between different stimuli, leading to either activation or tolerance. The initial paradigm of discrimination between self and non-self was proposed by Burnet in 1959 [2]. The need for a second signal or 'costimulation' for B [3] and T cell [4] activation was subsequently proposed. The T cell requirement for interaction with antigen presenting cells (APCs) (which themselves are not antigen-specific) did not fit readily with the self/non-self model of immune recognition. Janeway, in 1989, suggested that APCs could be activated via pattern recognition receptors (PRRs), which bind to specific molecules and foreign antigens, and is the key element of innate immunity recognizing and interacting with microbial pathogens (see Chapters 1 and 5) [5].

In order to incorporate a number of biological processes, including autoimmune diseases and foetal tolerance, Matzinger, in 1994, formulated the 'danger' model of immune activation [6]. This model suggests that the prime role of the immune system is to react to cellular stress or damage, as opposed simply to non-self [6]. 'Danger' signals from damaged or dying cells activate APCs (e.g. dendritic cells [DCs]) and macrophages which release proinflammatory cytokines (e.g. interferon-gamma [IFN-γ] and interleukin 12 [IL-12]), providing the required costimulation to activate T lymphocytes and adaptive immunity. The subsequent discovery of a number of endogenous 'danger' signals, including HSPs, RNA, DNA, hyaluron (a breakdown product of damaged vessels), uric acid, and IFN-α, have provided a mechanistic basis for this hypothesis [7]. In this model of immune activation, effective antitumour immunity will only develop if tumours possess unique or tumour-specific antigens, whose antigenic peptides are sampled by APCs and presented to $CD4^+$ and $CD8^+$ T cells (linked to class II and I molecules, respectively) (signal 1). For this to progress into an effective antitumour response, costimulatory interactions (e.g. DC, CD80/86; T cell, CD28) (signal 2) need to be reinforced by the crucial third signal provided by the danger signals (released by 'stressed' cancer cells) interacting with PRRs on DCs. 'Progressively' growing tumours are more likely to induce immune tolerance (lack of signal 3), whereas, areas of hypoxia and necrosis in some tumours may more readily activate the immune system through release of HSPs, etc. The balance of positive and negative signals received by DCs, within the tumour microenvironment, is likely to alter during the natural history of tumour progression and growth. According to Matzinger's hypothesis, successful antitumour immunotherapy will need to involve strong and effective 'danger' signals [8]. This is illustrated in Figure 4.1.

The 'danger' theory has been supported by documentation of spontaneous tumour regressions associated with preceding surgical interventions, infections, autoimmune

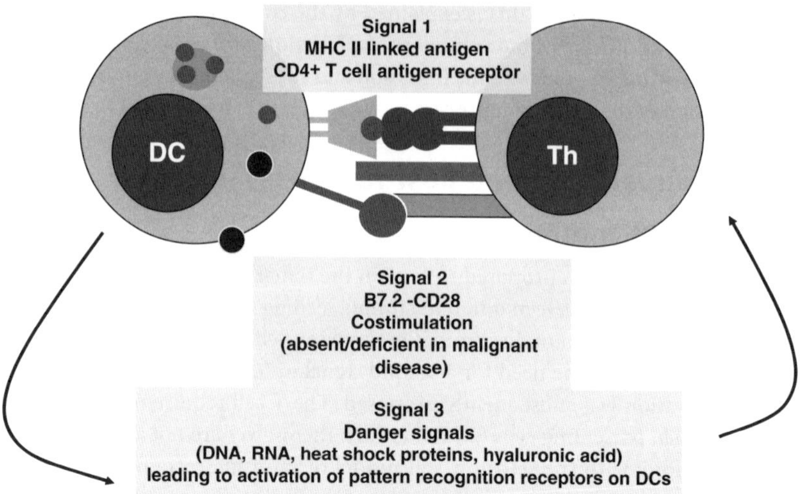

Fig. 4.1 An illustration of the 'danger signals' determining the nature of the CD4$^+$T helper (Th1 or Th2) cell response, which may be beneficial or detrimental to the host anticancer immune response. Signals 1 and 2 activate cells to proliferation effector function; signal 3 'tunes' the response to a Th1 or Th2 cytokine response ansd a more substantial and prolonged immune response. Small grey circles indicate tumour-associated antigens (TAAs) black circles pattern recognition receptors (PRRs). DCs, dendritic cells.

disturbances, administration of bacterial vaccines, transfusion reactions, and irradiation of a focus of disease and regression of metastases at distant nonirradiated sites [9]. In a series of 449 patients with regressing tumours after bacterial infection, regression was commonly associated with erysipelas [10]. In 1966, Everson and Cole reported a series of 176 spontaneous tumour regressions, and found that 40% had been preceded by operative interventions, including biopsies and partial resections [11]. These preceding factors may have provided the necessary 'danger' signals which contribute to activation of PRRs on DCs, resulting in the generation of CD4$^+$ T helper (Th) lymphocytes and CD8$^+$ cytotoxic T lymphocytes (CTLs), and an effective anticancer adaptive cell-mediated immunity (CMI). In modern oncological practice, intravesical instillation of the bacillus Calmette–Guérin (BCG) acts as a nonspecific inflammatory and immune stimulant (and probable 'danger' signal), and has been effective in reducing the recurrence of superficial bladder tumours [12].

Immune surveillance

Mouse models

Spontaneous tumour development in immunodeficient mice: An established approach for testing the role of the immune system in controlling tumour development is to remove specific components of the mouse immune system (knock-out mice) and monitor the mice for the subsequent development of tumours. Through the use of gene-targeted mice, this approach has demonstrated that a number of

Table 4.1 Spontaneous tumours in immunodeficient mice

Mouse strain	Immune defect (absence, deficiency)	Spontaneous tumours	References
SCID	T and B cells	T cell lymphomas	[13]
Rag2–/–	T and B cells	Intestinal and lung adenocarcinomas	[14]
Rag2–/–Stat1–/–	T and B cells, IFN-γ signalling	Breast and colonic adenocarcinomas	[14]
Perforin–/–	Perforin	B cell lymphomas	[15]
Ifng–/–	IFN-γ	T cell lymphomas	[16]
Perforin–/–Ifng–/–	Perforin, IFN-γ	B cell lymphomas	[16]
Perforin–/–B2 m–/–	Perforin, MHC class I	B cell lymphomas	[17]
Lmp2–/–	MHC class I	Endometrial adenocarcinomas	[18]
Trail–/–	TRAIL	B and T cell lymphomas	[19]
Gmcsf–/–Ifng–/–	GM-CSF, IFN-γ	Ovarian choriocarcinomas, teratomas	[20]
Ll12rb2–/–	IL-12R	Lung adenocarcinomas	[21]

immune effector cells and pathways are important for suppression of tumour development (Table 4.1). The latter have been a range of solid cancers and T and B cell lymphomas.

A role for the adaptive immune system in suppressing tumour growth is well established in various animal tumour models (carcinogen, viral-induced) [13]. This was further reinforced when it was shown that 129/Sv RAG2-deficient mice, which lack both B and T cells, developed spontaneous adenocarcinomas of the intestine and lung (35% and 15%, respectively, of all mice analysed) at 15–16 months of age, and an additional 50% of mice developed intestinal adenomas [14]. Interestingly, when *Rag2*$^{-/-}$mice were also deficient for STAT1, an important mediator of signalling induced by both type I and type II IFN, tumour incidence was increased further, and the spectrum of tumours broadened to include breast adenocarcinomas (~40% of mice), colon adenocarcinomas (~10% of mice), or both (~20% of mice) [14]. These results suggest that both the innate and the adaptive arms of the immune system are involved in the prevention of spontaneous tumours, as mice lacking both IFN-γ signalling and an adaptive immune system develop a broader spectrum of tumours, compared with mice lacking only an adaptive immune system.

The importance of both the innate and adaptive immune responses in immune surveillance was further highlighted in mice lacking T cell and natural killer (NK) cell cytotoxic effector pathways, which was associated with an enhanced incidence of spontaneous tumours. Mice that lacked perforin, a cytotoxic molecule used by cytotoxic cells (CD8$^+$ T cells and NK cells) to form membrane pores in target cells, developed lymphomas with progressive ageing. These spontaneous lymphomas were of B cell origin, developed in older mice (>1 year of age) and regardless of the mouse strain [15,16]. When transplanted into wild type (WT) mice, the lymphoma cells were rejected by $CD8^+$ CTLs [15]. B cell lymphomas also arise in mice lacking both perforin and β_2-microglobulin (β2M); tumour onset is earlier and occurs with increased prevalence compared with mice lacking only perforin. In addition, B cell lymphomas derived from mice lacking both perforin and β2M are rejected by either NK cells or γδ T cells (key cells in innate immunity) following transplantation into WT mice, rather than by MHC-restricted $CD8^+$ αβ T cells (as in tumours derived from mice lacking only perforin). These findings suggest that cell surface expression of MHC molecules by tumour cells is an important factor in determining which effector cells mediate immune protective effects [17]. Intriguingly, mutations in the gene encoding perforin have also been identified in a subset of lymphoma patients [22], although it is not clear whether this contributes to the initiation of the disease. Mice lacking the death-inducing molecule TNF-related apoptosis-inducing ligand (TRAIL) or expressing a defective mutant form of the death-inducing molecule Fas ligand (FasL) have also been shown to be susceptible to spontaneous late onset lymphomas [19,23]. These studies in ageing mice have clearly demonstrated a critical role for cytotoxic pathways in immunoregulation and/or immunosuppression of tumour development in mice, both for spontaneous solid cancers and for lymphomas.

Various cytokine-deficient mice also have developed spontaneous malignancies. In one study, approximately 50% of IFN-γ-deficient C57BL/6 mice were found to develop T cell lymphomas that were predominantly disseminated, although some cases of thymic lymphoma were also documented. The susceptibility of *Ifng*$^{-/-}$ mice to developing T cell lymphomas was shown to be strain dependent [24]. Furthermore, the spectra of tumours observed in IFN-γ and STAT1-deficient mice do not overlap, despite STAT1 being a crucial signalling molecule downstream of the IFN-γ receptor. These findings indicate that either these molecules have some nonoverlapping activities or that the background strain has a modifying influence on the tumour type developed. In addition, C57BL/6 mice lacking both IFN-γ and perforin displayed accelerated B cell lymphoma onset, compared with perforin-deficient-only mice [24], indicating that IFN-γ has an important role in modifying the progression to B cell lymphoma in perforin-deficient mice. IL-12 and IL-18 are important IFN-γ-inducing cytokines. However, studies with ageing mice have demonstrated that neither IL-12- nor IL-18-deficient mice have an increased incidence of tumours, compared with WT mice [24]. Thus, other, as yet, unrecognized factors play an important role in inducing spontaneous lymphomas in ageing mice. Spontaneous development of tumours in immunodeficient mice (variable components) is illustrated in Figure 4.2.

Inflammation and carcinogenesis: A possible link between tumour immunity and autoimmune or infection-induced inflammation has been raised by several studies. With increasing age, 50% of mice lacking the β2 subunit of the IL-12 receptor (IL-12Rβ2) develop plasmacytomas or lung carcinomas, as well as autoimmune-induced mesangial glomerulonephritis [21]. It is presently unclear why IL-12-deficient mice, with the same genetic background as the IL-12Rβ2-deficient mice, do not display either autoimmunity or spontaneous tumour development. Furthermore, mice deficient for both IFN-γ and granulocyte–macrophage colony stimulating factor (GM-CSF)

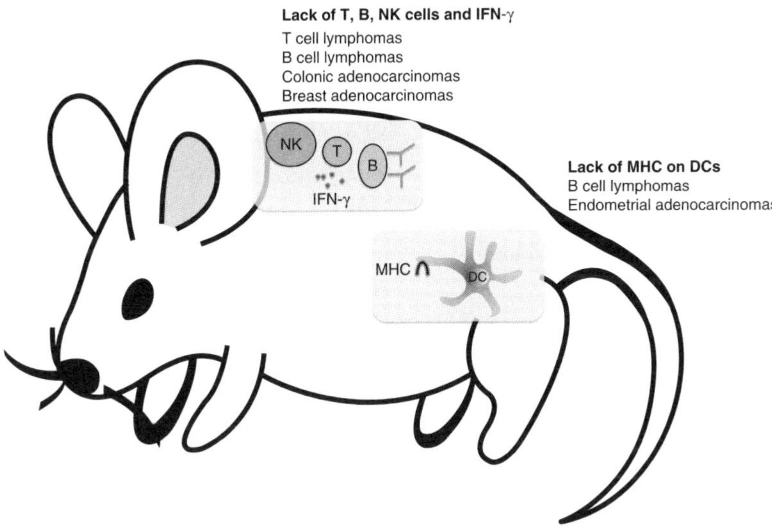

Fig. 4.2 Mouse model of spontaneous carcinogenesis in absence of various components of the immune response.

have also been found to develop tumours with advancing age. In these models, tumour development is associated with acute or chronic inflammatory lesions in a range of organs, and maintaining mice on the antibiotic enrofloxacin prevents (or at least delays) tumour onset [20]. Collectively, these findings suggest that the immune system under certain biological/pathological conditions may not suppress the establishment of tumours. The finding that antibiotic treatment could prevent tumour development in *Gm-csf*$^{-/-}$*Ifng*$^{-/-}$ mice raises the possibility that as well as directly eliminating tumour cells, the immune system might, in certain susceptible hosts, prevent tumour growth by the timely elimination of infections, thereby, aborting or restricting the inflammatory process, which is known to facilitate tumour development [25]. However, this finding is not universally applicable, as *Rag2*$^{-/-}$ and *Rag2*$^{-/-}$*Stat1*$^{-/-}$ mice, maintained on the same antibiotics and housed under strict specific pathogen-free conditions, developed malignancies. Such mice had increased tumour incidence despite testing negative for common pathogens with known links to malignancy and showing no signs of associated inflammation [14].

Experimental carcinogenesis in immunodeficient mice: In order to define more precisely the role of the immune system in tumorigenesis, researchers have studied various tumour models, including carcinogen-induced tumours. The two most commonly employed carcinogen-induced tumour models are fibrosarcomas induced by methylcholanthrene (MCA) and skin papillomas induced by a combination of 7,12-di-methylbenz[*a*]-anthracene (DMBA) and 12-*O*-tetradecanoyl-phorbol-13-acetate (TPA). To date, a number of mice with defined immunodeficiencies have been tested for their susceptibility to carcinogens (Table 4.2).

Table 4.2 Carcinogen-induced tumours in immunodeficient mice

Mouse strain	Immune defect (absence, deficiency)	Carcinogen-induced tumours	References
SCID	T and B cells	MCA-induced sarcomas	[26]
Rag2–/–	T and B cells	MCA-induced sarcomas	[14]
Ja18–/–	NK T cells	MCA-induced sarcomas	[27,28]
Ifngr–/–	IFN-γ receptor 1	MCA-induced sarcomas	[29]
Trail–/–	TRAIL	MCA-induced sarcomas	[30]
Perforin–/–Ifng–/–	Perforin, IFN-γ	MCA-induced sarcomas	[24]
Ifnar–/–	Type I IFN signalling	MCA-induced sarcomas	[31]
IL–12p40–/–	IL-12, IL-23	DMBA and TPA-induced squamous cell carcinomas	[18,28]
IL–12p35–/–	IL-12	Nitrosourea-induced lymphomas	[32]
CD80–/–CD86–/–	GM-CSF, IFN-γ	UV-induced squamous cell carcinomas	[33]

DMBA, 7,12-di-methylbenz[*a*]-anthracene; MCA, methylcholanthrene; TPA, 12-*O*-tetradecanoyl-phorbol-13-acetate.

Rag2$^{-/-}$ and SCID mice (both strains lack an adaptive immune system) have an increased susceptibility to tumour induction with MCA [14,26]; similar findings have been demonstrated in nude mice [34], which lack most T cell subsets. Both αβ T (adaptive immunity) and γδ T (innate immunity) cells were subsequently found to be important in suppressing MCA-induced tumours, as mice deficient for either of these T cell subsets had an increased incidence of tumour induction [35]. Interestingly, 40% of tumours derived from *Rag2*$^{-/-}$ mice were rejected when transplanted into WT recipients. However, they grew progressively in either *Rag2*$^{-/-}$ hosts or mice depleted of CD4$^+$ and CD8$^+$ T cells. Tumours derived from WT mice, on the other hand, grew readily when transplanted into either wild type or *Rag2*$^{-/-}$ hosts [14]. These observations are important because they show that not only are carcinogen-induced tumours seen more frequently in immunodeficient mice, but also that tumours derived in these immunodeficient mice are more immunogenic than those arising in mice with a normal immune system.

CD1d-restricted T (γδ T, NK T) cells, which bridge the innate and adaptive arms of the immune system, also have a role in suppressing MCA-induced fibrosarcomas. Mice that lack the T cell receptor (TCR) component Jα18 are unable to generate the semi-invariant Vα14-Jα18-containing TCR expressed by NK T cells, and show increased susceptibility to fibrosarcoma induction [27,28]. A portion of tumours arising in mice lacking Jα18 are rejected when transplanted into WT mice [36], indicating that they are immunogenic and that the absence of NK T cells might contribute to the increased incidence of tumours seen in *Rag2*$^{-/-}$ mice. Further evidence that the innate immune system is important in the suppression of MCA fibrosarcomas was provided in mice chronically depleted of NK cells, such mice having an increased incidence of tumours [28] (see Chapter 1 for discussion of NK, NK T, and γδ T cells).

To further understand how the immune system suppresses fibrosarcoma growth, a number of mice deficient for specific immune effector molecules and pathways have been examined, including mice lacking perforin [37], TRAIL [38], IL-12 [28], IFN-γ [29], IFNAR1 (component of type I IFN receptor) [31], and NK group 2 member D (NKG2D) [39]. Each of these mouse strains demonstrated enhanced susceptibility to fibrosarcoma induction, suggesting that cytotoxic cells (NK cells and $CD8^+$ CTLs) use these pathways to suppress tumour growth *in vivo*. Further investigation of these immune processes revealed that tumour cells are important targets for the antitumour effects of IFN-γ [40]. On the other hand, the host haematopoietic system is the target of the antitumour effects of type I IFN [31], suggesting that the ability of type I IFNs to induce antitumour activity in immune cells is probably an important mode of action for this cytokine family.

This interpretation of the role of IFN-γ in the prevention of MCA-induced fibrosarcomas has not been universally accepted. However, other researchers have proposed that IFN-γ contributed to the establishment of an inflammatory response that resulted in the encapsulation of injected MCA (a process referred to as a *foreign body reaction*), limiting its spread and, thereby, reducing its carcinogenic effects [41]. However, the finding that *Ifng*$^{-/-}$ mice are more susceptible to lymphomas induced by the soluble carcinogen *N*-methyl-*N*-nitrosourea, where encapsulation of the carcinogen does not occur, is at odds with this concept [32]. The finding that restoration of IFN-γ receptor 1 (IFN-γR1) expression in MCA-induced tumour lines from *Ifngr1*$^{-/-}$ mice leads to a delay in tumour growth or complete tumour rejection when such tumours are transplanted into WT mice also suggests IFN-γ is not merely a driver for initiation of inflammation and encapsulation of MCA.

A role for the immune system in regulating the development of DMBA/TPA-induced papillomas has also been investigated (Table 4.2). With the DMBA/TPA model, skin carcinomas are induced by the topical application of DMBA (the tumour initiator), followed by repetitive doses of TPA (the tumour promoter). In this model, lesions progress from benign papillomas through to metastatic squamous cell carcinomas, and the number and progression of the lesions is dependent on the mouse strain. While γδ T cells confer protection from DMBA/TPA-induced papillomas [35], αβ T cells seem to promote tumour progression in this model of carcinogenesis [42]. One mechanism by which γδ T cells might regulate tumour development is through NKG2D recognition of the stress ligand retinoic acid early transcript 1 (RAE1), expression of which is induced in the skin by DMBA/TPA treatment. NKG2D-expressing epidermal γδ T cells can kill RAE1-expressing targets *in vitro* [35], but in transgenic mice expressing RAE1 in the skin, NKG2D expression is down-modulated on lymphocytes and these mice are consequently more susceptible to papilloma induction than are WT mice [43]. Collectively, these data indicate that the NKG2D pathway is important in the control of carcinogen-induced tumours.

IL-23 and IL-12 are functionally related heterodimeric cytokines that both contain IL-12β (although paired with distinct subunits) and activate specific receptors that contain the IL-12Rβ1 subunit. Recently, Langowski *et al.* induced papillomas in mice that lacked either the IL-23-specific subunit that pairs with IL-12β or the IL-12-specific subunit that pairs with IL-12β [44]. Interestingly, mice that lacked functional IL-23 were resistant to tumour development, whereas mice that lacked functional IL-12 developed increased numbers of papillomas, compared with the WT mice. In a broad panel of human tumours, the authors also found substantial up-regulation of the mRNAs encoding both subunits of IL-23 and hypothesized that expression of IL-23 in human tumours has a causative role in promoting tumour development. Although the mechanisms by which IL-23 promotes tumour growth require further clarification, it has been found that carcinogen-treated IL-23-deficient mice produced less IL-17 (a cytokine with tumour growth-promoting activity) than did the WT controls [45,46]. Moreover, since the DMBA/TPA model of cancer is known to be dependent on a strong inflammatory response, more work is needed to explore the relative importance of inflammation versus immunoediting in other primary tumour models and whether these are distinct or overlapping processes. Tumours induced by physical carcinogens such as UV radiation also appear to be modulated by the immune system (Table 4.2) [47]. It is suggested that UV-induced immune suppression in the skin and subcutaneous tissues is an important factor in the development of UV-induced tumours. Also, UV-induced tumours are often immunogenic and rejected when transplanted into naive hosts but grow in immunosuppressed recipients or those depleted of $CD8^+$ T cells [48].

Human tumours

Tumour-infiltrating lymphocytes and role of T regulatory cells: Human tumours are infiltrated to a variable degree by cells involved in host defences. A correlation between the presence of tumour infiltrating lymphocytes (TILs) and an improved prognosis was first observed in melanoma patients. The presence of dense intratumoural (but not peritumoural) TILs, in the vertical growth phase of primary cutaneous melanomas, carried a favourable prognosis (reduced incidence of metastases, prolonged survival) [49–51]. The absence of TILs has subsequently been shown to predict sentinel lymph node metastasis in patients with cutaneous melanoma [50]. The presence of TILs and infiltration by $CD8^+$ T cells has now been shown to be a favourable independent predictor of survival for many tumour types (ovarian, colon, renal cell, non-small-cell lung cancers, and follicular lymphomas) [51,52]. A recent study investigated TILs in a large cohort of resected colorectal cancer specimens (TNM stage I–III), by *in situ* immunohistochemistry and gene expression profiling, followed by validation in two other patient populations [53]. The expression of genes associated with an adaptive cell-mediated immune response and increased cytotoxic and memory T cell infiltration correlated with reduced tumour recurrence. The prognostic value of the density, type, and location of immune cells was independent of, and superior to, classification by the UICC–TNM classification in predicting disease-free survival. The powerful predictive value of the TIL infiltrate in colorectal cancer suggests that the local adaptive immune response plays a key role in the prevention of tumour recurrence, and that the modulating effect of the immune system continues even when tumour growth progresses.

In addition to $CD8^+$ T cells, tumour-infiltrating NK cells have also been associated with a favourable prognosis in colorectal [54], gastric [55], and lung cancers [56]. The presence of tumour-reactive T cells in itself is not sufficient to confer a favourable prognosis. In patients with melanoma, melanoma-reactive T cells in the blood, in contrast to TILs, did not predict survival [57]. In a colorectal cancer study, intratumoural

T cell nests, in contrast to the presence of peritumoural T cells, carried prognostic significance [58].

In virtually all human cancers (e.g. liver, lung, breast, melanoma), DCs have been identified in tumour stromal infiltrates [59–61]. However, in these infiltrates the DCs are immature (poor APCs) and switched off by tumour cells inducing the DCs to secrete the immunosuppressive cytokine transforming growth factor-beta (TGF-β) [62].

Despite the number of convincing studies showing the positive prognostic value of TILs, not all TILs have a beneficial antitumour effect. Regulatory T cells (Tregs), a subset (10%) of $CD4^+$ T cells ($CD4^+$ $CD25^+$ $Foxp3^+$), actively inhibit $CD4^+$ T cells, $CD8^+$ T cells, NK, NK T, and B cells [63]. Tregs play a key role in maintaining self-tolerance and immune homeostasis. Tregs protect against the development of autoimmunity [64] (see Chapter 1). Increased tumour infiltration by Tregs correlated with a poorer prognosis in lung and ovarian cancers [65,66]. Tumour-induced expression of addressins on the surface of endothelial cells has recently been found to allow the selective migration of Tregs into human pancreatic tumours, providing a mechanistic explanation for tumour infiltration by Tregs, in addition to identifying a potential therapeutic target [67].

Studies of human TILs suggest that the immune system influences the pathological behaviour of established cancers, and that an adaptive antitumour immune reaction confers a favourable prognosis, albeit not necessarily preventing progressive tumour growth. The pivotal role of Tregs in tilting the balance towards immunity or tolerance and the implication for the host is illustrated in Figure 4.3.

In humans, high levels of Tregs have been identified in blood, lymph nodes, ascites, and tumours from different types of cancers (prostate, melanoma, gastric, pancreas, breast, liver, ovarian) [68–72]. Macrophages infiltrating the tumours (TIMs) (as well as the tumour cells themselves) release the chemokine CCL22 which chemoattracts and directs Tregs expressing CCR4 into the tumour microenvironment [72]. Tumour cells may also stimulate immature DCs in the tumour to secrete TGF-β and induce the conversion of naive T cells to Tregs [62]. The *in situ* Tregs secrete TGF-β, IL-10, and IL-35 and by direct cell contact substantially down-regulate the antitumour immune responses generated, suppressing the activity of DCs and TAA presentation, $CD4^+$ Th cells, and the generation of tumour specific $CD8^+$ CTLs, and inhibiting the cytotoxic activity of NK and NK T cells [73]. Another important mechanism, whereby tumour-infiltrating Tregs may suppress the generation of effective $CD8^+$ CTLs *in situ* is through inhibitory signalling via the cytotoxic T lymphocyte-associated antigen 4 (CTLA-4). This member of the immunoglobulin superfamily links the same ligands as CD28 on the CD 80/86 costimulatory receptors on DCs, thereby, downgrading DC activation and generation of $CD8^+$ T cells, by interfering with IL-2 production and T cell cycle progression [74,75].

Tumour-infiltrating macrophages: There is good clinical and experimental evidence that macrophages promote tumour induction and the early stages of tumourigenesis, by creating an inflammatory response which is mutagenic and growth-promoting. As the cancer progresses, macrophages enhance tumour cell growth, suppress anticancer host defences, and stimulate angiogenesis and tumour cell invasion. This tumour-promoting role is also seen at sites of tumour metastatic spread [76]. Within tumours they are also referred to as tumour-associated macrophages (TAMs).

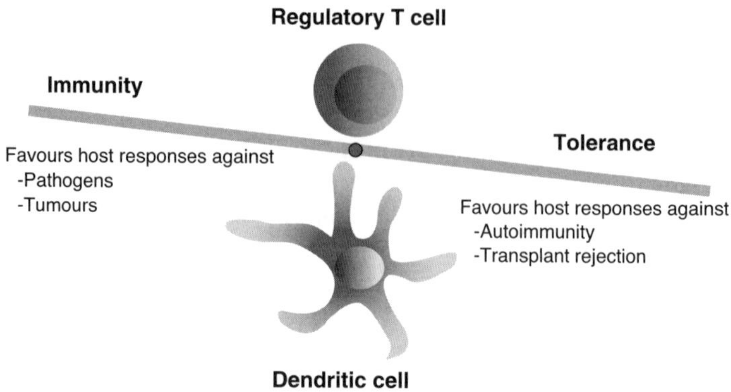

Fig. 4.3 Regulatory T cells (Tregs) are critical in determining the balance between immunity and tolerance in the host.

TIMs arise from circulating monocoytes infiltrating tumours. They are accompanied by a variable and heterogeneous group of other myeloid-derived suppressor cells (MDSCs)—see below. In human cancers the content of TIMs can vary from 10% to 40%. The TIMs are often not readily discernible on routine histological assessment (alteration of processes and distortion of normal morphology), but can be detected using specific monoclonal antibodies (MABs) and immunohistochemical staining techniques. They can both promote or inhibit tumourigenesis [76,77].

Macrophages are a heterogeneous population of cells and can be categorized into two major fractions: (1) M1 macrophages, stimulated by Toll-like receptor (TLR) ligands (e.g. LPS) and IFN-γ, are very efficient APCs. They have an increased expression of major histocompatability complex (MHC) class II antigens, and increased production of IL-12, tumour necrosis factor-alpha (TNF-α), and reactive oxygen species (ROSs). (2) M2 macrophages, activated by IL-4, IL-10, and IL-13 and are promoters of tumourigenesis [76,78]. During progressive tumour growth M2 TIMs produce prominent amounts of TGF-β which significantly suppresses the *in situ* anticancer immune responses and predispose to tumour cell dissemination and metastasis formation. This is associated with an inhibition of NF-κB activity within the TIMs [79]. Macrophages within tumours ingest necrotic or damaged tumour cells, express class II molecules, and show variable APC function. M2 TIMs are thought to compete with intratumoural DCs for tumour peptide presentation, thereby, inhibiting adaptive immunity (see 'Failure of cancer immune editing and immune escape', below).

It has been demonstrated in various types of cancers (breast [80], endometrium [81], and bladder cancer [82]) that a prominent infiltrate of the tumours by macrophages is associated with a poor prognosis. More than 80% of studies show a correlation between macrophage density and poor clinical outcome. A notable exception is the increased survival in pancreatic cancer. Macrophage differentiation, growth and chemotaxis is regulated by various factors—colony-stimulating factor-1 (CSF-1), GM-CSF, IL-3, vascular endothelial growth factor (VEGF), and CCL2 [76]. CCL2 is overexpressed in a large number of cancers and is associated with a poor prognosis in a range of solid tumours in humans. In animal models, inhibition of CSF-1 (antisense or antibodies), reduces macrophage recruitment and inhibits growth and dissemination of xenografts of human tumours [76]. CCL2 is expressed by tumour cells, fibroblasts, and endothelial cells in tumours, as well as TIMs [83].

MDSCs are a heterogeneous group of poorly defined leucocytes which have been documented in the circulation, secondary lymphoid compartments, and infiltrating tumours in mice and various cancers in humans. They are increased in a number of pathological conditions (e.g. infection, inflammation, trauma), apart from malignancy. GM-CSF and VEGF, produced by tumours, significantly increase the entry into and numbers of these cells in the tumour microenvironment. Prostaglandins (PGs) secreted by tumour cells up-regulate the production of PGE2, which stimulates the activity of nitric oxide synthetase and production of nitric oxide. MDSCs inhibit $CD4^+$ T and $CD8^+$ T lymphocytes via L-arginine metabolism. The depletion of L-arginine affects the production of ROSs with a switch from nitric oxide to superoxide (O_2^-) radicals. The latter are particularly toxic to T cell function and survival [84].

Multiple myeloma; natural progression: Multiple myeloma is a plasma cell malignancy in which immunoediting can be evaluated in a clinical setting [85]. The advantage of studying multiple myeloma is that several stages of the disease have been identified. The disease progresses from a premalignant state, known as monoclonal gammopathy of undetermined significance (MGUS), through to a terminal phase [86]. The ability to detect this premalignant phase of disease allows for immunological monitoring to assess the contribution of the immune system to preventing and/or inhibiting progression to multiple myeloma [87]. Such monitoring has revealed that T cells derived from the bone marrow of patients with MGUS mount strong responses to autologous premalignant cells; these responses are not detected in patients with multiple myeloma [87]. These findings are consistent with a T cell response keeping premalignant cells in check initially, followed subsequently by the failure of this response to control abnormal plasma cell clones, and resulting in the eventual transition to multiple myeloma (i.e. tumour escape) (see later sections).

Paraneoplastic syndromes: The neurological paraneoplastic syndromes are thought to be caused by cross-reactivity between an antitumour immune response and self antigens in the central or peripheral nervous system, and offer a unique opportunity to study the generation of antitumour immunity in humans [80] (see Chapter 8). Neurological paraneoplastic syndromes are characterized by both high titres of antibodies and lymphocytes reactive to antigens shared between the tumour and neural tissue [80]. The presentation of paraneoplastic syndromes can precede overt tumour occurrence by several years [81], implying that an antitumour immune response has been initiated in the early preclinical stages of tumour development. Rare cases in which spontaneous regression of an underlying tumour is reported, and cases in which an underlying tumour is never detected on follow-up, suggest that antitumour immune responses can be effective [82]. A paraneoplastic immune response can be generated without causing paraneoplastic symptoms. In a series of 196 patients with small-cell lung cancer, anti-Hu antibodies were detected in 32 patients, and were associated with a higher rate of complete response to treatment and increased overall survival [88].

Immunocompromised patients: Immunosuppression (caused by either primary or secondary immunodeficiencies) is often associated with an increased risk of developing malignancies. Immunosuppression to prevent transplant rejection is clearly associated with an increased risk (3- to 100-fold increase) of developing certain types of malignancies [89]. These diseases are predominantly lymphomas and squamous cell cancers in skin, which tend to be more aggressive (rapidly growing, spread to regional nodes). A range of solid tumours with no known viral association also occur with increased frequency [89,90]. In addition to these tumours in patients receiving immunosuppressive drugs, a number of tumours (especially lymphomas) also occur commonly in patients with primary and acquired immunodeficiencies; however, these are generally thought to have a viral aetiology [90]. In summary, although evidence from immunosuppressed patients supports the theory of immunoediting, further investigation in this area is warranted, as the contributions of viral infection, cytotoxic drugs, and persistent inflammation progressing to tumourigenesis in this setting must also be taken into consideration (see Chapter 3).

The modern concept of immunoediting

Introduction

Tumour immunoediting can be considered as consisting of three phases: designated elimination, equilibrium, and escape (Figure 4.4) [91]. The elimination phase of cancer immunoediting is exactly the same process as described in the original theory of tumour immune surveillance, whereby, the immune system detects and eliminates tumour cells that have arisen as a result of failed intrinsic tumour suppressor mechanisms. The elimination phase can be complete, when all tumour cells are destroyed and removed, or incomplete, when only a portion of the tumour cells are destroyed and eliminated. In the case of partial tumour elimination, the theory of immunoediting postulates that a temporary state of equilibrium can then develop between the antitumour host immune system and the residual tumour cell mass. During this period it is envisaged that tumour cells either remain dormant (possibly due to significant numbers of cancer progenitor or stem cells) or continue to multiply, accumulating further changes (such as DNA mutations or alterations in gene expression) that can modulate the tumour-specific antigens and stress-induced antigens that they express. As this process continues, the immune system induces selective tumour cell damage and eliminates susceptible tumour clones but with a variable degree of effectiveness. The resultant anticancer responses exerted by the immune system during this phase is sufficient to prevent or significantly restrict tumour progression. Eventually, however, the anticancer immune responses fail to completely eliminate or effectively control the tumour cells. This results in the selection of tumour cell variants that are able to resist, avoid, or suppress the antitumour immune response, leading to the escape phase. During the escape phase the anticancer host defences are no longer able to effectively control and contain the malignancy, and a progressively growing tumour results. This leads to tumour cell dissemination and the establishment of regional (lymph nodes draining the tumour) and distant (e.g. skeletal system, lungs, liver) tumour metastatic deposits.

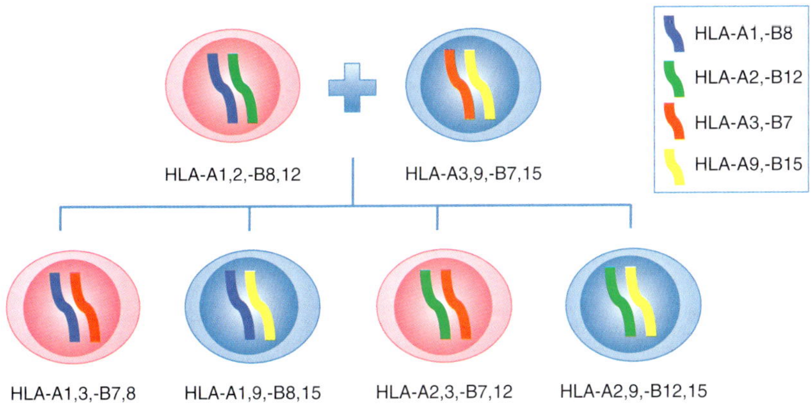

Plate 1 Mendelian inheritance of codominantly expressed HLA types. An individual inherits one copy (haplotype) of the full complement of MHC genes from each parent, and expresses them codominantly. Chromosomal crossover within the MHC is rare. There is a 25% chance that an individual will have a two-haplotype match with a sibling, a 25% chance of a two-haplotype mismatch, and a 50% chance of a one-haplotype match. HLA, human leucocyte antigen; MHC, major histocompatibility complex.

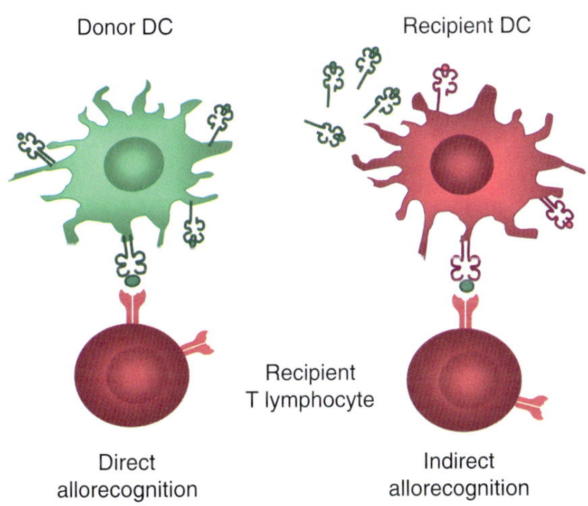

Plate 2 Two pathways of allorecognition. In direct allorecognition, recipient T lymphocytes recognize (by cross-reactivity) and respond to intact, non-self class I and class II HLA molecules expressed on donor-derived APCs. In indirect allorecognition, recipient $CD4^+$ T lymphocytes recognize and respond to donor HLA molecules that have been taken up and processed by recipient APCs, and presented as peptide fragments in the peptide binding cleft of recipient HLA class II molecules (recognition by MHC restriction). APC, antigen-presenting cell; DC, dendritic cell; HLA, human leucocyte antigen.

(a)

(b)

(c)

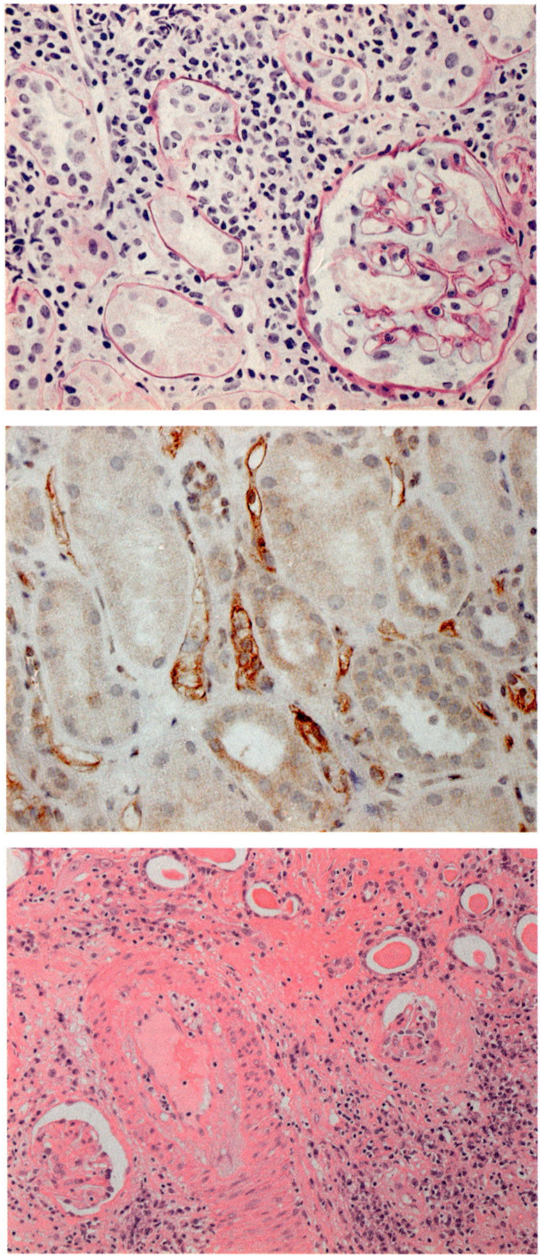

Plate 3 Pathology of renal allograft rejection: (a) Inflammatory infiltrate characteristic of acute cellular rejection. The tubules are separated by an interstitial infiltrate of lymphocytes, and lymphocytes have infiltrated the tubular epithelium (tubulitis). PAS ×400. (b) C4d deposition in a renal transplant with acute humoral rejection. C4d is demonstrated circumferentially in peritubular capillaries using immunohistochemistry (brown staining). ×400. (c) Characteristic appearance of graft vasculopathy in a renal transplant with chronic rejection. The wall of the interlobular artery is thickened by fibrosis and an infiltrate of lymphocytes and macrophages. There is associated atrophy of tubules and glomeruli. H&E ×200. Images kindly supplied by Dr Meryl Griffiths, Consultant Pathologist, Addenbrooke's Hospital, Cambridge.

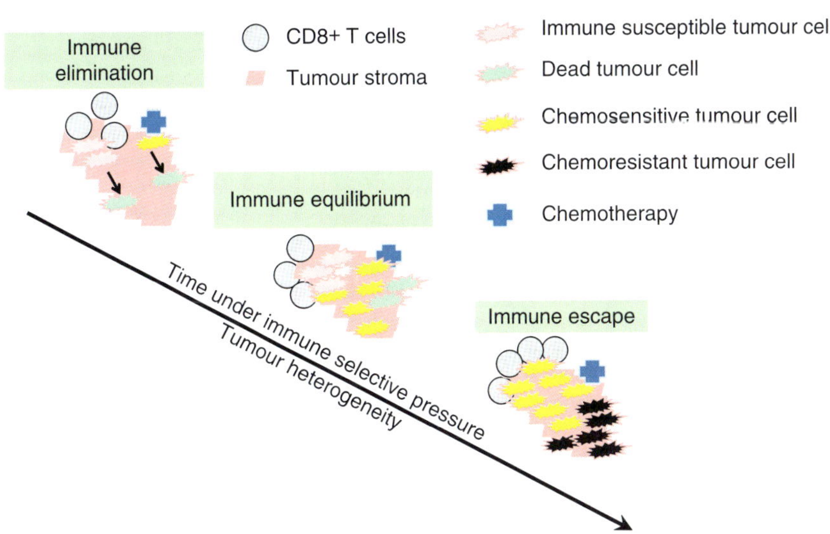

Plate 4 Extrinsic tumour suppression and control by the immune system. Transformed cells escaping intrinsic control are subjected to extrinsic tumour suppressor mechanisms that detect and eliminate growing cancer cells before they become clinically apparent. This is known as the elimination phase of a complex, multifactorial process that has been termed cancer immunoediting. Cancer immunoediting encompasses the concepts that the host defence system both protects the host against tumour development and promotes tumour growth. Cancer immunoediting is a process involving three phases: *elimination*, or cancer immune surveillance; *equilibrium*, a phase of tumour dormancy where tumour cells and immunity enter into a dynamic equilibrium that keeps tumour cell expansion in check; and *escape*, where tumour cells emerge that display reduced responsiveness to immune defences and/or resistance to chemotherapy, employ a large number of immunosuppressive mechanisms to inhibit antitumour immune responses, resulting in progressive tumour growth. These phases have been termed the '3 Es' of cancer immunoediting.

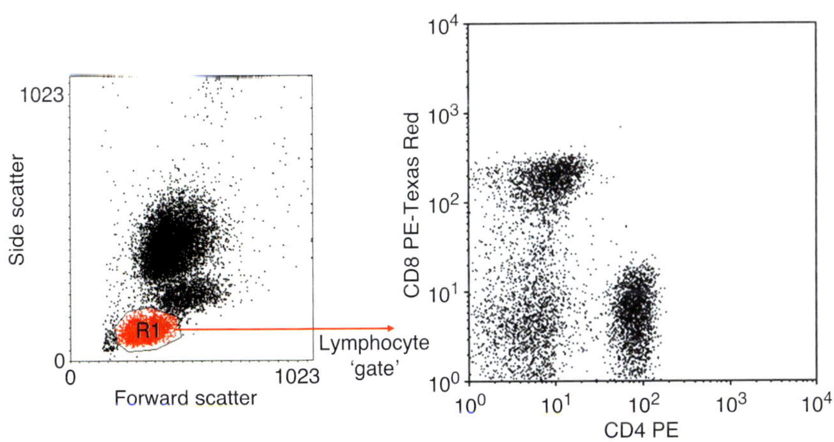

Plate 5 Analysis of human peripheral blood leucocytes. Forward (FS lin) and side (SS lin) scatter allows identification of the main leucocyte subsets. An example of 'gating' is shown, where the distribution of CD4 and CD8 staining is shown only for cells in the R1 region, defined as the lymphocyte gate.

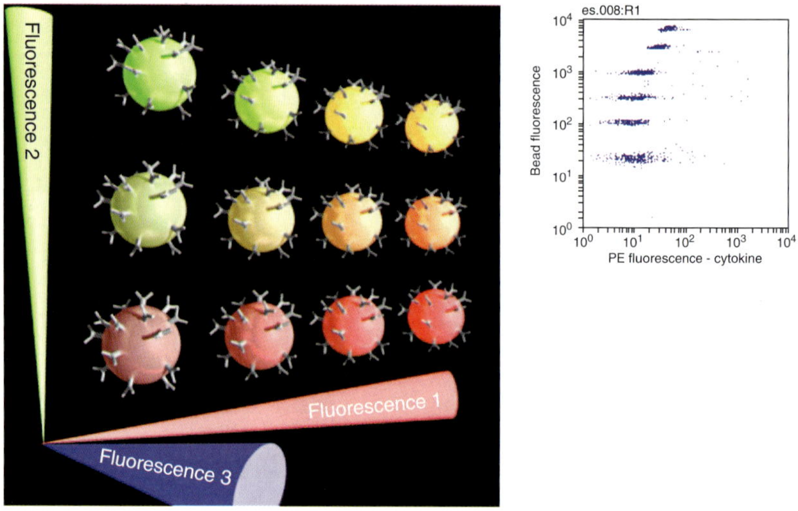

Plate 6 Principle of the bead immunoassay. One bead here represents many thousands of identically coloured beads in a real assay. Each defined mixture of fluorescence 1 and 2 within a bead set allows separation of different bead sets in two dimensions. Each bead set is coated in a different specific antibody. Once target antigen is bound (not shown) a second specific antibody, labelled with fluorescence 3, is bound to each target molecule. Thus, each cluster of beads can be identified and the level of fluorescence 3 on the beads indicates the level of antigen present in the sample, which can be compared with a standard curve for quantification. The insert plot shows actual results from a 6-plex assay.

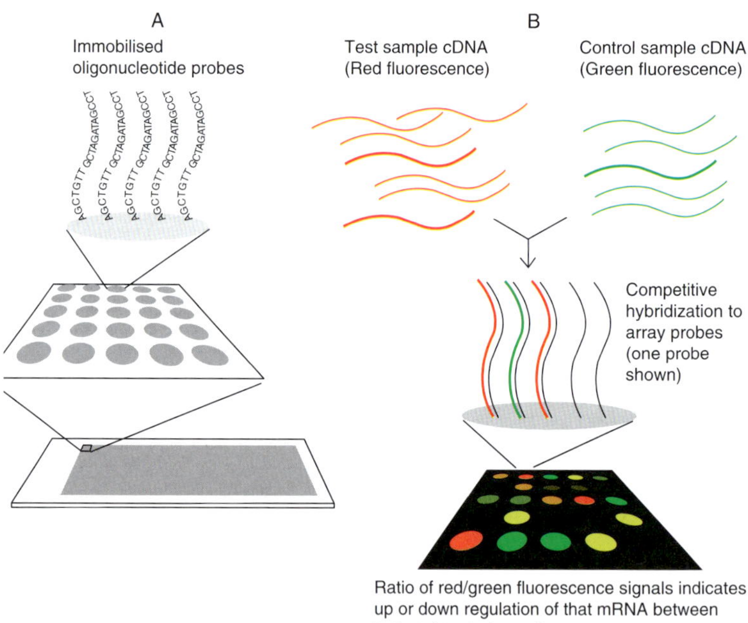

Plate 7 Principle of a dual-colour comparative transcriptome analysis. (A) Gene (mRNA) specific oligonucleotide probes are arrayed in extremely dense arrays across the surface of a solid support. (B) mRNA samples from a control sample (cells or tissue) are converted to cDNA, labelled with a fluorescent dye (shown in green). Test sample cDNA is labelled with a different dye (shown in red). Hybridization of equal quantities of each sample to the array results in proportional binding of cDNAs from both samples, if present. Quantification of each fluorescence bound to a probe feature allows comparison of gene expression between the samples.

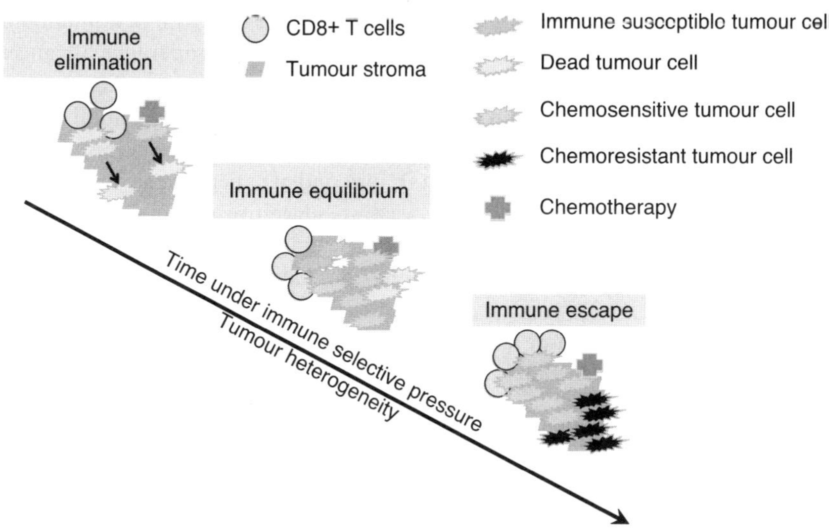

Fig. 4.4 Extrinsic tumour suppression and control by the immune system. Transformed cells escaping intrinsic control are subjected to extrinsic tumour suppressor mechanisms that detect and eliminate growing cancer cells before they become clinically apparent. This is known as the elimination phase of a complex, multifactorial process that has been termed cancer immunoediting. Cancer immunoediting encompasses the concepts that the host defence system both protects the host against tumour development and promotes tumour growth. Cancer immunoediting is a process involving three phases: *elimination*, or cancer immune surveillance; *equilibrium*, a phase of tumour dormancy where tumour cells and immunity enter into a dynamic equilibrium that keeps tumour cell expansion in check; and *escape*, where tumour cells emerge that display reduced responsiveness to immune defences and/or resistance to chemotherapy, employ a large number of immunosuppressive mechanisms to inhibit antitumour immune responses, resulting in progressive tumour growth. These phases have been termed the '3 Es' of cancer immunoediting (see also colour plate section).

Elimination

The elimination phase is equivalent to the original immunosurveillance concept. Based upon the 'danger' hypothesis of immune recognition [6], elimination is expected to be initiated by a 'danger' signal from newly emerging malignant cells. These signals may be multifactorial and due to factors inducing angiogenesis, cytokine production (e.g. IL-6) by tumour cells, and/or the expression of stress-induced molecules (e.g. HSPs) [7]. Cells of the innate and adaptive arms of the immune system are recruited, leading to an antitumour immune response. If successful, this process leads to the complete destruction and elimination of small clones of malignant cells developing during the early phase of tumour development.

Equilibrium

If the immune system fails to eliminate all cancer cells, the immunoediting model proposes a subclinical equilibrium phase. During this phase selective elimination of cancer cells continues, resulting in the survival of tumour cells with new mutations that favour resistance to anticancer host defences or a preponderance of cancer progenitor/stem cells. This process may take place over many years [1]. Direct proof of the existence of this equilibrium is difficult to provide, but there is clinical data to support it. Clinical observations of prolonged periods between the successful treatment of primary tumours and subsequent relapse, and of patients remaining disease-free despite evidence of micrometastatic disease, are suggestive of 'tumour dormancy.' For example, relapses after 15–20 years are well recognized after the treatment of primary breast cancer [92]. The equilibrium phase provides a plausible explanation of this oncological puzzle. Tumour vaccination models in mice have noted a correlation between the persistence of low levels of tumour cells in the bone marrow and long-term protective immune memory [93], with evidence that dormant tumour cells were kept under control by $CD8^+$ T cells [94]. Consistent with this is the finding that the proportion of memory T cells among the T cell population within the bone marrow of breast cancer patients, after treatment of the primary tumour, is higher than in normal controls [95]. In this group of patients, memory T cell levels were higher in the presence of micrometastatic disease in the bone marrow, detected by the nested polymerase chain reaction (PCR) [95]. There are cases in which donors have transmitted occult tumours in donated organs to recipients [96], suggesting tumour cell dormancy in the donor. Once transplanted, these tumour cells would have been removed from the previous immune control in the donor, and proliferation in the recipient occurs in the presence of added suppression of host defences by antirejection therapy (see Chapter 3).

Escape

During tumour escape, the balance between immunological control of the tumour and tumour progression shifts in favour of progressive tumour growth. Tumours can continue to grow in the presence of an antitumour immune response, as evidenced by the finding of TILs and of paraneoplastic syndromes in association with clinically detectable tumours. The previously discussed prognostic importance of TILs shows that, although during tumour escape the balance between immunological control and growth has moved in favour of progression, the immune system can still influence the rate and extent of tumour growth. Poorly immunogenic, newly formed aggressive tumours may enter the escape phase directly without a prior equilibrium phase.

Failure of cancer immune editing and immune escape

Tumour resistance to host defences and growth promotion

The concept of immunostimulation, whereby a host immune response against a cancer can promote tumour growth, was first proposed by Prehn in 1972. The original theory postulated that a 'weak' host immune response may promote tumour growth. There is murine data to support the concept that nonprotective host immune responses can support tumour growth. For example, chemical induction of tumours occurred more rapidly in irradiated, thymectomized mice who had been inoculated with lymphocytes to partially restore their immune system, compared with mice with a fully restored normal immune system [97]. Within the immunoediting hypothesis, tumour cell selection will be in favour not only of cells that evade the anticancer immune response but also of tumour cells that promote a tumour-growth-enhancing immune response. More recently, possible mechanisms by which the host immune response can promote tumour growth have been described [98,99].

Chronic inflammatory changes can promote tumour growth, with innate immune cells providing proliferation and angiogenic signals. Chronic inflammatory diseases are associated with an increased risk of cancer. Epidemiological studies have shown that the use of anti-inflammatory drugs in chronic inflammatory diseases reduces cancer risk [100]. Tumour infiltration by certain innate immune cells has been reported to be detrimental. For example, mast cells (containing multiple mediators of inflammation) [99], infiltrating lung cancers [101], and melanomas [102] are associated with a poor prognosis. Similarly, the infiltration of macrophages into breast [103], endometrial [104], and bladder cancers [105] is associated with a poor prognosis. Innate immune cells may promote cancer by multiple mechanisms, including free-radical release and resulting damage, angiogenesis, the suppression of adaptive immune responses, the production of growth factors, and ongoing tissue remodelling [98]. Proinflammatory cytokines, including VEGF, TNF-α and several chemokines [99], appear capable of promoting tumour growth and development. In contrast, other innate immune cells, such as NK cells, appear to have a protective role in immunosurveillance by inducing cancer cell lysis and the production of antiangiogenic mediators [106].

The innate immune system plays a key role in initiating the adaptive immune response. The innate inflammatory response, however, can also inhibit the development of a protective adaptive immune response [98]. For example, ovarian tumour-derived macrophages have been shown to produce a chemokine, CCL22, which enhances trafficking of Tregs into the tumour cell milieu [72]. Myeloid suppressor cells are innate immune cells whose immunosuppressive properties inhibit the development of specific antitumour immunity [107]. Also, evidence is emerging that persistent humoral or antibody-based adaptive immune responses can promote carcinogenesis [108].

Reduced/absent immunogenicity of the tumour

Immune recognition may lead to the emergence of tumour cell variants with a diminished capacity for T cell recognition, through either modulation of the binding of peptides to MHC molecules or the binding of TCRs to MHC–peptide complexes, in a process termed *antigenic drift* [109]. MHC class I down-regulation in tumour cells is well documented and reduces the sensitivity of malignant cells to CTL-mediated lysis [110]. MHC class I down-regulation may, however, make the cancer cells susceptible to NK-cell-mediated immunosurveillance, as NK cells are activated and attracted to the malignant cells lacking normal MHC class I antigens [110]. Resistance to immune-mediated killing has been documented in all of the major cytotoxic mechanisms. The release of perforin from cytolytic granules is a major pathway of cancer cell damage and destruction by $CD8^+$ CTLs and NK cells. Impaired binding of perforin to the tumour cell surface can prevent perforin-mediated killing [111]. The interaction between Fas and FasL is an alternative and important pathway of cytotoxicity, and down-regulation or mutation of Fas is present in some tumours [112]. Resistance to another immune killing mechanism has also been found, involving mutations in the TRAIL receptors 1 and 2 and defective apoptosis in tumours [113].

Impairment of anticancer host defences by the tumour

Many mechanisms have been documented by which malignancies inhibit the development of an effective anticancer immune response, as outlined below. According to the 'danger' model of immune activation, tumours that fail to produce the necessary signals (2 and 3) that optimally activate DCs will induce tolerance or anergy in any tumour-specific reactive T cells which may be generated [114]. The induction of $CD8^+$ T cell anergy results in the immune system regarding the tumour as 'self.' Suboptimal activation of DCs can also lead to the production of immunosuppressive $CD4^+$ $CD25^+$ T regs and the establishment of tumour tolerance [115]. Moreover, the down-regulation of vascular endothelial adhesion molecules will reduce immune cell infiltration into the tumour cell milieu [116].

Tumour expression of the enzyme indoleamine 2,3-dioxygenase results in tryptophan deficiency in the tumour microenvironment, inhibiting T cell activation and proliferation [117]. Malignancies secrete a range of soluble and very effective immunosuppressive mediators, including nitric oxide [118], TGF-β [119], and IL-10 [120], suppressing cell-mediated anticancer defences. Tumour cells expression of FasL can kill infiltrating immune reactive cells, while avoiding damage to the tumour [121]. Tumours also induce infiltration of a population of inflammatory leucocytes (MDSCs), which significantly inhibit $CD8^+$ CTLs, NK cell activity, and DC maturation [107].

All of these factors, in association with a defective anticancer immune response (suboptimal/tolerogenic, switched off/anergic, or dysfunctional), result in growth of cancer cells, their systemic dissemination, and the establishment of metastatic (incurable) disease.

Tumour microenvironment: role of TGF-β

Introduction: TGF-β significantly affects the various cell types that have been shown to influence the initiation and progression of cancer. TGF-β is a key immunosuppressive cytokine produced both by tumour cells and by immune cells and plays a critical role in inhibiting the generation of an effective anticancer response in the tumour microenvironment. TGF-β can suppress tumourigenesis, but its overproduction usually results in progressive tumour growth and tumour cell dissemination [122]. TGF-β inhibits the activity of innate immunity (DCs, NK cells, macrophages, neutrophils) and adaptive immunity ($CD4^+$ and $CD8^+$ cells). Blocking TGF-β by targeted inhibitors shows promise in cancer therapy [122].

TGF-β expression is usually up-regulated in human cancers. It is sequestered in the extracellular matrix (ECM) as an inactivate complex until activation. The latter can be induced by various molecules—integrin, cathepsin D, elastase, matrix metalloproteinase (MMP) 9, and ROSs. TGF-β signalling components (e.g. receptors) are often lost or mutated in human cancers with resultant enhanced up-regulation of the corresponding ligands. TGF-β can promote an epithelial to mesenchymal transition; this has been associated with increased tumour cell mobility, invasion and formation of metastasis [123].

Neutrophils: TGF-β is a very potent chemoattractant for neutrophils and inhibits their ability to suppress tumourigenicity [124]. Neutrophils are able to recognize and destroy FasL-expressing tumour cells. In the presence of TGF-β this neutrophil function is attenuated, thereby, providing a permissive environment for tumour growth [125]. These neutrophils promote tumour angiogenesis and metastatic dissemination of cancer cells [126].

NK cells and DCs: TGF-β down-regulates NKG2D expression (resultant inhibition of NK cell activity) and this has been documented in patients with lung and colorectal cancer with high levels of serum TGF-β [127]. TGF-β down-regulates expression of DC MHC class II molecules and costimulatory molecules (CD80/86), and reduces production of TNF-α, INF-α, and IL-12. The resultant immature and tolerogenic DCs promote the presence of Tregs, suppressing $CD4^+$ and $CD8^+$ T cells [128].

TIMs and MDSCs: TIMs and MDSCs within the tumour microenvironment produce significant amounts of TGF-β. The TIMs are strongly phagocytic and compete with DCs as APCs, further inhibiting the generation of CTLs, and are associated with reduced NF-κB. In skin cancer, recruitment of macrophages by TGF-β into the tumours changes a regressive tumour into a rapidly growing lesion [129]. TGF-β promotes the differentiation of monocytes to macrophages. It also inhibits the priming of macrophages by IFN-γ and attenuates the cytotoxic and cytostatic ability of TAMs to induce cancer cell damage and death. It downgrades the expression of key regulatory cytokines (e.g. IL-1, IL-8, GM-CSF and IL-10) in TAMs [123].

In tumour models and various human cancers (e.g. lung, breast, head and neck), increased infiltration by MDSCs occurs, with high levels of secretion of TGF-β, especially at the leading edge of the tumour. When cancer cells lose the ability to respond to TIMs/TAMs they up-regulate proinflammatory cytokines and chemokines and promote entry of MDSCs into the tumour microenvironment [123].

$CD4^+$ and $CD8^+$ T cells: TGF-β inhibits the generation of CTLs and their cytotoxic function (reduction of perforin, granzyme granules, secretion of IFN-γ and FasL) [130]. It inhibits $CD4^+$ Th cells and shifts the profile from Th1 to Th2 (less effective antitumour response) [131] and, very importantly, is involved in generating ($CD4^+$ $CD25^+$ $Foxp3^+$) Tregs. The precise mechanisms for this are unclear [72]. Good data, from animal tumour models and some human tumours, suggest that the degree of Treg infiltration correlates with tumour volume and dissemination [72, 132].

Tumour antigens

Introduction

Malignant transformation arises from normal cells and tissues in the host. It is a complex biological process associated with gene mutation, production of various oncogenes (e.g. *ras*, *myc*, *erb*, *fos*) and related proteins (growth factors/receptors, signal transducers, regulators of transcription, cell cycle control mechanisms) resulting in dysregulation of normal cell control and differentiation pathways and the development of the abnormal, uncontrolled cancer phenotype. The anticancer immune responses generated by the host against many of the antigens (new, previously repressed, or cryptic, e.g. oncofetal) expressed on these transformed cells are often ineffectual as a result of existing self-tolerance. However, there are several classes of antigens that have a restricted expression, or the expression pattern is characteristic of the malignant growths rather than healthy tissues and, thus, is not hindered by self-tolerance or prone to generate adverse autoimmune effects.

Some selected characteristics of tumour antigens that make them useful targets for immunotherapy are: (1) common expression on a variety of carcinomas, thus, making the vaccine more broadly applicable; (2) stable expression through different stages of tumour development so that stem cells, progenitor cells and mature tumour cells can all be targets of the elicited immune responses; (3) indispensable for tumour survival and, thus, not susceptible to immunoediting [133]. Many tumour antigens identified to date have these characteristics. They belong to several categories that include products of mutated genes, viral antigens, differentially expressed antigens, and tissue-restricted antigens. Most tumour antigens characterized so far are differentially expressed antigens and tissue-restricted antigens.

Repertoire of tumour antigens

Products of mutated oncogenes and tumour suppressor genes

Genetic alterations occur during the development of most malignancies. Since these mutations occur exclusively in tumours and not in normal tissues, such mutated gene products can be ideal targets for immunotherapy. However, mutated gene products have the potential disadvantage of not being displayed properly on the tumour cell surface because of the down-regulation of MHC class I molecules through the immune selection process as part of immune editing. Some of these mutated gene products are outlined in Table 4.3.

Tumour-specific expressed cellular proteins

Most tumour cells represent the clonal progeny of a single cancer stem cell and therefore express antigens present on only a few normal cells. CALLA (common acute lymphoblastic leukaemia antigen) in acute leukaemia and 17-1A epithelial antigen in colon cancer are cancer-specific examples. Universally overexpressed tumour antigens are human telomerase reverse transcriptase (hTERT) [134] and survivin [135], expressed by malignant cells and normal stem cells. The inherent hazard of targeting some of these antigens is the possible collateral damage to normal tissues expressing them. However, to date, this has not been documented with these two pantumour antigens.

Tumour antigens produced by oncogenic viruses

Abnormal proteins are also produced by cells infected with oncoviruses, e.g. Epstein–Barr virus (EBV) and human papillomavirus (HPV) [136]. Cells infected by these

Table 4.3 Mutated gene products as tumour-associated antigens

Mutated gene	Protein	Tumour
Chromosomal translocations		
BCR-ABL	Tyrosine kinase	Chronic myeloid and acute lymphoid leukaemias
H4-RET	Growth factor receptor	Thyroid carcinoma
L MYC-RLF	Transcription factor	Small cell lung carcinoma
TPR-MET	Growth factor receptor	Gastric carcinoma
Chromosomal deletions		
ERB-B	Growth factor receptor	Glioma
Chromosomal point mutations		
RB1	Tumour suppressor/cell cycle regulator	Pancreatic carcinoma, retinoblastoma, osteosarcoma
ras	GTP binding protein	Squamous cell skin carcinoma
p53	Tumour suppressor/cell cycle regulator	A large number of solid carcinomas (e.g. lung, colon, bladder)
ERB-B2	Growth factor receptor	Breast carcinoma

viruses contain latent viral DNA, which is transcribed; the resulting protein, expressed on the cell membrane linked to MHC class I molecules, can generate a peptide-specific $CD8^+$ CTL response.

Oncofoetal antigens

Oncofoetal antigens are differentiation antigens expressed during foetal development but not normally expressed, or expressed at very low levels, in adult life. Examples are alpha-fetoprotein (AFP) expressed by liver tumours (hepatomas), and carcinoembryonic antigen (CEA), expressed by colon and breast carcinomas (tumours arising from cells derived from the primitive gut).

Altered cell surface glycolipids and glycoproteins

Altered glycosylation is a feature of malignant tumours. This may give rise to carbohydrate epitopes with a protein backbone as tumour antigens, e.g. mucins which may be overexpressed in breast, pancreatic, and gastric carcinomas, rendering them potential immunotherapeutic targets.

Cell-type-specific differentiation antigens

A large number of antigens are expressed in malignant tumours and testis in adults but sparsely expressed in normal tissues. It is likely, therefore, that the malignant differentiation process itself leads to up-regulation of these antigens. Table 4.4 outlines some of these antigens.

Table 4.4 Tumour differentiation antigens and their expression in malignant and benign tissues

Differentiation antigen	Tumour expression	Normal tissue expression
Melanoma differentiation antigens		
MelanA/MART-1	Melanoma	Benign melanocytes
Tyrosinase		
gp75/TRP-1		
gp100/pmel-17		
Cancer testis antigens		
MAGE-1	Melanoma Lung carcinoma	Testis
MAGE-3		
GAGE		
BAGE		
NY-ESO		
Other differentiation antigens		
Prostate specific antigen	Prostate cancer	Normal prostate

Cancer and cellular immune mechanisms: innate and adaptive

Introduction

DCs can be considered the 'pacemakers' of the immune response as they activate both the innate and adaptive arms of the immune system by interacting with CD4$^+$Th cells, CD8$^+$CTLs, NK cells, NK T cells, macrophages, B cells, and eosinophils (see Chapter 1) (Figure 4.5). In order to initiate an antigen-specific immune response, the antigen has to be presented, in intimate combination with MHC (class I and II) molecules sited on the surface of DCs, to the peptide-specific TCR (peptide–MHC complex; signal 1). Associated with this, the appropriate second signal involves costimulatory molecules: DC CD80/86 interacting with CD4$^+$ or CD8$^+$ T cells (CD28); DC CD40 interacting with CD4$^+$ or CD8$^+$ T cells (CD40L) [8]. Tumour cells lack costimulatory molecules, and are therefore poor activators of T cells. Hence, tumour antigens need to be presented by professional APCs. DCs are the most effective of the APCs (DCs, macrophages, B cells) that prime naive T cells and play an important role in the induction of an immune response [137,138]. DCs present exogenous antigens (derived from lysed tumour cells or shed TAAs) incorporated into an MHC class II processing pathway and expressed with MHC class II molecules to activate CD4$^+$ Th lymphocytes. DCs present endogenous antigens (derived from viral vectors, carcinogens) by MHC class I molecules to CD8$^+$ CTLs. DCs are equally capable of processing exogenous antigens, loading them on to MHC class I molecules and presenting them to CTLs. This dual versatility of antigen presentation and lymphocyte priming by DCs is called

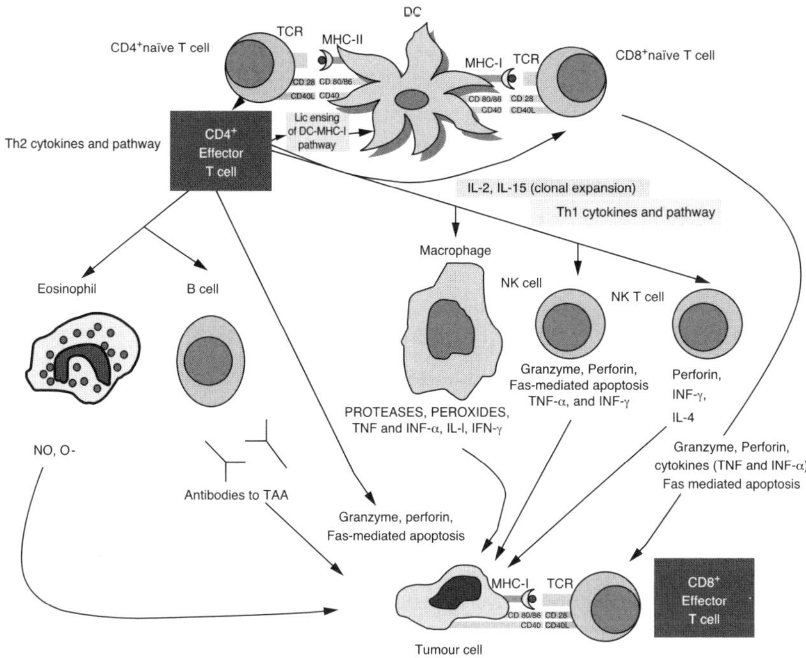

Fig. 4.5 The host's adaptive and innate immunity interacting with a tumour-associated antigen (TAA), leading to multiple pathways targeting the tumour cell. (see text for further details).

'cross-presentation' and 'cross-priming,' respectively [139]. This is essential for an amplified and a sustained antigen-specific immune response (see Chapter 1).

Dendritic cells

DCs are amongst the first cells to infiltrate the tumour microenvironment, where they recognize, capture (phagocytose), and process (digest and re-express) the putative antigens. There is published evidence that peripheral circulating DCs and tumour infiltrating DCs are significantly reduced in number and functional activity in various cancers [52]. Conversely, increased infiltration of cancers by DCs is associated with improved outcomes [140]. The presence of CD83$^+$ DCs at the edge of tumours (breast, colon) has been shown to be a good prognostic factor. Low levels of the chemokines CXCL14 in head and neck cancers has been shown to lead to low levels of tumour infiltration by DCs [84]. There is also evidence to suggest that the DCs are poorly differentiated and immature in patients with cancer. Such DCs not only fail to present antigens to naive T cells in lymphoid tissues (e.g. paracortical areas of regional tumour-draining lymph nodes), but also induce immune tolerance to the antigens they encounter. This is related to the milieu in which their differentiation and maturation occurs (see 'Human tumours', above). Tumour-derived inhibitory factors, implicated *in vitro* and confirmed *in vivo,* are IL-10 [141,142], IL-6 [143–145], GM-CSF [146,147],

VEGF [148–150], and TGF-β [122] (see 'Tumour microenvironment: role of TGF-β', above). Several other mediators have been recognized *in vitro* but, as yet, have not been confirmed *in vivo* to cause failure of DCs to differentiate and mature. As a consequence of the loss of the antigen presentation and tumour recognition by DCs, immune evasion occurs and cancer growth progresses.

An important mechanism in rendering DCs ineffective in generating an optimal $CD8^+$ CTL response is the presence of Tregs, macrophages, and myelosuppressive cells in the tumour microenvironment (see 'Human tumnours', above—TILs and TIMs).

Antigen-specific T cells (human vaccination)

In strategies designed to recognize and interact with TAAs the objective of cancer immunotherapy is tumour regression. However, this may not be readily apparent in large-volume tumours (primaries and metastatic deposits). A primary endpoint of this approach is the successful generation of TAA-specific CTLs by the immunotherapy. Immunotherapy using specific MHC class I compatible short peptides of the TAA (sequences of 8–10 amino acids) has the advantage of generating peptide-specific antitumour $CD8^+$ T lymphocytes in the circulation which can be monitored during the course of the vaccination. Novel approaches using tetrameric MHC molecules and semi-automated enzyme-linked immunosorbent spot (ELISPOT) to document CTLs in the circulation have been developed [151,152]. Tetramer analysis quantifies the numbers of peptide-specific $CD8^+$ cells induced by the vaccine. T cells recognize epitopes presented by MHC molecules on target cells. These MHC–peptide complexes can be expressed as recombinant proteins. In general, they are not recognized as monomer complexes. A group of four molecules labelled with a fluorescent dye is used as a 'bait' for antigen-specific T cells. Soluble recombinant MHC–peptide tetramer molecules are powerful tools for enumerating antigen-specific T cells *ex vivo*, without the need for *in vitro* manipulation. In general, data are expressed as $tetramer^+$ (i.e. antigen-specific) $CD8^+$ T cells. The principle of the tetramer assay is illustrated in Figure 4.6 and an illustrative tetramer analysis tracked during a vaccination programme is shown in Figure 4.7.

NK cells

NK cells reside in the large granulocyte lymphocyte (LGL) subpopulation in blood and are important cells of the innate immune system. They lack the characteristic TCR, but recognize lipids and glycolipids presented by CD1d molecules on cells, in a nonclassical MHC-restricted manner. They induce target cell death through the release of cytoplasmic granules (perforin, granzyme) causing damage to intracellular structures and cell membranes, resulting in apoptosis. They secrete a range of cytokines with important immune reactivities (e.g. IL-2, IL-12, IL-15, IL-18) and the chemokine CCL5 (see Chapter 1, Table 1.5).

Mice depleted of NK cells are more susceptible to MCA-induced sarcomas and, in this model, NK cells appear to use the NKG2D pathway to protect the host from tumour development [39] (see Chapter 1). Most human cancers appear to show low

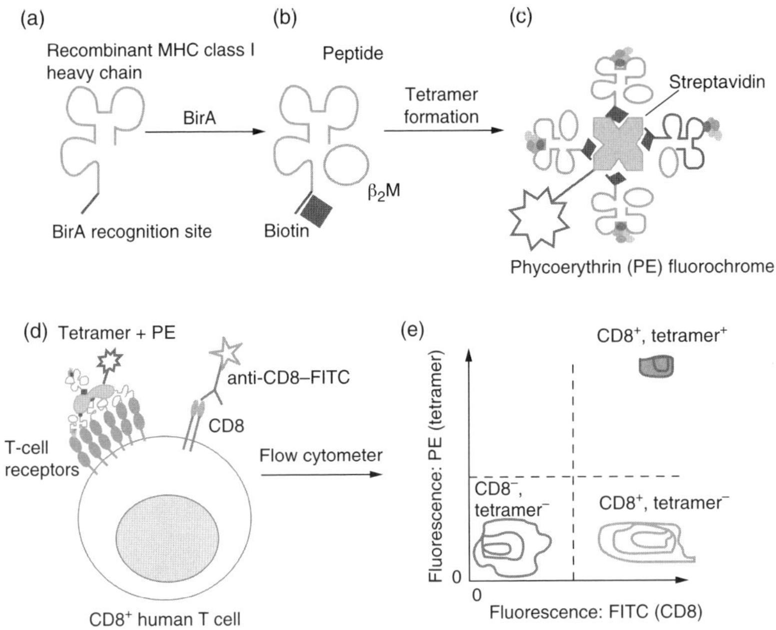

Fig. 4.6 Tetramer analysis to detect T cells that have peptide-specific T cell receptors on their cell surface. (a) Soluble versions of the heavy chain of MHC class I molecules are synthesized in *Escherichia coli* bacteria. (b) The molecules adopt an appropriate conformation following the addition of β2M and a synthetic peptide that represents the epitope that is recognized by the TCR of interest. This peptide binds to the MHC molecule. The enzyme BirA is used to attach a biotin molecule to the specific BirA-recognition sequence, which has been incorporated into the C-terminus of the MHC molecule. (c) Four MHC–biotin complexes are linked to a single streptavidin molecule, using the specific biotin–avidin interaction, to form a tetramer. The streptavidin molecule is 'tagged' with a fluorochrome, e.g. phycoerythrin (PE). (d) Tetramers are mixed with the cell population that is to be analysed (e.g. blood mononuclear cell populations or CD8$^+$ T lymphocytes). Only T cells that have TCRs that are capable of binding to the particular MHC–peptide combination that is present in the tetramer are able to bind the tetramer; thus, such cells will become labelled with the PE fluorochrome (shown in the graph in (e)). A monoclonal antibody (MAB) specific for the T cell marker, and tagged with a different fluorochrome (e.g. fluorescein isothiocyanate (FITC)), can also be used. (e) The cells are then analysed using flow cytometry; the proportion of the CD8$^+$ T cell population that stains positively with the tetramer can be determined (upper, outer quadrant).

levels of infiltration by NK cells. However, where tumours showed a prominent infiltration by NK cells, the prognosis was good (e.g. breast, gastric, and lung cancers). In humans, the paucity of NK cell-selective deficiencies has hampered the characterization of NK cell biological function *in vivo*, in general, and in antitumour immunesurveillance, in particular. However, an 11-year follow-up epidemiological survey has

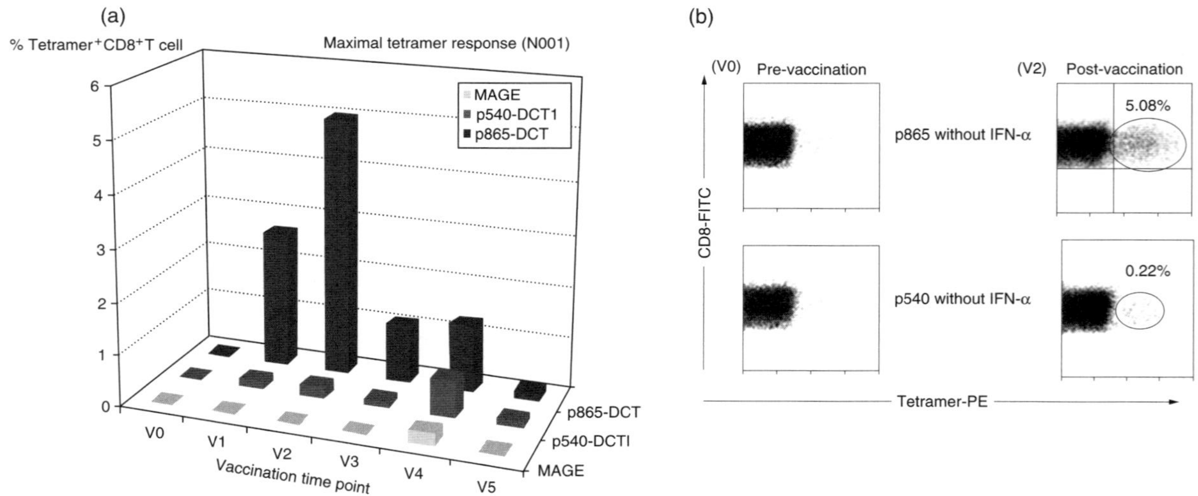

Fig. 4.7 (a) Maximal tetramer response (vaccine DCT vs vaccine DCTI): time course of tetramer response to vaccination in a patient who generated the highest level of tetramer$^+$CD8$^+$T cells after 2 courses (V2), compared with baseline (V0) The two class I peptides used were 9-mer p 540 and p 865 of hTERT (see 4.3.2). (b) Flowcytometry of peak tetramer response: tetramer flowcytometry plots for N001 at V0 and V2, 150 000 events were acquired and analysed.

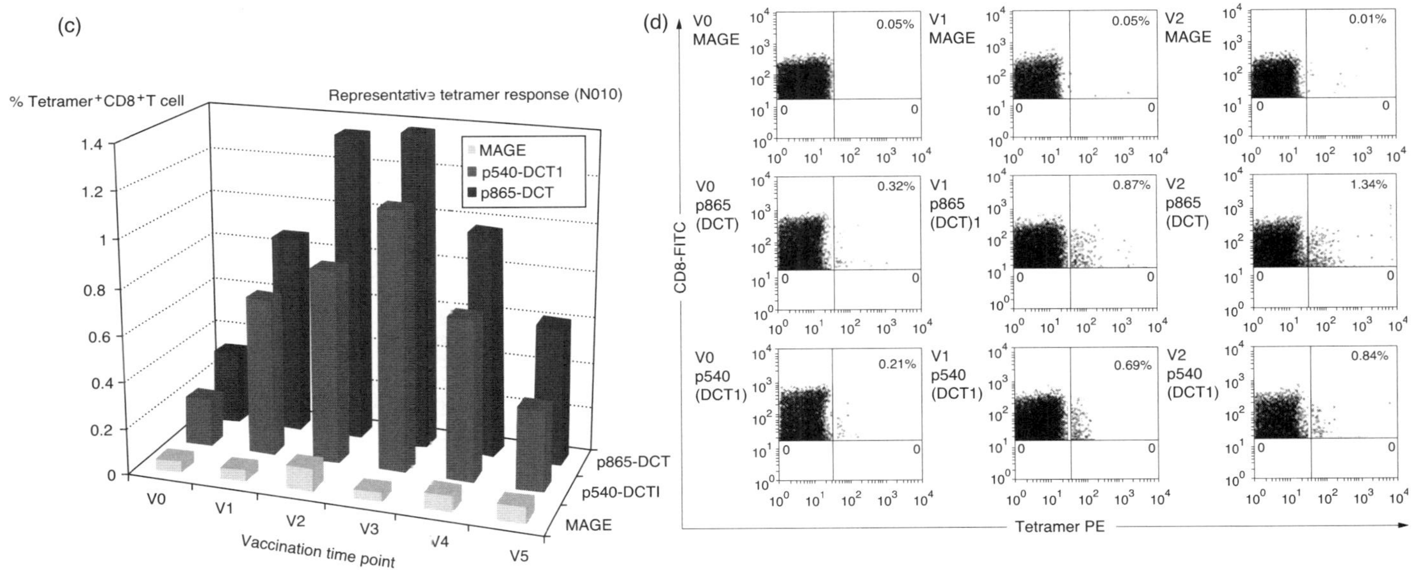

Fig. 4.7 *(continued)* (c) Representative tetramer response (vaccine DCT vs vaccine DCTI): time course of tetramer responses to vaccination in a representative patient who generated equivalent tetramer$^+$CD8$^+$T cell responses to DCT and DCTI. (d) Flow cytometry of representative tetramer response: tetramer flowcytometry plots for the patient at V0, V1, and V2. MAGE-3 was used as the control, non-TAA; 150 000 events were acquired and analysed. DCTI, autologous DCs generated *in vitro* from CD14$^+$monocytes with GM-CSF, IL-4, TNF-α, and IFN-α; DCT, autologous DCs generated *in vitro* from CD14$^+$monocytes with GM-CSF, IL-4, TNF-α [153].

shown that the extent of NK cell activity in peripheral blood is associated with cancer risk in adults; low NK cell activity is associated with an increased cancer risk [154]. Good manufacturing practice (GMP) grade production of NK cells for immunotherapy has been possible [155], and NK cell-mediated therapy after haematopoietic cell transplantation appears safe [156].

NK T cells

NK T cells are a relatively newly recognized member of the immune system, with important biological effects, despite their small numbers (0.2% of blood T and NK cells). They are T cells with a TCR (αβ) but, unlike conventional T cells that detect peptide antigens presented by conventional MHC molecules, NK T cells recognize lipid and glycolipid antigens presented by CD1d, a nonclassical MHC molecule. They are members of both the innate and adaptive immune systems and bridge the gap between the two immune systems. NK T cells respond rapidly by setting the parameters for subsequent immune responses. They share certain features with NK cells ($CD16^+$, $CD56^+$, perforin/granzyme production). They have both effector and regulatory roles in infectious and autoimmune diseases (see Chapter 1).

Subsets of NK T cells can have distinct and sometimes opposing roles. In cancer, type I NK T cells, defined by their invariant TCR using Vα14Jα18 in mice and Vα24Jα18 in humans, are mostly protective, by producing IFN-γ to activate NK and $CD8^+$ T cells and by activating DCs to make IL-12 [157]. In contrast, type II NK T cells, characterized by more diverse TCRs, recognizing lipids presented by CD1d, primarily inhibit tumour immunity [157]. Moreover, type I and type II NK T cells counter-regulate each other, forming a new immunoregulatory axis [157]. Because NK T cells respond rapidly, the balance along this axis can greatly influence other immune responses that follow. Therefore, learning to manipulate the balance along the NK T regulatory axis may be critical to designing successful immunotherapy protocols for cancer.

γδ T cells

Most mature T cells express the αβ TCR heterodimer, a small proportion express an alternative γδ TCR heterodimer [158,159]. Unlike αβ T cells, which recognize specific processed peptide antigens presented on MHC molecules by APCs, γδ T cells appear to directly recognize and respond rapidly to a variety of MHC-like stress-induced self antigens (CD1c) expressed by malignant cells, as well as to inflammatory signals, through activation of PRRs on γδ cells [150,160]. Thus, γδ T cells can recognize malignant cells through less specific mechanisms that require no prior antigen exposure or priming, a function that is shared by other innate immune cells such as macrophages and NK cells [158]. Although γδ T cells make up less than 10% of total peripheral blood T cells, they are present in substantially greater numbers within epithelial tissues [161], contrasting with αβ T cells, most of which either circulate in the peripheral blood or are resident in lymphoid organs. They are the primary source of neutrophil-attracting IL-17 in various models of infection and autoimmunity [160].

Several lines of evidence point to a role for γδ T cells in tumour immunesurveillance. It has recently been shown that mice lacking γδ T cells are highly susceptible to cutaneous carcinogenesis [162]. In clinical studies, γδ T cells have been shown to infiltrate a variety of tumours, including lung cancer [163], renal cell carcinoma [164], seminoma [165], and breast cancer [166]. *In vivo*, $V\gamma 9V\delta 2^+$ T cell amplification revealed disease stabilization/partial tumour regression with multiple myeloma and hormone-resistant disseminated prostate cancer [161].

Cancer and humoral immune mechanisms

Immunoglobulins

More than a century ago, surgeons commented on the apparent prominent lymph nodes found adjacent to a variety of solid cancers. Such alterations in size, shape, and consistency of the tumour-draining lymph nodes was regarded as a beneficial host response. Subsequent alterations in microarchitecture, histiocytosis, prominent follicles, and germinal centres (B lymphocyte compartment) and a variable expansion of the paracortical area (T lymphocyte compartment), were shown to be associated with increased populations of macrophages, B lymphocytes, and T lymphocytes, respectively. However, there is no conclusive evidence that the nodal responses detected were due to released TAAs or necessarily directed against the malignant tumours being drained.

Naturally occurring tumour-antigen-specific antibodies can have antitumour effects by interfering with the function of molecules which are crucial for the survival and proliferation of tumour cells. Almost all the tumour-specific antibodies which have been described are germ-line coded and belong exclusively to the IgM class [167,168]. Furthermore, they are all bound to carbohydrates on post-translationally modified cell surface receptors on malignant cells [167,168]. Much of the early attention on the immune effects of tumour antigen-specific MABs was on their ability to recruit innate mechanisms such as antibody-dependent cellular cytotoxicity (ADCC) (Figure 4.5). The highest titre of antibody is usually documented in the early phase of tumour growth. Interaction of tumour-specific antibody with TAA can lead to membrane redistribution and endocytosis of the immune complex of the tumour cell. This modulation of TAA may inhibit the generation of an effective cell mediated immune response. Also, shedding of antibody–TAA complex can lead to blocking of effector mechanisms. This is not well established in humans, but has been shown in experimental tumour models in animals. However, a growing body of evidence now suggests that antibodies may also have the capacity to recruit tumour-antigen-specific adaptive immunity [169,170].

DCs express Fcγ receptors and are efficient at uptake of opsonized TAAs, such as can be found on lethally damaged antibody-coated tumour cells [170]. Uptake of tumour cells by DCs can lead to the induction of either immunity or tolerance, depending on the context of the cell death, the nature of the phagocytic components, and other signals from the tumour microenvironment [171]. As various types of tumours do not express MHC II proteins, uptake of tumour antigens by APCs is also important for the induction of $CD4^+$ Th responses. Even in some settings when tumours express MHC class II molecules (as in the case of some haematological tumours), defects in MHC class II antigen processing can occur and this correlates with outcome [172]. Several studies with both human and murine DCs have now shown that the uptake of opsonized TAAs by DCs via Fcγ receptors leads to enhancement of cross-presentation and efficient generation of both tumour antigen-specific $CD4^+$ and $CD8^+$ T cell responses, both *in vitro* and *in vivo* [170,173].

Commercially available MABs have emerged as effective therapeutic agents for an increasing number of human malignancies. They have become some of the most important biological agents approved for the treatment of human cancer in the last decade [174] (comprehensively discussed in Chapter 1; see also Chapter 7).

Complement

Several studies of human cancers have established that chronic inflammation can promote the process of carcinogenesis and exacerbate the growth of existing tumours [175]. Conversely, acute inflammation appears to have the opposite effect [175]. Recent data indicate that this dualism in the role of inflammation in cancer is mirrored by the effects of the complement system on this disease process [176]. Current evidence suggests that complement proteins are thought to contribute to the immunesurveillance of malignant tumours. However, complement-based anticancer immunotherapies have not, as yet, been explored in humans.

Cytokines

Distinctive $CD4^+$ T cell subsets (Th1 or Th2) secrete unique repertoires of proinflammatory and anti-inflammatory cytokines. For example, Th1 cells produce IL-2 and IFN-γ and, therefore, directly enhance cell-mediated immune responses. Th2 cells, on the other hand, produce IL-4 and IL-10 and facilitate local humoral responses. In the circulation of patients with bladder and colorectal cancers, the number of Th1 cells, identified by intracellular production of IFN-γ or IL-2, was markedly reduced. The number of Th2 cells producing IL-4, IL-6, and/or IL-10 was significantly elevated, as compared with Th1 and Th2 levels in otherwise healthy populations [177,178]. Moreover, in human cervical carcinomas, $CD3^+$ TILs displayed enhanced Th2 cytokine profiles, with specifically increased IL-4 and reduced IFN-γ production [179].

Consistent with these findings, alterations in immune status (suppressed CMI and enhanced humoral immunity) have also been reported in chronic inflammatory diseases associated with increased incidence of developing cancer. For example, intestinal B cell responses have been observed in ulcerative colitis, a chronic inflammatory condition with a high risk for the development of colorectal cancer [180,181]. Decreased Th1/Th2 ratios in circulating blood lymphocytes have been reported in hepatitis C virus-related liver cirrhosis, a liver disease closely associated with the development of hepatocellular carcinoma. In Barrett's oesophagus, an intermediate step in the progression from reflux oesophagitis to oesophageal adenocarcinoma, infiltration of Th1 effector cells is largely replaced by Th2 effector cells (and associated IgG producing plasma cells and mast cells), when reflux oesophagitis progresses to Barrett's oesophagus [182]. Taken together, these interesting clinical findings indicate that pronounced humoral immunity may underlie the increased risk for neoplastic progression in tissues with chronic inflammatory disorders.

Molecular mechanisms by which cytokines impact on cancer initiation, promotion and progression are complex. Cytokines derived from neoplastic cells, activated resident stromal cells or infiltrating host TILs, TIMs, and MDSCs, can all regulate cancer growth by affecting angiogenesis, cell survival, death, or differentiation. Cellular immunity and Th1-generated cytokines, such as IFN-γ, tend to exhibit antiangiogenic bioactivities [183], whereas Th2-associated cytokines, such as IL-10, stimulate angiogenesis and are therefore protumourigenic [183]. Increased IL-10 expression in patients with gastric cancer correlated with tumour angiogenesis, attenuated CD8^{+} T cell infiltration, and poor prognosis [184]. Although IL-6 has been implicated in both Th1- and Th2-type responses, in several chronic inflammatory diseases and various types of cancers, IL-6 is better known to direct Th2-type responses and play a central role as a differentiation and growth factor of neoplastic epithelial cells [185,186].

IL-13 promotes survival and/or growth of selective tumour clones through direct action on neoplastic cells, in addition to suppressing cellular immunity [187]. IL-23, a cytokine produced by DCs and macrophages following bacterial exposure and TLR engagement, is also found highly expressed in various types of human carcinomas, compared with adjacent normal tissue, indicating a potentially important role in tumour development [44]. In a mouse model of chemical carcinogenesis, absence of IL-23 resulted in a significant reduction in local inflammatory responses in the tumour microenvironment that paralleled an increase in CTL infiltration, resulting in resistance to carcinogenesis [44]. Although, IL-23 is not generally regarded as a Th2 cytokine, it appears to exert Th2-like cytokine bioactivities by promoting inflammatory responses and inhibiting CTL responses. The degree to which IL-23 neutralization will translate to other mouse models of *de novo* carcinogenesis and/or human cancer development is yet to be defined.

Chemokines

Chemokines are part of a network of inflammatory mediators and are a key component in the recruitment of these mediators to the cancer microenvironment. They play a crucial role in recruitment of leucocytes, in particular TAMs, into tumours (primary and metastatic sites) [188]. They are small proteins secreted by neoplastic and associated stromal cells and constitute the largest human cytokine family. The chemokine system is highly promiscuous, in order to provide flexibility and specificity in leucocyte trafficking (see Chapter 1).

CCL2 and CCL5 are the major chemoattractants of TIMS and CXCL of MDSCs into tumours. Their levels correlate with degree of infiltration and tumour aggressiveness. CXCL8 is overexpressed in a range of solid tumours [189]. This is associated with a poor outcome.

NK cells are relatively infrequent in tumours. CX3CL1 is a key chemoattractant and high levels are associated with a better prognosis. CX3CL3 expression in gastric cancer shows a similar pattern of clinical outcome. TILs are recruited by a range of ligands; CXCL9 and CXCL10 are secreted by TAMs and CXCL16 by various tumours [190].

CXCL5 and CXCL8 are strong promoters of angiogenesis by interacting with their corresponding receptors (CXCR1/2) on endothelial cells. CXCL12 acts in concert with VEGF and further supports the establishment of an angiogenic network in tumours [188].

Tumour metastasis

Introduction

In the 1860s, the invasion of veins and lymphatics by tumour cells was documented histologically. Later, tumour cells were isolated from the venous circulation and subsequent post-mortem studies documented the presence of tumour emboli in lungs of patients who died from malignant disease. Numerous studies have detected the presence of significant numbers of tumour cells in the venous effluent from a variety of solid cancers, the numbers being enhanced substantially during anaesthesia and surgical procedures.

A century ago, Paget postulated the importance of the microenvironment in inducing the growth of entrapped tumour emboli, on the basis of his studies of the pattern of metastatic spread in patients with breast cancer. On the other hand, in the early part of the 20th century, Ewing stressed the importance of the vascular architecture and the haemodynamics of the circulation. Both pathophysiological mechanisms are believed to be important in determining the organ distribution and growth of metastatic deposits [191]. Host defence mechanisms are thought to play a crucial role at three anatomical sites: (1) The site of primary tumour cell growth and local haemolymphatic invasion; (2) the haemolymphatic compartments (vascular and lymphatic), including the 'filter' role of lymph nodes; (3) the *in situ* macrophages and leucocytes within individual organs of tumour cell arrest, e.g. liver, lungs, bone marrow.

Rapid cell proliferation is believed to be linked to alterations in the genome, with resultant enhanced and/or inappropriate expression of various proto-oncogenes and their secreted products, increased production of growth factors, and augmentation of their membrane receptors, resulting in increased mitogenicity and autocrine-driven cell growth, and cell replication. These metabolic abnormalities, as well as structural and functional changes in the cell membrane (e.g. overexpression of adhesion molecules and chemokine receptors), lead to enhanced tumour cell aggressiveness, loss of contact inhibition, and local invasion. The latter is associated with an increased attachment of the malignant cell to the basement membrane through laminin and other receptors and the increased release of various proteolytic enzymes (e.g. proteases, MMPs), causing breakdown of subepithelial collagen and disruption of surrounding ground substance. The acquisition of a tumour vasculature, induced by angiogenesis factors (e.g. VEGF), secreted by the malignant cells and associated macrophages, is crucial to the delivery of oxygen and essential nutrients to the rapidly expanding mass of neoplastic cells. Also, it is an important route for the eventual entry by invading tumour cells and their subsequent dissemination.

Another important route of tumour cell dissemination is via the regional tumour-draining lymphatic channels and lymph nodes. The tumour-draining lymph nodes, in particular those adjacent to the solid growth, undergo macro- and microarchitectural alterations suggestive of altered immune responses to filtered tumour cells and/or cellular products. Although in some animal models lymph nodes have been shown to inhibit tumour cell dissemination, in others their ability to function as a 'mechanical filter' has been shown to be inefficient. Transmigration of lymph nodes, even by large tumour cells, is well documented; the tumour cells eventually reach the venous system via the thoracic duct. Also, venous–lymphatic communications have been demonstrated within lymph nodes of some species and are thought to represent a further possible site of entry of malignant cells into the vascular compartment.

The presence of metastatic deposits within regional lymph nodes is a poor prognostic feature and is a biological indicator of more distal dissemination. Surgical removal of such involved nodes reduces the risk of local recurrence but probably does not influence overall survival. Conversely, removal of uninvolved lymph nodes (even where they have undergone hyperplastic changes) does not appear to compromise patient survival.

Probably less than 1% of the tumour cells that enter the venous circulation survive transport to distant organs. The mechanical stresses imposed on the tumour emboli by the blood flow are mainly responsible for this high death rate. Coating of tumour aggregates with fibrin and platelets probably provides protection from the stresses of blood flow, as well as from host defence mechanisms. Although the evidence in humans is inconclusive, substantial data have accumulated from a variety of animal studies that NK cells play a crucial role in preventing the establishment of tumour metastases. The latter studies suggest that NK cells are most effective in dealing with circulating tumour cells, especially in the early phase of tumour dissemination. Once metastatic disease is established, NK cells appear to be less efficacious as antitumour agents (see 'NK cells', above).

As mentioned previously, the 'soil' probably plays a crucial role in the establishment and progressive growth of tumour emboli. Paradoxically, many of the common sites of tumour metastatic growth—lungs, liver, lymph nodes, skeletal system—are rich in host defence cells. Induction of suppressor mechanisms by tumour cell products (e.g. PGE2) and enhancement of tumour cell growth by molecules released by tissue macrophages have been invoked to offer an explanation. These are discussed in more detail below.

TAMs, migration, and invasion

Tumour models, using intravital imaging and *in vivo* breast xenograft assays, have shown the crucial role played by TAMs in tumour cell migration and invasion. Tumour cells secrete CSF-1, which stimulates TAMs to produce epidermal growth factor which then activates tumour cell migration, the TAMs and tumour cells closely intertwined. Inhibition of either signal aborts the invasive process. Macrophage polarization to the invasive-promoting phenotype is up-regulated by $CD4^+$ Th secreted IL-4 [76]. TAMs on adjacent vessels encourage tumour cells to migrate down collagen fibrils towards the vessels where the tumour cells intravasate [192].

For effective tumour cell spread, degradation of components of the basement membrane and ECM needs to occur through the release of proteolytic enzymes (proteases, cathepsins, MMPs) by the TAMs. The presence of the latter has been correlated with metastatic potential in a variety of solid tumours, in particular with production of MMP9 [83]. Hypoxia is an effective signal in TAMs that up-regulates a number of genes encoding proteins that promote proliferation, invasion, and metastasis of tumour cells. TAMs accumulate in large numbers in hypoxic and/or necrotic areas in a range of solid cancers. Hypoxia inhibits expression of TAM CCR2, and CCR5, entrapping the cells and immobilizing the TAMs [193].

Angiogenesis

Tumour growths are restricted to a definitive size (2–3 mm^3) and are unable to metastasize unless they are associated with an appropriate tumour vasculature [194]. Hypoxic stress in the tumour mass promotes the recruitment of TIMs and their conversion to a M2 phenotype. There is a resultant secretion of various growth factors and cytokines (e.g. FGF, PDGF, VEGF, GM-CSF, IL-1 and IL-6, TGF-β) inhibiting anti-cancer immune responses, inducing tumour cell migration and the establishment of new blood vessels. TAM-derived proteases are essential for extracellular breakdown of ECM and release of various proangiogenic molecules bound to heparin sulphate and fragments of fibrin and collagen, which facilitate angiogenesis [83]. Studies in which TAMs are reduced in mammary tumours in mice show that it prevents the induction of the angiogenic switch [195]. Macrophages produce VEGF in both human and mouse tumours [195]. They also make it available through the production of MMPs which release VEGF from ECM depots.

Normal pericytes are embedded within the basement membrane of capillaries, as solitary or single cell layers, and coordinate intercellular signalling with endothelial cells and prevent leakage. They are postulated to be involved in tumour angiogenesis and metastasis formation [196]. In the initial stage of angiogenesis there is endothelial cell pericyte dissociation, followed by endothelial cell invasion and proliferation, subsequent tubulogenesis and vessel maturation [196]. Pericyte signalling is important for the growth phase of angiogenesis. VEGF and PDGF are important mediators of endothelial cell–pericyte ineractions. Under hypoxic conditions VEGF is secreted by pericytes. Following initial destabilization and new vessel growth, pericytes induce stability and maturation of the newly created vasculature [197]. In tumours, pericytes control the intravasation of tumour cells. However, this function is defective, resulting in immature and leaky vessels and raised interstitial pressure. All of this promotes entry of tumour cells into the vascular tree and formation of metastasis [196].

Metastatic tumour bed

In humans, intravasation, circulation and extravasation at a potential tumour metastatic site is a complex biopathological process. The fate of the many thousands of circulating cells is intravascular disruption and death, with very few embedding successfully and proliferating. Macrophages (and other leucocytes) are believed to play a crucial role in preparing distant premetastatic niches [198]. Tumour cells secrete myeloid cell chemoattractants. The resultant migratory cells secrete MMPs, release ECM-bound VEGF, and initiate angiogenesis. The niche provides a site for tumour cells to adhere and proliferate, supported by the associated myeloid-mononuclear cells which rapidly differentiate into macrophages (Figure 4.8) [76].

CXCR4 is the most frequently overexpressed chemokine receptor on a range of tumour cells. It is also expressed on vascular endothelial cells. CXCL12 induces

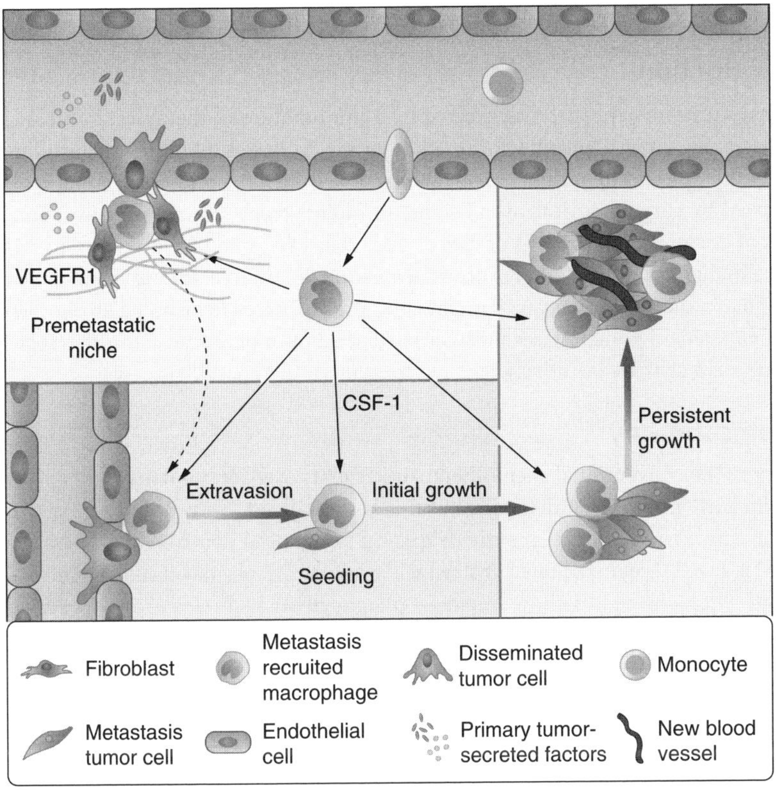

Fig. 4.8 Macrophages promote seeding and growth of metastatic cells; myeloid cells, most likely macrophages, are recruited to the premetastatic niche in response to secreted products from the primary tumour. The metastatic target organs contain fibroblasts and elaborate extracellular matrix consisting of fibronectin and collagen. These niches direct and enhance tumour cell seeding in sites distant from the primary tumour. Once the tumour cells arrive at the metastatic site and begin to extravasate, they recruit macrophages that are differentiated from blood borne monocytes. These macrophages enhance the ability of tumour cells to extravasate and promote their subsequent survival and growth. They continue to accumulate in metastatic lesions, where they stimulate the growth and survival of the metastatic cells. Several growth factors and signaling pathways are important for these macrophage functions, including vascular endothelial growth factor (VEGF) in the premetastatic site and colony stimulating factor-1 (CSF-1). Reproduced from Qian B-Z, Pollard JW, Macrophage diversity enhances tumour progression and metastasis. Cell 2010; 141: 39–51, with permission from Elsevier.

endothelial cell proliferation and migration to sites of metastatic disease by recruiting circulating or bone marrow endothelial cell precursors. Overexpression of CXCR4 is associated with metastatic tumour cell migration to the bone marrow or premetastatic niches, attracted by CXCL12 produced by *in situ* macrophages at those sites.

Nonsurgical treatment and host defences

Introduction

Primary tumours are currently treated by a combination of therapies. In most cases this involves surgery, possibly local radiotherapy, followed subsequently by adjuvant chemotherapy and/or antihormonal therapy. Even when the primary tumour has been removed by surgery or destroyed by chemo/radiotherapy, any residual micrometastases of dormant tumour cells or cancer stem cells may, in due course, lead to relapse of the malignant disease and result in therapeutic failure to eradicate the malignancy. Design of a successful anticancer therapeutic strategy needs to be based on eliminating disseminated micrometastases and associated progenitor or cancer stem cells. However, cancer stem cells are intuitively resistant to modern therapeutic strategies.

Chemotherapy

Many of the conventional chemotherapeutic agents used, at standard and high doses, significantly inhibit host defences, but this is short-lived. Neutrophils, in particular, are sensitive to chemotherapeutic drugs and substantial neutropenia (albeit short-lived) is a well recognized side effect, which in some patients may result in neutropenic sepsis. The neutrophils show impaired phagocytosis and release of lytic enzymes. Inhibitors of DNA synthesis reduce migration of monocytes to sites of inflammation. Inhibition of humoral immunity has been documented with adriamycin, cyclophosphamide, *cis*-platinum, and vinblastine, particularly if both the drug and immunizing antigen have been given concurrently. Natural cytotoxicity (NK cells) and ADCC (K cells) are also inhibited, albeit temporarily, by cyclophosphamide, adriamycin, vincristine, methotrexate, and mitomycin [199]. However, some of these agents (e.g. cyclophosphamide), when used at low and metronomic doses, have an immunomodulatory function. Cyclophosphamide, prescribed at low metronomic doses, is known to suppress Treg ($CD4^+CD25^+$ $Foxp3^+$) numbers and function [200–202]. Such metronomic therapy, in combination with cancer vaccination, is likely to be effective, especially in light of the findings that patients with low levels (<0.5%) of circulating Tregs are more likely to show a favourable response to immunotherapy [153].

A number of studies in humans and animals have documented augmentation of immune responses with chemotherapy. Humoral immunity is enhanced with melphalan, *cis*-platinum, and cyclophosphamide through reduction in Tregs and enhanced antigenicity of TAAs. Enhanced macrophage phagocytosis and cytotoxicity has been documented with *cis*-platinum, cyclophosphamide, and adriamycin. Also, some drugs have been shown to augment NK cell activity and K cell-mediated ADCC (5-FU and methotrexate). Immune-modulating effects of conventional chemotherapeutic agents used in cancer are discussed in more detail in Chapter 7.

Radiotherapy

Radiotherapy has a deleterious effect on bone marrow-derived stem cells and causes lymphopenia [203]. Both T and B lymphocytes are very radiosensitive, but the fall in T lymphocyte count is more prolonged; there is a differential susceptibility amongst the T cell subsets. Mature T cells are more resistant than circulating naive T cells.

$CD4^+$ Th and Tregs are said to be particularly radiosensitive. The critical factor inducing lymphopenia is the volume of blood irradiated. NK cells are also sensitive to radiotherapy, but their recovery is usually relatively rapid (several months). However, radiotherapy is known to increase antigen uptake by DCs and T cells homing into irradiated tumours, and reduces circulating Tregs [203,204]. Therefore, it appears that radiotherapy exerts its beneficial effects by immunomodulation, in addition to direct killing of malignant cells by radiation damage. More detailed studies on the immunomodulating effects of radiotherapy are required before it can be considered a synergistic adjuvant to anticancer vaccination (see Chapter 7).

Biological agents

Surgery, radiotherapy, and chemotherapy are the conventional treatment modalities for cancer. The long-term outcome achieved with these approaches has been limited in a number of solid cancers because of several factors such as micrometastases at time of presentation, chemoresistance to drugs, nonspecificity of drug action leading to tissue damage and toxicity, and unresectable malignant disease. To combat these problems, the concept of targeted therapy using immunotoxins was developed. Immunotoxins are chimeric proteins with a specifically cell-reactive ligand chemically linked or genetically fused to a toxin moiety. Ligands used are MABs or single-chain variable fragments directed against specific receptors or antigens; if these are fused with bacterial or plant toxins they are referred to as *immunotoxins*. Pseudomonas exotoxin, anthrax toxin, and diphtheria toxin are the commonly used bacterial toxins. An in-depth discussion of these therapies is outside the remit of this textbook and they have been reviewed elsewhere [205].

MABs targeted against tumour cell growth factors/receptors, receptors on tumour-associated blood vessels, immune inhibitory cytokines, and suppressor Tregs, as well as small-molecule inhibitors directed against various tyrosine kinases, are being used in clinical practice to suppress tumour cell growth and up-regulate antitumour defences (see Chapters 1 and 7 for a more detailed discussion).

Immunotherapy in malignant disease

Introduction

Cancer immunotherapy can be active or passive, based on the involvement of particular components of the host's immune system. Passive immunotherapy consists of administration of specific antitumour antibodies or activated $CD8^+$ CTLs targeted against cancer cells. In contrast, active immunotherapy involves empowering the host's immune system to orchestrate an efficient and comprehensive immune response (innate and adaptive) against cancer cells expressing TAAs.

Passive immunotherapy

Adoptive cellular transfer

Adoptive cellular transfer involves the identification and expansion *ex vivo* of autologous $CD8^+$ T lymphocytes (e.g. TILs) with antitumour activity, which are then infused

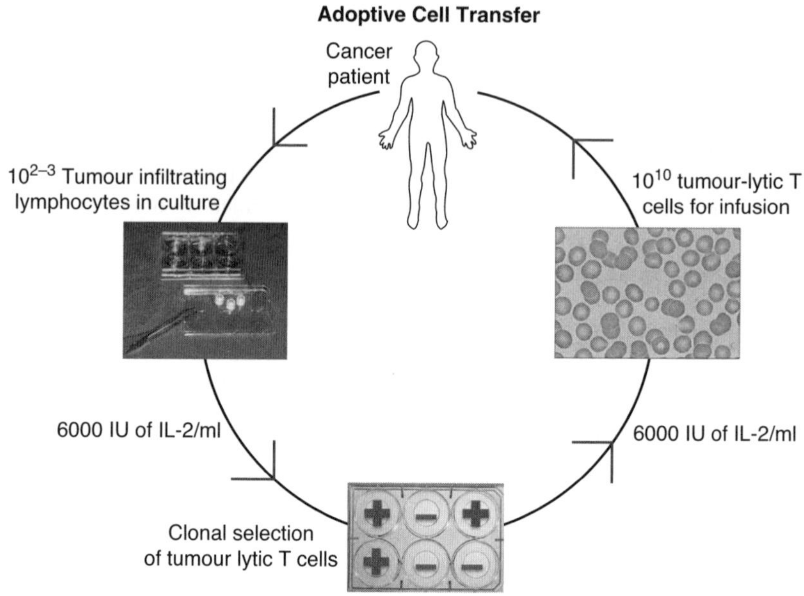

Fig. 4.9 An illustration of adoptive cell therapy using clonal expansion of tumour-lytic autologous TILs.

into cancer patients, often with appropriate growth factors (e.g. IL-2) to stimulate their survival and further expansion *in vivo* [206]. A small number of antitumour cells with the appropriate properties can be expanded substantively *ex vivo* by treatment with recombinant (r) IL-2 in a GMP grade laboratory. *In vitro* tests can identify the different populations generated and effector functions required for cancer regression, characterized and selected for expansion. This approach, illustrated in Figure 4.9, has proved to be highly effective for the treatment of experimental tumours in animals and in some patients with malignant melanoma and renal cell carcinoma [207].

Monoclonal antibodies

Passive vaccination with r-derived MABs has emerged as effective therapy for an increasing number of human malignancies. These MABs are frequently used as adjuvants in the treatment of early stage disease in combination with chemotherapy. MABs have become one of the commonest forms of new agents approved for the treatment of human cancer in the last two decades. Examples of some MABs available for therapeutic use in cancer are outlined in Table 4.5 (see Chapters 1 and 7 for a detailed discussion).

Active immunotherapy

Introduction

There are several methods that can be used to induce an active antitumour immune response. The mechanisms underlying the antitumour immune response are schematically outlined in Figure 4.5, and are comparable across a wide range of approaches.

Table 4.5 Examples of monoclonal antibodies approved for therapeutic use

Monoclonal antibody	Subtype	Cancer target	Cancer	Reference
Trastuzumab	IgG1	HER2/Neu	Breast	[208,209]
Rituximab	IgG1	CD20	Lymphoma	[210,211]
Cetuximab	IgG1	EGFR	Colorectal	[212]
Bevacizumab	IgG1	VEGFR	Lung, breast, colorectal	[213]
Alemtuzumab	IgG1	CD52	Chronic lymphocytic leukaemia	[214]

The TAA epitopes are small peptides (8–12 amino acids) and can be loaded on to APCs, for efficient presentation to TCRs on $CD8^+$ T lymphocytes. Antigens can be incorporated into autologous DC-based vaccines as small peptides, as well as proteins, mRNA, DNA, whole tumour cells, or tumour lysates (Table 4.6). These larger molecules are taken up by the DCs, processed, and the appropriate peptide re-expressed with MHC class I and II proteins. They can also be administered without *ex vivo* autologous DCs, relying on antigen uptake by DCs at the site of injection (e.g. Langerhans cells in the skin and dermal DCs) and subsequent presentation to naive T lymphocytes in the paracortical areas of regional lymph nodes. However, this approach may be inefficient as it is well established that DCs in cancer patients are 'switched off' and require to be 'switched on' *ex vivo* before they can be used in immunotherapy [51,215]. We have established a novel technique to switch on these DCs *ex vivo*, in order to render them effective in immunotherapy [216].

Vaccine adjuvants

Vaccination with TAAgs alone is insufficient to elicit a potent immune response. Adjuvants are frequently used to enhance the response. Adjuvants act through a wide

Table 4.6 TAA approaches, specificity and the risk of autoimmunity with various cancer vaccine preparations

TAA	Vaccine preparation	Tumour specificity	Risk of autoimmunity
Peptide	Immunodominant epitope administered directly or pulsed on DCs	++++	+
Proteins	Tumour-derived HSP or TAA fused to immunostimulatory molecules, by itself or pulsed on DCs	+++	++
mRNA	Virally or nonvirally transfected into DCs	+++	+
DNA	Virally or nonvirally transfected into DCs	+++	+
Tumour cell	Fusion with DCs by electroporation	++	+++
Tumour lysates	Irradiated DCs pulsed with tumour lysates	+	++++

range of mechanisms; from a depot action causing slow release of antigen to local inflammation causing enhanced recruitment of DCs to the injection site and then subsequent activation by stimulation of PRRs by released 'danger' signals [217,218]. Other adjuvants enable antigens to be directly delivered to the cytosol, facilitating cross-priming and mimicking a 'danger' signal [217,218]. An ideal cancer vaccine adjuvant should direct the immune response towards a Th1 response [217]. Stimulating combinations of appropriate innate receptors such as TLRs may achieve this effect [219]. GM-CSF has been shown to enhance cell-mediated and humoral immunity by several mechanisms and also facilitate cross-presentation [220,221]. Biodegradable microspheres, virus-like particles, HSPs, and various lipid-based chemical adjuvants (liposomes, QS21, and Montanide) promote cross-presentation of the antigen (see Chapter 1).

Peptide vaccines

One of the major challenges of tumour immunology is the identification of strongly immunogenic TAA peptides for vaccination. The characterization of the molecular structure of MHC and the anchor-residue sequence of the binding peptides has greatly increased the understanding of peptide avidity to MHC on DCs and TCR interactions with the MHC molecules (see Chapter 1). This has led to the identification of a vast repertoire of immunogenic peptide epitopes for any given tumour antigen by 'reverse immunology,' an evolving science amalgamating genomics and bioinformatics. This helps to predict and identify immunogenic peptide epitopes from the sequence of a gene product of interest and has been postulated to be a particularly efficient, high-throughput approach for tumour antigen documentation [222].

Advantages of using a peptide as a TAA is that immunogenicity can be enhanced by modification of the amino acid sequence; this is called *peptide enhancement*. Peptide vaccines are tumour specific and unlikely to trigger autoimmune damage of normal tissue. They have the ability to cause *epitope spreading*, whereby killed target cells release new antigenic epitopes that are taken up, processed, and presented to a new repertoire of naive CD8$^+$ T cells to generate further CTLs for further cancer cell lysis [223,224]. Moreover, they are relatively easy to synthesize and remain stable (lyophilysed) in storage for prolonged periods. However, there are limitations in using peptides for vaccination. First, individual peptides will be beneficial only in patients with the appropriate HLA haplotype capable of presenting that peptide. Secondly, unlike microbial pathogens, peptides by themselves cannot trigger a 'danger' signal. They require an adjuvant to enhance efficacy. The purpose of the adjuvant is to bring about DC activation in a manner analogous to microbial triggering of DCs through PRRs. Adjuvants such as GM-CSF, CD40L, IL-12, IL-15, Montanide, and Freund's adjuvant have been used for this purpose. Although most tumour peptides are highly specific for binding to MHC molecules on DCs and initiating a peptide-specific T cell response, peptides of HSPs are known to bind to DCs through TLRs, thus, triggering the innate immunity pathways (see Chapter 1).

Protein vaccines

Protein vaccines consist of a range of proteins that are expressed exclusively or predominantly by cancer cells. If expressed by normal cells, these proteins differ in the aminoacid sequence, structure or frequency of expression. They include mutated oncoproteins (K-ras, p53), aberrant glycoproteins like the MUC (mucin) family of proteins; CEA, which is overexpressed by many gastrointestinal tumours; AFP, which is overexpressed by most hepatocellular carcinomas and some germ cell tumours; PSA (prostate specific antigen), which is overexpressed by prostate cancers; melanocyte differentiation antigens such as MART-1, gp 100, and tyrosinase, HER2/neu, which is overexpressed in some breast and gastric cancers; cancer testis antigens such as MAGE-3, and VEGFR; and self-antigens that are overexpressed by the vast majority of cancers, such as hTERT and survivin.

Protein-based vaccines are more antigenic than peptide vaccines, but they have a lower specificity compared with a vaccine that is based on a peptide epitope of the same protein. Consequently, the risk of developing autoimmune tissue damage is higher.

Recombinant live viral vectors for gene transfer

Genetically recombinant viruses (adenovirus, vaccinia, and avipox) can be used to deliver tumour antigens such as CEA or PSA with immunostimulatory molecules and cytokines into tumour cells and DCs [225–228]. However, their development is still very rudimentary as a result of several limitations. Multiple vaccinations with recombinant viruses induce antiviral neutralizing antibodies. Prior systemic immunity can cause resistance, which can be overcome by mucosal immunization. Mucosal vaccination has been found to induce both mucosal and systemic immunity, but systemic vaccination may not induce mucosal immunity [229]. Viral vector antigens may be preferentially antigenic, compared with the TAAs they are designed to express. Moreover, there is no absolute guarantee of the safety of using recombinant 'live viruses'. There is a theoretical risk of viral mutation and resultant pathogenicity.

DNA and RNA plasmid vaccines

DNA and RNA plasmid sequences, respectively transcribing and translating TAAs, can be introduced into DCs. This is a novel therapeutic concept that has arisen from evidence that naked DNA plasmids, when injected *in vivo,* could generate immune responses [230,231]. These plasmids incorporate TAA genes into DC DNA, to enable the TAA to be expressed through both MHC class I and II pathways (cross-presentation), which may not be achievable through other vaccination approaches. Another advantage of this approach is the elimination of risks associated with a live viral vaccine. Moreover, the nucleic acids in their own right act as 'danger' signals to activate PRRs. However, designing a DNA or RNA plasmid requires elaborate knowledge of the TAA gene sequence, which can be time consuming and technically demanding. Large doses of DNA and RNA plasmids are required for a significant immunological response.

Tumour cell vaccines

Tumour cells, either irradiated or prepared as lysate, possess the broadest range of tumour antigenicity, as they comprise the whole repertoire of TAAs expressed by the tumour. They also stimulate the release of proinflammatory cytokines and 'danger' signals that activate PRRs. Their immunogenicity can be enhanced further by

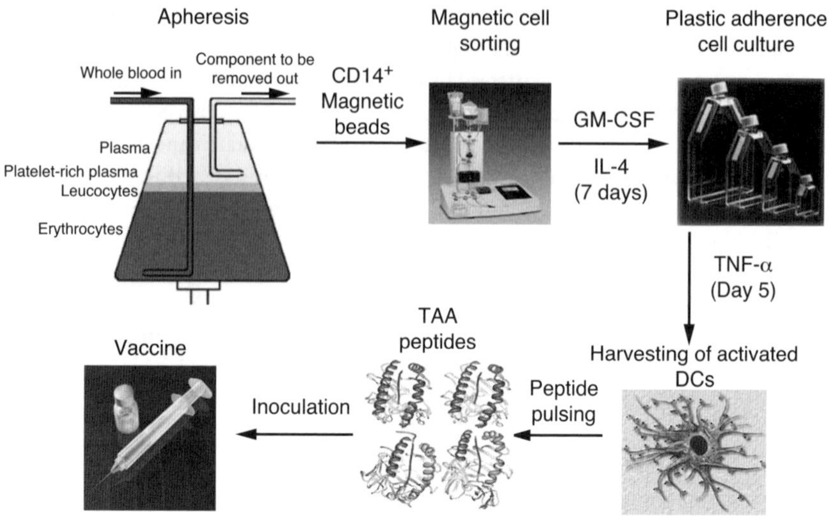

Fig. 4.10 An illustrative *ex vivo* dendritic cell vaccine generation protocol using autologous CD14$^+$ mononuclear cells in a GMP facility. Reproduced from Qian B-Z and Pollard JW (2010). Macrophage Diversity Enhances Tumor Progression and Metastasis. *Cell* **141**(1): 39–51, with permission from Elsevier.

adjuvants such as BCG or KLH. Vaccine preparations require autologous tumour cells. This approach is technically easier, as TAAs need not be defined. However, the broad antigenicity of this approach results in low specificity and a potential for triggering autoimmune responses, as some of the TAAs may be shared with nonmalignant cells.

DC-based vaccines

DCs are the most effective APCs capable of activating naive T cells. They constantly sample the tissue microenvironment for mutagenic antigens and transformed or premalignant cells. They capture, process, and present these antigens to naive T cells in secondary lymphoid compartments and prime these T cells to eliminate the antigen-bearing cancer cells. It is well established that DCs are immature and dysfunctional in patients with cancer [232]. Thus, the design of any DC-based vaccine should endeavour to reactivate and mature autologous DCs *ex-vivo* before they can be used for immunotherapy. The technique outlined in Figure 4.10 involves the harvesting of blood mononuclear cells by leucopheresis, followed by selective isolation of CD14$^+$ cells (DC precursors) and subsequent culture with different cytokines. All the vaccination approaches discussed above can be modified and be incorporated into a DC-based vaccine. There are a variety of ways to harness autologous DCs for use in immunotherapy: DCs can be pulsed with tumour lysates, tumour protein extracts, or synthetic epitopes of TAAs, or fused with irradiated tumour cells by electroporation. It is also feasible to incorporate DNA and RNA into DCs by recombinant viruses, inactive plasmids or by simple electroporation. The incorporation of DNA and RNA into DCs by these methods facilitates incorporation of costimulatory molecules and cytokines into DCs to enhance vaccine efficacy.

There are several limitations of using DC-based vaccines, such as the statutory requirement to culture and process the cells in a GMP-grade sterile environment; this can be labour intensive, time consuming, and expensive. As yet, there seems to be a lack of consensus on the optimal technique for producing activated and partially mature DCs. Also, there is no consensus on how best to load TAAs on to DCs. Using inadequately reactivated and immature DCs in a vaccine could lead to the induction of tolerance to the vaccinating tumour antigen(s). An illustrative *ex vivo* DC generation protocol in a GMP facility is depicted in Figure 4.10.

Evidence is emerging that activation and pulsing of *in situ* DCs (e.g. Langerhans cells in the skin and dermal DCs) is an effective method for vaccination with small GMP-grade peptides, provided there is concomitant injection of suitable adjuvants to deliver the necessary 'danger' signals, activation of PRRs (TLRs on DCs), thereby, ensuring the full range of signals (1–3) for optimal DC peptide uptake, activation, and generation of tumour-specific CTLs in secondary lymphoid compartments (see Chapter 1).

Cancer cachexia

What is cachexia?

Cachexia is a clinical state induced by a multifactorial process and characterized by progressive loss of body weight; it is often, but not always, accompanied by anorexia. It is a summation of various effects of the malignant disease on the host, which are not a direct result of mechanical interference with nutritional intake. Cancer therapies, including surgery, chemotherapy, and radiotherapy, can cause morbidity, with reduced food intake and further weight loss. The mechanisms responsible for the latter are different from that responsible for cancer cachexia. Depending on the tumour type, weight loss occurs in 30–80% of cancer patients and is severe (with loss of >10% of the initial body weight) in 15% of patients [233]. Patients with pancreatic or gastric cancer have the highest frequency of weight loss, while patients with non-Hodgkin's lymphoma, breast cancer, acute nonlymphocytic leukaemia, and sarcomas have the lowest frequency and extent of weight loss [233].

Role of cytokines

Many cytokines have an effect on appetite, including IL-1, IL-6, and TNF-α [234]. The cytokines are transported across the blood–brain barrier where they interact with the luminal surface of brain endothelial cells to release substances that affect appetite [235]. Receptors for TNF-α and IL-1 are found in the hypothalamic areas of the brain, which regulate food intake. Evidence for a role of IL-6 in the development of cancer cachexia has come mainly from studies using the murine colon-26 adenocarcinoma, where increasing levels of IL-6 correlated with the development of cachexia, and treatment with a neutralizing antibody to IL-6, but not TNF-α or IFN-α, attenuated the development of weight loss and other key parameters of cachexia [236]. IL-6 levels increase in blood gradually during the early stages of cachexia and then show a sudden and steep rise just before death [237].

A TGF-β superfamily member, macrophage inhibitory factor-1 (MIF-1), has recently been implicated in the process of anorexia and weight loss in cancer patients [238]. In patients with advanced prostatic cancer there was a direct correlation between serum levels of MIF-1 and weight loss, while in mice transplanted with prostate tumour xenografts there was a marked weight loss that was mediated through a decreased food intake [238].

Role of hormones (leptin)

Cancer anorexia may be a result of an imbalance between orexigenic signals, such as neuropeptide Y, and anorexigenic signals, such as proopiomelanocortin (POMC) [239]. Hypothalamic melanocortin, alpha-melanocyte stimulating hormone, (a product of POMC), is strongly implicated in the control of normal food intake and induces anorexia by activating melanocortin receptors in the hypothalamus [240]. Leptin plays a contributing role in the control of body fat stores by inhibiting food intake and increasing energy expenditure through a feedback loop involving the hypothalamus. Serum leptin concentration depends on the total amount of body fat. As fat levels decrease in cachexia, leptin levels fall correspondingly and are inversely related to the intensity of the inflammatory response [241].

Potential therapies

Agents affecting appetite

The most widely employed appetite stimulant is megestrol acetate (Megace), a synthetic progestin, which probably stimulates appetite via neuropeptide or by down-regulating the synthesis and release of proinflammatory cytokines. Ghrelin, a neuropeptide released from the stomach in response to fasting, stimulates food intake and is another appetite-enhancing agent, although results of efficacy are awaited from ongoing clinical trials.

Agents affecting cachectic mediators or signalling pathways

The primary effect of eicosapentanoic acid (EPA) may be to attenuate muscle atrophy by blocking signalling pathways leading to muscle catabolism. It has also been shown to be an appetite stimulant, although slightly inferior to megestrol acetate [242].

Thalidomide has been evaluated as a treatment for cachexia because of its ability to reduce production of TNF-α, by increasing the degradation rate of TNF-α mRNA. A small study in 10 patients with nonobstructing and inoperable oesophageal cancer, in which the patients received an isocaloric diet for 2 weeks followed by 2 weeks of thalidomide, showed that the patients lost both body weight and lean body mass while on the diet alone, but they gained both weight and lean body mass when receiving thalidomide [243].

Most patients with gastrointestinal cancer have an acute-phase response, which has been suggested to contribute to weight loss; therefore, if this is down-regulated, weight loss should also be attenuated. Thus, administration of nonsteroidal anti-inflammatory agents like ibuprofen to patients with nonresectable pancreatic cancer can reduce resting energy expenditure and retard weight loss due to acute inflammation [244].

Psychoneuroimmunological aspects of cancer

Psychosocial and psychiatric morbidity

In the last 30 years, it has been widely reported that the diagnosis and treatment of cancer are associated with high levels of psychosocial and psychiatric morbidity. Not only the illness itself, but treatments such as surgery, chemotherapy, hormone therapy, radiotherapy, and the biological response modifiers, can all cause wide-ranging problems, including anxiety, depression, sexual dysfunction, body image problems, fatigue, nausea, vomiting, pain and the Damocles syndrome (i.e. an inability to get on with life here and now because of a preoccupation with what may happen in the future) [245].

In the late 1970s, a random sample of 215 new admissions to three cancer centres in North America found a point prevalence of 47% for psychiatric morbidity, assessed using standardized criteria. In a study of almost 5 000 patients assessed between 1987 and 1993, Zabora *et al.* reported an overall point-prevalence of psychiatric morbidity of 35% [246]. Of the more common cancers, patients with lung cancer had the highest point-prevalence (43%) followed by cancers of the breast (33%), colon (32%), and prostate (31%). A more recent study of 269 women with early breast cancer reported that 50% were clinically anxious and 37% were clinically depressed (as assessed using a structured clinical interview) in the first 3 months after the diagnosis [247].

Although there is evidence that much psychiatric morbidity is preventable [245,248], it is clear that, despite considerable investment in information and support services, the diagnosis and treatment of cancer continue to be very stressful for many patients, and the incidence of psychiatric morbidity generally remains high. This is of importance not only on compassionate grounds, but because certain types of stress are known to affect the immune system. This inhibition of innate and adaptive immunity could have significant and detrimental consequences on anticancer immune responses.

Effects of stress on the immune system

It is well known that the central and peripheral nervous systems (CNS and PNS) can affect host defences via a number of pathways, including the hypothalamic–pituitary–adrenocortical (HPA) axis, the sympathetic–adrenal–medullary (SAM) axis, and direct innervation of lymphoid tissue [249,250] (see Chapter 1). It is not surprising, therefore, that psychosocial factors have been shown to be capable of influencing the immune system [251]. Exposure to enduring and severely stressful life events, such as the diagnosis and treatment of cancer, have predictable and measurable effects on the immune system. Generally, decreases in functional immune parameters, such as proliferative responses *in vitro* to mitogens and NK cell activity, have been observed, as well as a reduction in the percentages of circulating leucocytes, and immunoglobulin levels [249]. Published evidence suggest that acute stressors tend to enhance immune responses, but chronic (long-term) stressors are associated with suppressed immune function [252].

Striking evidence for the controlling effects of the CNS comes from studies of classically conditioned immune responses. For example, Bovjberg *et al.* found that women who had undergone chemotherapy for ovarian cancer had reduced proliferative responses to T cell mitogens, simply by being brought to the hospital where chemotherapy had been given previously [253].

Many studies have attempted to demonstrate causal relationships between the onset and progression of cancer on the one hand, and psychosocial factors such as the type C ('cancer-prone') personality, anxiety, mood, life events, and social support on the other [252,254]. There are numerous, and formidable, methodological problems in investigating these putative links, and not surprisingly, both positive and negative findings have been reported [249,255,256].

Perhaps the most consistent evidence comes from studies that have shown a negative relationship between depression and survival following the diagnosis of cancer [257,258]; a relationship has also been found in coronary heart disease [259]. Obviously a number of confounders might explain this association, for example the known negative relationship between depression and adherence to treatments such as chemotherapy. However, Walker *et al.* showed in women undergoing neoadjuvant chemotherapy for breast cancer that anxiety and depression scores independently predicted both clinical and pathological responses to chemotherapy [260]. Nevertheless, these studies have not demonstrated that the effects are mediated by psychoneuroimmunological mechanisms.

Because of the methodological difficulties noted above, a number of studies have examined the effects of psychosocial factors on surrogate immunological markers of survival. Recent studies have suggested that higher levels of circulatory VEGF predicted poorer survival in various cancers, including colorectal and ovarian cancers [261,262]. Sharma *et al.* found that cancer-related concerns and depression were independent predictors of preoperative and postoperative VEGF-A levels in patients with newly diagnosed colorectal cancer [261]. Lutgendorf *et al.* found that women with ovarian carcinoma, who reported higher levels of social well being, had lower levels of VEGF [262]. Conversely, individuals who reported greater helplessness had higher VEGF levels. These are potentially important observations. However, correlation and causation are not the same, and stronger evidence for the causal influence of psychosocial factors comes from randomized controlled trials.

Effects of psychosocial and related interventions on host defences

Given that the diagnosis and treatment of cancer are stressful, it is not surprising that substantial efforts have been made to develop interventions to help patients to cope more effectively. In addition to evaluating psychosocial outcomes, some of these studies have also documented the effects of these interventions on host defences.

Most work has been carried out in early breast cancer, and most studies have included an intervention to promote relaxation. Andersen *et al.* randomized 227 women with stage 2 or stage 3 breast cancer to a group intervention consisting of progressive muscular relaxation training, problem solving, education, and lifestyle advice. A number of beneficial psychological and behavioural changes were observed, and lymphocyte proliferation to mitogens *in vitro* was higher in the intervention group [263].

Six weeks after surgery, Green *et al.* randomized 183 women with early breast cancer to foot reflexology, scalp massage, or self-initiated support (SIS). Both reflexology and massage had beneficial effects on quality of life and mood. Blood lymphocyte phenotyping showed that $CD25^+$ cells were significantly higher in the massage group than in the SIS group. The percentage of T cells, and more specifically the Th subset producing IL-4, decreased significantly in the massage group, compared with the SIS group. This change was accompanied by an increase in the percentage of $CD8^+$ T CTLs producing IFN-γ in the massage group. NK and LAK cell cytotoxicity measurements, serum levels of cortisol, prolactin, and growth hormone, and flow cytometric assessment of their corresponding receptors all revealed no significant differences between the three groups of patients [264].

The psychoneuroimmunological effects of a 'mindfulness stress reduction programme' was evaluated by Carlson *et al.* [265]. They randomized 49 patients with early breast cancer and 10 patients with prostate cancer. In the intervention group, there was enhanced production of IL-4 but reduced IFN-γ; NK cell production of IL-10 was decreased.

Patients with locally advanced breast cancer have also been studied. Eremin *et al.* randomized 80 women with locally advanced breast cancer to a high level of support, with or without relaxation and guided imagery. Compared with women in the control group, patients who received the psychological intervention had significantly better quality of life, mood, and coping, during the 37-week protocol. In addition, the intervention resulted in increased levels of LAK cell activity, a higher proportion of total T cells ($CD2^+$), activated T cells ($CD25^+$), and NK cells (CD 56^+) [266].

Intervention studies have found changes in other types of cancers. Fawzy *et al.* randomized 68 patients with newly diagnosed malignant melanoma to a psychoeducational programme (including relaxation training) or routine care. Patients in the intervention group had an increased percentage of LGLs and NK cells, as well as an increase in NK cell activity and a decrease in the percentage of circulating $CD4^+$ cells [267]. However, subsequent studies have been less definitive. A review by Ben-Eliyahu *et al.* concluded that there appeared to be promising associations between stress, NK cells, and cancer, but that neuroendocrine and immunological mediators of stress need further careful assessment in patients with cancer to support or refute this postulate [268].

These and various other studies show that a range of psychosocial interventions can produce alterations in various parameters of host defences. However, although some of these immunological changes could be beneficial in patients with cancer, no study, to date, has demonstrated that intervention-induced changes translate into improved survival.

Overview

Despite considerable investment in information services, communication skills training, and psychosocial support, many patients find the diagnosis and treatment of cancer to be stressful, and the incidence of psychiatric morbidity generally remains high. There is a substantial literature showing that certain types of stress result in reduced functional immune parameters, such as *in vitro* proliferative responses to mitogens and NK cell activity, as well as a reduction in the percentages of circulating leucocytes.

On the other hand, a number of psychosocial interventions have been found to improve coping and to compensate for stress-induced immunosuppression. None of these studies, however, has demonstrated that the immunological changes have translated into improved survival. Although psychosocial interventions can enhance coping and improve quality of life, it is important that patients are not given unrealistic expectations about their effects in terms of cancer prognosis.

Future research should address individual differences in psychoneuroimmunological responses to psychosocial interventions, as there is good evidence that 'one size does not fit all'. Targeting interventions towards individuals with particular psychobiological characteristics could prove particularly fruitful [254,269].

Summary and conclusions

Occurrence of cancer invariably elicits a variable degree of immune response in the host. This immune response may be effective and able to eliminate the cancer but in many patients it is inadequate. Even if the host immune response is optimal, most cancers eventually counteract the host defences and escape the host anticancer responses by immune editing, leading to immune escape and eventual disease progression.

New and rapidly expanding knowledge about the complex interactions between the innate and adaptive immunity and the cancer cells in the tumour microenvironment is providing a better understanding of the factors responsible for progressive tumour growth and formation of metastasis.

Conventional anticancer therapies like chemotherapy and radiotherapy also have an immune modulating effect. Highly selective, toxin-based anticancer biological therapies are being evaluated at present. MABs (against growth factors, VEGFRs, host immune cells, and cytokine production) are showing promise.

Harnessing the immune system is an exciting therapeutic option and has seen important developments in the last decade through active and passive immunotherapy trials. The efficacy of immunotherapy is constantly improving as the factors responsible for cancer-induced immune dysregulation are being discovered and addressed. Cancer immunotherapy is likely to deliver optimal clinical benefit, if combined with other available therapeutic options.

Cancer cachexia is a cytokine/hormone-mediated nutritional disorder seen in many cancers. Its treatment is evolving through blocking mechanisms inducing cachexia and improving appetite.

The diagnosis and treatment of cancer is associated with a significant psychological and psychiatric morbidity. The close interaction between the central and peripheral nervous systems and host defences has resulted in the rise of psychoneuroimmunological interventions to both improve the quality of life and, hopefully, treatment outcomes.

References

1. Dunn GP, Bruce AT, Ikeda H, Old LJ, Schreiber RD. Cancer immunoediting: from immunosurveillance to tumor escape. *Nat Immunol* 2002; **3**: 991–998.

2. Burnet F. *The clonal selection theory of acquired immunity*. Vanderbilt University Press, Nashville, TN, 1959.
3. Bretscher P, Cohn M. A theory of non self discrimination. *Science* 1970; **169**: 1042–1049.
4. Lafferty KJ, Cunningham AJ. New analysis of allogeneic interactions. *Austral J Exp Biol Med Sci* 1975; **53**: 27–42.
5. Janeway CA Jr. Approaching the asymptote? Evolution and revolution in immunology. *Cold Spring Harb Symp Quant Biol* 1989; **54**: 1–13.
6. Matzinger P. Tolerance, danger and the extended family. *Annu Rev Immunol* 1994; **12**: 991–1045.
7. Gallucci S, Matzinger P. Danger signals: SOS to the immune system. *Curr Opin Immunol* 2001;**13**: 114–119.
8. Matzinger P. The danger model: a renewed sense of self. *Science* 2002; **296**: 301–305.
9. Nathanson L. Spontaneous regression of malignant melanoma: a review of the literature on incidence, clinical features, and possible mechanisms. *Natl Cancer Inst Monogr* 1976; **44**: 67–76.
10. Nauts HC. *The beneficial effects of bacterial infection on host resistance to cancer: end results in 449 cases*, 2nd ed. Cancer Research Institute, New York, 1980.
11. Everson TC. *Spontaneous regression of cancer*. W.B Saunders, London, 1966.
12. Alexandroff AB, Jackson AM, O'Donnell MA, James K. BCG immunotherapy of bladder cancer: 20 years on. *Lancet* 1999; **353**: 1689–1994.
13. Bosma GC, Custer RP, Bosma MJ. A severe combined immunodeficiency mutation in the mouse. *Nature* 1983; **301**: 527–530.
14. Shankaran V, Ikeda H, Bruce AT *et al.* IFNgamma and lymphocytes prevent primary tumour development and shape tumour immunogenicity. *Nature* 2001; **410**: 1107–1111.
15. Smyth MJ, Thia KYT, Street SEA, MacGregor D, Godfrey DI, Trapani JA. Perforin-mediated cytotoxicity is critical for surveillance of spontaneous lymphoma. *J Exp Med* 2000; **192**: 755–760.
16. Street SEA, Trapani JA, MacGregor D, Smyth MJ. Suppression of lymphoma and epithelial malignancies effected by interferon gamma. *J Exp Med* 2002; **196**: 129–134.
17. Street SEA, Hayakawa Y, Zhan YF *et al.* Innate immune surveillance of spontaneous B cell lymphomas by natural killer cells and gamma delta T cells. *J Exp Med* 2004; **199**: 879–884.
18. Hayashi T, Faustman DL. Development of spontaneous uterine tumors in low molecular mass polypeptide-2 knockout mice. *Cancer Res* 2002; **62**: 24–27.
19. Zerafa N, Westwood JA, Cretney E *et al.* Cutting edge: TRAIL deficiency accelerates hematological malignancies. *J Immunol* 2005; **175**: 5586–5590.
20. Enzler T, Gillessen S, Manis JP *et al.* Deficiencies of GM-CSF and interferon gamma link inflammation and cancer. *J Exp Med* 2003; **197**: 1213–1219.
21. Airoldi I, Di Carlo E, Coco C *et al.* Lack of Il12rb2 signaling predisposes to, spontaneous autoimmunity and malignancy. *Blood* 2005; **106**: 3846–3853.
22. Clementi R, Locatelli F, Dupre L *et al.* A proportion of patients with lymphoma may harbor mutations of the perforin gene. *Blood* 2005; **105**: 4424–4428.
23. Davidson WF, Giese T, Fredrickson TN. Spontaneous development of plasmacytoid tumors in mice with defective Fas-Fas ligand interactions. *J Exp Med* 1998; **187**: 1825–1838.

24. Street SEA, Cretney E, Smyth MJ. Perforin and interferon-gamma activities independently control tumor initiation, growth, and metastasis. *Blood* 2001; **97**: 192–197.
25. Coussens LM, Werb Z. Inflammation and cancer. *Nature* 2002; **420**: 860–867.
26. Engel AM, Svane IM, Rygaard J, Werdelin O. MCA sarcomas induced in scid mice are more immunogenic than MCA sarcomas induced in congenic, immunocompetent mice. *Scand J Immunol* 1997; **45**: 463–470.
27. Nishikawa H, Kato T, Tawara I *et al.* Accelerated chemically induced tumor development mediated by CD4(+)CD25(+) regulatory T cells in wild-type hosts. *Proc Natl Acad Sci U S A* 2005; **102**: 9253–9257.
28. Smyth MJ, Thia KYT, Street SEA *et al.* Differential tumor surveillance by natural killer (NK) and NK T cells. *J Exp Med* 2000; **191**: 661–668.
29. Kaplan DH, Shankaran V, Dighe AS *et al.* Demonstration of an interferon-gamma dependent tumour surveillance system in immunocompetent mice. *Proc Natl Acad Sci U S A* 1998; **95**: 7556–7561.
30. Cretney E, Takeda K, Yagita H, Glaccum M, Peschon JJ, Smyth MJ. Increased susceptibility to tumor initiation and metastasis in TNF-related apoptosis-inducing ligand-deficient mice. *J Immunol* 2002; **168**: 1356–1361.
31. Dunn GP, Bruce AT, Sheehan KCF *et al.* A critical function for type I interferons in cancer immunoediting. *Nat Immunol* 2005; **6**: 722–729.
32. Liu JG, Xiang ZY, Ma XJ. Role of IFN regulatory factor-1 and IL-12 in immunological resistance to pathogenesis of N-methyl-N-nitrosourea-induced T lymphoma. *J Immunol* 2004; **173**: 1184–1193.
33. Loser K, Scherer A, Krummen MBW *et al.* An important role of CD80/CD86-CTLA-4 signaling during photocarcinogenesis in mice. *J Immunol* 2005; **174**: 5298–5305.
34. Svane IM, Engel AM, Nielsen MB, Ljunggren HG, Rygaard J, Werdelin O. Chemically induced sarcomas from nude mice are more immunogenic than similar sarcomas from congenic normal mice. *Eur J Immunol* 1996; **26**: 1844–1850.
35. Girardi M, Oppenheim DE, Steele CR *et al.* Regulation of cutaneous malignancy by gamma delta T cells. *Science* 2001; **294**: 605–609.
36. Crowe NY, Smyth MJ, Godfrey DI. A critical role for natural killer T cells in immunosurveillance of methylcholanthrene-induced sarcomas. *J Exp Med* 2002; **196**: 119–127.
37. van den Broek ME, Kagi D, Ossendorp F *et al.* Decreased tumor surveillance in perforin-deficient mice. *J Exp Med* 1996 Nov 1; **184**: 1781–90.
38. Takeda K, Smyth MJ, Cretney E *et al.* Critical role for tumor necrosis factor-related apoptosis-inducing ligand in immune surveillance against tumor development. *J Exp Med* 2002; **195**: 161–169.
39. Smyth MJ, Swann J, Cretney E, Zerafa N, Yokoyama WM, Hayakawa Y. NKG2D function protects the host from tumor initiation. *J Exp Med* 2005; **202**: 583–588.
40. Kaplan DH, Shankaran V, Dighe AS *et al.* Demonstration of an interferon gamma-dependent tumor surveillance system in immunocompetent mice. *Proc Natl Acad Sci U S A* 1998; **95**: 7556–7561.
41. Qin ZH, Kim HJ, Hemme J, Blankenstein T. Inhibition of methylcholanthrene-induced carcinogenesis by an interferon gamma receptor-dependent foreign body reaction. *J Exp Med* 2002; **195**: 1479–1490.
42. Girardi M, Glusac E, Filler RB *et al.* The distinct contributions of murine T cell receptor (TCR)gamma delta(+) and TCR alpha beta(+) T cells to different stages of chemically induced skin cancer. *J Exp Med* 2003; **198**: 747–755.

43. Oppenheim DE, Roberts SJ, Clarke SL *et al.* Sustained localized expression of ligand for the activating NKG2D receptor impairs natural cytotoxicity in vivo and reduces tumor immunosurveillance. *Nat Immunol* 2005; **6**: 928–937.

44. Langowski JL, Zhang X, Wu L *et al.* IL-23 promotes tumour incidence and growth. *Nature* 2006; **442**: 461–465.

45. Numasaki M, Fukushi J, Ono M *et al.* Interleukin-17 promotes angiogenesis and tumor growth. *Blood* 2003; **101**: 2620–2627.

46. Tartour E, Fossiez F, Joyeux I *et al.* Interleukin 17, a T-cell-derived cytokine, promotes tumorigenicity of human cervical tumors in nude mice. *Cancer Res* 1999; **59**: 3698–3704.

47. Norbury KC, Kripke ML. Ultraviolet carcinogenesis in T cell depleted mice. *J Natl Cancer Inst* 1978; **61**: 917–921.

48. Ward PL, Koeppen HK, Hurteau T, Rowley DA, Schreiber H. Major histocompatibility complex class-I and unique antigen expression by murine tumors that escaped from CD8$^+$ T-cell dependant surveillance. *Cancer Res* 1990; **50**: 3851–3858.

49. Clark WH, Jr., Elder DE, Guerry DT *et al.* Model predicting survival in stage I melanoma based on tumor progression.[see comment]. *J Natl Cancer Inst* 1989; **81**: 1893–1904.

50. Clemente CG, Mihm MC Jr, Bufalino R, Zurrida S, Collini P, Cascinelli N. Prognostic value of tumor infiltrating lymphocytes in the vertical growth phase of primary cutaneous melanoma. *Cancer* 1996; **77**: 1303–1310.

51. Hodi FS, Dranoff G. The biologic importance of tumor-infiltrating lymphocytes. *J Cutan Pathol* 2010; **37**(Suppl 1): 48–53.

52. Aloysius MM TA, Robins A, Eremin O. Dendritic cell biology, dysfunction and immunotherapy in gastrointestinal cancers. *The Surgeon* 2006; **4**: 195–210.

53. Galon J, Costes A, Sanchez-Cabo F *et al.* Type, density, and location of immune cells within human colorectal tumors predict clinical outcome. *Science* 2006; **313**: 1960–1964.

54. Coca S, Perez-Piqueras J, Martinez D *et al.* The prognostic significance of intratumoral natural killer cells in patients with colorectal carcinoma. *Cancer* 1997; **79**: 2320–2328.

55. Ishigami S, Natsugoe S, Tokuda K *et al.* Prognostic value of intratumoral natural killer cells in gastric carcinoma. *Cancer* 2000; **88**: 577–583.

56. Takanami I, Takeuchi K, Giga M. The prognostic value of natural killer cell infiltration in resected pulmonary adenocarcinoma. *J Thorac Cardiovasc Surg* 2001; **121**: 1058–1063.

57. Haanen J, Baars A, Gomez R *et al.* Melanoma-specific tumor-infiltrating lymphocytes but not circulating melanoma-specific T cells may predict survival in resected advanced-stage melanoma patients. *Cancer Immunol Immunother* 2006; **55**: 451–458.

58. Naito Y, Saito K, Shiiba K *et al.* CD8($^+$) T cells infiltrated within cancer cell nests as a prognostic factor in human colorectal cancer. *Cancer Res* 1998; **58**: 3491–3494.

59. Cai XY, Gao Q, Qiu SJ *et al.* Dendritic cell infiltration and prognosis of human hepatocellular carcinoma. *J Cancer Res Clin Oncol* 2006; **132**: 293–301.

60. Bergeron A, El-Hage F, Kambouchner M, Lecossier D, Tazi A. Characterisation of dendritic cell subsets in lung cancer micro-environments. *Eur Respir J* 2006; **28**: 1170–1177.

61. Treilleux I, Blay JY, Bendriss-Vermare N *et al.* Dendritic cell infiltration and prognosis of early stage breast cancer. *Clin Cancer Res* 2004; **10**: 7466–7474.

62. Ghiringhelli F, Puig PE, Roux S *et al.* Tumor cells convert immature myeloid dendritic cells into TGF-beta-secreting cells inducing CD4$^+$CD25$^+$ regulatory T cell proliferation. *J Exp Med* 2005; **202**: 919–929.

63. Beyer M, Schultze JL. Regulatory T cells in cancer. *Blood* 2006; **108**: 804–811.

64. Taams LS, Smith J, Rustin MH, Salmon M, Poulter LW, Akbar AN. Human anergic/suppressive CD4(+)CD25(+) T cells: a highly differentiated and apoptosis-prone population. *Eur J Immunol* 2001; **31**: 1122–1131.

65. Petersen RP, Campa MJ, Sperlazza J *et al.* Tumor infiltrating Foxp3$^+$ regulatory T-cells are associated with recurrence in pathologic stage I NSCLC patients. *Cancer* 2006 Dec 15; **107**(12): 2866–72.

66. Wolf D, Wolf AM, Rumpold H *et al.* The expression of the regulatory T cell-specific forkhead box transcription factor FoxP3 is associated with poor prognosis in ovarian cancer.[see comment]. *Clin Cancer Res* 2005; **11**: 8326–8331.

67. Nummer D, Suri-Payer E, Schmitz-Winnenthal H *et al.* Role of tumor endothelium in CD4(+)CD25(+) regulatory T cell infiltration of human pancreatic carcinoma. *J Natl Cancer Inst* 2007; **99**: 1188–1199.

68. Viguier M, Lemaître F, Verola O *et al.* Foxp3 expressing CD4$^+$CD25(high) regulatory T cells are overrepresented in human metastatic melanoma lymph nodes and inhibit the function of infiltrating T cells. *J Immunol* 2004 Jul 15; **173**: 1444–53.

69. Kawaida H, Kono K, Takahashi A *et al.* Distribution of CD4$^+$CD25high regulatory T-cells in tumor-draining lymph nodes in patients with gastric cancer. *J Surg Res* 2005; **124**: 151–157.

70. Liyanage UK, Moore TT, Joo HG *et al.* Prevalence of regulatory T cells is increased in peripheral blood and tumor microenvironment of patients with pancreas or breast adenocarcinoma. *J Immunol* 2002; **169**: 2756–2761.

71. Miller AM, Lundberg K, Ozenci V *et al.* CD4$^+$CD25high T cells are enriched in the tumor and peripheral blood of prostate cancer patients. *J Immunol* 2006; **177**: 7398–7405.

72. Curiel TJ, Coukos G, Zou L *et al.* Specific recruitment of regulatory T cells in ovarian carcinoma fosters immune privilege and predicts reduced survival.[see comment]. *Nat Med* 2004; **10**: 942–949.

73. Nishikawa H, Sakaguchi S. Regulatory T cells in tumor immunity. *Int J Cancer* 2010; **127**: 759–767.

74. Walunas TL, Bakker CY, Bluestone JA. CTLA-4 ligation blocks CD28-dependent T cell activation. *J Exp Med* 1996; **183**: 2541–2550.

75. Greenwald RJ, Oosterwegel MA, van der Woude D. CTLA-4 regulates cell cycle progression during a primary immune response. *Eur J Immunol* 2002; **32**: 366–373.

76. Qian BZ, Pollard JW. Macrophage diversity enhances tumor progression and metastasis. *Cell* 2010; **141**: 39–51.

77. Mantovani A, Sica A, Allavena P, Garlanda C, Locati M. Tumor-associated macrophages and the related myeloid-derived suppressor cells as a paradigm of the diversity of macrophage activation. *Hum Immunol* 2009; **70**: 325–330.

78. Martinez FO, Helming L, Gordon S. Alternative activation of macrophages: an immunologic functional perspective. *Annu Rev Immunol* 2009; **27**: 451–483.

79. Mantovani A, Sica A. Macrophages, innate immunity and cancer: balance, tolerance, and diversity. *Curr Opin Immunol* 2010; **22**: 231–237.

80. Posner JB. Immunology of paraneoplastic syndromes: overview. *Ann N Y Acad Sci* 2003; **998**: 178–186.

81. Mathew RM, Cohen AB, Galetta SL, Alavi A, Dalmau J. Paraneoplastic cerebellar degeneration: co-expressing tumor revealed after a 5-year follow-up with FDG-PET. *J Neurol Sci* 2006; **250**: 153–155.

82. Darnell RB, Deangelis LM. Regression of small cell lung carcinoma in patients with paraneoplastic neuronal antibodies *Lancet* 1993; **341**: 21–22.
83. Siveen KS, Kuttan G. Role of macrophages in tumour progression. *Immunol Lett* 2009; **123**: 97–102.
84. Talmadge JE, Donkor M, Scholar E. Inflammatory cell infiltration of tumors: Jekyll or Hyde. *Cancer Metastasis Rev* 2007; **26**: 373–400.
85. Dhodapkar MV. Immune response to premalignancy—insights from patients with monoclonal gammopathy. *Ann N Y Acad Sci* 2005; **1062**: 22–28.
86. Kyle RA, Therneau TM, Rajkumar SV *et al.* A long-term study of prognosis in monoclonal gammopathy of undetermined significance. *N Engl J Med* 2002; **346**: 564–569.
87. Dhodapkar MV, Krasovsky J, Osman K, Geller MD. Vigorous premalignancy-specific effector T cell response in the bone marrow of patients with monoclonal gammopathy. *J Exp Med* 2003; **198**: 1753–1757.
88. Graus F, Dalmau J, Rene R *et al.* Anti-Hu antibodies in patients with small-cell lung cancer: Association with complete response to therapy and improved survival. *J Clin Oncol* 1997; **15**: 2866–2872.
89. Buell JF, Gross TG, Woodle ES. Malignancy after transplantation. *Transplantation* 2005; **80**: S254–264.
90. Penn I. Tumors of the immunocompromised patient. *Annu Rev Med* 1988; **39**: 63–73.
91. Dunn GP, Old LJ, Schreiber RD. The three Es of cancer immunoediting. *Annu Rev Immunol* 2004; **22**: 329–360.
92. Karrison TG, Ferguson DJ, Meier P. Dormancy of mammary carcinoma after mastectomy. *J Natl Cancer Inst* 1999; **91**: 80–85.
93. Khazaie K, Prifti S, Beckhove P *et al.* Persistence of dormant tumor cells in the bone marrow of tumor cell-vaccinated mice correlates with long-term immunological protection. *Proc Natl Acad Sci U S A* 1994; **91**: 7430–7434.
94. Schirrmacher V. T-cell immunity in the induction and maintenance of a tumour dormant state. *Semin Cancer Biol* 2001; **11**: 285–295.
95. Feuerer M, Rocha M, Bai LH *et al.* Enrichment of memory T cells and other profound immunological changes in the bone marrow from untreated breast cancer patients. *Int J Cancer* 2001; **92**: 96–105.
96. Myron Kauffman H, McBride MA, Cherikh WS, Spain PC, Marks WH, Roza AM. Transplant tumor registry: donor related malignancies. *Transplantation* 2002; **74**: 358–362.
97. Prehn RT. Immunostimulation of chemical oncogenesis in mouse. *Int J Cancer* 1977; **20**: 918–922.
98. de Visser KE, Eichten A, Coussens LM. Paradoxical roles of the immune system during cancer development. *Nat Rev Cancer* 2006; **6**: 24–37.
99. Ichim CV. Revisiting immunosurveillance and immunostimulation: Implications for cancer immunotherapy. *J Transl Med* 2005; **3**: 8.
100. Dannenberg AJ, Subbaramaiah K. Targeting cyclooxygenase-2 in human neoplasia: rationale and promise. *Cancer Cell* 2003; **4**: 431–436.
101. Imada A, Shijubo N, Kojima H, Abe S. Mast cells correlate with angiogenesis and poor outcome in stage I lung adenocarcinoma. *Eur Resp J* 2000; **15**: 1087–1093.

102. Ribatti D, Ennas MG, Vacca A *et al.* Tumor vascularity and tryptase-positive mast cells correlate with a poor prognosis in melanoma. *Eur J Clin Invest* 2003; **33**: 420–425.
103. Leek RD, Lewis CE, Whitehouse R, Greenall M, Clarke J, Harris AL. Association of macrophage infiltration with angiogenesis and prognosis in invasive breast carcinoma. *Cancer Res* 1996; **56**: 4625–4629.
104. Salvesen HB, Akslen LA. Significance of tumour-associated macrophages, vascular endothelial growth factor and thrombospondin-1 expression for tumour angiogenesis and prognosis in endometrial carcinomas. *Int J Cancer* 1999; **84**: 538–543.
105. Hanada T, Nakagawa M, Emoto A, Nomura T, Nasu N, Nomura Y. Prognostic value of tumor-associated macrophage count in human bladder cancer. *Int J Urol* 2000; **7**: 263–269.
106. Smyth MJ, Crowe NY, Godfrey DI. NK cells and NK T cells collaborate in host protection from methylcholanthrene-induced fibrosarcoma. *Int Immunol* 2001; **13**: 459–463.
107. Gallina G, Dolcetti L, Serafini P *et al.* Tumors induce a subset of inflammatory monocytes with immunosuppressive activity on CD8(+) T cells. *J Clin Invest* 2006; **116**: 2777–2790.
108. Tan TT, Coussens LM. Humoral immunity, inflammation and cancer. *Curr Opin Immunol* 2007; **19**: 209–216.
109. Bai XF, Liu JQ, Li O, Zheng P, Liu Y. Antigenic drift as a mechanism for tumor evasion of destruction by cytolytic T lymphocytes. *J Clin Invest* 2003; **111**: 1487–1496.
110. Bubenik J. MHC class I down-regulation: tumour escape from immune surveillance? *Int J Oncol* 2004; **25**: 487–491.
111. Lehmann C, Zeis M, Schmitz N, Uharek L. Impaired binding of perforin on the surface of tumor cells is a cause of target cell resistance against cytotoxic effector cells. *Blood* 2000 Jul; **96**: 594–600.
112. Real LM, Jimenez P, Kirkin A *et al.* Multiple mechanisms of immune evasion can coexist in melanoma tumor cell lines derived from the same patient. *Cancer Immunol Immunother* 2001; **49**: 621–628.
113. Shin MS, Kim HS, Lee SH *et al.* Mutations of tumor necrosis factor-related apoptosis-inducing ligand receptor 1 (TRAIL-R1) and receptor 2 (TRAIL-R2) genes in metastatic breast cancers. *Cancer Res* 2001; **61**: 4942–4946.
114. Kowalczyk DW. Tumors and the danger model. *Acta Biochim Pol* 2002; **49**: 295–302.
115. Elpek KG, Lacelle C, Singh NP, Yolcu ES, Shirwan H. $CD4^+CD25^+$ T regulatory cells dominate multiple immune evasion mechanisms in early but not late phases of tumor development in a B cell lymphoma model. *J Immunol* 2007; **178**: 6840–6848.
116. Ryschich E, Schmidt J, Hammerling GJ, Klar E, Ganss R. Transformation of the microvascular system during multistage tumorigenesis. *Int J Cancer* 2002 Feb; **97**: 719–25.
117. Uyttenhove C, Pilotte L, Theate I *et al.* Evidence for a tumoral immune resistance mechanism based on tryptophan degradation by indoleamine 2,3-dioxygenase. *Nat Med* 2003; **9**: 1269–1274.
118. Zhang XM, Xu Q. Metastatic melanoma cells escape from immunosurveillance through the novel mechanism of releasing nitric oxide to induce dysfunction of immunocytes. *Melanoma Res* 2001; **11**: 559–567.
119. Beck C, Schreiber H, Rowley DA. Role of TGF-beta in immune-evasion of cancer. *Microsc Res Tech* 2001; **52**: 387–395.

120. Kawamura K, Bahar R, Natsume W, Sakiyama S, Tagawa M. Secretion of interleukin-10 from murine colon carcinoma cells suppresses systemic antitumor immunity and impairs protective immunity induced against the tumors. *Cancer Gene Ther* 2002; **9**: 109–115.
121. Whiteside TL. Tumor-induced death of immune cells: its mechanisms and consequences. *Semin Cancer Biol* 2002; **12**: 43–50.
122. Flavell RA, Sanjabi S, Wrzesinski SH, Licona-Limón P. The polarization of immune cells in the tumour environment by TGFbeta. *Nat Rev Immunol* 2010; **10**: 554–567.
123. Bierie B, Moses HL. Transforming growth factor beta (TGF-beta) and inflammation in cancer. *Cytokine Growth Factor Rev* 2010; **21**: 49–59.
124. Reibman J, Meixler S, Lee TC *et al.* Transforming growth factor beta 1, a potent chemoattractant for human neutrophils, bypasses classic signal-transduction pathways. *Proc Natl Acad Sci U S A* 1991; **88**: 6805–6809.
125. Chen JJ, Sun Y, Nabel GJ. Regulation of the proinflammatory effects of Fas ligand (CD95L). *Science* 1998; **282**: 1714–1717.
126. Nozawa H, Chiu C, Hanahan D. Infiltrating neutrophils mediate the initial angiogenic switch in a mouse model of multistage carcinogenesis. *Proc Natl Acad Sci U S A* 2006; **103**: 12493–12498.
127. Lee JC, Lee KM, Kim DW, Heo DS. Elevated TGF-beta1 secretion and down-modulation of NKG2D underlies impaired NK cytotoxicity in cancer patients. *J Immunol* 2004; **172**: 7335–7340.
128. Li MO, Wan YY, Sanjabi S, Robertson AK, Flavell RA. Transforming growth factor-beta regulation of immune responses. *Annu Rev Immunol* 2006; **24**: 99–146.
129. Byrne SN, Knox MC, Halliday GM. TGF-beta is responsible for skin tumour infiltration by macrophages enabling the tumours to escape immune destruction. *Immunol Cell Biol* 2008; **86**: 92–97.
130. Thomas DA, Massagué J. TGF-beta directly targets cytotoxic T cell functions during tumor evasion of immune surveillance. *Cancer Cell* 2005; **8**: 369–380.
131. Knutson KL, Disis ML. Tumor antigen-specific T helper cells in cancer immunity and immunotherapy. *Cancer Immunol Immunother* 2005; **54**: 721–728.
132. Yamazaki S, Iyoda T, Tarbell K *et al.* Direct expansion of functional $CD25^+$ $CD4^+$ regulatory T cells by antigen-processing dendritic cells. *J Exp Med* 2003; **198**: 235–247.
133. Dunn GP, Old LJ, Schreiber RD. The immunobiology of cancer immunosurveillance and immunoediting. *Immunity* 2004; **21**: 137–148.
134. Shay JW, Bacchetti S. A survey of telomerase activity in human cancer. *Eur J Cancer* 1997; **33**: 787–791.
135. Kim EK, Cho HI, Yoon SH *et al.* Efficient generation of survivin-specific cytotoxic T lymphocytes from healthy persons in vitro: quantitative and qualitative effects of $CD4^+$ T cells. *Vaccine* 2008; **26**: 3987–3997.
136. Stanley M, Gissmann L, Nardelli-Haefliger D. Immunobiology of human papillomavirus infection and vaccination - implications for second generation vaccines. *Vaccine* 2008; **26**(Suppl 10): K62–67.
137. Banchereau J, Steinman RM. Dendritic cells and the control of immunity. *Nature* 1998 Mar 19; **392**(6673):245–52.
138. Belardelli F, Ferrantini M. Cytokines as a link between innate and adaptive antitumor immunity. *Trends Immunol* 2002; **23**: 201–208.

139. Heath WR, Carbone FR. Cross-presentation, dendritic cells, tolerance and immunity. *Annu Rev Immunol* 2001; **19**: 47–64.

140. Shurin M, Gabrilovich D. Regulation of dendritic cell system by tumour. *Cancer Res Ther Control* 2001; **11**: 65–78.

141. Allavena P, Piemonti L, Longoni D *et al.* IL-10 prevents the differentiation of monocytes to dendritic cells but promotes their maturation to macrophages. *Eur J Immunol* 1998; **28**: 359–369.

142. Buelens C, Verhasselt V, De Groote D, Thielemans K, Goldman M, Willems F. Interleukin-10 prevents the generation of dendritic cells from human peripheral blood mononuclear cells cultured with interleukin-4 and granulocyte/macrophage-colony-stimulating factor. *Eur J Immunol* 1997; **27**: 756–762.

143. Menetrier-Caux C, Montmain G, Dieu MC *et al.* Inhibition of the differentiation of dendritic cells from CD34($^+$) progenitors by tumor cells: role of interleukin-6 and macrophage colony-stimulating factor. *Blood* 1998; **92**: 4778–4791.

144. Park SJ, Nakagawa T, Kitamura H *et al.* IL-6 regulates in vivo dendritic cell differentiation through STAT3 activation. *J Immunol* 2004 Sep 15; **173**: 3844–54.

145. Ratta M, Fagnoni F, Curti A *et al.* Dendritic cells are functionally defective in multiple myeloma: the role of interleukin-6. *Blood* 2002; **100**: 230–237.

146. Pak AS, Wright MA, Matthews JP, Collins SL, Petruzzelli GJ, Young MR. Mechanisms of immune suppression in patients with head and neck cancer: presence of CD34($^+$) cells which suppress immune functions within cancers that secrete granulocyte-macrophage colony-stimulating factor. *Clin Cancer Res* 1995; **1**: 95–103.

147. Young MR, Wright MA, Lozano Y *et al.* Increased recurrence and metastasis in patients whose primary head and neck squamous cell carcinomas secreted granulocyte-macrophage colony-stimulating factor and contained CD34$^+$ natural suppressor cells. *Int J Cancer* 1997; **74**: 69–74.

148. Almand B, Clark JI, Nikitina E *et al.* Increased production of immature myeloid cells in cancer patients: a mechanism of immunosuppression in cancer. *J Immunol* 2001; **166**: 678–689.

149. Almand B, Resser JR, Lindman B *et al.* Clinical significance of defective dendritic cell differentiation in cancer. *Clin Cancer Res* 2000; **6**: 1755–1766.

150. Kusmartsev S, Nefedova Y, Yoder D, Gabrilovich DI. Antigen-specific inhibition of CD8$^+$ T cell response by immature myeloid cells in cancer is mediated by reactive oxygen species. [erratum appears in J Immunol 2004; 172: 4647]. *J Immunol* 2004; **172**: 989–999.

151. Altman JD MP, Goulder PJR. Phenotypic analysis of antigen specific T lymphocytes. *Science* 1996; **274**: 94–96.

152. Herr W LB, Leister N, Wandel E, Meyer zum Buschenfelde KH, Wolfel T. The use of computer-assisted video image analysis for quantification of CD8$^+$T lymphocytes producing tumour necrosis factor alpha spots in response to peptide antigens. *J Immunol Meth* 1997; **203**: 141–252.

153. Aloysius MM, Mc Kechnie AJ, Robins RA *et al.* Generation in vivo of peptide-specific cytotoxic T cells and presence of regulatory T cells during vaccination with hTERT (class I and II) peptide-pulsed DCs. *J Transl Med* 2009; **7**: 18–46.

154. Imai K, Matsuyama S, Miyake S, Suga K, Nakachi K. Natural cytotoxic activity of peripheral-blood lymphocytes and cancer incidence: an 11-year follow-up study of a general population. *Lancet* 2000; **356**: 1795–1799.

155. McKenna DH, Jr., Sumstad D, Bostrom N *et al.* Good manufacturing practices production of natural killer cells for immunotherapy: a six-year single-institution experience. *Transfusion* 2007; **47**: 520–528.

156. Miller JS, Soignier Y, Panoskaltsis-Mortari A *et al.* Successful adoptive transfer and in vivo expansion of human haploidentical NK cells in patients with cancer. *Blood* 2005; **105**: 3051–3057.

157. Berzofsky JA, Terabe M. A novel immunoregulatory axis of NK T cell subsets regulating tumor immunity. *Cancer Immunol Immunother* 2008; **57**: 1679–1683.

158. Boismenu R, Havran WL. An innate view of gamma delta T cells. *Curr Opin Immunol* 1997; **9**: 57–63.

159. Havran WL, Boismenu R. Activation and function of gamma delta T cells. *Curr Opin Immunol* 1994; **6**: 442–446.

160. Bonneville M, O'Brien RL, Born WK. Gamma delta T cell effector functions: a blend of innate programming and acquired plasticity. *Nat Rev Immunol* 2010;**10**: 467–478.

161. Boismenu R, Havran WL. Modulation of epithelial cell growth by intraepithelial gamma delta T cells. *Science* 1994; **266**: 1253–1255.

162. Girardi M. Immunosurveillance and immunoregulation by gamma delta T cells. *J Invest Dermatol* 2006; **126**: 25–31.

163. Ferrarini M, Heltai S, Pupa SM, Mernard S, Zocchi R. Killing of laminin receptor-positive human lung cancers by tumor infiltrating lymphocytes bearing gammadelta(+) T-cell receptors. *J Natl Cancer Inst* 1996; **88**: 436–41.

164. Choudhary A, Davodeau F, Moreau A, Peyrat MA, Bonneville M, Jotereau F. Selective lysis of autologous tumor cells by recurrent gamma delta tumor-infiltrating lymphocytes from renal carcinoma. *J Immunol* 1995; **154**: 3932–3940.

165. Zhao X, Wei YQ, Kariya Y, Teshigawara K, Uchida A. Accumulation of gamma/delta T cells in human dysgerminoma and seminoma: roles in autologous tumor killing and granuloma formation. *Immunol Invest* 1995; **24**: 607–618.

166. Bagot M, Heslan M, Dubertret L, Roujeau JC, Touraine R, Levy JP. Antigen-presenting properties of human epidermal cells compared with peripheral blood mononuclear cells. *Br J Dermatol* 1985; **113**(Suppl 28): 55–60.

167. Gnjatic S, Old LJ, Chen YT. Autoantibodies against cancer antigens. *Methods Mol Biol* 2009; **520**: 11–19.

168. Vollmers HP, Brandlein S. Natural antibodies and cancer. *Nat Biotechnol* 2009; **25**: 249–298.

169. Amigorena S. Fc gamma receptors and cross-presentation in dendritic cells. *J Exp Med* 2002; **195**: F1–3.

170. Dhodapkar KM, Dhodapkar MV. Recruiting dendritic cells to improve antibody therapy of cancer. *Proc Natl Acad Sci U S A* 2005; **102**: 6243–6244.

171. Dhodapkar MV, Dhodapkar KM, Palucka AK. Interactions of tumor cells with dendritic cells: balancing immunity and tolerance. *Cell Death Differ* 2008; **15**: 39–50.

172. Chamuleau ME, Souwer Y, Van Ham SM *et al.* Class II-associated invariant chain peptide expression on myeloid leukemic blasts predicts poor clinical outcome. *Cancer Res* 2004; **64**: 5546–5550.

173. Dhodapkar KM, Krasovsky J, Williamson B, Dhodapkar MV. Antitumor monoclonal antibodies enhance cross-presentation of cellular antigens and the generation of myeloma-specific killer T cells by dendritic cells. *J Exp Med* 2002; **195**: 125–133.

174. Weiner LM, Surana R, Wang S. Monoclonal antibodies: versatile platforms for cancer immunotherapy. *Nat Rev Immunol* 2010; **10**: 317–327.
175. Morgan BP, Harris CL. Complement therapeutics; history and current progress. *Mol Immunol* 2003; **40**: 159–170.
176. Markiewski MM, Lambris JD. Is complement good or bad for cancer patients? A new perspective on an old dilemma. *Trends Immunol* 2009; **30**: 286–292.
177. Agarwal A, Verma S, Burra U, Murthy NS, Mohanty NK, Saxena S. Flow cytometric analysis of Th1 and Th2 cytokines in PBMCs as a parameter of immunological dysfunction in patients of superficial transitional cell carcinoma of bladder. *Cancer Immunol Immunother* 2006; **55**: 734–743.
178. Kanazawa M, Yoshihara K, Abe H *et al.* Effects of PSK on T and dendritic cells differentiation in gastric or colorectal cancer patients. *Anticancer Res* 2005; **25**: 443–449.
179. Sheu BC, Lin RH, Lien HC, Ho HN, Hsu SM, Huang SC. Predominant Th2/Tc2 polarity of tumor-infiltrating lymphocytes in human cervical cancer. *J Immunol* 2001; **167**: 2972–2978.
180. Dalgleish AG, O'Byrne KJ. Chronic immune activation and inflammation in the pathogenesis of AIDS and cancer. *Adv Cancer Res* 2002; **84**: 231–276.
181. Brandtzaeg P, Carlsen HS, Halstensen TS. The B-cell system in inflammatory bowel disease. *Adv Exp Med Biol* 2006; **579**: 149–167.
182. Moons LM, Kusters JG, Bultman E *et al.* Barrett's oesophagus is characterized by a predominantly humoral inflammatory response. *J Pathol* 2005; **207**: 269–276.
183. Qin Z, Blankenstein T. $CD4^+$ T cell—mediated tumor rejection involves inhibition of angiogenesis that is dependent on IFN gamma receptor expression by nonhematopoietic cells. *Immunity* 2000; **12**: 677–686.
184. Sakamoto T, Saito H, Tatebe S *et al.* Interleukin-10 expression significantly correlates with minor $CD8^+$ T-cell infiltration and high microvessel density in patients with gastric cancer. *Int J Cancer* 2006; **118**: 1909–1914.
185. Rose-John S, Scheller J, Elson G, Jones SA. Interleukin-6 biology is coordinated by membrane-bound and soluble receptors: role in inflammation and cancer. *J Leukoc Biol* 2006; **80**: 227–236.
186. Riedel F, Zaiss I, Herzog D, Gotte K, Naim R, Hormann K. Serum levels of interleukin-6 in patients with primary head and neck squamous cell carcinoma. *Anticancer Res* 2005; **25**: 2761–2765.
187. Terabe M, Park JM, Berzofsky JA. Role of IL-13 in regulation of anti-tumor immunity and tumor growth. *Cancer Immunol Immunother* 2004; **53**: 79–85.
188. Mantovani A, Savino B, Locati M, Zammataro L, Allavena P, Bonecchi R. The chemokine system in cancer biology and therapy. *Cytokine Growth Factor Rev* 2010; **21**: 27–39.
189. Xie K. Interleukin-8 and human cancer biology. *Cytokine Growth Factor Rev* 2001; **12**: 375–391.
190. Ludwig A, Schulte A, Schnack C *et al.* Enhanced expression and shedding of the transmembrane chemokine CXCL16 by reactive astrocytes and glioma cells. *J Neurochem* 2005; **93**: 1293–1303.
191. Schirrmacher V. Cancer metastasis: experimental approaches, theoretical concepts, and impacts for treatment strategies. *Adv Cancer Res* 1985; **43**: 1–73.
192. Wyckoff JB, Wang Y, Lin EY *et al.* Direct visualization of macrophage-assisted tumor cell intravasation in mammary tumors. *Cancer Res* 2007; **67**: 2649–2656.

193. Hu H, Sun L, Guo C *et al.* Tumor cell-microenvironment interaction models coupled with clinical validation reveal CCL2 and SNCG as two predictors of colorectal cancer hepatic metastasis. *Clin Cancer Res* 2009; **15**: 5485–5493.
194. Folkman J. Tumor angiogenesis. *Adv Cancer Res* 1985; **43**: 175–203.
195. Lin EY, Li JF, Gnatovskiy L *et al.* Macrophages regulate the angiogenic switch in a mouse model of breast cancer. *Cancer Res* 2006; **66**: 11238–11246.
196. Raza A, Franklin MJ, Dudek AZ. Pericytes and vessel maturation during tumor angiogenesis and metastasis. *Am J Hematol* 2010; **85**: 593–598.
197. Gerhardt H, Betsholtz C. Endothelial-pericyte interactions in angiogenesis. *Cell Tissue Res* 2003 Oct; **314**: 15–23. Epub 2003 Jul 22.
198. Kaplan RN, Riba RD, Zacharoulis S *et al.* VEGFR1-positive haematopoietic bone marrow progenitors initiate the pre-metastatic niche. *Nature* 2005; **438**: 820–827.
199. Brittenden J, Heys SD, Ross J, Park KG, Eremin O. Natural cytotoxicity in breast cancer patients receiving neoadjuvant chemotherapy: effects of L-arginine supplementation. *Eur J Surg Oncol* 1994; **20**: 467–472.
200. Ghiringhelli F, Menard C, Puig PE *et al.* Metronomic cyclophosphamide regimen selectively depletes $CD4^{+}CD25^{+}$ regulatory T cells and restores T and NK effector functions in end stage cancer patients. *Cancer Immunol Immunother* 2007; **56**: 641–648.
201. Hermans IF, Chong TW, Palmowski MJ, Harris AL, Cerundolo V. Synergistic effect of metronomic dosing of cyclophosphamide combined with specific antitumor immunotherapy in a murine melanoma model. *Cancer Res* 2003; **63**: 8408–8413.
202. Lord R, Nair S, Schache A *et al.* Low dose metronomic oral cyclophosphamide for hormone resistant prostate cancer: a phase II study. *J Urol* 2007; **177**: 2136–2140; discussion 40.
203. Zitvogel L, Apetoh L, Ghiringhelli F, Kroemer G. Immunological aspects of cancer chemotherapy. *Nat Rev Immunol* 2008; **8**: 59–73.
204. Lissoni P, Brivio F, Fumagalli L *et al.* Effects of the conventional antitumor therapies surgery, chemotherapy, radiotherapy and immunotherapy on regulatory T lymphocytes in cancer patients. *Anticancer Res* 2009; **29**: 1847–1852.
205. Mathew M, Verma RS. Humanized immunotoxins: a new generation of immunotoxins for targeted cancer therapy. *Cancer Sci* 2009; **100**: 1359–1365.
206. Rosenberg SA, Spiess P, Lafreniere R. A new approach to the adoptive immunotherapy of cancer with tumor-infiltrating lymphocytes. *Science* 1986; **233**: 1318–1321.
207. Rosenberg SA, Restifo NP, Yang JC, Morgan RA, Dudley ME. Adoptive cell transfer: a clinical path to effective cancer immunotherapy. *Nat Rev Cancer* 2008; **8**: 299–308.
208. Cobleigh MA, Vogel CL, Tripathy D *et al.* Multinational study of the efficacy and safety of humanized anti-HER2 monoclonal antibody in women who have HER2-overexpressing metastatic breast cancer that has progressed after chemotherapy for metastatic disease. *J Clin Oncol* 1999; **17**: 2639–2648.
209. Romond EH, Perez EA, Bryant J *et al.* Trastuzumab plus adjuvant chemotherapy for operable HER2-positive breast cancer. *N Engl J Med* 2005; **353**: 1673–1684.
210. McLaughlin P, Grillo-Lopez AJ, Link BK *et al.* Rituximab chimeric anti-CD20 monoclonal antibody therapy for relapsed indolent lymphoma: half of patients respond to a four-dose treatment program. *J Clin Oncol* 1998; **16**: 2825–2833.

211. Kaminski MS, Estes J, Zasadny KR *et al.* Radioimmunotherapy with iodine (131)I tositumomab for relapsed or refractory B-cell non-Hodgkin lymphoma: updated results and long-term follow-up of the University of Michigan experience. *Blood* 2000; **96**: 1259–1266.

212. Foon KA, Yang XD, Weiner LM *et al.* Preclinical and clinical evaluations of ABX-EGF, a fully human anti-epidermal growth factor receptor antibody. *Int J Radiat Oncol Biol Phys* 2004; **58**: 984–990.

213. Hurwitz H, Fehrenbacher L, Novotny W *et al.* Bevacizumab plus irinotecan, fluorouracil, and leucovorin for metastatic colorectal cancer. *N Engl J Med* 2004; **350**: 2335–2342.

214. Lundin J, Kimby E, Bjorkholm M *et al.* Phase II trial of subcutaneous anti-CD52 monoclonal antibody alemtuzumab (Campath-1H) as first-line treatment for patients with B-cell chronic lymphocytic leukemia (B-CLL). *Blood* 2002; **100**: 768–773.

215. Satthaporn S, Aloysius MM, Robins RA *et al.* Ex vivo recovery and activation of dysfunctional, anergic, monocyte-derived dendritic cells from patients with operable breast cancer: critical role of IFN-alpha. *BMC Immunol* 2008; **9**: 32.

216. Satthaporn S, Robins A, Vassanasiri W *et al.* Dendritic cells are dysfunctional in patients with operable breast cancer. *Cancer Immunol Immunother* 2004; **53**: 510–518.

217. Dredge K, Marriott JB, Todryk SM, Dalgleish AG. Adjuvants and the promotion of Th1-type cytokines in tumour immunotherapy. *Cancer Immunol Immunother* 2002; **51**: 521–531.

218. Tartour E, Benchetrit F, Haicheur N, Adotevi O, Fridman WH. Synthetic and natural non-live vectors: rationale for their clinical development in cancer vaccine protocols. *Vaccine* 2002; **20**(Suppl 4): A32–39.

219. Napolitani G, Rinaldi A, Bertoni F, Sallusto F, Lanzavecchia A. Selected Toll-like receptor agonist combinations synergistically trigger a T helper type 1-polarizing program in dendritic cells.[see comment]. *Nat Immunol* 2005; **6**: 769–776.

220. Arina A, Tirapu I, Alfaro C *et al.* Clinical implications of antigen transfer mechanisms from malignant to dendritic cells. exploiting cross-priming. *Experimental Hematology* 2002 Dec; **30**(12):1355–64.

221. Mellstedt H, Fagerberg J, Frodin JE *et al.* Augmentation of the immune response with granulocyte-macrophage colony-stimulating factor and other hematopoietic growth factors. *Curr Opin Hematol* 1999; **6**: 169–175.

222. Viatte S, Alves PM, Romero P. Reverse immunology approach for the identification of CD8 T-cell-defined antigens: advantages and hurdles. *Immunol Cell Biol* 2006; **84**: 318–330.

223. Butterfield LH, Ribas A, Dissette VB *et al.* Determinant spreading associated with clinical response in dendritic cell-based immunotherapy for malignant melanoma. *Clin Cancer Res* 2003; **9**: 998–1008.

224. Vanderlugt CL, Miller SD. Epitope spreading in immune-mediated diseases: implications for immunotherapy. *Nat Rev Immunol* 2002; **2**: 85–95.

225. Marshall JL, Hoyer RJ, Toomey MA *et al.* Phase I study in advanced cancer patients of a diversified prime-and-boost vaccination protocol using recombinant vaccinia virus and recombinant nonreplicating avipox virus to elicit anti-carcinoembryonic antigen immune responses. *J Clin Oncol* 2000; **18**: 3964–3973.

226. Zhu MZ, Marshall J, Cole D, Schlom J, Tsang KY. Specific cytolytic T-cell responses to human CEA from patients immunized with recombinant avipox-CEA vaccine. *Clin Cancer Res* 2000; **6**: 24–33.

227. Hodge JW, Sabzevari H, Yafal AG, Gritz L, Lorenz MG, Schlom J. A triad of costimulatory molecules synergize to amplify T-cell activation. *Cancer Res* 1999; **59**: 5800–5807.

228. Oh S, Hodge JW, Ahlers JD, Burke DS, Schlom J, Berzofsky JA. Selective induction of high avidity CTL by altering the balance of signals from APC. *J Immunol* 2003; **170**: 2523–2530.

229. Belyakov IM, Moss B, Strober W, Berzofsky JA. Mucosal vaccination overcomes the barrier to recombinant vaccinia immunization caused by preexisting poxvirus immunity. *Proc Natl Acad Sci U S A* 1999; **96**: 4512–17.

230. Tang DC, DeVit M, Johnston SA. Genetic immunization is a simple method for eliciting an immune response. *Nature* 1992; **356**: 152–154.

231. Ulmer JB, Donnelly JJ, Parker SE *et al.* Heterologous protection against influenza by injection of DNA encoding a viral protein.[see comment]. *Science* 1993; **259**: 1745–1749.

232. Gabrilovich D. Mechanisms and functional significance of tumour-induced dendritic-cell defects. *Nat Rev Immunol* 2004; **4**: 941–952.

233. Calman K, Fearon K. Weight loss and nutritional abnormalities in cancer patients: incidence, severity and significance. In: Calman KC, Fearon KCH, eds, *Clinics in Oncology*. W.B. Saunders, London, 1986, pp. 115–126.

234. Plata-Salaman CR, Oomura Y, Kai Y. Tumor necrosis factor and interleukin-1 beta: suppression of food intake by direct action in the central nervous system. *Brain Res* 1988; **448**: 106–114.

235. Banks WA. Anorectic effects of circulating cytokines: role of the vascular blood-brain barrier. *Nutrition* 2001; **17**: 434–437.

236. Strassmann G, Fong M, Kenney JS, Jacob CO. Evidence for the involvement of interleukin 6 in experimental cancer cachexia. *J Clin Invest* 1992; **89**: 1681–1684.

237. Iwase S, Murakami T, Saito Y, Nakagawa K. Steep elevation of blood interleukin-6 (IL-6) associated only with late stages of cachexia in cancer patients. *Eur Cytokine Netw* 2004; **15**: 312–316.

238. Johnen H, Lin S, Kuffner T *et al.* Tumor-induced anorexia and weight loss are mediated by the TGF-beta superfamily cytokine MIC-1. *Nat Med* 2007; **13**: 1333–1340.

239. Davis MP, Dreicer R, Walsh D, Lagman R, LeGrand SB. Appetite and cancer-associated anorexia: a review. *J Clin Oncol* 2004; **22**: 1510–1517.

240. Fan W, Boston BA, Kesterson RA, Hruby VJ, Cone RD. Role of melanocortinergic neurons in feeding and the agouti obesity syndrome. *Nature* 1997; **385**: 165–168.

241. Aleman MR, Santolaria F, Batista N *et al.* Leptin role in advanced lung cancer. A mediator of the acute phase response or a marker of the status of nutrition? *Cytokine* 2002; **19**: 21–26.

242. Jatoi A, Rowland K, Loprinzi CL *et al.* An eicosapentaenoic acid supplement versus megestrol acetate versus both for patients with cancer-associated wasting: a North Central Cancer Treatment Group and National Cancer Institute of Canada collaborative effort. *J Clin Oncol* 2004; **22**: 2469–2476.

243. Khan ZH, Simpson EJ, Cole AT *et al.* Oesophageal cancer and cachexia: the effect of short-term treatment with thalidomide on weight loss and lean body mass. *Aliment Pharmacol Ther* 2003; **17**: 677–682.

244. Wigmore SJ, Falconer JS, Plester CE *et al.* Ibuprofen reduces energy expenditure and acute-phase protein production compared with placebo in pancreatic cancer patients. *Br J Cancer* 1995; **72**: 185–188.

245. Walker LG, Walker MB, Sharp DM. The organisation of psychosocial support within palliative care. In: Lloyd-Williams M, eds. *Psychosocial issues in palliative care.* Oxford University Press, Oxford, 2003, pp. 49–66.

246. Zabora J, BrintzenhofeSzoc K, Curbow B, Hooker C, Piantadosi S. The prevalence of psychological distress by cancer site. *Psychooncology* 2001; **10**: 19–28.

247. Hall A, A'Hern R, Fallowfield L. Are we using appropriate self-report questionnaires for detecting anxiety and depression in women with early breast cancer? *Eur J Cancer* 1999; **35**: 79–85.

248. Walker LG. Psycho-science: where do we go from here? *Eur J Cancer* 2009; 45(Suppl 1): 455–456.

249. Walker LG, Green VL, Greenman J, Walker AA, Sharp DM. PNI and chronic malignant disease: cancer. In Irwin M, Vedhara V, eds, *Human psychoneuroimmunology.* Oxford University Press, New York, 2005, pp. 137–163.

250. Tracey KJ. Reflex control of immunity. *Nat Rev Immunol* 2009; **9**: 418–428.

251. Zachariae R. Psychoneuroimmunology: a bio-psycho-social approach to health and disease. *Scand J Psychol* 2009; **50**: 645–651.

252. Dhabhar FS, McEwen BS. Acute stress enhances while chronic stress suppresses cell-mediated immunity in vivo: a potential role for leukocyte trafficking. *Brain Behav Immun* 1997; **11**: 286–306.

253. Bovbjerg DH, Redd WH, Maier LA *et al.* Anticipatory immune suppression and nausea in women receiving cyclic chemotherapy for ovarian cancer. *J Consult Clin Psychol* 1990; **58**: 153–157.

254. Walker LG. Hypnotherapeutic insights and interventions: a cancer odyssey. *Contemp Hypn* 2004; **21**: 35–45.

255. Anderson J, Walker LG. Psychological factors and cancer progression: involvement of behavioural pathways. Chapter 7 in Lewis CE, O'Brien R, Barraclough J, eds, *The psychoimmunology of cancer,* 2nd ed. Oxford University Press, Oxford, 2002, pp. 235–257.

256. Garssen B. Psychological factors and cancer development: evidence after 30 years of research. *Clin Psychol Rev* 2004; **24**: 315–338.

257. Ratcliffe MA, Dawson AA, Walker LG. Eysenck Personality Inventory L-scores in patients with Hodgkin's disease and non-Hodgkin's lymphoma. *Psychooncology* 1995; **4**, 39–45.

258. Satin JR, Linden W, Phillips MJ. Depression as a predictor of disease progression and mortality in cancer patients: a meta-analysis. *Cancer* 2009; **115**: 5349–5361.

259. Barth J, Schumacher M, Herrmann-Lingen C. Depression as a risk factor for mortality in patients with coronary heart disease: a meta-analysis. *Psychosom Med* 2004; **66**: 802–813.

260. Walker LG, Heys SD, Walker MB *et al.* Psychological factors can predict the response to primary chemotherapy in patients with locally advanced breast cancer. *Eur J Cancer* 1999; **35**: 1783–1788.

261. Sharma A, Greenman J, Sharp DM, Walker LG, Monson JR. Vascular endothelial growth factor and psychosocial factors in colorectal cancer. *Psychooncology* 2008; **17**: 66–73.

262. Lutgendorf SK, Johnsen EL, Cooper B *et al.* Vascular endothelial growth factor and social support in patients with ovarian carcinoma. *Cancer* 2002; **95**: 808–15.

263. Andersen BL, Farrar WB, Golden-Kreutz DM *et al.* Psychological, behavioral, and immune changes after a psychological intervention: a clinical trial. *J Clin Oncol* 2004; **22**: 3570–3580.

264. Green VL, Alexandropoulou A, Walker MB *et al.* Alterations in the Th1/Th2 balance in breast cancer patients using reflexology and scalp Massage. *Exp Therapeut Med* 2009; **1**: 97–108.

265. Carlson LE, Speca M, Patel KD, Goodey E. Mindfulness-based stress reduction in relation to quality of life, mood, symptoms of stress, and immune parameters in breast and prostate cancer outpatients. *Psychosom Med* 2003; **65**: 571–581.
266. Eremin O, Walker MB, Simpson E *et al.* Immuno-modulatory effects of relaxation training and guided imagery in women with locally advanced breast cancer undergoing multimodality therapy: a randomised controlled trial. *Breast* 2009; **18**: 17–25.
267. Fawzy FI, Kemeny ME, Fawzy NW *et al.* A structured psychiatric intervention for cancer patients. II. Changes over time in immunological measures. *Arch Gen Psychiatry* 1990; **47**: 729–735.
268. Ben-Eliyahu S, Page GC and Schleifer SJ. Stress, NK cells, and cancer: still a promissory note. *Brain Behav Immun* 2007; **21**: 881–887.
269. Editorial. The emergence of a new science of the mind: Immunology benefits the mind. *Mol Psychiatry* 2010; **15**, 337–338.

Chapter 5

Sepsis and the immune response

Rajan K. Thakkar, Xin Huang, Joanne Lomas-Neira, Daithi Heffernan, and Alfred Ayala

Key summary points

- Sepsis is defined as the systemic inflammatory response to infection, manifested by two or more of the SIRS criteria.
- Innate immunity provides the first line of defence against pathogens (PAMPS) and danger signals (DAMPS) released from damaged tissue via PRRs, and epithelial barriers.
- Cytokines (e.g. IL-1, IL-6, IFN-γ, TNF-α) and chemokines (e.g. IL-8), components of SIRS, are believed to mediate many of the systemic and local proinflammatory effects of sepsis.
- Anti-inflammatory cytokines (e.g. IL-10, TGF-β) appear to tolerize or suppress leucocyte function during sepsis. This response often develops concomitantly with SIRS in the septic patient.
- Complement and the coagulation cascades are phylogenetically related and appear to contribute to the septic immune, vascular, and/or organ dysfunction.
- Monocytes/macrophages are significant producers of pro-/anti-inflammatory mediators; they have important regulatory and effector roles in the septic response.
- Neutrophils (short-lived effector cells of the innate immune response) have been shown to be dysfunctional in bacterial handling; their apoptotic response is suppressed while their respiratory burst activity and cell adherent capacity are potentiated during sepsis, contributing to cell and organ injury.
- Sepsis appears to differentially activate NK cells and various regulatory lymphoid T cell subsets; however, their significance is unclear.
- Sepsis induces the apoptotic loss of T and B lymphocytes along with DCs. This may contribute to immune suppression and the inability to overcome the septic challenge.
- The vascular endothelium helps to maintain a balance locally between pro-/anti-inflammatory mediators and between pro-/anticoagulant factors.

- Current hypotheses proposed to explain the pathogenesis, morbidity and mortality of sepsis include: (1) overzealous (dysfunctional) SIRS; (2) inability to properly respond to septic pathogens due to development of immune dysfunction or suppression; (3) inappropriate induction of apoptosis in immune and/or nonimmune cells; (4) altered vascular–leucocyte interactions.
- Age, gender, and nutritional status are all important components and play a differential role in the pathogenesis of sepsis.
- The septic animal's immune response is determined at local tissue, organ, and systemic levels, not only by interactions with immune and nonimmune cells but also via interactions with the neuroendocrine system.
- Numerous animal models are available to mimic aspects of the inflammatory, cardiovascular, and metabolic responses observed in humans with sepsis.
- Source control and early empiric antibiotics remain essential in the management of sepsis.
- Despite successful animal studies, clinical trials with various anti-inflammatory agents have not been successful. Only the PROWESS trial, using activated protein C in patients with severe sepsis, has shown a significant decrease in mortality.

Background and basic concepts in sepsis

Until 1992, no clear consensus definition of sepsis had been formulated and documented in the literature to provide an accurate assessment of patients with this form of inflammatory response. Bone and colleagues convened a consensus conference to define this commonly used clinical term [1]. They determined that sepsis is the systemic response to infection. However, since a similar, or even identical, response can arise in the absence of infection a new term, systemic inflammatory response syndrome (SIRS), was introduced. SIRS was defined as being manifested by two or more of the following conditions:

- Temperature >38° C or <36° C
- Heart rate >90 beats/minute
- Respiratory rate >20 breaths/minute or $PaCO_2$ <32 mmHg
- White blood cell count >12 000 cells/mm^3, or <4000 cells/mm^3, or >10% immature (band) cells in the peripheral blood smear.

Sepsis was then defined to be the systemic response to infection, manifested by two or more of the SIRS criteria. The term *septic shock* was characterized as sepsis associated with hypotension despite adequate fluid resuscitation, along with the presence of perfusion abnormalities that may include, but not limited to lactic acidosis, oliguria, or an acute change in mental status. Subsequently, the term *severe sepsis* came to be associated with organ dysfunction, hypoperfusion, or hypotension. Lastly, the term *multiple organ dysfunction syndrome* (MODS) was described as the presence of altered organ function in an acutely ill patient such that homeostasis cannot be maintained without intervention. These terms provided definable phases for the continuum of severity that an infection may pose to an individual patient [1] (see Figure 5.1).

Through multiple epidemiological studies, sepsis has been found to be common, fatal, and expensive. It is estimated that there are over 750 000 cases annually in the USA, with an associated mortality ranging from 18% to 44% [2–4]. As a consequence of this common and fatal disease process, the USA spends an estimated $17 billion annually on dealing with this major and very serious problem [2]. One promising trend is that, although the incidence is increasing along with the number of deaths, the mortality rate is decreasing, perhaps as much as 1% per year [4].

Given the importance of this disease, the causes and pathogenesis of sepsis remain an area of very active research. The causes are complex, but can include practically any infectious organism. These organisms, which include bacteria, viruses, parasites, and fungi, contain a limited number of unique cellular substances not found in mammalian animals. These substances are referred to as pathogen-associated molecular patterns (PAMPs) (see Figure 5.2). On the host side, the initial responses to these pathogens are from the innate immune system. The initial host response during infection is through different classes of pattern recognition receptors (PRRs), which bind to the conserved PAMPs of the microbe.

Several investigators have found that these exogenous signals (PAMPs) are not the only trigger of this initial inflammatory response. In fact, in response to cellular injury, endogenous mediators termed danger-associated molecular patterns (DAMPs) and/or alarmins, which include heat shock proteins (HSPs), fibrinogen, fibronectin, hyaluran, biglycans, and high mobility group box-1 (HMGB-1), are released to activate innate immunity through augmentation of PRR expression [5] (see Figure 5.2).

Importantly, what is becoming clear is that in many ways it is the patient's (or animal's) own immune response to these mediators that appears to contribute to not

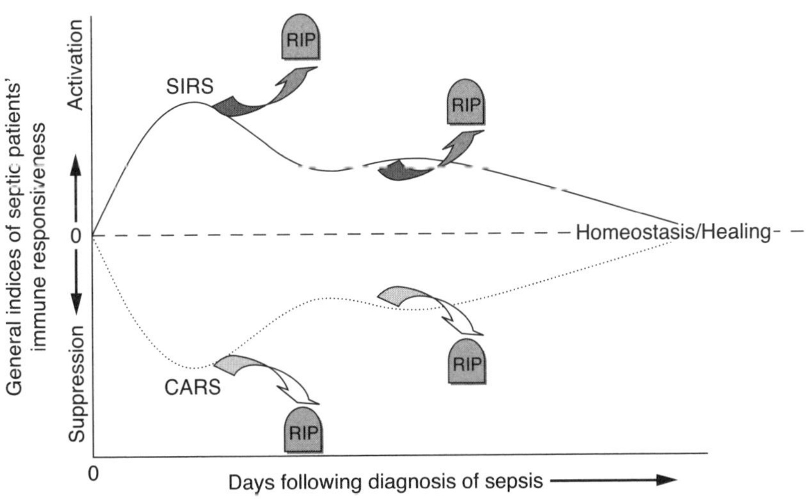

Fig. 5.1 General SIRS/CARS response over time, relative to the normal homeostatic/healed state of the patient in response to septic insults; RIP represents points at which patients might die. CARS, compensatory anti-inflammatory response syndrome; SIRS, systemic inflammatory response syndrome.

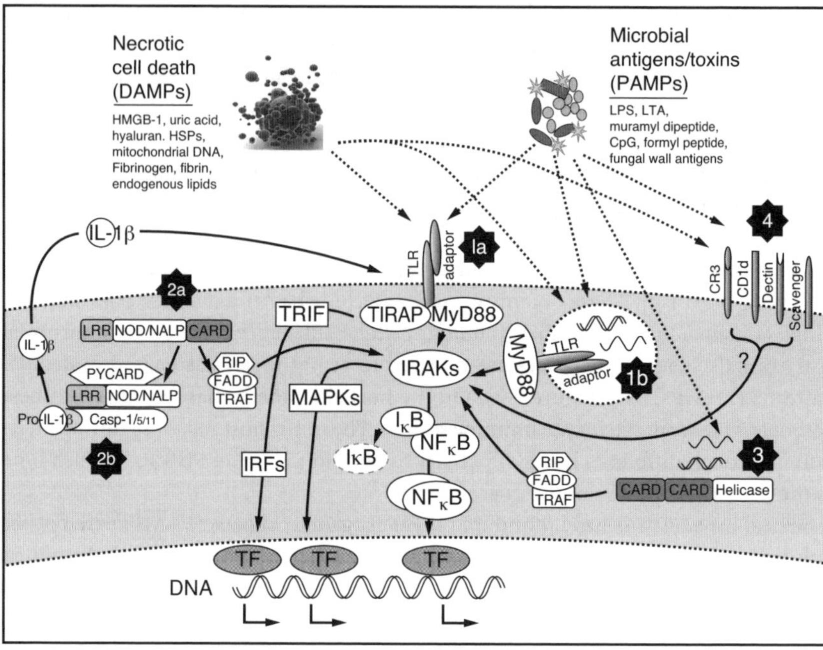

Fig. 5.2 PAMPs, DAMPs, and primary PPRs families: 1a, cell surface TLRs; 1b, endosomal TLRs; 2a, NOD/NALP cytoplasmic sensing; 2b, NOD/NALP-inflammasome/IL-1β; 3, helicase-RIG cytoplasmic RNA-DNA sensing; 4, various other potential PRRs, e.g. dectin, C3b, scavenger receptors, CD1d. CpG, cytosine phosphate–guanine; DAMP, danger/damage-associated molecular pattern; HMGB-1, high mobility group box-1 (protein); HSP, heat shock protein; IRAK, interleukin receptor-associated kinase; LPS, lipopolysaccharide; LTA, leukotriene A; NOD, nucleotide-oligomerization domain; PAMP, pathogen-associated molecular pattern; PRR, pattern recognition receptor; RIG, retinoic acid-inducible gene 1; TF, tissue factor; TLR, Toll-like receptor.

only the development of the septic state, but more significantly, to the condition of severe septic shock and MODS. In this chapter we attempt to delineate not only how elements of the innate and adaptive immune response may contribute to the altered immune response to septic stimuli but also how they are reshaped by insult (or how various predispositional states may actually increase the individual's chances of developing sepsis), and how such aberrations in immune responsiveness translate into severe tissue damage and MODS.

Innate immunity and sepsis

Introduction

Innate immunity provides the first line of defence against pathogens, both in its role as a barrier (via cells of the epithelium—mucosa and skin) and its ability to be activated immediately upon challenge by a pathogen or noxious agent. As already mentioned, cells of the innate immune system recognize foreign pathogens or endogenous 'danger signals' via PRRs, which readily activate an inflammatory response.

Innate immune response in sepsis

PPRs and SIRS

To date, primarily three families of PRRs have been described: (1) Toll-like receptors (TLRs); (2) nucleotide-oligomerization domain leucine-rich repeat (NOD-LRR) proteins; and (3) cytoplasmic caspase activation and recruiting domain helicases such as retinoic acid-inducible gene I (RIG-I)-like helicases (RLHs) (see Figure 5.2). Together, they sense danger signals through direct or indirect antigen binding, stimulate specific signaling pathways, and trigger activation of NF-κB and other transcription factors and gene regulatory systems that up-regulate the expression of proinflammatory mediators. The extent of this pathway activation appears to be, in large part, dependent on the expression levels of various TLRs on the surface of cells involved in innate immunity—neutrophils, macrophages, natural killer (NK) cells, dendritic cells (DCs), and vascular endothelial cells. In this respect, TLR expression is significantly upregulated in experimental models of sepsis and in patients with sepsis [6]. Alternatively, cytoplasmic PRRs exist to detect invasive intracellular pathogens. However, the NOD proteins also recognize common fragments of bacterial peptidoglycan (see Figure 5.2). In sepsis, multiple positive feedback loops between DAMPs and their multiple receptors are thought to temporally and spatially drive the process of an imbalanced inflammatory response [6]. In tissues, cells are concomitantly exposed to multiple stimuli that act in synergy leading to the production of further inflammatory mediators, which include cytokines, chemokines, and complement proteins, as well as cell surface adhesion molecules. Inflammatory and immune cells are activated in response to these inflammatory mediators, they in turn release powerful secondary mediators, such as reactive oxygen species (ROSs) and reactive nitrogen species (RNSs) that are thought to further amplify the inflammatory process.

Compensatory anti inflammatory response syndrome

A compensatory anti-inflammatory response syndrome (CARS) is initiated (sometimes concomitantly during the initiation of SIRS) in an attempt to damp the ongoing inflammatory response (see Figure 5.1). The CARS is not thought to be as generalized a pathophysiological process as SIRS, but rather appears to drive a reprogramming of many leucocyte subpopulations (this is sometimes also called tolerance, immune suppression, or anergy). CARS was initially purported to be an adaptive compartmentalized response with the proposed purpose of switching off acute proinflammatory genes leading to resolution of the inflammatory immune response, while maintaining the possible expression of genes involved in the anti-infectious process. However, this appears to depend on the context and compartment (blood versus tissues), the type of insult (primary or secondary), and the nature of the mediators and leucocytes that are involved (see Chapter 2).

Pro- and anti-inflammatory mediators in sepsis

Cytokines and chemokines

Tumour necrosis factor-alpha (TNF-α and interleukin-1 (IL-1) are historically the best studied and appear to be major proinflammatory cytokines produced during the initial and early phase of the inflammatory response and the SIRS. They have been shown in both *in vivo* animal models and *in vitro* cell cultures to be able to activate target cells and induce the production of numerous proinflammatory mediators, such as cytokines (e.g. interferon-gamma [IFN-γ], IL-6, IL-8, IL-12, IL-17, macrophage inhibitory factor [MIF]), chemokines (IL-8, macrophage inflammatory protein [MIP-1, -2], monocyte chemotactic protein [MCP-1], thymus activation-regulated chemokine (TARC); ROSs; RNSs; eicosanoids; and proteolytic enzymes. Target cells include virtually all leucocytes, endothelial cells, epithelial cells, and organ-specific cell types such as hepatocytes and fibroblasts. As already mentioned, during the course of inflammation, an anti-inflammatory CARS response develops, made up of anti-inflammatory cytokines and mediators, such as IL-10, transforming growth factor-beta (TGF-β), IL-1 receptor antagonist (IL-1Ra), soluble TNF receptors (sTNFRs), glucocorticoids, and eicosanoids, which are capable of inhibiting the production of IL-1 and TNF-α. Cytokines produced by local immune cells like macrophages and DCs can increase the local production of antimicrobial products that provide host defence at skin and epithelial cell surfaces.

Many cell types, including lymphocytes, fibroblasts, and monocytes, produce IL-6. This cytokine has a variety of biological effects including activation of B and T lymphocytes, proliferative effects, and induction of acute-phase protein production in the liver. Many studies in humans have demonstrated that plasma IL-6 concentrations in sepsis correlate closely with severity and outcome of the sepsis [7]. However, although IL-6 appears to show promise as a prognostic or diagnostic marker in the critically ill septic animal or patient [8], the infusion of IL-6 into human volunteers and experimental animals does not induce a sepsis-like state, as seen with infusion of TNF-α and IL-1β [9]. This reduces its significance as a potential causative explanation for the pathophysiological changes seen in the septic state.

MIF is a special regulatory cytokine with a unique protein structure and its receptor is distinct from other cytokine receptor families. It is constitutively expressed and stored in intracellular pools and does not require *de novo* synthesis before secretion. It is produced by a wide spectrum of cells, including DCs, monocytes, macrophages, lymphocytes, neutrophils, eosinophils, basophils, and mast cells, in virtually all non-immune mucosal cell types and tissues that are in direct contact with the external environment, such as cells lining the respiratory, gastrointestinal, and genitourinary tracts, and the skin. MIF antagonizes glucocorticoids and sustains the inflammatory response through enhanced production of cytokines, nitric oxide (NO), matrix metalloproteinases (MMPs), and prostaglandins (PGs) [10,11].

IL-10 is a potent anti-inflammatory cytokine that mediates leucocyte deactivation during sepsis. It is produced by an activated T helper 2 (Th2) subset of $CD4^+$ and T regulatory cells (Tregs), B cells, monocytes, and several structural nonimmune cells. IL-10 can upregulate other regulatory molecules and/or receptors, including IL-1ra, CD32, and chemokine receptor 1 (CCR1) and CCR5 expression. During sepsis, while the expression of early inflammatory response cytokines is often rapid and transient, the expression of IL-10 is more prolonged and often sustained. Monocytes isolated from septic patients retain their ability to produce IL-10, even though their ability to produce proinflammatory cytokines appears impaired. Moreover, elevations of blood monocyte IL-10 mRNA expression or plasma IL-10 levels may be of prognostic significance, as high IL-10 expression is associated with worse outcomes in paediatric patients with sepsis [12].

IL-17A, the first described member of the IL-17 family, is produced by Th17 cells, neutrophils, $CD8^+$ T cells, NK cells, other Th cell subsets, and $\gamma\delta$ T cells. It can trigger the production of many other cytokines, such as IL-1β, IL-6, and TNF, thus, providing cross-talk between lymphocytes and phagocytes. It has been shown that increased IL-17A levels have adverse effects during experimental sepsis; however, it is not yet known whether levels of IL-17A are increased in patients with sepsis [13].

The CXC chemokine IL-8 (the homologues of which are MIP-2 and KC in the mouse as well as cytokine-induced neutrophil chemoattractant [CINC] in the rat) is produced by mononuclear phagocytes, neutrophils, lymphocytes, endothelial cells, epithelial cells, and a variety of mesothelial cell types in response to various stimuli, including endotoxin, IL-1β and TNF-α. The primary function of IL-8 is to activate and chemoattract neutrophils to the site of tissue damage and inflammation. Neutrophils respond to IL-8 by changing shape, adhering (due to the up-regulation of various adhesion molecules) to endothelial cells and increasing production of ROSs. However, although the infusion of IL-8 into human volunteers does not cause septic shock, it does induce recruitment and activation of neutrophils (as access in an *ex vivo* setting). This latter aspect, which is often referred to as *neutrophil priming* and has been proposed as a mechanism that could lead to tissue damage, assuming the granulocytes see appropriate secondary stimuli *in vivo*. In septic patients, the plasma concentration of IL-8 has been reported to peak at 3–4 hours after the initial diagnosis of severe septic shock and the concentrations of circulating IL-8 appeared to correlate with worse outcomes [14].

Certain chemokines, particularly chemokines belonging to the CC chemokine family, have been causally linked to impaired leucocyte responsiveness. For example; TARC (CCL17) and the macrophage-derived chemokine MDC/CCL22 are reported to be expressed in high concentrations by alternatively activated macrophages (cells activated by IL-4 and IL-13) and can thus serve as markers of this alternatively activated phenotype in macrophages [15]. It has also been shown that shedding of key activating chemokine receptors by various leucocyte subpopulations in sepsis may lead to impaired chemokine responsiveness of these cells [16].

HMGB-1, which has been described as a DAMP and/or alarmin, has been recently shown to be a weak proinflammatory mediator [17]. However, the effects of HMGB-1 can be strengthened by binding various other molecules, such as the bacterial lipid molecule CpG-DNA [17], which appear to potentiate the actions of both mediators' effects on the immune cell target. Alternatively, when HMGB-1 is released in large quantities into the extracellular environment, it becomes a lethal mediator of systemic inflammation. This relates to its better-described role as a DAMP or alarmin, released from necrotic or late apoptotic-necrotic dying cells (see Figure 5.2). Importantly, HMGB-1 plasma levels in intensive care patients correlated with the disseminated intravascular coagulation (DIC) score and sepsis-related multiple organ failure (MOF). HMGB-1 is produced by stressed, damaged, or dying cells (via apoptosis and necrosis, resulting in cellular disintegration and possibly autophagy), and in some cases by macrophages and other immune cells, where it is thought to be actively secreted [18]. It also induces DC maturation and migration of cells of the immune system to the site of injury, as well as stimulates their release of cytokines and other inflammatory mediators [19].

It is worth noting that the number and nature of known endogenous host cell molecules that can serve as endogenous DAMPs and alarmins is growing rapidly. Some examples are uric acid, hyaluran, some of the HSP family members, fibrinogen, fibronectin, and certain endogenous lipids (see Figure 5.2). The challenge from an immunological as well as from a septic organ injury perspective will be to determine how these endogenous DAMPs and alarmins, which often share the same stimulatory PRRs, TLRs, etc., can define and interact with a foreign pathogenic challenger [20].

Complement and coagulation cascade

Complement and coagulation, major components of the plasma cascades, are phylogenetically related and both contribute to inflammation. They are activated in a sequential manner by common stimuli and mutually interact at several biological steps.

Complement acts as both a PRR system and an effector system. Generally, the antibacterial properties of complement may be divided into three categories: (1) opsonization, which contributes to phagocytosis and subsequent killing of the pathogens via the membrane attack complex (MAC); (2) promotion and expansion; (3) coordination of inflammatory events by the anaphylatoxins C3a and C5a.

Tissue factor (TF) is a key initiator of the coagulation cascade and is produced in response to proinflammatory cytokine activation of endothelial cells and mononuclear cells. The release of thrombin further amplifies the production of proinflammatory mediators. In addition, the function of anticoagulation pathways that prevent systemic activation of coagulation under normal conditions appears also to be impaired during sepsis, further perpetuating inflammation-induced activation of coagulation. Thus, activation of coagulation in critical illness often leads to DIC. Binding of coagulation proteases to protease-activated receptors (PARs) is thus an important mechanism in the modulation of inflammation by coagulation. For instance, binding of thrombin and TF–factor VIIa complex to their respective PARs enhances production of proinflammatory cytokines. Conversely, thrombomodulin and activated protein C exhibit marked anti-inflammatory properties. The latter is thought to be a basis for some of the protective effects of activated protein C (APrC) in the severely ill patient in septic shock [21].

Thrombin can cleave C3 and C5 of the complement cascade. C5a, in turn, can amplify the expression of TF. One complement component, mannan-binding serine protease 2, can also promote the conversion of prothrombin to thrombin. The binding of coagulation proteases or anticoagulant proteins to their receptors on mononuclear cells or vascular endothelium may affect cytokine production, as well as inflammation-induced apoptosis.

Defensins and antimicrobial peptides

Antimicrobial peptides are defined as ribosomal-derived proteins containing 12–50 amino acids, with 2–9 positively charged lysine (Lys) or arginine (Arg) residues and up to 50% hydrophobic amino acids, that have microbicidal activity [22]. They show an exceptionally broad spectrum of activity, ranging from Gram-negative and Gram-positive bacteria to fungi and viruses. In humans, two major classes of antimicrobial peptides, defensins and cathelicidin, have been described. hCAP-18/LL-37, the only endogenous human cathelicidin-18 identified to date, is a major protein of the specific granules in neutrophils. It also occurs in monocytes, human keratinocytes, and airway epithelia. Defensins make up 30–50% of the granule proteins in human neutrophils and can structurally be defined as α- and β-defensins; α-defensins are mainly produced by neutrophils and intestinal Paneth cells, whereas β-defensins are primarily expressed by epithelial cells of the skin, urinary tract, and tracheobronchial lining. There is constitutive production of β-defensins at sites such as epithelial tissues that are steadily exposed to potentially infectious microbes, i.e. the external milieu. Secretion is induced by the contact of cells with microbes and proinflammatory mediators.

Lipid mediators

High density lipoprotein (HDL), low density lipoprotein (LDL), and very low density lipoprotein (VLDL) can bind and neutralize the bioactivity of bacterial components, such as lipopolysaccharide (LPS) and lipoteichoic acid (LTA). However, during sepsis, circulating levels of HDL decline dramatically, resulting in elevated circulating LPS levels. This is thought to be due not only to the loss of the inhibitory effects of the LPS–HDL interaction, but also as LPS has been shown to bind alternatively to LDL and VLDL. Native HDL also can suppress the inhibitory activity of LPS binding protein (LBP), which may contribute to its proinflammatory property by enhancing monocyte responses to LPS [23].

Reactive oxygen species and reactive nitrogen species

ROSs and RNSs are pivotal to the defence against invading pathogens. However, overwhelming production of ROSs and RNSs results in oxidative and nitrosative stress, respectively; key elements in the deleterious processes of sepsis. Increased activity of xanthine oxide, one important contributor to ROS production, has been reported to be elevated in adult and paediatric patients with sepsis. Depleted levels of reduced glutathione, an important intramitochondrial antioxidant, in combination with excess generation of ROSs and RNSs, severely inhibit oxidative phosphorylation and ATP generation. Proinflammatory mediators can also activate NADP oxidase to produce superoxide radicals (O_2^-). Myeloperoxidase from neutrophil azurophilic granules produces hypochlorous acid from hydrogen peroxide (H_2O_2) and chloride anions (Cl^-) are released during the respiratory burst. These free radicals are highly cytotoxic and, thus, neutrophils use them to damage and destroy pathogens. O_2^- in the presence of NO generates peroxynitrite ($ONOO^-$), which can cause DNA strand breakage and initiate lipid peroxidation, changing the functions of ion channels, cell signalling proteins, receptors, enzymes, and transcription factors; it is, therefore, thought to play an important role in the pathogenesis of sepsis [5].

NO is produced as a proinflammatory mediator in response to inflammatory stimuli. NO has an uneven number of electrons but is relatively unreactive in physiological concentrations. NO maintains normal homeostasis by reducing leucocyte adhesion, platelet aggregation, relaxation of vascular smooth muscle, and preservation of mucosal integrity. At high concentrations, NO is harmful because it generates vasodilation and increases vascular permeability. NO inhibits mitochondrial respiration which leads to decreased ATP synthesis, which may trigger apoptosis. Unfortunately, although the experimental case for these molecules in the pathogenesis of tissue injury appears quite strong, neither antioxidant nor antinitrosative approaches have, as yet, shown any efficacy in patients with sepsis.

Small molecules

Excessive depletion of ATP along with the concordant rise of adenosine levels has been suggested to impact significantly not only on cellular metabolic and physiological homeostasis and cell death but also on leucocyte function, as well as inflammation in response to various experimental septic stimuli. It is thought to play a role in both immune and nonimmune organ dysfunction via activation of a diverse family of purogenic receptors. Here again, neither inhibitors of the effects of adenosine nor supplementation with ATP has shown significant clinical relevance [24].

Cellular components of innate immune response in sepsis

Monocytes and macrophages

Circulating monocytes can, according to their phenotype and external stimuli, either migrate to the site of inflammation, differentiate into DCs, or colonize different organs as tissue macrophages. Monocytes and macrophages are the most effective producers of pro- and anti-inflammatory mediators—cytokines, chemokines, defensins, lipid mediators, ROSs, and RNSs (see Figure 5.3). The characteristics of circulating monocytes are greatly influenced by the margination and sequestration of any activated cells and the enhancement of haematopoiesis. The status of monocytes appears to be modified during sepsis and SIRS, as assessed by *ex vivo* functional measurements, such as oxidative burst capacity, cytokine production, or HLA-DR expression at the cell surface. Oxidative burst in monocytes from the circulation exposed to phorbol myristate acetate (PMA) is significantly attenuated in septic patients. Also, the altered *ex vivo* cytokine production (upon *in vitro* activation) of circulating monocytes in septic patients has been well documented. Blood monocytes from such patients demonstrate a diminished capacity to release TNF-α, IL-1α, IL-1β, IL-6, and IL-12. Importantly, the impaired capacity of these monocytes to produce inflammatory cytokines in response to LPS has been described in numerous clinical settings, including different types of bacterial, viral, and parasitic infections, SIRS, or severe organ dysfunction. However, the capacity of blood monocytes from septic patients to produce and secrete other cytokines (IL-1ra, IL-10, MIF) is not changed, and may even be enhanced, with or without other stimuli instead of LPS. Thus, there is likely no global cellular defect in the *ex vivo* cytokine production, but rather a specific alteration of the production of some inflammatory cytokines in response to select

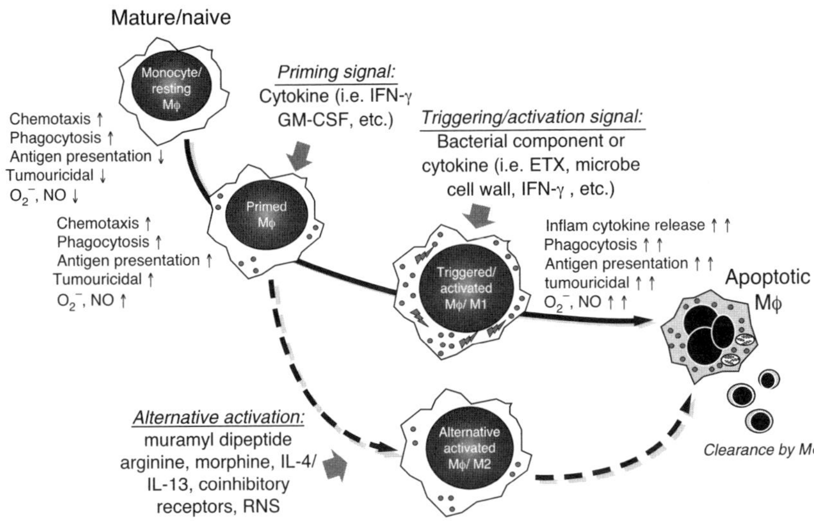

Fig. 5.3 Postulated steps at which the process of immune cell activation/differentiation might be inhibited by various agents associated with the resolution of a response to foreign antigen in a macrophage (Mφ) and/or lead to alternative macrophage activation. AG, antigen; ETX, endotoxin; GM-CSF, granulocyte-macrophage colony stimulating factor; RNS, reactive nitrogen species.

stimuli. The term *reprogramming* is therefore often used to define these modifications more appropriately [25].

The reduced expression of major histocompatability complex (MHC) class II (HLA-DR) molecules on monocytes is also a hallmark of the response to sepsis and SIRS and has been reported to correlate directly with the severity of sepsis. The down-regulation is more pronounced in superinfected trauma patients and is associated with a poor outcome. Decreased HLA-DR expression is found in a number of other cell types, as well as in the amount of HLA-DR expressed per cell. Furthermore, even though the decreased HLA-DR expression appears universal in septic patients, its evolution over time can distinguish between survivors and nonsurvivors. Continued decrease in HLA-DR expression is most evident in the nonsurvivors group [26,27] (see Figure 5.3).

Several recent studies in animal models of sepsis and patients suggest that while HLA-DR/MHC class II molecules appear to decline on these cells, much like the situation with cytokine production, these cells may be up-regulating the expression of various coinhibitory (but not so much costimulatory) molecules, such as cytotoxic T lymphocyte antigen-4 (CTLA-4), PD-1, and CD47. The rise in these latter ligands has been documented in monocytes and other cells in severely septic and/or injured patients and animals [27–29]. Although the significance of these changes is not clear, they may be indicative or diagnostic of the developing dysfunction and anergy in host immune defences, as often described in both animals and patients with severe sepsis.

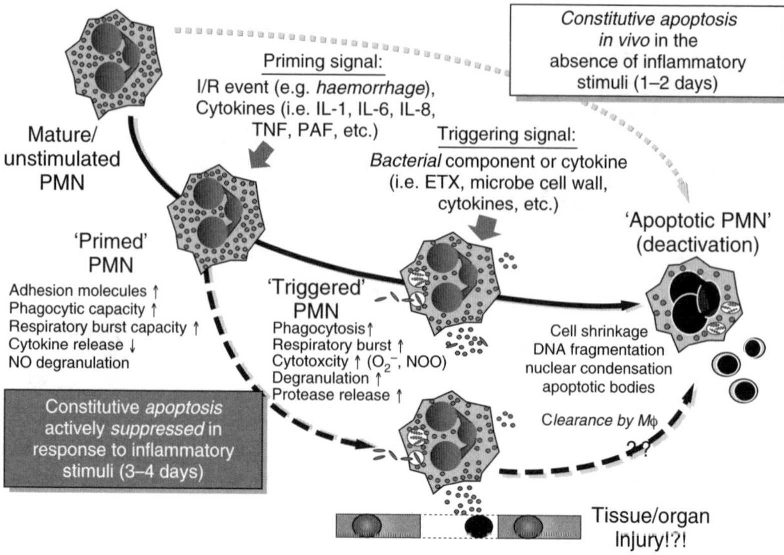

Fig. 5.4 Postulated steps at which the process of immune cell activation/differentiation might be inhibited by various agents associated with the resolution of a response to foreign antigen in neutrophils (PMN). ETX, endotoxin; PAF, platelet activating factor; TNF, tumour necrosis factor.

Neutrophils

Neutrophils are the major cellular contributors to the early and active innate immune response elicited in sepsis (see Figure 5.4). Their capacity for phagocytosis of foreign pathogens and molecules exceeds that of macrophages, but their capacity for synthesizing RNA and proteins is quite low. Neutrophils possess numerous granules and vesicles rich in antimicrobial proteins, proteases, and enzymes which can be used for degradation of cellular structures during migration and subsequent lodgement in various tissues. They are also short-lived cells, which mature in blood and are programmed to die typically within 24–48 hours after leaving the bone marrow. They also favour a procoagulant state and are rich in membrane receptors utilized in phagocytosis and membrane trafficking. Neutrophils are the major source of oxidants including ROSs and RNSs, which are highly cytotoxic (see Figure 5.4).

Since infection is associated with marked stimulation of haematopoiesis, the functions of circulating neutrophils in septic patients can be suppressed, enhanced, and/or 'primed'. Alteration in neutrophil phenotype, similar to those observed in monocytes and macrophages described above, can be observed during sepsis. Some of the specific defects reported in neutrophils isolated from septic animal models include impairments in migration, adherence, inflammatory cytokine (e.g. IL-1β, IL-1ra, IL-8) production and H_2O_2 generation. In humans with sepsis, functionally significant down-regulation of the chemokine receptor CXCR2 has been observed [25].

The highly proapoptotic nature of neutrophils is also pivotal for maintaining a balance between antimicrobial effectiveness and the antimicrobial-associated damage (see Figure 5.4). The reduced apoptosis of neutrophils is a hallmark of sepsis and SIRS, potentially contributing to cell and organ damage and dysfunction [25]. Neutrophils from patients with sepsis manifest markedly prolonged survival *in vitro* in association with evidence of cellular activation and/or 'priming' for enhanced oxidant production. Such capacity may contribute to the destruction of foreign pathogens; if misdirected and not regulated, this results in injury to host tissues where the neutrophils migrate to and reside (see Chapter 2).

Dendritic cells

DCs are critical cells bridging the generation between the innate and adaptive immune responses elicited. They are not only affected (dysfunctional, destroyed) by SIRS but also contribute to the development of immune suppression seen during sepsis (see Figure 5.5). It has been shown that DCs are required for mice to survive sepsis and this is supported by two clinical observations indicating that a decrease in DCs is associated with a poor outcome. Apoptosis may be one fundamental mechanism of DC loss. Evidence delineating the extent to which the DCs also serve as an important bridge between innate and adaptive immune responses in sepsis is limited. The up-regulation of inhibitory IL-10 production and down-regulation of stimulating IL-12 secretion seen in DCs derived from septic mice points to a potential mechanism of suppression by humoral mechanisms [30].

NK cells

NK cells have a cytotoxic function and the ability to produce cytokines and chemokines. Although they can recognize danger signals through PRRs, their processing and full activation depends on signals derived from accessory cells, such as DCs, monocytes, and macrophages. Activated NK cells are one of the main sources of IFN-γ during acute septic shock [19]. IFN-γ potentiates the ability of macrophages, monocytes and DCs for production of inflammatory cytokines (e.g. TNF-α, IL-1, IL-12, IL-18) that can feed back and further stimulate NK cells. In patients with septic shock, increased cytotoxic cell function has been correlated with an increasing mortality rate and deteriorating organ function.

Innate regulatory $\gamma\delta$ T and NK T cells

$\gamma\delta$ T cells and natural killer T (NK T) cells are usually classified as innate regulatory T lymphocytes and are often considered to be a component of the first line of defence against infection because they can respond to a select group of highly defined antigens, via their PPRs (see Figures 5.2 and 5.6). $\gamma\delta$ T cells recognize antigens presented by MHC class I-like molecules such as CD1 (see Figures 5.2 and 5.6), which does not require formal cellular antigen presentation and processing (see Chapter 1). PAMPs, LPS, TNF-α, or superantigens can also activate $\gamma\delta$ T cells. Once localized in tissues (primarily in the GIT, lungs, and skin), $\gamma\delta$ T cells (resident and/or recruited) appear to play a major role, not only in the development of a regional mucosal immune response through the induction of a local proinflammatory response but also via the recruitment of neutrophils. The observation that $\gamma\delta$ T cell deficiency can have divergent effects on mortality in studies of polymicrobial sepsis in mice suggests that the contribution of these cells to the immune response in sepsis may be different in the earlier

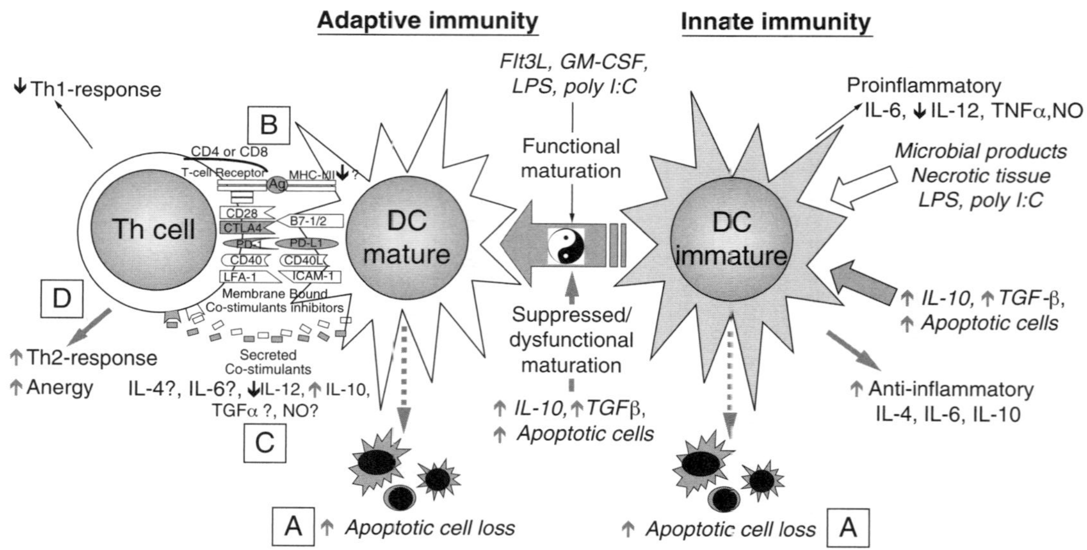

Fig. 5.5 The DC:T cell interaction plays a major role in determining the type of T lymphocyte immune response to be developed after an antigen challenge. This is highly dependent on initial stimuli present at the time of DC maturation. On the one hand, inflammatory stimuli such as microbial products may induce proinflammatory cytokine production by DCs (IL-12) as well as up-regulation of costimulatory receptors on their surface (B7–1/2). This may lead to a shift towards the Th1 type of immune response. On the other hand, anti-inflammatory/deactivating stimuli may induce incomplete maturation of DCs, their production of anti-inflammatory cytokines (IL-10) and expression of regulatory receptors such as PD-L1 at their surface. This type of stimulation may rather induce a Th2 type of immune response; this latter quiescent/suppressive state is the default condition for the DC normally. After sepsis, DCs exhibit several alterations of both their phenotype and function: (A) increased apoptosis of both mature and immature DCs; (B) changes in surface molecule expressions; (C) changes in cytokine production, and; (D) impairment in capacity to induce Th1 type/proinflammatory T cell activation. DC, dendritic cell; Flt-3L, Fms-like tyrosine kinase ligand 3; GM-CSF, granulocyte-macrophage colony stimulating factor; LPS, lipopolysaccharide.

than in the later phases of this response, and may also be dependent on the strength of the injury. Therefore, it is unclear at this point how the balance of immunoprotective versus immunopathogenic effects of $\gamma\delta$ T cells after sepsis and tissue damage relates to eventual clinical outcomes, and whether these cells can eventually become a useful clinical therapeutic target in the future.

In contrast to conventional cytotoxic T lymphocytes (CTLs), the majority of NK T cells express invariant T cell receptor alpha (TCR-α) chains associated with a variety of β-chains, and the most widely studied is the Va14/Ja281 subset in mice and Va24/JaQ in humans. As such, these cells are often referred to as 'invariant NK T cells'. NK T cells recognize and kill target cells expressing lipid antigens presented by the MHC I-like molecule designated as CD1d (see Figure 5.2). Thus, they recognize antigens usually ignored by conventional effector $\alpha\beta$ T cells. The type of invariant NK T cell response after an antigenic stimulation varies depending on the strength of the antigenic signal and the cytokine background in which the antigen is presented (see Chapter 1). The potential of NK T cells to produce pro- and anti-inflammatory cytokines provides them with the capacity to either promote or inhibit immune responses during sepsis. The results of the few studies published in animal models, to date, suggest that NK T cells appear to play a deleterious role in sepsis and might participate in the induction of immune dysfunction [31].

Nonprofessional immune cell effectors

Vascular endothelium is heterogeneous and its morphology and function is different in different organs—pulmonary and brain capillaries, hepatic and splenic sinusoids. Vascular endothelium can produce and be activated by inflammatory mediators. It also secretes vasoactive mediators to regulate vascular tone and permeability. The endothelium is anticoagulated under normal conditions. Thus, it maintains the local balance between pro- and anti inflammatory mediators as well as the balance between pro- and anticoagulant factors. During infection, activation of the endothelium induces increased leucocyte adhesiveness, a procoagulant surface, and reduced barrier function. Thus, it plays a critical role in recruitment of leucocytes from the blood to extravasate to sites of infection and tissue damage. (see Chapter 2).

Adaptive immune response in sepsis

$CD4^+/CD8^+$ T and B cells

As described above, relative to $\gamma\delta$ T and NK T cells, various lymphocyte populations are influenced by and contribute to diverse aspects of immune (innate) activation and the immunosuppressive effects seen in sepsis (see Figure 5.6). Regarding immune suppression, this effect may be directly due to a decrease in lymphocyte numbers (via apoptosis) and/or the active suppression of function, or indirectly due to changes in antigen presenting function (see Figure 5.7). Sepsis results in a substantial drop in the number of circulating lymphocytes. Lymphopenia develops early after the onset of sepsis and the persistence and magnitude of the lymphopenia can be correlated with the risk of nosocomial infection and death [32]. A substantial loss of splenic B cells, $CD4^+$ T cells, and follicular DCs has been observed in nonsurviving septic patients.

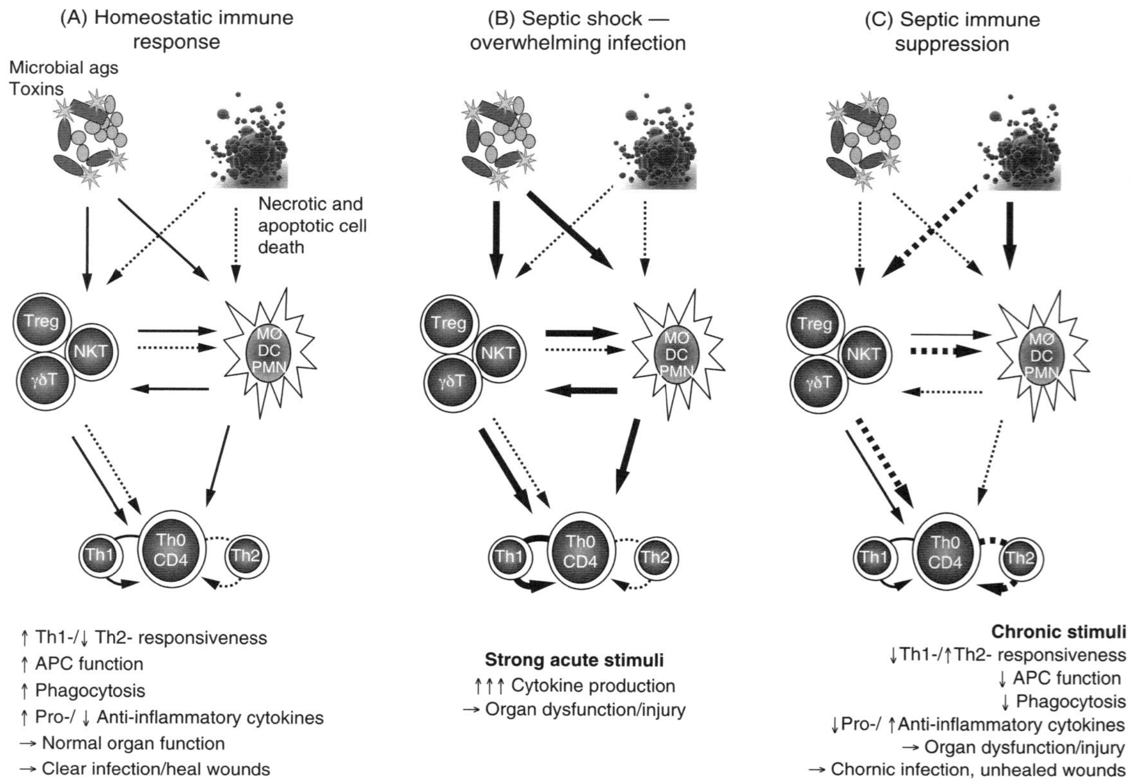

Fig. 5.6 Hypothetical mechanisms by which Treg, γδT, and NK T cell activation, in response to the diverse signal(s) derived from tissue injury and infectious microbial agents, leads to either: (A) clearance of the septic challenge (infection) and wound healing; (B) overzealous activation of innate immunity via overt NK T cell and/or Treg activation; or (C) immune suppression of $CD4^{+}$ Th1 cells via anergic/chronic stimulation of Tregs and/or NK T cells, and/or loss of γδ T cells. Solid lines indicate potentiation of immune response; dotted lines indicate regulation of immune response. APC, antigen-presenting cell; see text for definition of other abbreviations.

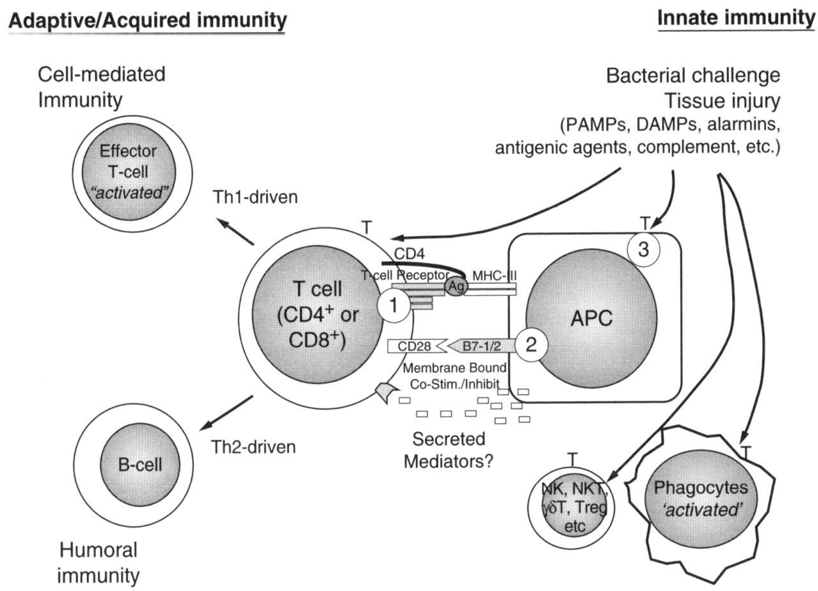

Fig. 5.7 Aspects of the process of T cell activation (signals 1–3) in the development of acquired immunity (either cell-mediated and/or humoral) in response to foreign antigen presented by an APC. APC, antigen-presenting cell; DAMP, danger/damage-associated molecular pattern; MHC, major histocompatibility complex; PAMP, pathogen-associated molecular pattern; see text for definition of other abbreviations.

The significance of such lymphocyte losses is indirectly supported by the observation of Hotchkiss *et al.* that *Rag*-deficient mice, which lack both mature and functional B and T cells, succumb rapidly to an experimental septic challenge [32].

However, studies have also consistently shown that sepsis results in anergy in patients and experimental animals as well as a shift in T cell cytokine responses, favouring a Th2, rather than Th1 phenotype response (at least in mice) [33,34]. It has also been shown that the effector/memory $CD8^+/CD45RO^+$ T lymphocyte subset in nonsurviving septic patients produced significantly less IFN-γ compared with that documented in survivors. *Ex vivo* T cell proliferative responses and cytokine production (IL-2, TNF-α) have also been found to be significantly depressed in patients with abdominal sepsis, as compared with healthy controls, and the degree of suppression of cytokine production directly correlated with patients' outcome. Some studies have also shown that the proportion of Th2 cells is increased in patients with sepsis, but not in nonseptic critically ill patients and healthy subjects [35]. Given the importance of the Th1 phenotype in maintaining an adequate adaptive response in immunity against pathogens, the shift from a predominantly Th1 to a Th2 phenotype has obvious implications for antimicrobial host immunity.

T regulatory cells

Tregs function as suppressors of $CD4^+$ and $CD8^+$ T cells, resulting in negative regulation of both innate and acquired immune responses. An increase in the percentage (but not absolute number) of Tregs ($CD4^+$ $CD25^+$ $FoxP3^+$) has been found in the blood, lymphatics, and spleen in septic mice, and in humans with sepsis. However, documenting their actual impact on survival in septic patients and animal models has proved controversial, with some studies showing no role and some indicating they are deleterious or protective [31].

Pathogenesis of septic shock and multiple organ failure

Introduction

Despite the intense research focus on sepsis, there is still no clearly defined aetiology explaining why some patients progress along the disease spectrum to MOF and eventual death while others, with seemingly equivalent condition(s) and/or preconditions, do not do so. Historically, the oldest hypotheses postulated that the septic individual's maladaptive response to the infectious agent and/or its components and toxins is central to the pathogenesis of sepsis. Clearly, the concept of removal of the septic source, as well as the efficacy provided by appropriate antibiotic therapy, focuses on the role of infection in the critically ill septic patient. However, over the years it has become clear that while many individuals benefit from such therapy, there remain those who do not. Upwards of 40% of critically ill and severely injured patients, defined as being septic and with MOF, do not exhibit overt evidence of infection and do not appear to benefit from the typical broad-spectrum antibiotics prescribed. Further, while therapies against microbial toxins, such as endotoxin and bacterial permeability factor, have been developed with the intention of inhibiting the progression of sepsis, none has yet proved efficacious clinically. However, in considering these microbial and/or toxin-driven hypotheses, it became clear experimentally that these agents also induced a substantial host response that could, via the actions of the host's own defence cells and associated mediators, produce a deleterious effect on organ function and survival. Thus, it was proposed that an exaggerated, hyperinflammatory systemic response occurs, which allows for uncontrolled inflammation-induced organ damage and sequential death. Here again, although numerous questions can be raised about clinical trial design in sepsis, the relative failure of anti-inflammatory agents, particularly inhibitors of TNF-α and IL-1β, to produce clear clinical benefit in septic patients has led researchers to question the theory that morbidity and mortality occurring in these patients is simply a result of an overactive hyperinflammatory response [36]. One feature of critically ill or severely injured patients, as well as aged individuals, who develop sepsis with or without MOF, is that while they exhibit aspects of inflammation, many of them often show substantial evidence of depression in the functions of both the innate and adaptive immune responses (see Figure 5.1). This paradox has led investigators to postulate that this decline in immune function leaves the patient vulnerable not only to developing sepsis but also to succumbing to it. This is similar to the situation in patients with AIDS or granulocytopenic disorders, or following active immune suppressive therapies [37]. However, as yet no therapies have been developed based on this hypothesis that have had overt clinical benefit. Thus, alternative explanations, including inappropriate activation of apoptosis, autophagy, various cellular dysfunctions, and coagulopathy, have all been proposed. Many of these concepts derive aspects of their genesis from the early hypotheses concerning infective agents and toxins, hyperinflammation, or immune suppression and anergy.

Multiple organ failure and mortality as a result of hyperinflammation

The predominant theory has been that sepsis causes an exuberant inflammatory response, which spirals out of control unchecked, with a resulting 'cytokine storm' that induces inflammation-associated organ damage. This postulate was based on initial observations of septic patients having elevated levels of various proinflammatory cytokines and animal model data that suggested this pathogenesis [38,39]. Success in blocking the various mediators in these animal models [40] made the hyperinflammatory theory even more promising as a possible new therapeutic strategy, mainly in terms of blocking TNF-α and IL-1β. Unfortunately, clinical trials using TNF-α blocking agents, as well as IL-1 receptor antagonists (IL-1ras), in humans with sepsis have largely been shown to be unsuccessful [41].

Multiple organ failure and mortality as a result of hypoinflammation

After the initial surge in release of proinflammatory mediators, as sepsis persists, a shift in the immune response occurs that is predominantly anti-inflammatory or even immunosuppressive [33]. It was noted in an early study that whole blood from patients with sepsis stimulated *ex vivo* with lipopolysaccharide (LPS) failed to mount a release of proinflammatory mediators (TNF-α, IL-1, and IL-6), as compared with healthy controls [42]. Related to this observation, it has been shown that septic patients who failed to mount an *ex vivo* LPS inflammatory response (producing TNF-α and IL-6) showed a significant increase in the amount of days on the ventilator, associated infections, and mortality [43]. Also, *ex vivo* stimulation of whole blood from septic patients versus healthy controls produced no difference in production of IL-10, an anti-inflammatory cytokine [44]. In fact, there have been several reports of increased levels of circulating IL-10 in septic patients [45]. The immunosuppressed state in sepsis is further strengthened by the observation that septic patients often succumb to hospital-acquired infections from organisms that are not so virulent to individuals with a normal immune system. Given these findings of an immunosuppressed state, clinical investigators have postulated that the use of immunostimulatory agents may improve outcomes in septic patients. One such multicentre double blind placebo-controlled study in over 700 patients with sepsis resulted in no harmful effects; however, there was no improvement in survival [46].

Multiple organ failure and mortality as a result of dysfunctional regulation of apoptosis

Another area of active research regarding the pathogenesis of sepsis includes the hypothesis that it is the inappropriate induction of apoptosis, leading to critical immune and, to a lesser extent nonimmune cell death, that may contribute to the development of the septic state and subsequently MOF. Several studies using animal models of sepsis have demonstrated the significance of apoptotic cell death [47]. An important study that demonstrated this effect in humans was based on autopsy studies in patients who died from sepsis, compared with those who died from other causes. This study showed an increase in apoptotic cell death in most organs along with lymphocytes and intestinal epithelial cells [48]. Perhaps more importantly, when this data was further analysed, the types of cells that were observed to be undergoing apoptosis were B cells, $CD4^+$ T cells, and DCs [32,49]. The loss of such key effector cells along with APCs during sepsis compromises both the innate and adaptive immune responses. Another potential link between immunosuppression and apoptosis is based on studies demonstrating that clearance of apoptotic cells by macrophages and DCs stimulates the release of IL-10 and TGF-β, along with suppressing the release of proinflammatory cytokines [50]. Given the evidence of apoptotic cell death being involved in experimental sepsis, investigators have tried to use this as a potential therapeutic target. In a murine model of sepsis, using caecal ligation and puncture, it was found that inhibition of Fas and/or caspase-8 by small interfering RNA (siRNA) significantly improved survival [51]. The complex pathways of apoptosis, along with the involvement of both the innate and adaptive immune response during the clearance of apoptotic cells, create a multifaceted network of mediators that may be therapeutically targeted.

Predispositional components

The multifaceted inflammatory response of sepsis is difficult to model, and when patient factors are considered as well it makes the whole experimental design even more complex.

As our population ages and our patients present with more severe illnesses, we will need to address age in our modelling of sepsis. Elderly patients are at increased risk of acquiring infections for various reasons, including but not limited to immunosenescence, general physiological decline, decreased mobility, and dementia. As well as their susceptibility to infections, older people have an increased risk of developing shock in response to a septic challenge as they have a decreased cardiopulmonary reserve, are more likely to be malnourished, and have a prolonged proinflammatory response leading to SIRS. Older patients also tend to have underlying medical problems, which makes the diagnosis more difficult and even leads to a delay in diagnosis and eventual treatment [52].

Another factor to consider in sepsis modelling is gender. Our understanding of the influences of sex hormones on immunity and tolerance to developing shock and MOF has continued to improve. Experimentally, it has been shown that female mice have a significant improvement in survival following a caecal ligation and puncture model of sepsis [53]. The initial suggestions from this data are that the differences between male and female hormonal profiles account for this. However, this is somewhat controversial, as clinical outcomes analysis has failed to consistently support some of these hypotheses. In a recent large study of trauma patients, female gender was found to be protective in both premenopausal and postmenopausal women, as regards the development of MOF and nosocomial infections [54]. This would imply that although a gender effect may be evident it might not be due to the beneficial effects of sexual hormones after trauma and/or sepsis (see Chapter 2).

It is well known in the surgical literature that poor preoperative nutritional status is associated with poorer postoperative outcomes [55]. Malnutrition and its relationship to immunity has been well studied and includes deficiencies in humoral and cell-mediated immunity, phagocytosis, complement system, cytokine production, coagulation dysfunction, and wound healing [56]. Numerous experimental studies have been done assessing the contribution of various nutritional components and supplements (e.g. ω-3 fatty acids, L-glutamine, zinc, probiotics), which document a potential role. These findings have been used to produce several immune-supportive diets (e.g. Impact, Immune-Aid™), for the clinical setting. While having no deleterious effect in critically ill septic or injured patients, they have as yet demonstrated no substantial benefit. Thus, the impact of malnourishment on the critically ill patient's immune response provides another possible confounding variable which needs to be considered in the development and pathogenesis of sepsis (see Chapter 6).

Another factor to consider, given its growing prevalence in the Western world, is obesity. Obesity has been evaluated in critically ill, septic patients as it relates to outcomes. Obese patients who have been admitted to the intensive care unit (ICU) have been found to have increased rates of developing sepsis, longer stays in the ICU, and more days on the ventilator [57,58]. Obesity has been found to be associated with a chronic low-grade inflammatory state with an increase in acute-phase reactants and proinflammatory cytokine release [59]. Adipose tissue is composed of various cell types, including macrophages. It is these macrophages that are thought to be responsible for high levels of TNF-α and IL-6 in obese patients [60]. Leptin, a protein secreted by adipose tissue, has been shown to protect lymphocytes from apoptosis and regulate their differentiation and cytokine production, along with effecting monocyte activation and phagocytosis [61]. Given these observations, it was attractive to suggest that leptin might play a central role in regulating the inflammatory state seen in adipose tissue associated with obesity. Thus, several clinical studies set out to determine if a correlation existed between leptin levels and septic mortality. Unfortunately, the data are conflicting; early studies demonstrated that higher circulating levels of leptin were seen in patients who succumb to sepsis [62], but a later study found it not to be independent of mortality in SIRS and MODS [63]. Hence, further studies are needed to properly evaluate the complexity of obesity, its impact on inflammation and immune responsiveness, and its contribution to septic morbidity and mortality (see Chapter 6).

Haemodynamic and vascular dysfunction in sepsis

Disseminated intravascular coagulation

Vascular endothelial cells are crucial to optimal vascular function and blood flow; they serve to regulate haemostasis, vasculogenesis, and angiogenesis. Importantly, increased endothelial cell apoptosis has been reported during sepsis and is believed to play an important role in the mortality of septic patients [64,65]. In the evolution of the inflammatory response, endothelial cells interact with cells of the innate immune system and their mediators in the circulation and respond by releasing and expressing proteins that mediate vascular endothelial cell permeability and adhesiveness, direct migrating leucocytes to inflamed tissues, and activate inflammation-induced coagulation. This latter response, while important in containing invading pathogens, is seen as playing an important role in the development of DIC, a significant complication of sepsis [66,67]. DIC is an inflammation-mediated syndrome associated predominately with vessels of the microcirculation. Schouten *et al.* give a clear and detailed review of our current understanding of the mechanisms and mediators effecting the endothelium and coagulation in sepsis [68].

In general, under normal, noninflammatory conditions the endothelium expresses an antithrombotic, anticoagulant phenotype. However, in a septic environment, this phenotype is altered; expression and exposure of TF by activated or damaged endothelial cells is one recognized explanation [69–71]. TF on endothelial cells (and circulating monocytes) complexes with factor VIIa in the blood and forms an enzyme that generates platelet-activating thrombin that also converts fibrinogen to fibrin. This cascade results in deposition of fibrin on vessel walls, formation of microthrombi, necrosis, MOD and, for some critically ill septic patients, death [66,72].

This scenario presents a complex set of issues in the treatment of the septic patient, and our progress in understanding the pathology of sepsis, with DIC and inflammation as components, appears contingent on preventing or suppressing vascular endothelial dysfunction and, as a result, microvascular dysfunction (see also Chapter 2 for coagulopathy and fibrinolysis in trauma patients).

Endothelial interface

The vascular endothelium is the interface between circulating systemic mediators and the tissues they perfuse. In response to inflammatory stimuli from the environment (TNF-α, IL-6, and IL-1) endothelial cells produce chemotactic proteins (chemokines such as IL-8 and MIP-1), that activate and direct localized recruitment of circulating leucocytes to infected and damaged tissue sites. Adhesion molecules, L-selectins (expressed on blood leucocytes), E-selectins, platelet activating factor (PAF), and P-selectin (on the surface of endothelial cells), and integrins and their respective ligands, serve to capture leucocytes and orchestrate their transmigration into the tissues. Leucocyte transmigration involves coordinated breaking and reforming of integrin and selectin bonds that serve to slow/tether and capture circulating neutrophils that traffic along chemokine gradients to sites of inflammation.

Most leucocytes appear to migrate between endothelial cells (paracellular migration), but a small percentage migrate through an individual cell (transcellular migration) [73]. This involves cytoskeletal rearrangements in the migrating cell to coordinate directional migration towards the junctions between endothelial cells and emigration to the apical surface of the endothelium [74]. A consequence of this process is augmentation of vascular permeability, with ensuing increases in tissue oedema and complement proteins, further aiding host defences [75].

In sepsis, however, these responses become proportionally amplified and dysregulated, interfering both with a functional immune response to infection and inflammation and, as observed in patients with DIC, with microvascular function.

Neuroimmune regulation of the septic response

Neuroendocrine–immune regulation

During infection, leucocyte responses are modulated by an integrated neuroimmune network that potentiates innate immunity, controls potential harmful effects (has anti-inflammatory effects), and also addresses metabolic and nutritional modifications supporting immune function. Communication between the neuronal and immune system is bidirectional, occurs between neurons and immune cells, and is based on the secretion of neurotransmitters, hormones, neuropeptides, and cytokines.

The neural system influences the immune system through two major pathways, the neuroendocrine axis and the autonomic nervous system (sympathetic and parasympathetic nerves). The stress-initiated neuroendocrine response substantially affects inflammatory and immune responses by activating the hypothalamic–pituitary–adrenal (HPA), somatotropic, hypothalamic–pituitary–gonadal (HPG), and hypothalamic–pituitary–thyroid (HPT) axes with subsequent secretion of neurotransmitters such as catecholamines, acetylcholine, vasoactive intestinal peptide (VIP), substance P (SP), and calcitonin-gene-related peptide (CGRP). Neurotransmitters have variable effects on immune cell activation and cytokine production. Catecholamines, including adrenaline (epinephrine) and noradrenaline (norepinephrine), are elaborated during the neuroendocrine response in sepsis and other conditions of severe stress. Catecholamines can inhibit inflammatory cytokine production from blood mononuclear cells while stimulating the release of IL-10. It has been suggested that a critical balance exists between hormones—growth hormone (GH), prolactin (PRL), glucocorticoids (GCs), catecholamines, insulin, leptin—and proinflammatory cytokines (mainly IL-1, IL-6 and TNF-α) involving nervous, endocrine, and immune organs (such as the thymus) and so-called 'target' tissues (i.e. adipose and muscle tissue). The balance of these agents can influence the immune response and, consequently, the course of the infection and severity of the disease, as well as host metabolism and growth, during the inflammatory process. Corticosteroids and catecholamines both individually and cooperatively induce a shift of T cell cytokine balance, reducing Th1 and favouring Th2 type cytokine production [76]. The effect is mediated, in part, through the inhibition of IL-12 production by monocytes, but also by a direct action on Th1 cells.

Many other neuromediators may also be responsible for the reduced reactivity of circulating leucocytes. For example, several hormones—GCs, GH, insulin-like growth factor-1 (IGF-1), leptin, Zn-thymulin—and their receptors have been identified in immune tissues and appeared to participate in the development, differentiation, and regulation of the immune response [77]. In addition, astrocytes and microglia in the brain can also produce cytokines—IFN-α, IFN-γ, IL-1, IL-2, IL-6, and TNF-α. Moreover, the hypothalamus and pituitary glands can endogenously produce IL-1, IL-6, TGF-β, leukaemia inhibitor factor, MIF, IL-10, and IL-18. Along with cytokines and chemokines produced at peripheral inflammatory sites, these cells can serve to modulate brain function and hormonal secretion by endocrine glands. The main cytokines involved in the immune system–nervous system communication appear to be TNF-α, IFN-γ, IL-1, IL-2, IL-6, IL-10, and IL-12. During antigen-mediated activation, $CD4^+$ and $CD8^+$ lymphocytes are also able to produce hormones such as GH, PRL, adrenocorticotropic hormone (ACTH), thyroid stimulating hormone (TSH), and gonadotropins. Thus, the nervous, immune, and endocrine systems share in the production of the same proteins that are able to act as immunomodulators as well as metabolic regulators. Importantly, and to be discussed in the later sections on therapeutic approaches to the septic patient, many of the supportive therapies presently being employed in the clinic use catecholamines, insulin, and GCs. While these hormones impact on various organ functions during therapy, suboptimal cardiovascular and pulmonary function, adrenal insufficiency, etc., may be supported by appropriate drugs. However, it is unclear how these agents may impact on the associated concurrent immune and inflammatory processes occurring in these septic individuals [77].

Inflammatory reflex

Neural pathways (sympathetic and parasympathetic innervations) have also recently been shown to regulate the septic animal's innate immune responses at regional, local, and systemic levels through neurotransmitters (catecholamines, acetylcholine, and neuropeptides, VIP, SP, and CGRP). Importantly, the sympathetic and parasympathetic nervous systems have been shown to inhibit inflammation at a regional level through innervation of lymphoid organs. This 'inflammatory reflex' has been defined as a response to an initial inflammatory stimulus, which activates afferent signals to the nucleus tractus solitarius in the brain. This in turn leads to subsequent activation of vagus efferent activity and inhibition of cytokine synthesis through direct stimulation of acetylcholine receptors on macrophages [78]. Moreover, it has recently been shown that signals transmitted via the vagus nerve appear to significantly attenuate the release of HMGB-1 and other cytokines involved in inflammation, and are believed to be associated with experimental sepsis in animals and in humans with sepsis.

Experimental models of sepsis (acute versus chronic)

Introduction

Animal models have enabled scientists to design controlled and reproducible studies of host defence mechanisms in sepsis, not feasible in the heterogeneous human patient population. The various animal models described here are used to mimic specific early and late phase cardiovascular and metabolic responses observed in humans with sepsis. In addition to enabling researchers to closely examine the mechanisms of immune response to sepsis, these animal studies are important models in the development of *in vivo* therapeutic targets and interventions for the treatment of sepsis.

Endotoxin and superantigen (exotoxin) challenge

Toxin challenge models in the study of sepsis allow for the examination of host defence mechanisms to specific bacterial proteins; for example, Gram-negative (LPS) or bacterial superantigens (*Staphylococcus aureus* enterotoxins, *Streptococcus pyogenes* pyrogenic exotoxins) [79,80]. However, this model does not reflect naturally occurring scenarios, as host responses to live bacteria involves a cascade of physiological events not reproduced by bacterial toxins alone. Also, response patterns and cardiovascular and vascular manifestations have been shown to be distinct from bacterial infection [81,82].

Intoxication, as opposed to infection, typically involves a bolus injection of bacterial protein (acute) [83–85] or slow continuous infusion, as delivered by an implanted osmotic pump (chronic) [86–88]. Animal models include rodents, dogs, cats, pigs, rabbits, and primates [81,89,90]. These species, however, vary considerably in their immune responses and sensitivities; rodents and rabbits in particular require presensitization with dead bacteria to induce enhanced immune responses to LPS [84,91].

Monospecific microbial challenge

Monospecific bacterial challenge, unlike endotoxin and exotoxin challenge, reproduces more of the pathophysiological characteristics associated with the development of sepsis in the clinical setting, such as changes in cardiac output and late systemic and pulmonary hypotension [92–94]. In this model, various animals (mice, dogs, baboons, pigs, sheep, cows [81,82]) are given live aerobic bacteria such as *Escherichia coli* [95], *Pseudomonas aeruginosa* [96], or *Streptococcus pneumonia* [97] as intravenous bolus injections (acute) [96,98] or low-dose subcutaneous injections over time (chronic) [95]. However, in reality, significant numbers of bacteria do not suddenly appear in the systemic environment, and lack of colonization or focus of infection, and intensity of initial host inflammatory response to the dose of bacteria delivered (complement specifically), are significant considerations in the model [99,100].

Bacterial strain and growth phase, route of administration, the site of the infection, the compartment involved (e.g. lung, peritoneal cavity), and bacterial load all present challenges in models of sepsis using exogenous bacteria [81,101].

Peritoneal cavity inoculation with faecal material

Peritoneal faecal soilage has been used as an experimental animal model for the study and treatment of fully developed polymicrobial sepsis [102–105]. This model has been shown to produce a lethal septicaemia, useful for investigating the hyperdynamic and hypermetabolic phase of sepsis (rats) [102], and to assess the efficacy of possible therapeutic agents (pigs) [104,105]. The model has some disadvantages; an individual/animal's tolerance to its own faecal flora necessitates the use of pooled inoculums [102,104,105] or human faecal inoculums [106]. Also, bacterial dose, species, and strain variability effect reproducibility between experiments and model species [107].

Pulmonary infection and sepsis

Dissemination of bacteria from the lungs to the bloodstream is associated with the development of sepsis [108–111]. This model, primarily used in rodents, allows for the investigation of factors that enable bacteria to evade the primary innate host defence mechanisms in the lungs and infect the systemic compartment. Bacteria is delivered to the lungs, via the intranasal or intratracheal route, resulting in infection and bacterial dissemination to the bloodstream. Recent experiments in this model have examined virulence factors associated with infectious versus noninfectious strains of *Streptococcus pneumonia* [109,110], the role of IFN-γ in clearance of bacteria in the lung [108], and *Yersinia pestis* virulence factors associated with the development of pneumonic plague [111].

Caecal ligation and puncture

The caecal ligation and puncture (CLP) model of sepsis is believed to best mimic the pathology of clinical sepsis and the CLP technique is regarded as manageable and highly reproducible. The severity of infection is controlled by the number and size of the caecum puncture and the quantity of faecal material extruded. In this model, the release of polymicrobial flora, as in peritonitis or perforated bowel, creates a focus of infection and necrotic tissue (ligated caecum), and replicates the biphasic pattern—early hyperdynamic and proinflammatory, late and hypodynamic/suppressed cardiac and vascular function—seen in patients with sepsis [101,112,113]. Cytokine responses, apoptosis, organ injury, and mortality have been shown to be similar in their intensity and severity, compared with patients with sepsis [47,82,114]. Animals can and do survive this model (~40%) by walling off the infection and forming an abscess [100,101]. Animal models for CLP include rodents [47,101,115], dogs [116], and sheep [117].

GIT or colon ascendens stent peritonitis (CASP)

The colon ascendens stent peritonitis (CASP) model is used, predominately in mice, to study the pathogenesis of sepsis. CASP produces a persistent leakage of faecal material from the colon into the peritoneal cavity as a source of infection [100,118]. The inserted stent, while presenting a technical surgical challenge, is a highly standardized and reproducible bacterial delivery system into the peritoneal cavity where sepsis develops. The diameter of the stent inserted provides a means of controlling the severity of the sepsis and associated mortality [100,118,119]. This model, in contrast to CLP, does not produce an abscess in resolving ongoing sepsis. However, removal of the stent allows for control of the infection focus, allowing for identification of critical-event time points during the course of sepsis [100,118]. This model has been shown to produce high levels of proinflammatory cytokines and bacteria in the blood [100].

Treatment strategies for sepsis

Historical background

Historically, therapy was designed to restore the proper balance of the four humours—blood, phlegm, black and yellow bile [120]. Sentinel advances in the treatment of sepsis span from Ignaz Semmelweiss's hand-washing with soap, water, and chlorine [121]; Joseph Lister's use of carbolic antiseptic dressings; Edward Jenner's cowpox pus to develop an effective smallpox vaccine; to Pasteur and Koch's demonstration of the pathogenicitiy of microorganisms. Paul Ehrlich's use of a parenteral arsenic derivative, salvarsan, to treat syphilis provided the basis for Alexander Fleming's 1928 seminal discovery of penicillin. Following World War II, penicillin and sulphonamides greatly diminished the severity of Gram-positive infections.

Source control

The surgical management of infections and sepsis dates to antiquity. Infections within a body cavity invariably require effective source control to avoid mortality. Inadequate source control may be associated with a more than sevenfold increase in mortality [122]. The innate immune system functions to bring cells, predominantly neutrophils, to the site of the infectious focus. As alluded to earlier, changes in both the recruited neutrophils as well as endothelial cell adhesion molecules favour neutrophil localization, emigration, and persistence within the tissues at the sites of infection. A combination of coagulation factors, macrophage-derived cytokines, reduced endothelial anticoagulant activity. and up-regulation of TF, coupled with bacteria and cellular debris, all combine to form an abscess.

The fibrous capsule effectively isolates the microbial challenge from the circulatory system, as well as a further influx of host immune cells or antibiotics. However, the resultant abscess continues to drive an ongoing immune response in a vain effort to clear the infection, with unfortunately resulting in ongoing profound systemic inflammation.

Definitive source control follows three principles: (1) drainage of the abscess; (2) debridement of nonviable tissue; (3) definitive management of the anatomical anomaly which was responsible for the ongoing microbial contamination, with restoration of functional anatomy.

Seminal work on source control includes Grunau's study of 48 postoperative intra-abdominal infections documenting a mortality of 19% where source control was achieved, compared with 100% in those without source control [123]. Further, in Solomkin *et al.*'s series of intra-abdominal infection, regardless of the antibiotic regimen, the mortality was 45% for inadequate source control, compared with 6% for patients in whom the site of infection was contained or eradicated [124].

Antibiotics

Early empiric antibiotics are essential in the management of the patient with sepsis. Any delay in the initiation of antibiotics significantly increases mortality [125]. Failure to administer early broad-spectrum empiric antibiotics, encompassing Gram-positive and Gram-negative organisms, is also associated with a worse mortality [126]. Consideration should also be given to fungal infections, the institutional specific organisms, local antibiograms, and the clinical circumstances.

Furthermore, many antibiotics are known to have immunomodulating properties. The predominance of the evidence pertains to the effects of macrolides and the fluoroquinolones. Ciprofloxacin has been shown to decrease IL-6 mRNA and increase IL-8 mRNA expression in a human endothelial cell line [127]. Williams *et al.* demonstrated that clarithromycin altered IL-4 content in $CD3^+$ T lymphocytes [128]. Both moxifloxacin and ciprofloxacin dose-dependently decreased IFN-γ and IL-4 production by T lymphocytes [128]. Following treatment with ciprofloxacin, in a murine model of LPS-induced acute lung injury, bronchoalveolar lavage concentrations of TNF, IL-1, and MIP-2 were significantly lowered, coupled with improvements in survival [129].

Steroids

The role of the adrenal glands in the body's response to severe infection was first demonstrated by Waterhouse (1911) and Friderichsen (1918) who described the association between severe infections, peripheral vascular collapse, and adrenal haemorrhage [130,131]. By the 1930s Rich demonstrated characteristic histological changes in the adrenal cortex in cases of severe meningococcal, streptococcal, and diphtheria infections, when associated with cardiovascular collapse. Corticosteroids have been proposed as a treatment strategy for sepsis since the 1940s [132], but the use of steroids remains controversial. Two recent reviews advocate abandoning steroids in sepsis [133,134], whereas the '2008 Surviving Sepsis Campaign' guidelines [135] advocate the use of steroids in a select patient population.

GCs are lipophilic and readily cross the cell membrane into the cell cytoplasm. The essence of steroid therapy lies in their ability to reduce the proinflammatory cytokine production, hopefully without causing immunosuppression. Binding of GC to its receptor (GCR), results in translocation of the GC–GCR complex to the cell nucleus. The GC response elements (GRE) bind to the promoter region of specific GC-responsive genes. Transcription and expression of several anti-inflammatory proteins then occurs [136]. Down-regulation of inflammatory mediators such as cytokines, adhesion molecules, and enzymes may also occur in the presence of the GC–GCR complex. This occurs through effects on transcription factors such as NF-κB and activator protein-1 (AP-1). Production of TNF-α and IL-6 are also altered by steroids at the mRNA level [137] (see Chapter 7).

It is proposed that impaired adrenal function accounts, in part, for decreased sensitivity of the cardiovascular system to medications such as noradrenaline in severe sepsis. Thus, steroids are believed to enhance vascular endothelial responsiveness to catecholamines. Although the mechanism is unknown, current data suggests that alterations in the PG or NO pathway, or changes in the adrenoceptor, may be involved [138,139].

Anticytokine therapies

The cytokine–receptor interaction can be blocked using either soluble receptors or monoclonal antibodies (MABs) directed against these receptors. By preventing transduction of the appropriate biological signal in a given immune and nonimmune target cell, it is proposed that the deleterious effects attributed to excessive cytokine release (frequently seen in cases of sepsis) would be mitigated. Although several studies have described MABs that block cellular cytokine receptors in preclinical animal models and could serve as anticytokine therapies, there has, unfortunately, been little clinical success with these agents.

As TNF is elevated in almost all patients with sepsis, it initially received the most attention with the development of MABs, specifically to TNF-α. A primate model of sepsis demonstrated improved mortality [140]. However, subsequent humans studies have failed to show a mortality benefit [141–144]. The initial NORASEPT study involved 971 patients with SIRS in 31 centres treated with MABs to TNF-α. There was no improvement in all-cause mortality at 28 days. Although it did not reach statistical significance, there appeared to be a trend towards improvement in patients with septic shock [142]. The NORASEPT II study was a randomized double-blind controlled trial using MABs to TNF-α, which enrolled 1879 septic patients over 105 centres. Again this study failed to show any mortality benefit at 28 days (40.3% versus 42.8%), although there was a notable improvement in coagulopathy in septic patients who received treatment [141].

The INTERSEPT study used a mouse MAB to recombinant human (rh) TNF-α, in patients with sepsis. This involved 553 patients over 14 countries, who were randomized to receive placebo versus high or low dose MAB. There was no difference in 28-day mortality (39.5% versus 31.5% versus 42.4%). However, the study did demonstrate a faster time to reversal of shock as well as delay in onset of first organ failure. Furthermore, patients receiving treatment had a lower number of organs that failed [143].

IL-1ra is a human monocyte-macrophage-derived, 17-kDa plasma protein that functions as a specific inhibitor of the proinflammatory cytokine IL-1 [145]. IL-1ra binds to type I and type II IL-Rs on target cells, yet fails to initiate signal transduction of IL-1 message, thus sterically generating a functional blockade of IL-1 action at the receptor level [146,147]. Animal models of IL-1ra demonstrated a highly significant mortality benefit [148]. Unfortunately, akin to the findings with TNF-α, two large clinical trials failed to reveal any improvement in mortality for patients with sepsis treated with IL-1ra [149,150]. Fisher *et al.* enrolled 893 patients in a multicentre, multinational placebo-controlled trial [149]. While there was no mortality benefit to patients who received rhIL-1ra, there was an increase in survival time with rhIL-1ra treatment among patients with sepsis and dysfunction of one or more organs.

Opal *et al.* enrolled 696 patients in a phase III multicentre, multinational clinical trial assessing the efficacy of two different doses (1.0 and 2.0 mg/kg per hour), compared with placebo in patients with sepsis [150]. There was no improvement in 28-day, all-cause mortality between the groups; 34% in the placebo, 31% in the low dose and 29% in the high dose treatement group ($p = 0.23$).

Antagonists to proinflammatory mediators such as platelet activating factor receptor (PAFR) have also been the subject of clinical trials [151–153]. Specifically, the PAFR antagonist BN 52021 (ginkgolide B) has been assessed for potential therapeutic value in patients with sepsis. Although no overall improvement in mortality was found, the data revealed that mortality in patients with Gram-negative sepsis was reduced from 57% in patients who received placebo down to 33% in patients who received the PAFR antagonist [151]. Vincent *et al.* utilized the PAFR antagonist BB-882 in 152 septic patients [153]. Again, there was no difference in 28-day mortality; it was 45% in the placebo and 53% in the treatment group.

These are the most notable studies, although other agents have also been investigated. To date, there has been very little clinical success despite some promising animal studies. Further, the uses of anti-inflammatory cytokines have been investigated in animal studies. Both IL-10 and IL-13 have shown some preliminary positive results, which have not been supported by human data [154,155]. One hypothesis that has been put forward to explain the lack of efficacy of single-mediator-targeted therapies is that the immune system is full of redundancy for many of these mediators and, thus, it is not surprising that alteration of a single cytokine does not have a large impact on mortality in the biological complexity of human beings. Heterogeneity, and/or a lack of understanding as to how genetic factors affect the response to sepsis, may also have played a significant role in inhibiting the ability to translate the findings made in preclinical studies to the clinical state seen in patients [156,157].

Activated protein C

In the response to severe infection, the inflammatory response and the coagulation cascade are intricately linked. Monocytes and endothelial cells are stimulated to release TF, thus activating the coagulation cascade, in response to infectious agents like endotoxin, as well as in response to cytokines such as TNF-α and IL-1β. Up-regulation of TF leads to the formation of thrombin and a fibrin clot. Cytokines are capable of activating coagulation and inhibiting fibrinolysis. Thrombin is capable of stimulating several inflammatory pathways, which often results in a widespread injury to the vascular endothelium. Protein C, a vitamin K-dependent serine protease, is an endogenous protein that promotes fibrinolysis while inhibiting thrombosis and inflammatory responses.

It has also been proposed that APrC exerts an antithrombotic effect by limiting the generation of thrombin, thus decreasing thrombin levels. The thrombin-mediated inflammatory, procoagulant, and antifibrinolytic response is thereby attenuated. Further, APrC has been shown to inhibit monocyte production of TNF-α, IL-1β, and IL-6, and limits monocyte and neutrophil adhesion to the endothelium. *In vitro* studies of LPS-stimulated human neutrophils have shown that APrC can decrease chemotaxis and IL-6 production while leaving other neutrophil functions unaffected [158]. It has also been shown that APrC decreases NF-κB binding at target sites in cultured endothelial cells, suppresses expression of p50 and p52 NF-κB subunits and blocks downstream targets, including vascular cell adhesion molecule-1 and E-selectin [159]. Further, APrC modulates the endothelial apoptosis pathway, including the Bcl-2 homologue protein and inhibitor of apoptosis protein, resulting in the ability of APrC to inhibit the induction of apoptosis by the potent inducer staurosporine. Thus, APrC may have some novel effects on inflammation and vascular function that may be independent of its anticoagulant activities.

Reduced levels of protein C have been reported in the majority of patients with sepsis and are associated with an increased risk of death. Supplementation of APrC levels was proposed to be a potentially beneficial therapeutic manoeuvre in the septic animal and patient. The PROWESS trial of APrC in patients with severe sepsis demonstrated a significant reduction in mortality [160]. However, benefit seemed to be restricted to only the sickest of patients, with APACHE II scores of 25 or greater. Surprisingly, trials of other agents that act on the coagulation system (such as TF pathway inhibitor and antithrombin) have yet to show a survival benefit [161,162]. Hence, further trials are needed to demonstrate the most effective roles for APrC in less severe forms of sepsis.

Unintentional immunomodulation of other ICU care and medications

Opioids

Opioids exert both a direct and an indirect immunomodulatory effect. The indirect effect is via the HPA axis. Morphine, for example, can increase plasma concentrations of ACTH and GCs [163]. The direct action of opioids, particularly morphine, is thought to be predominantly at the μ_3 receptor, which is expressed predominantly on macrophages, and other immune cells. Binding to the μ_3 receptor induces immunosuppression by transcription factor stabilization of NF-κB and AP-1. This occurs via an increase in cAMP levels [164]. These effects are most notable in T cells (see Chapter 7).

Statins

Both human and animal models reveal that statins modulate the immune response to sepsis. However, only observational data currently exist, but these data suggests improved survival in critically ill and injured patients. The beneficial effects are believed, in part to involve NO synthase III [165]. Dobesh *et al.* assessed the impact of statin use in patients with severe sepsis requiring ICU care. The statin group had a 35% relative reduction in mortality, compared with the nonstatin group (mortality rate 31.7% versus 48.4%). Most of the mortality reduction attributed to statins occurred in patients with APACHE II scores higher than 24 [166].

Summary and conclusions

While the overall mortality rate has decreased over the last few decades, due to state-of-the-art supportive care, appropriate tailoring of antibiotics, and aggressive operative intervention, sepsis remains one of the leading causes of death in critically ill patients in trauma/surgical ICUs in the USA and Europe. This is due, in part, not only to the heterogeneous nature of the population that is being treated with what is broadly defined as sepsis or severe septic shock, but also due to our incomplete understanding of the immune-pathological responses which underpin the development of this serious condition. In this chapter we have provided an overview of some of the more salient aspects of what is known about the innate and, to a lesser extent, the adaptive immune response alterations and contributions in clinical and experimental sepsis. We describe how both the SIRS response and aspects of the anti-inflammatory and immune suppressive state appear to coexist in these patients and animals. Also, we have reviewed what appear to be the central mediators, pathways, and cellular components involved. Importantly, while much of the data points to sequelae of proinflammation as an important contributor to septic morbidity and mortality, there is inability to translate this information into clinically useful antiseptic therapies. This implies that the roles of other processes such as dysfunctional regulation of cell death, vascular abnormalities, the impact of comorbid states, etc, all need to be better understood if we are going to be able to apply successfully immuno-molecular biological approaches to the treatment of sepsis.

Acknowledgements

We are grateful to Ms Courtney Coto for her assistance in the transcription of the references for this manuscript. This work was funded in part by NIH GM 46354, GM 53209 and HL 73525(A.A.) as well as the Armand D. Versaci Research Scholar in Surgical Sciences Award (R.K.T.).

References

1. Bone RC, Balk RA, Cerra FB. Definitions for sepsis and organ failure and guidelines for the use of innovative therapies in sepsis. *Chest* 1999; **101**: 1644–1655.
2. Angus DC, Linde-Zwirble WT, Lidicker J, Clermont G, Carcillo J, Pinsky MR.Epidemiology of severe sepsis in the United States: analysis of incidence, outcome, and associated costs of care. *Crit Care Med* 2001; **29**: 1303–1310.
3. Martin GS, Mannino DM, Eaton S. The epidemiology of sepsis in the United States from 1979 through 2000. *N Engl J Med* 2003; **16**: 1546–1554.
4. van Ruler O, Schultz MJ, Reitsma JB. Has mortality from sepsis improved and what to expect from new treatment modalities: review of current insights. *Surg Infect* 2009; **10**: 339–348.

5. Cinel I, Opal SM. Molecular biology of inflammation and sepsis. *Crit Care Med* 2009; **37**: 291–304.
6. Tsujimoto H, Ono S, Efron PA, Scumpia PO, Moldawer LL. Role of toll-like receptors in the development of sepsis. *Shock* 2008; **29**: 315–321.
7. Spittler A, Razenberger M, Kupper HM *et al.* Relationship between interleukin-6 plasma concentration in patients with sepsis, monocyte phenotype, monocyte phagocytic properties, and cytokine production. *Clin Infect Dis* 2000; **31**: 1338–1342.
8. Osuchowski MF, Welch K, Siddiqui J, Remick DG. Circulating cytokine/inhibitor profiles reshape the understanding of the SIRS/CARS continuum in sepsis and predict mortality. *J Immunol* 2006; **177**: 1967–1974.
9. Dinarello CA. Proinflammatory and anti-inflammatory cytokines as mediators in the pathogenesis of septic shock. *Chest* 1997; **112**: 321S–329S.
10. Calandra T, Roger T. Macrophage migration inhibitory factor: a regulator of innate immunity. *Nat Rev Immunol* 2003; **3**: 791–800.
11. Flaster H, Bernhagen J, Calandra T, Bucala R. The macrophage migration inhibitory factor-glucocorticoid dyad: regualtion of inflammation and immunity. *Mol Endocrinol* 2007; **21**: 1267–1280.
12. Lyn-Kew K, Standiford TJ. Immunosuppression in sepsis. *Curr Pharm Des* 2008; **14**: 1870–1881.
13. Rittirsch D, Flierl MA, Ward PA. Harmful molecular mechanisms in sepsis. *Nat Rev Immunol* 2008; **8**: 776–787.
14. Boontham P, Chandran P, Rowlands B, Eremin O. Surgical sepsis: dysregulation of immune function and therapeutic implications. *Surgeon* 2003; **1**: 187–206.
15. Gordon S, Taylor PR. Monocyte and macrophage heterogeneity. *Nat Rev Immunol* 2005; **5**: 953–964.
16. Cummings CJ TR Martin, CW Frevert *et al.* Expression and function of the chemokine receptors CXCR1 and CXCR2 in sepsis. *J Immunol* 1999 **162**: 2341–2346.
17. Zimmerman K, Volkel D, Pable S *et al.* Native versus recombinant high mobility group B1 proteins: functional activity in vitro. *Inflammation* 2004; **28**: 221–229.
18. Ulloa L, Tracey KJ. The 'cytokine profile': a code for sepsis. *Trends Mol Med* 2005; **11**: 56–63.
19. Castellheim A, Brekke OL, Espevik T, Harboe M, Mollnes TE. Innate immune responses to danger signals in systemic inflammatory response syndrome and sepsis. *Scand J Immunol* 2009; **69**: 479–491.
20. Chen GY, Tang J, Zheng P, Liu Y. CD24 and siglec-10 selectively repress tissue damage-induced immune responses. *Science* 2009; **323**: 1722–1725.
21. Levi M, van der Poll T. Two-way interactions between inflammation and coagulation. *Trends Cardiovasc Med* 2005; **15**: 254–259.
22. Hirsch T, Metzig M, Niederbichler A, Steinau HU, Eriksson E, Steinstraesser L. Role of host defense peptides of the innate immune response in sepsis. *Shock* 2008; **30**: 117–126.
23. Adib-Conquy M, Cavaillon J-M. Stress molecules in sepsis and systemic inflammatory response syndrome. *FEBS Lett* 2007; **581**: 3723–3733.
24. Carre JE, Singer M. Cellular energetic metabolism in sepsis: the need for a systems approach. *Biochim Biophys Acta* 2008; **1777**: 763–771.
25. Adib-Conquy M, Cavaillon JM. Compensatory anti-inflammatory response syndrome. *Crit Thromb Haemost* 2009; **101**: 36–47.

26. Tschaikowsky K, Hedwig-Geissing M, Schiele A, Bremer F, Schywalsky M, Schüttler J. Coincidence of pro- and anti-inflammatory responses in the early phase of severe sepsis: Longitudinal study of mononuclear histocompatibility leukocyte antigen-DR expression, procalcitonin, C-reactive protein, and changes in T-cell subsets in septic and postoperative patients. *Crit Care Med* 2002; **30**: 1015–1023.
27. Monneret, G, Lepape A, Voirin N *et al.* Persisting low monocyte human leukocyte antigen-DR expression predicts mortality in septic shock. *Intensive Care Med* 2006; **32**: 1175–1183.
28. Huang, X, Venet F, Wang YL *et al.* PD-1 expression by macrophages plays a pathologic role in altering microbial clearance and the innate inflammatory response to sepsis. *Proc Natl Acad Sci U S A* 2009; **106**: 6303–6308.
29. Bandyopadhyay, G, De AK, Laudanski K *et al.* Negative signaling contributes to T-cell anergy in trauma patients. *Crit Care Med* 2007; **35**: 794–801.
30. Wen H, Schaller MA, Dou Y, Hogaboam CM, Kunkel SL. Dendritic cells at the interface of innate and acquired immunity: the role for epigenetic changes. *J Leukoc Biol* 2008; **83**: 439–446.
31. Venet F, Chung CS, Monneret G *et al.* Regulatory T cell populations in sepsis and trauma. *J Leukoc Biol* 2007; **83**: 523–535.
32. Hotchkiss RS, Tinsley KW, Swanson PE Jr *et al.* Sepsis-induced apoptosis causes progressive profound depletion of B and CD4+ T lymphocytes in humans. *J Immunol* 2001; **166**: 6952–6963.
33. Lederer JA, Rodrick ML, Mannick JA. The effects of injury on the adaptive immune response. *Shock* 1999; **11**: 153–159.
34. Ayala A, Deol ZK, Lehman DL, Herdon CD, Chaudry IH. Polymicrobial sepsis but not low dose endotoxin infusion causes decreased splenocyte IL-2/IFN-gamma release while increasing IL-4/IL-10 production. *J Surg Res* 1994; **56**: 579–585.
35. Ferguson NR, Galley HF, Webster NR. T helper subset ratios in patients with severe sepsis. *Intensive Care Med* 1999; **1**: 106–109.
36. Marshall J. Clinical trials of mediator-directed therapy in sepsis: what have we learned? *Intensive Care Med* 2000; **26**: S75–S83.
37. Ward N, Casserly B, Ayala A. The compensatory anti-inflammatory response (CARS) in critically ill patients. *Clin Chest Med* 2008; **29**: 617–625.
38. Waage A, Halstensen A, Espevik T. Association between tumor necrosis factor in serum and fatal outcome in patients with meningococcal disease. *Lancet* 1987; **i**: 355–357.
39. Remick DG. Acute in vivo effects of human recombinant tumor necrosis factor. *Lab Invest* 1987; **56**: 583–590.
40. Beutler B, Milsark IW, Cerami A. Passive immunization against cachectin/tumor necrosis factor protects mice from lethal effect of endotoxin. *Science* 1985; **229**: 869–871.
41. Remick DG. Cytokine therapeutics for the treatment of sepsis: why nothing has worked. *Curr Pharm Des* 2003; **9**: 75–82.
42. Ertel W. Downregulation of proinflammatory cytokine release in whole blood from septic patients. *Blood* 1995; **85**: 1341–1347.
43. Heagy W, Nieman K, Hansen C. Lower levels of whole blood LPS-stimulated cytokine release are associated with poorer clinical outcomes in surgical ICU patients. *Surg Infect* 2003; **4**: 171–180.
44. Rigato O, Salomao R. Impaired production of interferon-gamma and tumor necrosis factor-alpha but not of interleukin 10 in whole blood of patients with sepsis. *Shock* 2003; **19**: 113–116.

45. Gogos CA. Pro- versus anti-inflammatory cytokine profile in patients with severe sepsis: a marker for prognosis and future therapeutic options. *J Infect Dis* 2000; **181**: 176–180.
46. Root RK, Lodato RF, Patrick W. Multicenter, double-blind, placebo-controlled study of the use of filgrastim in patients hospitalized with pneumonia and severe sepsis. *Crit Care Med* 2003; **31**: 367–373.
47. Wesche DE, Lomas-Neira JL, Perl M, Chung CS, Ayala A. Leukocyte apoptosis and its significance in sepsis and shock. *J Leukoc Biol* 2005; **25**: 325–337.
48. Hotchkiss RS, Swanson PE, Freeman BD *et al.* Apoptotic cell death in patients with sepsis, shock and multiple organ dysfunction. *Crit Care Med* 1999; **27**: 1230–1251.
49. Hotchkiss RS, Tinsley KW, Swanson PE *et al.* Depletion of dendritic cells, but not macrophages, in patients with sepsis. *J Immunol* 2002; **168**: 2493–2500.
50. Albert, ML. Death-defying immunity: do apoptotic cells influence antigen processing and presentation? *Nat Rev Immunol* 2004; **4**: 223–231.
51. Wesche-Soldato DE, Chung CS, Lomas-Neira JL, Doughty LA, Gregory SH, Ayala A. In vivo delivery of caspase 8 or Fas siRNA improves the survival of septic mice. *Blood* 2005; **106**: 2295–2301.
52. Opal SM. The immunopathogenesis of sepsis in elderly patients. *Clin Infect Dis* 2005; **41**: S504–S512.
53. Zellweger R, Wichmann MW, Ayala A, Stein S, DeMaso CM, Chaudry IH. Females in proestrus state maintain splenic immune functions and tolerate sepsis better than males. *Crit Care Med* 1997; **25**: 106–110.
54. Sperry JL. Characterization of the gender dimorphism after injury and hemorrhagic shock: are hormonal differences responsible. *Crit Care Med* 2008; **36**: 1838–1845.
55. Gibbs J. Preoperative serum albumin levels as a predictor of operative morbidity and mortality. *Arch Surg* 1999; **134**: 36–42.
56. Mora RJF. Malnutrition: organic and functional consequences. *World J Surg* 1999; **23**: 530–535.
57. Yaegashi M. Outcomes of morbid obesity in the intensive care unit. *J Intensive Care Med* 2005; **20**: 147–154.
58. Bercault N. Obesity-related excess mortality rate in adult intensive care unit: a risk adjusted matched cohort study. *Crit Care Med* 2004; **32**: 998–1003.
59. Vachharajani V. Obesity and sepsis. *J Intensive Care Med* 2006; **21**: 287–295.
60. Weisberg SP. Obesity is associated with macrophage accumulation in adipose tissue. *J Clin Invest* 2003; **112**: 1796–1808.
61. Fantuzzi G. Leptin in the regulation of immunity, inflammation, and hematopoiesis. *J Leukoc Biol* 2000; **68**: 437–446.
62. Arnalich F. Relationship of plasma leptin to plasma cytokines and human survival in sepsis and septic shock. *J Infect Disease* 1999; **180**: 908–911.
63. Papathanassoglou EDE. Serum leptin levels are higher but not independently associated with severity or mortality in the multiorgan dysfunction/systemic inflammatory response syndrome: a matched case control and longitudinal study. *Clin Endocrinol* 2001; **54**: 225–233.
64. Matsuda N, Yamamoto S, Takano K-I *et al.* Silencing of Fas-associated death domain protects mice from sepsis lung inflammation and apoptosis. *Am J Respir Crit Care Med* 2009; **179**: 806–815.
65. Zhou M, Simms HH, Wang P. Adrenomedullin and adrenomedullin binding protein - 1 attenuate vascular endothelial cell apoptosis in sepsis. *Ann Surg* 2004; **240**: 321–330.

66. Levi M, van der Poll T. Inflammation and coagulation. *Crit Care Med* 2010; **38**: S26–S34.
67. Gando S, Saitoh D, Ogura H *et al.* Disseminated intravascular coagulation (DIC) diagnosed based on the Japanese Association for Acute Medicine criteria is a dependent continuum to overt DIC in patients with sepsis. *Thrombosis Res* 2009; **123**: 715–718.
68. Schouten M, Wiersinga WJ, Levi M, van der Poll T. Inflammation, endothelium, and coagulation in sepsis. *J Leukoc Biol* 2008; **83**: 536–545.
69. Camerer E, Kolsto AB, Prydz H. Cell biology of tissue factor, the principle initiator of blood coagulation. *Thromb Res* 1996; **81**: 1–41.
70. Opal SM, Esmon CT. Bench-to-bedside review: functional relationships between coagulation and the innate immune response and their respective roles in the pathogenesis of sepsis. *Crit Care* 2003; **7**: 23–38.
71. Aird WC. Endothelium as a therapeutic target in sepsis. *Curr Drug Targets* 2007; **8**: 501–507.
72. Levi M, Keller TT, van Gorp E, Ten Cate H. Infection and inflammation and the coagulation system. *Cardiovasc Res* 2003; **60**: 26–39.
73. Schenkel AR, Mamdouh Z, Chen X, Liebman RM, Muller WA. CD99 plays a major role in the migration of monocytes through endothelial junctions. *Nat Immunol* 2002; **3**: 143–150.
74. Lorant DE, McEver RP, McIntyre TM, Moore KL, Prescott SM, Zimmerman GA. Activation of polymorphonuclear leucocytes reduces their adhesion to p-selectin and causes redistribution of ligands for p-selectin on their surfaces. *J Clin Invest* 1995; **96**: 171–182.
75. Ley K, Reutershan J. Leukocyte-endothelial interactions in health and disease. *Handb Exp Pharmacol* 2006; **176**: 97–133.
76. Panina-Bordignon P, Mazzeo D, Lucia PD *et al.* Beta2-agonists prevent Th1 development by selective inhibition of interleukin 12. *J Clin Invest* 1997; **100**: 1513–1519.
77. Borghetti P, Saleri R, Mocchegiani E, Corradi A, Martelli P. Infection, immunity and the neuroendocrine response. *Vet Immunol Immunopathol* 2009; **130**: 141–162.
78. Oke SL, Tracey KJ. The inflammatory reflex and the role of complementary and alternative medical therapies. *Ann N Y Acad Sci* 2009; **1172**: 172–180.
79. Bohach GA Fast DJ, Nelson RD, Schlievert PM. Staphylococcal and streptococcal pyrogenic toxins involved in toxic shock syndrome and related illnesses. *Crit Rev Microbiol* 1990; **17**: 251–272.
80. Dinges MM, Orwin PM, Schlievert PM. Exotoxins of *Staphylococcus aureus*. *Clin Microbiol Rev* 2000; **13**: 16–34.
81. Fink MP, Heard SO. Laboratory models of sepsis and septic shock. *J Surg Res* 1990; **49**: 186–196.
82. Deitch EA. Animal models of sepsis and shock: a review and lessons learned. *Shock* 1998; **9**: 1–11.
83. Sparwasser T. Macrophages sense pathogens via DNA motifs: induction of tumor necrosis factor-a-mediated shock. *Eur J Immunol* 1997; **27**: 1671–1679.
84. Kawa K, Tsutsui H, Uchiyama R *et al.* IFN-γ is a master regulator of endotoxin shock syndrome in mice primed with heat-killed *Propionibacterium acnes*. *Int Immunol* 2010; **22**: 157–166.
85. Rajagopalan G, Asmann YW, Lytle AK *et al.* Cyclooxygenase 2 pathway and its therapeutic inhibition in superantigen-induced toxic shock. *Shock* 2008; **30**: 721–728.
86. Yang S, Zhou M, Chaudry IH, Wang P. The role of lipopolysaccharide in stimulating adrenomedullin production during polymicrobial sepsis. *Biochim Biophys Acta* 2001; **1537**: 167–174.

87. Zhou M, Jacob A, Ho N *et al.* Downregulation of protein disulfide isomerase in sepsis and its role in tumor necrosis factor-alpha release. *Crit Care* 2008; 12: R100.
88. Weber P, Wang P, Maddens S *et al.* VX-166: a novel potent small molecule caspase inhibitor as a potential therapy for sepsis. *Crit Care* 2009; 13: R146.
89. Sakaue Y, Nezu Y, Komori S, Hara Y, Tagawa M, Ogawa R. Evaluation of hepatosplanchnic circulation and intestinal oxygenation in dogs with a condition that mimicked septic shock induced by continuous infusion of a low dose of lipopolysaccharide. *Am J Vet Res* 2004; **65**: 1347–1354.
90. Lindsey DC, Emerson TE, Thompson TE *et al.* Characterization of an endotoxemic baboon model of metabolic and organ dysfunction. *Circ Shock* 1991; **34**: 298–310.
91. Michie HR. The value of animal models in the development of new drugs for the treatment of sepsis syndrome. *J Antimicrob Chemother* 1998; **41**: 47–49.
92. Lagoa CE, Poli de Figueiredo LF, Cruz RJ, Silva E, Rocha e Silva M. Effects of fluid resuscitation on splanchnic perfusion in a canine severe sepsis model. *Crit Care* 2004; **8**: 221–228.
93. Dehring DJ, Crocker SH, Wismar BL, Steimberg SM, Lowery BD, Cloutier CT. Comparison of live bacteria infusions in a porcine model of acute respiratory failures. *J Surg Res* 1983; **34**: 151–158.
94. Giantomasso DD, May CN, Bellomo R. Vital blood flow during hyperdynamic sepsis. *Chest* 2003; **124**: 1053–1059.
95. Hargrove DM, Lang CH, Bagby GJ, Spitzer JJ. Epinephrine-induced increase in glucose turnover is diminished during sepsis. *Metabolism* 1989; **38**: 1070–1076.
96. Postel J, Schloerb PR, Furtado D. Pathophysiologic alterations during bacterial infusions for the study of bacteremic shock. *Surg Gynecol Obstet* 1975; **141**: 683–692.
97. Rubins JB, Pomeroy C. Role of γ-interferon in the pathogenesis of bacteremic pneumococcal pneumonia. *Infect Immun* 1997; **65**: 2975–2977.
98. Taylor FB. Staging of the pathophysiologic responses of the primate microvasculature to *Escherichia coli* and endotoxin: examination of the elements of the compensated response and their links to the corresponding uncompensated lethal variants. *Crit Care Med* 2001; **29**: 78–89.
99. Cross AS, Opal SM, Sadoff JC, Gemski P. Choice of bacteria in animal models of sepsis. *Infect Immun* 1993; **61**: 2741–2747.
100. Maier S, Traeger T, Entleutner M. Cecal ligation and puncture versus colon ascendens stent peritonitis: two distinct animal models for polymicrobial sepsis. *Shock* 2004; **21**: 505–511.
101. Wichterman KA, Baue AE, Chaudry IH. Sepsis and septic shock - A review of laboratory models and a proposal. *J Surg Res* 29; 1980: 189–201.
102. Lang CH GJ Bagby, GH Bornside, LJ Vial, and JJ Spitzer. Sustained hypermetabolic sepsis in rats: Characterization of the model. *J Surg Res* 1983; **35**: 201–210.
103. Lang CH, Bagby GJ, Ferguson JL, Spitzer JJ. Cardiac output and redistribution of organ blood flow in hypermetabolic sepsis. *Am J Physiol* 1984; **246**: R331–R337.
104. Barth E, Bassi G, Maybauer DM. Effects of ventilation with 100% oxygen during early hyperdynamic porcine fecal peritonitis. *Crit Care Med* 2008; **36**: 495–503.
105. Hauser B, Barth E, Bassi G *et al.* Hemodynamic, metabolic, and organ function effects of pure oxygen ventilation during established fecal peritonitis-induced septic shock. *Crit Care Med* 2009; **37**: 2465–2469.

106. King DW, Gurry JF, Ellis-Pegler RB, Brooke BN. A rabbit model of perforated appendicitis with peritonitis. *Br J Surg* 1975; **62**: 642–644.
107. Parker SJ, Watkins PE. Experimental models of Gram-negative sepsis. *Br J Surg* 2001; **88**: 22–30.
108. Moore TA, Perry ML, Getsoian AG, Newstead MW, Standiford TJ. Divergent role of gamma interferon in a murine model of pulmonary versus systemic *Klebsiella pneumoniae* infection. *Infect Immun* 2002; **70**: 6310–6318.
109. Mizrachi-Nebenzahl Y, Lifshitz S, Teitelbaum R *et al.* Differential activation of the immune system by virulent *Streptococcus pneumoniae* strains determines recovery or death of the host. *Clin Exp Immunol* 2003; **134**: 23–31.
110. Kadioglu, A, Brewin H, Hartel T *et al.* Pneumococcal protein PavA is important for nasopharyngeal carriage and development of sepsis. *Mol Oral Microbiol* 2010; **25**: 50–60.
111. Doyle TM, Matuschak GM, Lechner AJ. Septic shock and nonpulmonary organ dysfunction in pneumonic plague: the role of *Yersinia pestis* pCD1- vs. *pgm*- virulence factors. *Crit Care Med* 2010; **38**: 1574–1583.
112. Ayala A, Chaudry IH. Immune dysfunction in murine polymicrobial sepsis: mediators, macrophages, lymphocytes and apoptosis. *Shock* 1996; **6**: S27–S38.
113. Chung CS, Xu YX, Wang W, Chaudry IH, Ayala A. Is Fas ligand or endotoxin responsible for mucosal lymphocyte apoptosis in sepsis? *Arch Surg* 1998; **133**: 1213–1220.
114. Wesche-Soldato DE, Lomas-Neira J, Perl M, Jones L, Chung C-S, Ayala A. The role and regulation of apoptosis in sepsis. *J Endotoxin Rese* 2005; **11**: 375–382.
115. Gordon SA, Hoffman RA, Simmons RL, Ford HR. Induction of heat shock protein 70 protects thymocytes against radiation-induced apoptosis. *Arch Surg* 1997; **132**: 1277–1282.
116. Stahl TJ, Alden PB, Ring WS, Madoff RC, Cerra FB. Sepsis-induced diastolic dysfunction in chronic canine peritonitis. *Am J Physiol* 1990; **258**: H625–H633.
117. Gnidec AG, Sibbald WJ, Cheung H, Metz CA. Ibuprofen reduces the progression of permeability edema in an animal model of hyperdynamic sepsis. *J Appl Physiol* 1988; **65**: 1024–1032.
118. Zantl N, Uebe A, Neumann B *et al.* Essential role of gamma interferon in survival of colon ascendens stent peritonitis, a novel murine model of abdominal sepsis. *Infect Immun* 1998; **66**: 2300–2309.
119. Emmanuilidis K, Weighardt H, Maier S *et al.* Critical role of Kupffer cell-derived IL-10 for host defense in septic peritonitis. *J Immunol* 2001; **167**: 3919–3927.
120. Castiglione A. *A history of medicine*. Knopf, New York, 1941, p. 159.
121. Wangensteen O, Wangensteen S.*The rise of surgery from empiric craft to scientific discipline.* Dawson Publishing, Inglewood, CA, 1979, pp. 414–452.
122. Schein M, Marshall J.*Source control.* Springer, Heidelberg, 2003.
123. Grunau G, Heemken R, Hau T. Predictors of outcome in patients with post-operative intra-abdominal infection. *Eur J Surg* 1996; **162**: 619–625.
124. Solomkin J, Dellinger R. Results of a multicenter trial comparing imipenem/cilastatin to tobramycin/clindamycin for intra-abdominal infections. *Ann Surg* 1990; **212**: 581–591.
125. Iregui M, Ward S, Sherman G, Fraser V, Kollef M. Clinical importance of delays in the initiation of appropriate antibiotic treatment for ventilator associated pneumonia. *Chest* 2002; **122**: 262–268.

126. Garnacho-Montero, J, Ortiz-Leyba C, Herrera-Melero I. Mortality and morbidity attributable to inadequate empirical antimicrobial therapy in patients admitted to the ICU with sepsis: a matched cohort study. *J Antimicrob Chemother* 2008; **61**: 436–441.

127. Galley H, Dhillon J, Paterson R, Webster N. Effect of ciprofloxacin on the activation of the transcription factors nuclear factor kappaB, activator protein-1 and nuclear-factor-interleukin-6 and interleukin-6 and interleukin-8 mRNA expression in a human endothelial cell line. *Clin Sci* 2000; **99**: 405–410.

128. Williams A, Galley H, Watt A, Webster N. Differential effects of three antibiotics on T-helper cell cytokine expression. *J Antimicrob Chemother* 2005; **56**: 502–506.

129. Huang, H, Shieh C, Yu W. Comparing the protective effects of ciprofloxacin, moxifloxacin and levofloxacin in mice with lipopolysaccharide induced acute lung injuries. *Respirology* 2008; **13**: 47–52.

130. Waterhouse R. Case of suprarenal apoplexy. *Lancet* 1911; **i**: 577.

131. Friderichsen C. Nebennierenapoplexie bei kleinen Kindern. *Jb Kinderheilk* 1918; **87**: 109.

132. Perla D, Marmorston J. Suprarenal cortical hormone and salt in the treatment of pneumonia and other severe infections. *Endocrinology* 1940; **27**: 367–374.

133. Lefering R, Neugebauer EA. Steroid controversy in sepsis and septic shock: a meta-analysis. *Crit Care Med* 1995; **23**: 1294–1303.

134. Cronin L, Cook D, Carlet J. Corticosteroids treatment for sepsis: a critical appraisal and meta-analysis of the literature. *Crit Care Med* 1995; **23**: 1430–1439.

135. Dellinger R, Carlet J, Masur H. Surviving sepsis campaign guidelines for management of severe sepsis and septic shock. *Crit Care Med* 2004; **32**: 858–873.

136. Barnes P. How corticosteroids control inflammation: quintiles prize lecture. *Br J Pharmacol* 2006; **148**: 245–254.

137. Quante T, Ng Y, Ramsay E. Corticosteroids reduce IL-6 in ASM cells via up-regulation of MKP-1. *Amer J Resp Cell Mol Biol* 2008; **39**: 208–217.

138. Annane D. Glucocorticosteroids in the treatment of severe sepsis and septic shock. *Curr Opin Crit Care* 2005; **11**: 449–453.

139. Annane, D, Sebille V, Charpentier C *et al.* Effect of treatment with low doses of hydrocortisone and fludrocortisone on mortality in patients with septic shock. *JAMA* 2002; **288**: 862–871.

140. Tracey KJ, Fong Y, Hesse DG *et al.* Anti-cachectin/TNF monoclonal antibodies prevent septic shock during lethal bacteremia. *Nature* 1987; **330**: 662–664.

141. Abraham E, Anzueto A, Guiterrez G. Double-blind randomized controlled trial of monoclonal antibody to human tumour necrosis factor in treatment of septic shock. *Lancet* 1998; **351**: 929–933.

142. Abraham E, Wunderink R, Silverman H *et al.* Efficacy and safety of monoclonal antibody to human tumor necrosis factor alpha in patients with sepsis syndrome. A randomized, controlled, double-blind, multicenter clinical trial. TNF-alpha MAb Sepsis Study Group. *JAMA* 1995; **273**: 934–941.

143. Cohen J, Carlet J. INTERSEPT: an international, multicenter, placebo-controlled trial of monoclonal antibody to human tumor necrosis factor-alpha in patients with sepsis: International Sepsis Trial Study Group. *Crit Care Med* 1996; **24**: 1431–1440.

144. Reinhart K, Menges T, Garlund B. Randomized, placebo-controlled trial of the anti-tumor necrosis factor antibody fragment afelimomab in hyperinflammatory reponse during severe sepsis: the RAMSES study. *Crit Care Med* 2001; **29**: 765–769.

145. Arend, W Interleukin-1 receptor antagonist, a new member of the interleukin-1 family. *J Clin Invest* 1991; **88**: 1445–1451.
146. Arend W, Welgus H, Thompson R. Biological properties of recombinant human monocyte-derived interleukin-1 receptor antagonist. *J Clin Invest* 1990; **85**: 1694–1697.
147. Granowitz EV, Clark BD, Mancilla J, Dinarello CA. Interleukin-1 receptor antagonist competitively inhibits the binding of interleukin-1 to the type II interleukin-1 receptor. *J Biol Chem* 1991; **266**: 14147–14150.
148. Ohlsson K, Björk P, Bergenfeldt M, Hageman R, Thompson RC. Interleukin-1 receptor antagonist reduces mortality from endotoxin shock. *Nature* 1990; **348**: 550–552.
149. Fisher C, Dhainaut J, Opal S. Recombinant human interleukin 1 receptor antagonist in the treatment of patients with sepsis syndrome. Results from randomized, double-blind, placebo-controlled trial. Phase III rhIL-1ra Sepsis Syndrome Study Group. *JAMA* 1994; **271**: 1836–1843.
150. Opal S, Fisher C, Dhainaut J. Confirmatory interleukin-1 receptor antagonist trial in severe sepsis: a phase III, randomized, double-blind, placebo-controlled, multicenter trial. The interleukin-1 receptor antagonist sepsis investigator group. *Crit Care Med* 1997; **25**: 1115–1124.
151. Dhainaut JFA, Tenaillon A, Le Tulzo Y *et al.* Platelet-activating factor receptor antagonist BN 52021 in the treatment of severe sepsis: A randomized double-blind, placebo-controlled, multicenter clinical trial. *Crit Care Med* 1994; **22**: 1720–1728.
152. Opal S, Laterre P, Abraham E. Recominant human platelet-activating factor acetylhydrolase for treatment of severe sepsis: results of a phase III, multicenter, randomized, double-blind, placebo-controlled clinical trial. *Crit Care Med* 2004; **32**: 332–341.
153. Vincent J, Spapen H, Bakkar J, Webster N, Curtis L. Phase II multicenter clinical study of the platelet-activating factor receptor antagonist BB-882 in the treatment of sepsis. *Crit Care Med* 2000; **28**: 638–642.
154. Muchamuel, T, Menon S, Pisacane P, Howard M, Cockayne D. IL-13 protects mice from lipopolysaccharide-induced lethal endotoxemia: correlation with down-modulation of TNF-alpha, IFN-gamma and IL-12 production. *J Immunol* 1997; **158**: 2903.
155. Scumpia P, Moldawer L. Biology of interleukin-10 and its regulatory roles in sepsis syndrome. *Crit Care Med* 2005; **33**: S468–S471.
156. Cavaillon J-M, Adrie C, Fitting C, Adib-Conquy M. Reprogramming of circulatory cells in sepsis and SIRS. *J Endotoxin Res* 2005; **11**: 311–320.
157. Namath A, Patterson A. Genetic polymorphisms in sepsis. *Crit Care Clinics* 2009; **25**: 835–856.
158. Galley H, El Sakka N, Webster N, Lowed D, Cuthbertson B. Activated protein C inhibits chemotaxis and interleukin-6 release by human neutrophils without affecting other neutrophil functions. *Br J Anaesth* 2008; **100**: 815–819.
159. Joyce DE, Gelbert L, Ciaccia A, DeHoff B, Grinnell BW. Gene expression and profile of antithrombotic protein c defines new mechanisms modulating inflammation and apoptosis. *J Biol Chem* 2001; **276**: 11199–11203.
160. Bernard GR, Vincent J-L, Laterre P-F *et al.* Efficacy and safety of recombinant human activated protein C for severe sepsis. *N Engl J Med* 2001; **344**: 699–709.
161. Abraham E, Reinhart K, Opal S. Efficacy and safety of tifacogin (recombinant tissue factor pathway inhibitor) in severe sepsis: a randomized controlled trial. *JAMA* 2003; **290**: 238–247.

162. Warren B, Eid A, Singer P. Caring for the critically ill patient. High dose antithrombin III in severe sepsis: a randomized controlled trial. *JAMA* 2001; **286**: 1869–1878.

163. Cabot P. Immune-derived opioids and peripheral antinociception. *Clin Exp Pharmacol Physiol* 2001; **28**: 230–232.

164. Wang J, Barke R, Roy S. Transcriptional and epigenetic regulation of interleukin-2 gene in activated T cells by morphine. *J Biol Chem* 2007; **282**: 7164–7171.

165. McGown C, Brown N, Hellewell P, Reilly C, Brookes Z. Beneficial microvascular and anti-inflammatory effects of pravastatin during sepsis involves nitric oxide synthase III. *Br J Anaesth* 2010; **104**: 183–190.

166. Dobesh P, Klepser D, McGuire T, Morgan C, Olsen K. Reduction in mortality associated with statin therapy in patients with severe sepsis. *Pharmacotherapy* 2009; **29**: 621–630.

Chapter 6

Nutrition and immunity

Steven D. Heys, Manuel Garcia-Caballero, and Klaus W.J. Wahle

Key summary points

- Specific nutrients modulate key aspects of inflammation, metabolic processes, and a variety of immune functions.
- Dysregulation of immune, metabolic and inflammatory processes can occur when there is either protein–energy malnutrition or obesity.
- Probiotics and prebiotics can beneficially modify GIT bacterial populations and both GALT and general immune functions, but their specific role as treatment or prevention of GIT disorders (e.g. CDAD) in clinical practice requires further clarification.
- Micronutrients play a key role in the regulation of the immune system, wound healing, and antioxidant defence mechanisms, and also modulate numerous metabolic processes as components of specific enzymes.
- Amino acids, in particular, L-arginine, L-glutamine, and branched chain amino acids, stimulate a variety of aspects of immune, inflammatory and metabolic functions.
- Saturated, monounsaturated, and the ω-3 and ω-6 LCPUFAs can influence immune functions, particularly inflammatory processes, in different, often opposing, ways.
- Saturated fatty acids activate TLR4 receptors and the stress-related NF-κB inflammatory cascade in immune cells and adipocytes. ω-3 LCPUFAs attenuate this pathway and reduce proinflammatory cytokine and eicosanoid formation.
- CLAs and ω-3 LCPUFAs can alter immunoglobulin synthesis and secretions in animals and humans.
- Th1 and Th2 cytokine profiles and NK cell activities can be significantly modulated by fatty acids *in vivo* and *in vitro* in animals and humans.
- Vitamins (fat and water soluble) have important biological effects on the immune system, albeit the mechanistic effects are poorly defined. Vitamin A deficiency can inhibit innate immunity and inhibit Th2 responses. Vitamin A is

important for T and B cell homing to the GIT. In GALT, vitamin A regulates IgA production (both T cell dependent and independent). Vitamin E supplementation has shown variable effects (inhibition and enhancement). Vitamin D is generally inhibitory, whilst vitamin C enhances neutrophil function. Vitamin D inhibits the differentiation, proliferation and activity of DCs. Vitamin D suppresses Th1 and Th17 cell function and corresponding INF-α and IL-6 and IL-23 production, respectively.

- Prolonged and excessive alcohol intake can alter immune reaction, T cell and NK cell numbers, and activity; elevated IgE production and enhanced secretion of Th1 and Th2 cytokines have been documented.
- Nutritional supplementation with an individual nutrient, while modifying immune function has, in general, not been shown to have clinical benefit to date. However, combinations of amino acids, fatty acids, and micronutrients have been shown to have clinical benefits by reducing infectious complications in severely ill patients.

Protein–energy malnutrition and the immune system

Protein–energy malnutrition (PEM) or protein–calorie malnutrition, occurs when the intake or absorption of proteins and calories is insufficient to meet the body's biological requirements. Alternatively, it may occur due to excessive catabolic states, as occurs in the systemic inflammatory response syndrome (SIRS), for example, or when there is inadequate intake to compensate for these losses. Usually, in most clinical situations, there is a deficiency of both protein and energy but under certain circumstances it is possible for the diet to contain adequate energy but have insufficient protein content.

The clinical manifestations are well recognized and include muscular weakness, reduced cardiac and pulmonary function, reduced muscle mass, biochemical and functional impairments, but there are also effects on several aspects of the immune system leading to immune dysfunction. In PEM there is a generalized atrophy of lymphoid tissues with a decrease in size of the thymus gland, and reductions in the number of lymphoid cells in both the spleen and lymph nodes. There are marked biological effects on lymphocytes in general, with a decrease in the proliferative response of lymphcocytes to mitogenic stimulation *in vitro* and a reduction in delayed-type hypersensitivity *in vivo*. In some individuals there may be little or no response to antigens. In addition, T lymphocyte subsets are also affected with a reduction in $CD4^+$ T helper (Th) cells accompanied by a smaller, but still significant, reduction in $CD8^+$ cytotoxic T lymphocytes (CTLs) [1]. This dysfunction is proportional to the severity of the PEM and is reversible with appropriate nutritional repletion.

In terms of B cell function, antibody production and humoral responses are less affected and there appears to be little impact in association with PEM. However, if the humoral response is dependent on T cell function then there is a reduced responsiveness. PEM does have an inhibitory effect on secretory IgA antibody levels, which are reduced, and this may be important in inhibiting the defensive capabilities at mucosal surfaces [2].

The activity of phagocytic cells and their ability to ingest and destroy microorganisms is impaired with PEM, possibly because of a reduction in lysosomal enzymes. This also may be related, at least in part, to reduced levels of opsonins and reductions in both the levels and activities of several complement (C) components required, including C3 and C5. Furthermore, there are reductions in the levels of cytokines produced including interferon-gamma (INF-γ) and interleukins (ILs) -1 and -2; macrophage inhibition factor is also decreased [3].

Obesity and the immune system

Obesity is an increasing problem in Western industrialized populations, largely because of the attendant consequences leading to the increased susceptibility of affected individuals for developing metabolic syndrome, insulin resistance, type-2 diabetes mellitus, cardiovascular disease, and cancer. Excessive food intake resulting in gross obesity can impact on the immune system, as occurs with PEM. There are, however, specific differences between the two conditions [4–6].

It has been recognized that obesity constitutes a low-grade inflammation of the white adipose tissue (WAT), particularly visceral WAT. This is characterized by chronic activation of inflammatory pathways in both adipocytes and monocytes/macrophages within adipose tissue. In the majority of obese individuals, WAT shows an elevated production of inflammatory cytokines, especially tumour necrosis factor-alpha (TNF-α) and IL-6. These not only influence WAT metabolism but also elicit systemic effects in other organs and tissues, in particular in the heart, peripheral blood vessels, liver, and kidneys [4–6].

It has been suggested that a high proportion of the WAT-associated inflammatory molecules are derived from infiltrating monocytes and tissue macrophages. Weight loss results in a decrease in lymphocyte and monocyte numbers, together with a reduction in the ongoing inflammatory response [4–6].

The role of adipocytes in the inflammation associated with WAT activation is still controversial, but evidence indicates that preadipocytes may act as monocytes, have the capacity for phagocytosis, can activate complement, and can secrete inflammatory cytokines. Furthermore, genes that encode transcription factors involved in inflammatory cell signalling and in fatty acid (FA) transport mechanisms are functionally expressed in adipocytes and monocytes/macrophages, suggesting that both cell types are important for the inflammatory milieu associated with obesity [4–6].

The inflammation in obese WAT is partly due to saturated FAs activating Toll-like receptors (TLRs) on both adipocytes and infiltrating monocytes and resident macrophages. This leads to activation of the stress signalling pathways (NF-κB, activator protein 1 [AP-1], c-Jun N-terminal kinase [JNK]) and increased production of proinflammatory molecules including cytokines, adipokines, and IL-6-elicited hepatic C-reactive protein (CRP). The resultant increase in nonesterified FAs in blood in obese individuals, due to an inability of insulin-resistant adipocytes to esterify FAs, exacerbates inflammatory signalling [6].

Interestingly, adipose tissue IL-6 content is higher in obese individuals who present with increased CRP, and these individuals have an approximate twofold increase in the risk of developing type 2 diabetes. Eventually, persistent inflammation can result in insulin resistance in these cells, as well as in liver and muscle tissues, resulting in hyperglycaemia and an increased risk of type 2 diabetes.

Obesity also results in significant changes in adipose-specific energy regulating factors, like leptin and adiponectin, that are also implicated in the regulation of specific immune responses in animals and humans. Leptin is overexpressed in obese subjects and is implicated, in part, in the increased TNF-α production and macrophage activation associated with increased fat deposition. Leptin receptors, expressed in different cells including several immune cells, belong to the cytokine class I receptor family; hyperleptinaemia increases inflammatory cytokines even in nonobese individuals.

Adiponectin is highly expressed in WAT and has been shown to enhance the production of the proinflammatory cytokine TNF-α, reduce hepatic gluconeogenesis and promote FA oxidation in skeletal muscle. Human adipocyte adiponectin mRNA expression is reduced by TNF-α and IL-6, indicating another mechanism whereby these inflammatory cytokines can induce insulin resistance [4–6].

Thus, apart from the physical and gross anatomical problems encountered by the surgeon during operations in obese patients, it is important to recognize that most of these individuals have a pre-existing low-grade inflammation which may be exacerbated perioperatively by the trauma and tissue damage associated with surgery (see Chapter 2).

Probiotics and prebiotics

Probiotics

A probiotic is defined as a live microbial food ingredient that is beneficial to health. They are live microorganisms which are provided either as a direct supplement or as part of the normal diet, and have a variety of effects which are thought to be beneficial to health, but in ways other than their direct nutritional value [7]. These benefits include stimulating the gut-associated lymphoid tissue (GALT), interference with and prevention of colonization of the gastrointestinal tract (GIT) by pathogenic bacteria (including their adherence to the mucosal receptors (Rs) and mucosal invasion). In addition, probiotics probably also have a direct antibacterial effect. Some of these antibacterial effects are mediated via the production of bacteriocin and related molecules [8].

Clearly, there are some basic prerequisites for probiotics to be used in humans. These include their human origin and the need to have undergone extensive safety assessments. Furthermore, to be effective they must be stable in gastric acid and bile. At present, the two most common microorganisms used as probiotics are the lactic acid bacteria, lactobacillus and bifidobacterium. Other bacteria which have been used include lactococcus and nonpathogeneic strains of *Escherichia coli* [9]. These microorganisms have a variety of effects on the immune system, both in the GIT and systemically. These have been evaluated *in vitro* and *in vivo* in both animal and human studies. However, it is important to note that there appear to be different effects in normal healthy volunteers, compared with individuals presenting with various disease states. Also, the effects on the immune system depend on the immune status of the individual, e.g. if they are atopic or have other disorders of immune function.

Studies *in vitro* have demonstrated that probiotics can decrease lymphocyte proliferation in response to mitogens together with decreasing cytokine production by T cells and phagocytic cells. This occurs to varying degrees and is dependent on the microorganism involved and on the quantity of organisms present. Specifically, in terms of effects on cytokine production by T helper (Th) cells, probiotic bacteria appear to increase production of proinflammatory Th1 cytokines (IL-2, IL-12) whilst decreasing anti-inflammatory Th2 cytokines (IL-4, IL-10) [10]. In the mucosa of the GIT, probiotics also reduce the expression of NF-κB which results in a further reduction of GALT immune responses, already suboptimal due to decreased cytokine production and eicosanoid synthesis (see Box 6.1).

Studies *in vitro* with human cells have shown that probiotics can stimulate dendritic cells (DCs), (crucial antigen presenting cells [APCs]) to mature and produce a variety of important regulatory cytokines (IL-10, IL-12) and increase the expression of major histocompatability complex (MHC) class II antigens, which play a key role in regulating immune responses [11]. This is significant because DCs are constituents of GALT, which is an important site of action of probiotics.

In human volunteer studies, the administration of probiotics has been shown to increase the phagocytic activity of polymorphonuclear granulocytes and monocytes (as well as decreasing their release of proinflammatory cytokines), and to stimulate the activity of natural killer (NK) cells in peripheral blood. In addition, increased Th1 cytokine production has been documented together with increased levels of GALT production of IgA (Box 6.1). Other studies, on the other hand, have revealed conflicting results on the immune system and suggest that the end-effects are dependent on the type of probiotic administered. Therefore, good-quality, randomized, controlled trials are required to fully elucidate the potential impact that probiotics can have on GALTs and systemically [12]. (Box 6.1)

Probiotics have also been evaluated in patients, e.g. in children with rotavirus infections [13]. In this latter study, the administration of probiotics resulted in an increase in systemic levels of IgA and antibody-producing cells. Furthermore, there was an increased production of IgA within the GALT. Although this study was in children it

Box 6.1 Enhanced immunological effects of lactobacilli on aspects of immune function

- Monocyte and macrophage phagocytic activity
- NK cell cytotoxicity
- B cell numbers and IgA production
- Th1 cell cytokine production (but reduced Th2 cytokines)
- IgA levels in faeces

may have an important application in clinical practice in adults, given the increasing occurrence of *Clostridium difficile* infections in hospitalized patients receiving antibiotic treatment. Some initial studies have confirmed this by suggesting that certain probiotics will significantly reduce *C. difficile-associated diarrhoea* (CDAD), although the mechanisms are not fully understood [14]. In patients with inflammatory bowel disease probiotics may also reduce the severity of symptoms, but further well-controlled trials are required to confirm these findings.

Prebiotics

Prebiotics have recently become the focus of considerable research interest with regard to their specific effects in competitively regulating the existing beneficial GIT microbial populations to the detriment of pathogenic bacterial growth and adhesion to mucosal surfaces. Prebiotics include a number of plant-derived, soluble fibre compounds such as inulin, fructo-oligosaccharides, galacto-oligosaccharides, and manno-oligosaccharides. They provide substrates for the specific growth advantage of the various beneficial GIT bacteria, such as lactobacilli and bifidobacteria (probiotics), thereby enabling the beneficial effects of probiotics to occur. The place of prebiotics in clinical practice remains to be defined, but maintenance of a healthy GIT microflora is of vital importance for the general health of patients of all ages.

Micronutrients

Zinc

Zinc is an essential micronutrient which is necessary for appropriate functioning of the immune system, together with playing a key role in several physiological processes that are important in patients undergoing surgery. Zinc is also vital in would healing, antioxidant defence mechanisms, and glucose homeostasis. Zinc plays a key role in modulating intracellular processes by regulating the function of many enzymes, transcription and replication factors [15,16]. Although chronic zinc deficiency states can occur, patients who are critically ill have transiently lowered plasma levels which return to normal with recovery.

Zinc is necessary for the development and function of both the innate and adaptive immune systems and ensuring that immune function is optimal. Zinc is important for the healthy development of the immune system and is required for T and B cell maturation. In the presence of zinc deficiency there is a failure of thymic development and associated lymphopenia. The latter is due to an increased apoptosis of pre-T and pre-B cells [17]. Furthermore, normal function and activity of NK cells, monocytes, macrophages, and neutrophils is also dependent on zinc. In the absence of zinc, antimicrobial lytic and phagocytic function, together with intracellular mechanisms, are impaired. Another effect of zinc, although not directly modulating immune function, is its central role in key intracellular antioxidant defence mechanisms. These effects are mediated via its role as a cofactor for the copper/zinc superoxide dismutase (SOD) that reduces reactive oxygen species (ROS) and the damage they cause to a variety of macromolecules within the cell [18].

The mechanisms by which these changes occur have not been fully elucidated. However, these may be mediated, at least in part, by a reduction in the secretion of key cytokines produced by Th1 cells (IFN-γ, TNF-α and IL-2). There is, however, no effect on production of cytokines by Th2 cells (IL-4 and IL-10) [19]. Zinc also has a direct effect on the expression of IL-2 and IL-2R genes and causes a reduction in the ability of the stress-activated nuclear factor NF-κB to bind to DNA. This attenuates the stress cascade leading to decreased inflammatory cytokine production [20]. Another possible mechanism involving zinc is its role as a cofactor for thymulin, produced by the thymus, which regulates many aspects of the immune function. Zinc is also implicated as a cofactor in essential FA (EFA) metabolism and prostaglandin (PG) synthesis; zinc and EFA deficiencies present with similar clinical features.

While it is essential to ensure that daily requirements are met, the role of supplementation with additional zinc in patients undergoing surgery remains uncertain. A recent systematic review indicated that in patients with critical illness (e.g. trauma, head injury, major burns) the benefits were unclear and there may be toxicity associated with high levels of zinc supplementation. Zinc supplementation, therefore, is not recommended in surgical patients at the present time [21].

Selenium

Selenium is deficient in the diets of a large section of the adult population in Scotland and other selenium-deficient countries/regions such as New Zealand and Keshan province in China. This has been suggested as a possible causal factor in a number of disease states in these regions. Selenium is incorporated into a variety of selenoproteins necessary for normal cellular function and, in particular, the maintenance of immune function and regulation of intracellular redox activity. This protects macromolecules such as DNA, lipids, proteins, and cell membranes against oxidative damage. Examples of key selenoproteins whose functions are well documented are the glutathione peroxidases, thioredoxin reductases, and iodothyronine deiodinases. In total, more than 30 seleno-proteins have been isolated but the functions of the others are less well understood.

Glutathione peroxidase is necessary for the reductive degradation of a variety of oxidative-stress-derived molecules (hydrogen peroxide and lipid peroxides), which are produced when the cell undergoes normal metabolism and oxidative stress. This may occur during inflammation, as a result of the release of inflammatory mediators from neutrophils, monocytes, and macrophages, as part of their respiratory burst. Thioredoxin reductases also have a key role because they regulate several molecules involved in the stress pathways, including reducing the oxidative-stress-activated NF-κB transcription factor. This is important because NF-κB binds to DNA of specific genes resulting in activation and expression of other proinflammatory cytokines, heat shock proteins (HSPs), and adhesion molecules. In selenium deficiency, several changes in the immune system can be detected. For example, neutrophil, monocyte, and macrophage cytotoxic activity and chemotaxis are reduced, there are reductions in $CD8^+$ CTL activity and in $CD4^+$ Th cell numbers, and decreased activity of NK and lymphokine-activated killer (LAK) cell activities. B cell function is also impaired with reductions in circulating levels of both IgG and IgM antibodies, together with reduction in the constituents of the complement system [22–24].

Studies in humans have shown that even in the presence of apparently normal selenium levels, supplementation with selenium can enhance various aspects of the immune system, independent of effects on redox enzyme systems. Given these effects on the immune system and antioxidant defence mechanisms, it is not surprising that clinical trials of supplemental selenium on clinical outcomes in patients with critical illness have been carried out. However, a recent analysis of 10 such trials (>1000 patients) found that there were no clinical benefits, either in terms of reduction in mortality or reduction in infectious complications [25]. Therefore, at present, supplementation with selenium is not recommended. Further studies with precise assessment of selenium status, redox enzyme expression, and oxidative ROS levels in patients are required before definitive guidelines are produced and applied to selenium supplementation in patients.

Copper

Copper is important in the development, maturation, and function of the immune system. Although deficiency of copper in humans is rare, it can be encountered in patients with severe malabsorption and in those who are receiving long-term parenteral nutritional support. Like other trace elements, copper also plays a role in intracellular antioxidant defences because it is a component of the enzyme SOD and is important in protecting against oxidative damage [26].

Copper has been shown to have an effect on the function of neutrophils, macrophages, and T cells, in particular. For example, in animal studies, copper deficiency results in a reduction in the numbers of T lymphocytes, especially within the $CD4^+$ T cells, together with a less marked reduction in $CD8^+$ T cells [27]. Other aspects of T cell function *in vitro* which appear to be reduced in copper deficiency are responses of T cells to mitogens, antigen processing, and presentation. Neutrophils are also affected in copper deficiency with reductions in numbers, respiratory burst, and cytotoxic activity being documented.

The effects of copper on the human immune system have been less well studied. However, copper supplementation given to healthy volunteers does increase responsiveness of T cells to mitogens, but does not affect numbers of neutrophils, macrophages, T cell subsets, or NK cell and macrophage activity [28]. With high intakes of copper in healthy individuals, there appears to be an elevation of proinflammatory cytokines, such as IL-6, and reduction in circulating neutrophils, possibly because high levels of this metal can result in oxidative stress. Therefore, further work is required to define more fully the role of copper and its effects on immunity in patients undergoing surgery. There is no indication for supplementation above the recommended intake.

Magnesium

Magnesium is an important trace element which, in addition to its variety of metabolic functions, also plays a role in the regulation of immune responses. Animal studies have shown that magnesium deficiency will lead to an increase in the number, and an enhanced activation, of neutrophils (increased respiratory burst and production of ROSs). Macrophage phagocytosis is increased and there is an involution of the thymus with a reduction in $CD8^+$ T cells. Magnesium deficiency also results in an increased production of the inflammatory cytokines IL-6 and TNF-α, accompanied by an inflammatory response, although the underlying mechanisms are unknown [29]. Although these effects occur in animal studies, the role of magnesium on the human immune system is less clear; in one study of magnesium supplementation in athletes there was no effect on neutrophil function or the inflammatory response occurring after exercise [30].

Iron

Iron is essential for several metabolic processes and electron transport systems, and is a key component of haem and myeloperoxidase enzymes. It also plays a vital role in the regulation of the immune system and is essential for its optimal functioning. Interestingly, it has been estimated that large percentages of the populations in all countries throughout the world are iron deficient, and almost one-half of pregnant women are deficient in iron, despite its key physiological importance.

The effects of a deficiency of iron on the immune system have been well documented in both human and animal studies. The function of neutrophils, macrophages, T and B lymphocytes, NK cell activity, antibody production, and cytokine secretion are all affected [31,32]. These effects are summarized in Table 6.1. When iron deficiency is reversed, immune function is restored. A less common condition than iron deficiency is iron overload, which may occur in conditions such as B-thalassaemia, sickle cell anaemia, and haemachromatosis, resulting in increased amounts of iron within the

Table 6.1 Immunological effects of iron deficiency and iron excess

Effects on the immune system	Iron deficiency	Iron excess
Neutrophil function	Intracellular killing reduced due to lower levels of myeloperoxidase and reduced respiratory burst, reduced neutrophil migration, reduced phagocytosis	Reduced myeloperoxidase activity and intracellular killing
T cells	Decreased response to mitogens; decreased Th and CTL numbers	Deceased response to mitogens; decreased $CD4^+$ T cells, reduction in $CD4^+/CD8^+$ ratio, decreased CTLs
B cell function	Reduced circulating antibody levels	Not altered
NK cell activity	Reduced cytotoxicity	Not altered
Macrophage cytotoxicity	Minor reduction of lytic activity	May be reduced
Cytokines	Decreased secretion of Th1 and Th2 cytokines	Increased levels of IL-4, IL-6, IL-10

body tissues. However, this will also result in impairment in a wide range of immune functions and these are shown in Table 6.1. The mechanisms underlying these effects have not been clarified and are not discussed further here.

Amino acids

In recent years interest has focused on amino acids and the biological effects that they have on the immune system, in addition to their central roles in many metabolic processes. The role of the important amino acids is discussed in more detail below, with a focus on aspects of the immune system that are important in the patient undergoing surgery.

L-Glutamine

L-Glutamine is a nonessential amino acid which is synthesized from branched chain amino acids (BCAAs) by transamination requiring the enzyme glutamine synthase. L-Glutamine makes up approximately 50–60% of the free amino acids within cells, but less than 10% of the structural protein within skeletal muscle. During conditions such as stress and trauma it is released in large quantities by the skeletal muscle into the blood and intracellular concentrations are decreased significantly. Under these circumstances, L-glutamine becomes an essential amino acid [33].

L-Glutamine is a most important substrate for energy production by a variety of rapidly proliferating cells, such as those of the immune system and enterocytes, and is also necessary for the production of nucleotides. L-Glutamine is metabolized to glutamate, aspartate, lactate, and pyruvate and is a substrate for the production of glutathione which is important in antioxidant intracellular defence mechanisms.

L-Glutamine has been shown to have a variety of effects on different components of the immune system (Table 6.2), in particular on aspects of lymphocyte and macrophage function. Initial studies have demonstrated that it stimulates the proliferation of T lymphocytes *in vitro* in response to mitogenic stimuli. Other *in vitro* studies have shown that it can prevent lymphocytes from entering into apoptosis and stimulates the production of antibodies. In addition, in animal studies, L-glutamine is able to stimulate NK and LAK cells, increasing numbers and activity in the liver and spleen, respectively. L-Glutamine has been shown to regulate the expression of a variety of cluster of differentiation (CD) markers such as CD25 and CD45RO (necessary for the regulation of immune function) on the surface of lymphocytes [34,35]. In the GIT, L-glutamine has a specific role in the maintenance of GALT and the secretion of IgA by the lymphoid cells in GALT. Both of these are important in the surgical patient, in preventing bacterial translocation across the GIT barrier.

Macrophage and monocyte phagocytic activity are dependent on L-glutamine, as is neutrophil phagocytosis and bactericidal activity. The production of a variety of immunoregulatory cytokines, by both lymphocytes and monocytes/macrophages, has been shown to be modulated by L-glutamine *in vitro*. For example, the production of IL-1, IL-6, IL-8, IFN-γ, and TNF-α are all dependent on an adequate supply of intracellular L-glutamine.

L-Glutamine modulates the expression of receptors which are essential for phagocytic activity. In particular, it is important for the expression of the high-affinity

Table 6.2 Effects of L-glutamine and L-arginine on the immune system

Effects on the immune system	L-Glutamine	L-Arginine
Neutrophil function	Increased phagocytosis and bactericidal activity	Not established
T cells	Increased proliferation, decreased apoptosis	Essential for normal cellular development, increased numbers and proliferation
B cell function	Increased antibody production, increased IgA secretion by GALT	Increased cell numbers and antibody production
NK cell activity	Increased numbers and activities of NK and LAK cells	Increased numbers and activities of NK and LAK cells
Macrophage cytotoxicity	Increased phagocytosis and increased cell surface receptors for phagocytosis, increased production of HSPs	Increased phagocytic activity, increased cytokine release, increased superoxide production
Cytokine release	IL-1,IL-6,IL-8, IFN-γ, and TNF-α	Not established

receptors for IgG and the complement components C3 and C4, and is necessary for the expression of the intercellular adhesion molecule 1 (I-CAM1). A further key biochemical process within macrophages is the production of arginine from glutamine leading to nitric oxide (NO) synthesis by activated macrophages. Finally, macrophages and lymphocytes express HSPs under conditions of stress which enable cells to survive. L-Glutamine plays an important role in modulating their expression. In the presence of low levels of L-glutamine, the ability to induce HSPs is inadequate and will result in cell death [36].

L-Arginine

L-Arginine is a basic amino acid which is synthesized from proline, glutamine, or glutamate. In addition, a major source of L-arginine in the body is its synthesis from citrulline. This is produced by the small intestine and then converted in the kidney into L-arginine. However, although the body is normally able to synthesize adequate amounts of L-arginine, in stress, an individual's dietary requirements are increased and this synthetic pathway is often insufficient to meet the body's needs. L-Arginine is therefore termed a *semi-essential* or *conditional* amino acid. L-Arginine has a variety of metabolic functions including that of precursor for the synthesis of NO, proline, creatinine, and polyamines and is an essential component of the urea cycle [37]. NO has an important role in causing vasodilatation and thus affects cardiac, pulmonary, and vascular function. Also, NO is produced by many cells of the immune system including macrophages, monocytes, NK cells, and Kupffer cells (see Table 6.2).

The key enzyme involved in the production of NO from L-arginine is NO synthase (NOS). This has a constitutive form expressed in a variety of tissues and an inducible form.

It is the inducible form of NOS (iNOS) that plays an important role in immunity. In addition to these effects, it has been well recognized for many years that L-arginine will stimulate the secretion of hormones such as prolactin, growth hormone, and insulin-like growth factor 1 (IGF-1). Hence, understanding the physiological and metabolic effects of L-arginine is complex because these hormones have stimulatory effects on a variety of anabolic and immune processes. For example, growth hormone will stimulate the thymus to increase the numbers of T lymphocytes and has similar effects on the bone marrow, whilst prolactin increases the production of IFN-γ, IL-2, and IL-12 by Th1 lymphocytes. IGF-1 has effects on the immune system similar to those of growth hormone [35].

The biological effects of L-arginine on the immune system were initially demonstrated in a series of *in vitro* and animal studies. L-Arginine was required for normal lymphocyte development and dietary supplementation resulted in an increase in thymic weight and cellularity, together with an increased activity of lymphocytes isolated from the spleen. Following these initial studies, more detailed examinations of the effects of L-arginine on the immune system demonstrated that many indices of immune function were modulated, including lymphocyte responses to mitogens, effects on macrophages, stimulation of NK cell cytotoxicity, and an increased expression of the IL-2Rs on T lymphocytes [38]. More recently, it has become apparent that physiological levels of L-arginine may actually modulate a component of the T cell receptor (TCR) that is necessary for maintenance of integrity and function.

Studies *in vitro* initially demonstrated that peripheral blood lymphocytes exhibited an enhanced response to mitogens when cultured with L-arginine. This led to subsequent studies *in vivo* where both healthy human volunteers and patients with different types of cancer had their normal diet supplemented with L-arginine. When these volunteers and patients were given 3 days of L-arginine supplementation (30 g/day) there was an increase in the number of T and B lymphocytes, an enhanced response to mitogenic stimulation, and a significant and substantial increase in NK and LAK cell cytotoxicity [39,40]. L-Arginine supplementation also could reduce the postoperative immune suppression that normally occurs following surgery. However, these enhancing effects on immune function appeared to be limited to patients who had some degree of malnutrition before surgery. This highlights the need to consider each patient's immune status, and to ensure optimum immune function before surgery in all patients through presurgical dietary supplementation, where necessary.

L-Arginine supplementation in animal studies has demonstrated optimal macrophage function—enhanced macrophage cytotoxicity, superoxide production, phagocytic activity, and cytokine release. Furthermore, macrophage cytotoxicity against tumour cells was also enhanced. In subsequent human studies, it was demonstrated *in vitro* that cytotoxicity mediated by monocytes was also enhanced by supplementation with L-arginine.

L-Arginine supplementation and effects on circulating B lymphocytes and production of immunoglobulins have been investigated both in patients with cancer and in those who have been involved in trauma. Supplementation with 30 g of L-arginine for periods of up to 7 days has shown that there was an enhanced response of lymphocyte mitogenic stimulation *in vitro*, increased circulating levels of IgM and IgG antibodies, and increased numbers of circulating B lymphocytes.

Another area of importance in critically ill patients, and in patients undergoing GIT surgery, is the effect of L-arginine on intestinal function and bacterial translocation. The initial evidence for this came from animal studies demonstrating that after a burn injury, supplementation reduced bacterial translocation across the GIT and increased the antibacterial activity of phagocytic cells. Similarly, in experimentally induced bacterial peritonitis in animal models, dietary supplementation with L-arginine substantially reduced subsequent mortality. This clearly has important implications for patients who are critically ill or are undergoing major GIT surgery [41].

L-Arginine, therefore, has a wide range of effects on the immune system which are important for the surgical patient both pre- and perioperatively. Although the mechanisms underlying these biological effects remain to be fully clarified, some of these may be mediated via increased release of key hormones, modulation of NO synthesis, and changes in polyamine production.

Branched chain amino acids

The BCAAs, L-leucine, L-isoleucine, and L-valine, are essential amino acids but they also have key properties which differentiate them from other amino acids: they are metabolized to a large extent in skeletal muscle (a key source of fuel during stress and infection) and they play a role in the regulation of protein synthesis in muscle and adipose tissue. These latter effects are thought to be mediated through leucine-induced activation of mTOR (mammalian target of rapamycin, a serine/threonine protein kinase), a pathway which is a key regulator of protein synthesis and breakdown.

BCAAs also act as a carbon skeleton donor for the synthesis of a variety of other amino acids including L-glutamine. During times of stimulation and activation of the immune system the uptake of these amino acids is increased substantially by a variety of cells of the innate and adaptive immune systems, and they are a vital source of energy.

In vitro studies using a variety of cell types, including immune cells, showed that if BCAA levels were reduced in the culture medium the ability of lymphocytes to respond to a mitogenic stimulus was substantially reduced and this was probably due to a reduction of protein synthesis. Others have confirmed that deficiencies in the supply of BCAAs result in reduced lymphocyte proliferation. However, the provision of increased amounts of amino acids did not result in an enhanced response of lymphocytes to mitogenic stimulation. Therefore, it has been suggested that a certain level of BCAAs is required for optimal immune function, but increasing above that level is not beneficial [42,43].

Studies *in vivo* in animals elucidated the role of BCAAs on the immune system. It was found that if intake was reduced (up to 50%) then specific indices of immune function, such as NK cell activity, were decreased. Conversely, with increased intake of BCAAs, the activity of CTLs and NK cells was increased. Moreover, the different BCAAs had different effects in that L-leucine was more potent than either L-isoleucine or L-valine. Importantly, this was translated into potential clinical relevance because reduction in BCAA intake resulted in increased susceptibility to infection (with reduced levels of circulating antibodies and complement) and increased mortality due to sepsis. For example, when BCAA ingestion in the diet of mice was reduced by 50% there was an increase in mortality due to sepsis when mice were challenged with *Salmonella typhimurium* [44].

Clinical studies have also tried to provide an insight into the effects of BCAAs on the immune system. Dietary supplementation in volunteers (healthy athletes) with BCAAs demonstrated enhanced *ex vivo* isolated lymphocyte proliferation *in vitro* in response to mitogenic stimulation, increased levels of IL-4, and reduced levels of IFN-γ and TNF-α. Similarly, in patients undergoing major surgery, intravenous supplementation of standard nutritional support with BCAAs also resulted in an enhanced immune function (lymphocyte response to mitogens and delayed type hypersensitivity to certain antigens) [45].

Methionine and cysteine (sulphur amino acids)

The sulphur-containing amino acids, methionine and cysteine, occupy a central role in metabolism. Methionine is an essential amino acid, but cysteine can be derived from methionine and so is considered to be semi-essential. Cysteine is used in the synthesis of glutathione which is a key molecule protecting against the damaging effects on DNA and other molecules by free radicals and ROSs (see 'Selenium' section above) [46]. Another role for cysteine is as a precursor for taurine, which is the most abundant amino acid within leucocytes, and may itself have an immunomodulatory and antioxidant role, although its functions remain unclear.

The biological and metabolic role of these sulphur-containing amino acids on the immune system has not been as comprehensively investigated as the amino acids discussed earlier in this chapter. However, increasing dietary intake of either methionine or cysteine resulted in an enhancement of T cell responses to mitogens *in vitro* and circulating antibody levels in experimental animal studies. When ingested in large amounts, however, immunity was impaired due to the toxic effects of the metabolic products of these amino acids. In studies in patients with sepsis and in patients with HIV infection, either oral intake or intravenous administration of a cysteine precursor was shown to enhance various aspects of immune function (lymphocyte response to mitogens, NK cell activity), and to elicit some clinical benefit through improved respiratory function [47]. However, further studies are required to fully understand the overt actions and underlying mechanisms of these amino acids on immune functions in humans.

Glutathione, a product of methionine metabolism and very closely related to the sulphur amino acids, also has beneficial effects on the immune system. Under normal circumstances, intracellular glutathione exists as a reduced (GSH) and an oxidized (GSSG) form. The ratio of GSH:GSSG is a good indicator of the redox state of the cell/tissue. If the intracellular concentrations of GSH decreases (increased oxidative state) then lymphocyte proliferation and the production of CTLs is reduced. Conversely, increased levels of glutamine leads to increased intracellular levels of GSH and increased cell proliferation. Clearly, the redox state of cells involved in immune reactivity affects their function and this might be a simple biomarker of immune competence.

Table 6.3 Effects of other amino acids on immune function

Amino acid	Effects on the immune system
Tryptophan	Inhibits T cell proliferation
Glycine	Decreases plasma levels of TNF-α and IL-1β, and increases IL-10 production
Homocysteine	Increases activation of monocytes, Th1 cell function
Histidine	Histamine produced from histidine and stimulates release of Th2 cell activity Histamine receptors present on many types of immune cells and have a role in inflammation and immunity (not fully clarified) Histidine prevents apoptosis and stimulates antibody production by lymphocytes
Lysine	Stimulates lymphocyte proliferation; if deficient in diet results in reduced T cell function
Phenylalanine	Regulates nitric oxide function in leucocytes Breakdown product (tyrosine) is a precursor for a variety of key hormones (e.g. catecholamines, thyroxine) which have immunomodulatory roles

Other amino acids

It is beyond the scope of this chapter to discuss in detail the other individual amino acids, some of which do have variable effects on the immune system. However, the impact of these amino acids is poorly characterized and has been assessed predominantly in *in vitro* studies. For example, tryptophan, glycine, histidine, and lysine all have varying modulating activities on immune function and the most important of these have been summarized in Table 6.3.

Fatty acids

FAs are major constituents of dietary fats, mainly triacylglycerols but also phospholipids, and can have significant effects on various aspects of immune function, dependent mainly on the type of FA contained in the fat (acylated to glycerol, sphingosine, or phosphatidic acids), its concentration, and existing physiological and immunological status. FAs modulate numerous functions of the cells of the immune system, are a source of energy, and constitute structural elements of membranes, including rafts which are important in cell signalling. They also can act as signalling molecules directly influencing gene expression (through FA response elements in specific gene promoters) and are precursors of the cell regulatory eicosanoids prostaglandins (PGs), prostacyclins (PIs), thromboxanes (TXs), leukotrienes (LTs), and hydroxy FAs. More recently, they have been shown to form anti inflammatory derivatives termed resolvins and protectins, particularly when aspirin-like compounds are present The effects of fatty acids on immune function are summarized in Table 6.4.

FAs are a diverse group of hydrocarbon compounds of differing chain length and varying degrees of unsaturation (number of double bonds). They are either ingested

Table 6.4 Important effects of the different classes of fatty acids on immune function in animals and humans

Class of fatty acid	Dietary sources	Important effects
Short-chain (volatile) FAs	Butter, milk, soluble fibre fermentations	**Decrease:** Inflammatory cytokines, eicosanoids, NF-κB expression; carcinogen activity and cell proliferation
Saturated FAs	Animal fats, particularly ruminant fats, hydrogenated plant oils	**Increase:** Inflammation, TLR activation, NF-κB activation, COX-2, 5-LOX expression, inflammatory cytokines and eicosanoid formation Tumour growth and metastasis dissemination
MUFAs	Plant oils olive, rapeseed, corn, animal fats	**Decrease:** Spleen lymphocyte proliferation, NK cell activity in animals Inflammatory cytokine formation in animals Effects in humans are generally neutral
ω-6 LCPUFAs	Most foods containing fats, plant oils, margarines, animal fats, hydrogenated fats	Can have both pro- and anti-inflammatory effects depending on concentrations **Increase:** NF-κB expression, inflammation, cytokines, eicosanoids, COX, LOX Tumour growth, metastasis in animals
ω-3 LCPUFAs	Plant oils, animal tissues, fish products, fish oil	**Decrease:** TLR activation by LPS, saturated FAs, inflammatory cytokines, eicosanoids, HSPs, NF-κB activation, MHC class II expression **Increase:** Resolvins, protectins
CLAs	Ruminant fats, hydrogenated plant oils	**Decrease:** NF-κB expression, cytokine and eicosanoid formation, COX, LOX expression Tumour growth and metastasis in animals

5-LOX, 5-lipooxygenase; CLA, conjugated linoleic acid; COX-2, cyclooxygenase-2; FA, fatty acid; HSP, heat shock protein; LCPUFA long-chain polyunsaturated fatty acid; LPS, lipopolysaccharide; MUFA, monounsaturated fatty acid; TLR, Toll-like receptor.

in the diet as plant or animal-derived macronutrients (fats and oils) or they can be synthesized *in situ* from two-carbon precursors (mainly in liver and adipose tissue) from carbohydrate, protein, and lipid catabolism. They are characterized by a terminal methyl group (CH_3) at the omega (ω) or n- end of the chain and a reactive carboxylic acid group (COOH) at the carboxylic or delta (δ)-end. The chain length of

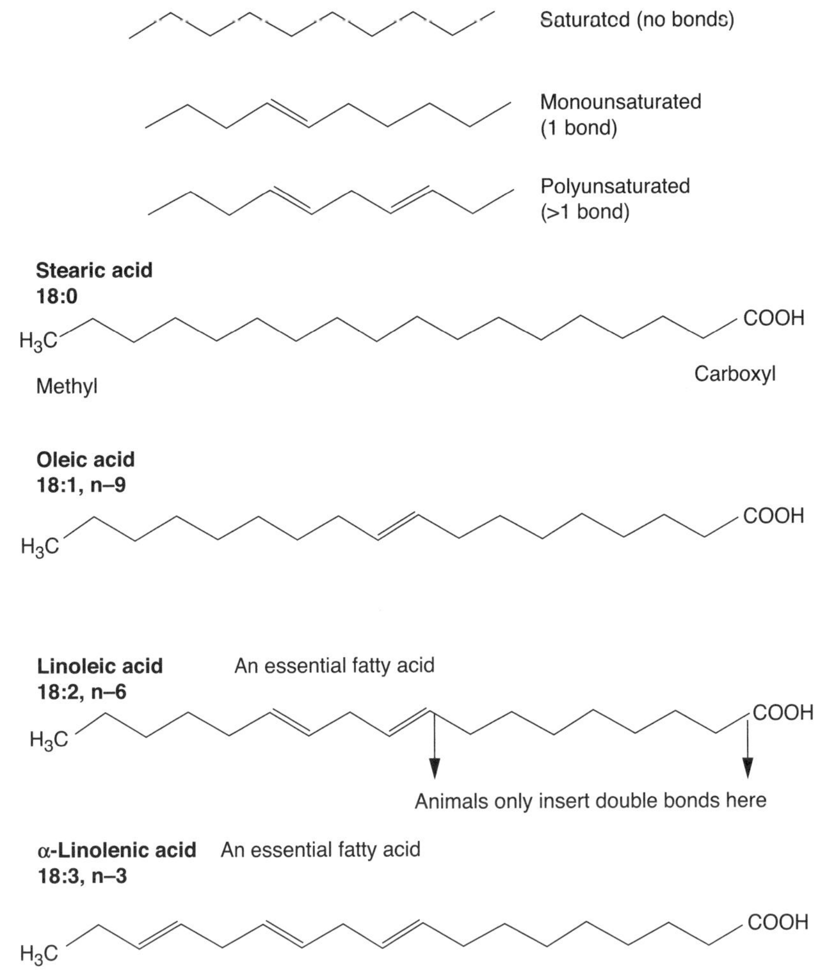

Fig. 6.1 Basic structures of physiologically important FAs in humans. Linoleic (18:2n-6) and α-linolenic (18:3n-3) acids are EFAs and must be ingested in the diet for optimum health since humans can only insert a double bond between an existing bond and the carboxyl end of the chain; n-3 and n-6 bonds are inserted only in plants. EFA, essential fatty acid; FA, fatty acid.

the most important and most common FAs found in human and mammalian tissues range from the saturated (no double bonds) two-carbon volatile FA (acetic acid) to the 24-carbon FAs with six double bonds (Figure 6.1). Other longer-chain and more unsaturated FAs occur in nature but are not regarded as important in human or animal physiology.

FAs can be grouped into three main families: saturated (no double bonds), monounsaturated (MU: one double bond; ω-7 or ω-9) and polyunsaturated (PU: two or more double bonds; ω-3 and ω-6) families, each of which has a number of subgroupings (Figure 6.1).

Saturated fatty acids

Short-chain, volatile FAs (C-2, acetate; C-3, propionate; C-4, butyrate) are produced from various forms of undigested nonstarch fibres derived from plant cell-walls (often termed prebiotics), such as polysaccharides and hemicelluloses, by microbial anaerobic fermentation in the colon of mammals, including humans. They have been implicated in maintaining colonic health, in that they can reduce the inflammatory cascade in mucosal cells through inhibition of NF-κB. Similar benefits are seen in the systemic cardiovascular system through attenuation of cytokine-induced adhesion molecule expression on vascular endothelium, again due to inhibition of NF-κB up-regulation by the inflammatory cytokines and pro-oxidative conditions [48].

This explains, at least in part, why prebiotics and probiotics are important for a healthy GIT, as well as general health. Inhibition of vascular endothelial adhesion molecules will reduce the metastatic spread of tumours, since adherence of cancer cells to the endothelial surfaces is impaired. These short-chain FAs, particularly butyrate (C-4), are also regarded as possibly being anticarcinogenic in the colon where they can inhibit cell cycle and cell proliferation. The medium- and long-chain saturated FAs—lauric (C-12), myristic (C-14), palmitic (C-16), and stearic (C-18)—are synthesized predominantly from metabolically derived two-carbon but also three- and four-carbon precursors (acetate, propionate, and butyrate).

All mammalian systems have the capability of introducing a double bond (desaturation) into a saturated FA at the δ-9 position to form a MUFA derivative due to activity of a δ-9 desaturase enzyme (SCD1), found in many tissues and cells, including host defence cells (see below). This allows the body a degree of regulation of the composition and fluidity of its cellular membranes since one double bond has a marked effect on the physicochemical characteristics of membranes. It is the position of the first double bond from the methyl end in the carbon chain that characterizes the FAs family as either ω-7 and ω-9 (MUFAs) or ω-3 and ω-6 (PUFAs) (Figure 6.1).

Saturated FAs have recently been implicated as causal factors in the increased systemic inflammatory state found in obese individuals due to their potentiation of ligand-activated proinflammatory pathways linked through TLRs, particularly TLR4, in monocyte-macrophages and adipocytes [49,50] (Figure 6.2). TLR4 activation, commonly elicited by bacterial lipopolysaccharide (LPS) ligands, has been shown to up-regulate the stress-related NF-κB pathway with subsequent induction of a variety of stress-response factors, including enhancement of COX-2 and 5-LOX expression and increased inflammatory cytokine and eicosanoid production (TNF-α, IL-1, PGs, LTs) [51].

Importantly, from a health and FA nutrition standpoint, TLR4 activation in monocytes and macrophages by saturated FAs is inhibited by ω-3 long-chain (LC) PUFAs, such as eicosapentaenoic acid (EPA) and docosahexaenoic acid (DHA) (Figure 6.2). Saturated FAs cannot compete in the chain elongation/desaturation reactions with the ω-3 LCPUFA. Therefore, in their presence, the ω-6 LCPUFAs are unrestricted in their metabolism. This suggests that the type of dietary fat consumed can determine responsiveness to inflammatory stimuli such as bacterial LPS or oxidative stress (Figure 6.2).

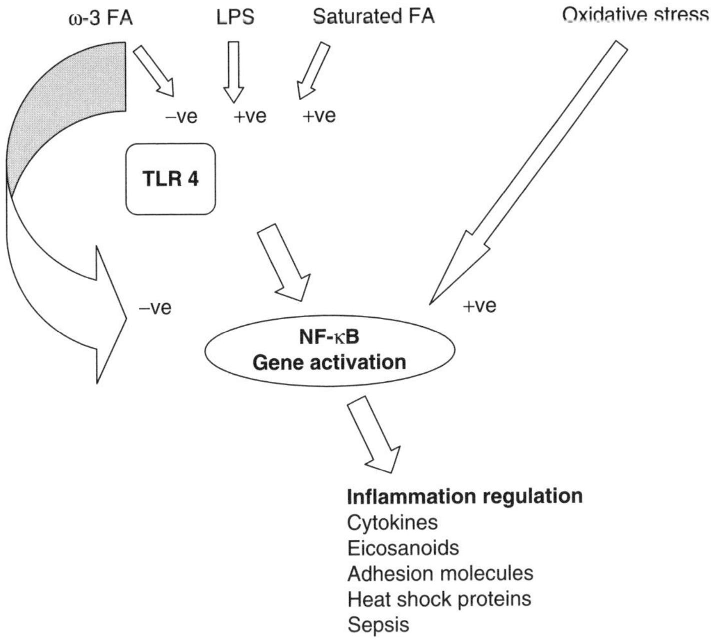

Fig. 6.2 Differential modulation of inflammatory cells by ω-3 and saturated FAs. Activation of NF-κB through receptors, including TLRs, results in increased transcriptional activity in stress-response genes leading to increased inflammatory mediator expression; ω-3 FAs (EPA and DHA) inhibit this pathway. DHA, docosahexaenoic acid; EFA, essential fatty acid; EPA, eicosapentaenoic acid; FA, fatty acid; LPS, lipopolysaccharide; TLR, Toll-like receptor.

ω-9 fatty acids

The MUFA members have one double bond in their chain and are mainly represented in the diet by oleic acid (18:1 ω-9) (Figure 6.1) and palmitoleic acid (16:1 ω-7). They are nonessential because they can be synthesized in the body. Oleic acid is a major component of olive oil and is implicated, at least in part, in the health benefits ascribed to the 'Mediterranean diet'. The presence of one double bond, removal of two hydrogen atoms from the chain, changes the physical characteristics of the FA from a solid form at room temperature (i.e. lard, mainly stearic acid) to that of an oil (i.e. olive oil, mainly oleic acid). Incorporation of MUFA into membranes of mammalian cells, including cells of the immune system, alters their physicochemical properties and functions. This is one of the underlying reasons for their health benefits; rigid membranes are less sensitive to stimuli and consequently less reactive.

MUFAs appear to elicit suppressive effects on immune function in animal studies, as demonstrated by suppression of spleen lymphocyte proliferation, NK cell activity, and inhibition of inflammatory cytokine production [52]. Slight effects of MUFA intake in healthy middle-aged men were evident at 2 months but not at 1 month duration of ingestion. However, MUFA intake in humans did not suppress lymphocyte

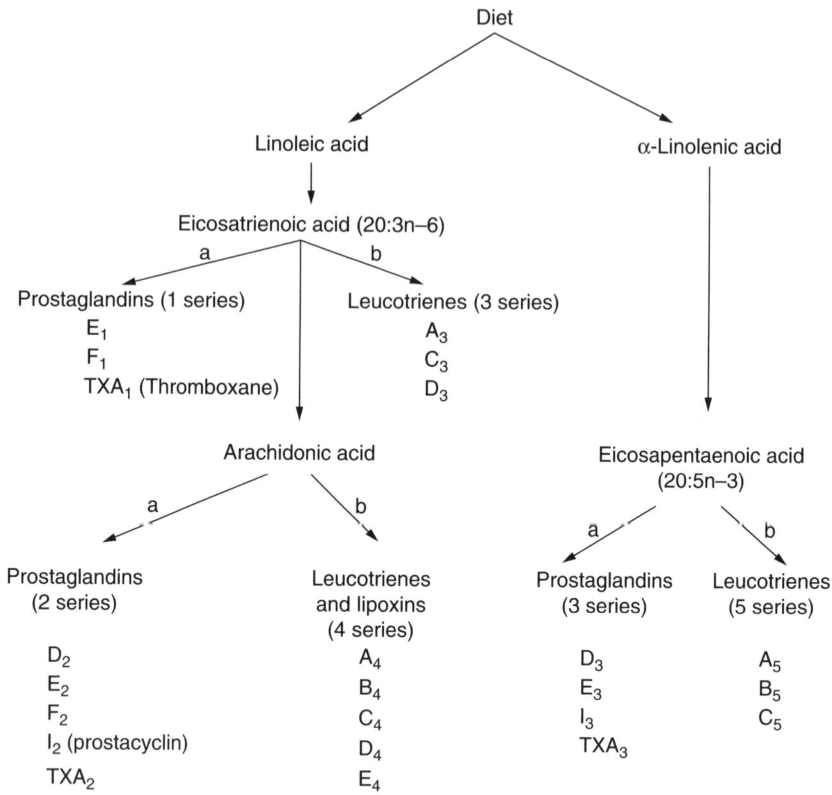

Fig. 6.3 Pathways for eicosanoid synthesis from ω-3 and ω-6 fatty acids. Eicosanoids are involved in the regulation of important cell mechanisms including inflammation and cell proliferation.

proliferation [53]. This differs from observations in animals and is thought to be largely due to the high levels of MUFA in the animal studies. High MUFA levels appear to act mainly through the reduction of available ω-6 in the diet and in cell membranes. MUFA ingestion in humans is generally regarded as neutral in relation to the ω-3 and ω-6 LCPUFAs that are precursors of the eicosanoids (Figure 6.3) utilized in parenteral nutrition formulations. In such formulations they are not thought to suppress immune cell proliferation and function [52].

ω-6 fatty acids

ω-6 LCPUFAs are usually polyunsaturated (i.e. they have more than one double bond) (Figure 6.1). The first member of the family is the plant-derived (corn oil, soya oil) linoleic acid (18:2n-6) from which the potent, longer-chain derivatives can be synthesized *in vivo* by the same elongating and desaturating enzymes that metabolize ω-3 LCPUFAs (Figure 6.4) (see below for ω-3). Linoleic acid (18:2n-6), like linolenic acid (18:3n-30 (see below), is termed an essential FA and has to be ingested in the diet because it cannot be produced in the mammalian body. It is vital for normal

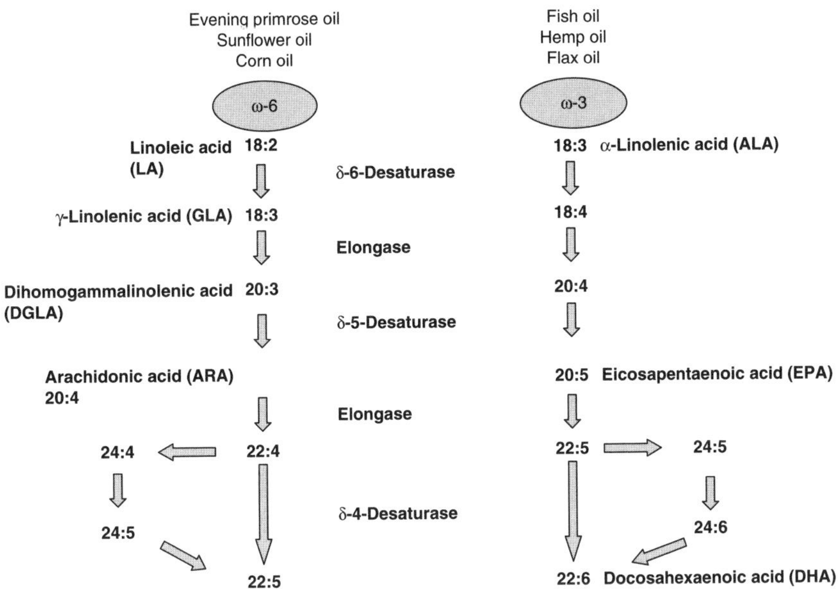

Fig. 6.4 Formation of the important long chain polyunsaturated derivatives of the parent ω-6 and ω-3 fatty acids by a series of desaturation and elongation reactions in human tissues.

function, particularly being the precursor of cell regulatory eicosanoids (see below); it also influences membrane and membrane raft composition and structure and, consequently, the activity of various cells, including those involved in immune reactivity.

The most important n-6 LCPUFA is the C-20 arachidonic acid (20:4n-6; ARA) (Figures 6.3 and 6.4) which plays a structural role in most cell membranes acylated to various phospholipids. ARA is also the precursor of cell-regulating, proinflammatory series 2 eicosanoids (PGE2), as well as the series 4 LTs (Figure 6.3). These eicosanoids are key mediators and regulators of inflammatory processes in cells and tissues and consequently appear to be involved in cardiovascular disease and cancer. The proinflammatory effects of PGE2 include increased vascular permeability, oedema and vasodilation. In animal models of cancer, PGE2 is implicated in tumour growth, progression, and the development of metastases.

Similarly to PGE2, LTB4 also increases vascular permeability, is important for enhanced chemotactic activity of leucocytes, and increases lysosomal enzyme release and the generation of ROS. Furthermore, it leads to an increase in proinflammatory cytokines such as TNF-α, IL-1β, and IL-6 through the NF-κB transcription factor pathway. LTC4, LTD4, and LTE4, produced by 5-LOX (lipooxygenase) action, are bronchoconstrictors involved in asthma. They also promote hypersensitivity and increase vascular permeability similar to PGE2.

Inflammatory conditions result in increased phospholipase activity and increased release of ARA-derived eicosanoids from membrane phospholipids. This leads to further enhancement of the inflammation. Increased concentrations of these eicosanoids are detectable in blood and tissues of patients with acute and chronic inflammatory conditions. Intriguingly, PGE2 can also inhibit the expression/activity of 5-LOX while inducing that of 15-LOX, thereby, promoting the synthesis of lipoxins from ARA which have strong anti-inflammatory effects. This is one explanation for the observations that ARA and its eicosanoid derivatives (PGs, LTs, lipoxins) are capable of eliciting both pro- and anti-inflammatory effects in cells and tissues. However, the overriding effect of ω-6 LCPUFA at various concentrations appear to be pro-inflammatory [54,55].

In inflammatory bowel disease the intestinal mucosa expresses elevated levels of inflammatory eicosanoids derived from n-6 ARA, such as LTB4, suggesting its involvement in the pathogenesis. The role of PGE2 in inflammatory bowel disease is less certain and, paradoxically, it has been suggested that PGE2 may be protective since inhibitors of cyclooxygenase (COX) which should reduce synthesis actually exacerbated inflammatory bowel disease. It has been suggested that low levels of PGE2 are important for normal cell function to occur and that excessive production, as in inflammatory conditions, leads to the pathological effects. It is well documented that PGE2 derived from constitutive, noninducible COX-2 activity is necessary for normal cell functions, whereas that produced by inducible COX-2 is involved in inflammation.

Inhibition of LT synthesis decreased colonic LTB4 but increased PGE2. Recent observations have shown that PGE2 can also have anti-inflammatory actions by inhibiting 5-LOX and reducing LT4 synthesis, while inducing 15-LOX and the synthesis of anti-inflammatory lipoxins. PGE2 can induce COX-2 expression in cultured cells involved in immune reactivity and thereby up-regulate its own production, which will further induce the production of inflammatory IL-6 in macrophages and exacerbate the inflammation [54,55]. Clearly, the effects of n-6 LCPUFAs can be both pro- and anti-inflammatory and this may be related to the level of their dietary intakes and concentration in cell membranes. It has been suggested that diets in the major industrialized countries contain excessive amounts of ω-6 LCPUFAs and insufficient amounts of ω-3 LCPUFAs. Ratios of dietary intake should be around 5:1 but are currently about 15–20:1. This enhances the ARA pool in cell membranes and increases the likelihood of the more inflammatory ω-6 eicosanoids being produced.

Relative proportions of eicosanoids synthesized in cells involved in immune reactivity appear to be dependent on cell type. PGE2 and PGF2 are produced predominantly in monocytes and macrophages, while neutrophils produce moderate amounts of PGE2 and mast cells PGD2. Similarly, monocytes, macrophages, and neutrophils produce LTB4, through the 5-LOX pathway, while mast cells, basophils, and eosinophils generally synthesize LTC4, LTD4, and LTE4 [54,55]. In animal models, feeding n-6 LCPUFAs enhances tumour growth and metastasis formation while the opposite is true for n-3 LCPUFAs.

In recent years, a great deal of interest has been shown in the activity of unsaturated FAs that are related to ω-6 linoleic acid and are termed conjugated linoleic acids (CLAs). They are also components of the human food chain but are present mainly in dairy products. CLAs are derived from linoleic acid by specific partial hydrogenation reactions in the rumen of cattle, goats, and sheep, and appear to elicit similar effects on immune-inflammatory processes to those observed for ω-3 LCPUFAs. They also have beneficial effects on obesity, cardiovascular disease, and cancer, similar to those observed for ω-3 LCPUFAs. In animal models of prostate and breast cancer, dietary ingestion of CLAs resulted in tumour necrosis and reduced growth and suppression of angiogenesis. Most observations with these FAs are in cell cultures and animal models, but modulation of cytokine production and immunoglobulin formation occurs in humans [56].

ω-3 fatty acids

ω-3 LCPUFAs, mainly EPA (20:5n-3) and DHA (22:6n-3) (Figure 6.4), are associated with a number of important health benefits in humans and animals that are thought to be related to their ability to attenuate elements of the inflammatory processes that underlie many disease states in industrialized areas of the world (Figure 6.2).

The only 'essential' ω-3 LCPUFA in mammals, including humans, is the C-18 α-linolenic acid (18:3n-3), present in many edible plants and oils extracted from these plants. It has to be ingested in the diet because humans have lost the ability to introduce the first ω-3 (n-3) double bond into the carbon chain. All subsequent double bonds can be inserted to produce the metabolic important longer-chain derivatives (i.e. EPA and DHA) by a series of desaturation and two-carbon elongation reactions *in vivo* (Figure 6.4). However, many studies have shown that the rate of conversion in humans of 18:3n-3 to EPA is limited, and to DHA is negligible, due largely to the high ω-6 EFA content in the diet. Consequently, preformed EPA and DHA need to be ingested in order to obtain anti-inflammatory and other health benefits attributed to these nutrients.

The richest natural sources of EPA and DHA are oily fish, although numerous commercial products are now available as dietary supplements [57]. EPA and DHA can inhibit the expression of a number of inflammatory cytokines through their attenuation of the stress-induced NF-κB transcription pathway, stimulation of which leads to a variety of stress responses including increased cytokine, eicosanoid and HSP production [57] (Figure 6.2).

ω-3 LCPUFAs, both EPA and DHA, can suppress the agonist-induced activation, i.e. LPS-induced activation, of TLRs in monocytes, macrophages, DCs, and adipocytes. The up-regulation of DC costimulatory molecules (CD80, CD86) and MHC class II expression, the secretion of proinflammatory cytokines (TNF-α, IL-1β,IL-6), and T cell activation is inhibited by ω-3 LCPUFAs [58,59]. EPA has been shown to inhibit the binding of LPS to its TLR [51].

The reciprocal regulation of innate and adaptive immune responses by saturated and ω-3 LCPUFAs demonstrates the close links between nutrition and immunity, and appears to be regulated, at least partly, through the TLRs and the NF-κB signalling system (Figure 6.2). This also offers an explanation for the detrimental health effects, such as increased obesity, metabolic syndrome, cardiovascular disease and cancer, ascribed to high saturated FA intake in Western populations.

ω-3 LCPUFAs, particularly EPA but also DHA, can reduce the inflammatory process by attenuating the excessive production of inflammatory eicosanoids (PGE2, PI2, TXA2, LTB4) derived from the ω-6 LCPUFA, ARA-20:4n-6, as documented in *in vitro* cell cultures and in *in vivo* animal and healthy volunteer studies (Figure 6.3) [60]. This can occur by the ω-3 PUFAs displacing ARA from cell-membrane phospholipids or inhibition of COX-2 and LOX-5 expression/activity, as well as enhanced competition with ARA for the relevant enzymes, which results in production of the 3-series of PGs and the 5-series of LTs, which are biologically less active than ARA derivatives and can have anti-inflammatory effects [60].

A novel group of EPA and DHA derivatives termed the E- and D-series, resolvins and protectins, have recently been identified that attenuate acute leucocyte responses and, as their name suggests, facilitate the resolution of inflammation in tissues and cells in the presence of aspirin compounds [61].

Nutritional support

In patients with acute respiratory distress syndrome (ARDS) and receiving enteral nutrition that included ω-3 LCPUFAs, the numbers of total white blood cells and neutrophils in alveolar fluid declined significantly, compared with appropriate controls. Similarly, IL-8, TNF-α, and LTB4 tended to be present in lower levels in the group receiving ω-3 LCPUFAs. Arterial oxygenation was also improved with a concomitant decreased requirement for oxygen. Furthermore, total hospital stay was shorter in the ω-3 group compared with controls, and fewer patients developed organ failure [62]. Clearly, ω-3 LCPUFAs can modulate the inflammatory mechanisms that underlie a number of pathological conditions in humans including cardiovascular disease, rheumatoid arthritis, sepsis and ARDS, and cancer (see Chapters 2 and 5).

The detrimental role of excessive inflammatory responsiveness, which is manifested by excess production of various cytokines, including TNF-α, IL-1β, IL-6, IL-8 and downstream ARA-derived inflammatory eicosanoids, is well recognized in trauma patients as a probable causal factor in the development of sepsis. In animal studies, these excess inflammatory responses can be replicated by simple bacterial LPS administration. The ability of ω-3 LCPUFAs (fish oil) to attenuate the production of these inflammatory mediators, in animals and humans, has been well documented and indicates their possible usefulness in controlling SIRS and ARDS. These beneficial effects have also been incorporated in the development of total parenteral nutrition (TPN) for clinical patients unable to ingest food orally and undergoing management for trauma and cancer [60,62,63] (see Chapters 2 and 4).

Lipid emulsions of many different compositions have been used previously for TPN, particularly in patients with serious intestinal disorders. The early objective was to increase the caloric intake of the patients to counter anorexia and cachexia, although the FA content of the products and their metabolic effects was not a primary consideration, and may have predisposed to inflammation and impairment of immune function. Later, nontoxic emulsions based on soybean oil, with its high content of the ω-6 LCPUFA (linoleic acid, 18:2 n-6) and low content of ω-3 LCPUFAs, (18:3n-3 or longer derivatives) were introduced. However, use of these soy-based lipid emulsions gave conflicting results in clinical trials, with some showing immune suppression while others have demonstrated no effects on immune function [62].

In recent years, based on the health benefits ascribed to ω-3LCPUFAs in healthy volunteer and animal studies, varying amounts of ω-3 LCPUFAs have been used in lipid emulsion preparations in TPN. This has generally resulted in similar anti-inflammatory benefits (reduced TNF-α, IL-6, and LTB4) and preservation of immune function (monocyte expression of HLA-DR and IFN-γ production) as those observed with enteral ω-3LCPUFA ingestion in healthy volunteers and patients [60–63]. In patients with sepsis receiving ω-3 LCPUFAs in their TPN, anti-inflammatory effects included reduced blood leucocyte counts, reduced systemic CRP concentration, reduced inflammatory cytokine production, and enhanced LTB5 formation *in vitro* by isolated, endotoxin-stimulated mononuclear cells and neutrophils. Liang *et al.* reported that patients undergoing surgery for colorectal cancer, receiving TPN containing a soybean: fish oil ratio of 5:1, had significantly reduced levels of serum IL-6, compared with a control group of patients [63]. Furthermore, the ratio of $CD4^+$ T:$CD8^+$ T cells also significantly increased with the supplementation, and there was a shorter postoperative hospital stay.

Both enteral and parenteral formulations contain a number of nutrients, apart from ω-6 and ω-3 LCPUFAs, that are also considered to be immunomodulatory (e.g. L-arginine and other amino acids, and trace elements). Preoperative oral L-arginine and n-3 FA supplementation reduced postoperative infectious complications and duration of SIRS ($p<0.05$), and increased $CD4^+$ T cell counts on preoperative day 1 and postoperative day 7 ($p<0.05$), compared with the control group [64]. Consequently, the observed immunomodulatory effects of these formulations cannot be ascribed to the ω-3 LCPUFAs alone. As in other nutritional studies, a matrix of nutrients emulating a balanced diet is probably more beneficial than any single component alone; it appears that there are beneficial interactions and synergies between various components in the nutrient matrix.

Alcohol

The effects of alcohol on the immune system have been difficult to separate from those caused by malnutrition, which is frequently present in individuals consuming an excess amount of alcohol. However, prolonged and excessive alcohol intake does appear to result in immune alterations and an increased risk of developing infections such as pneumonia, hepatitis C, and HIV. The reasons for this have not been fully clarified, but abnormalities in T cells have been described. For example, there are reductions in the numbers of T cells and responses to endotoxin, reductions in number and activity of NK cells, and abnormalities in APCs [65].

B cell functions have been shown to be altered in some studies in patients with chronic alcohol consumption. More specifically, increased levels of immunoglobulins, in particular IgE and IgA, have been documented in people with an excess alcohol intake. Increased IgA levels in serum are found with and in the absence of significant liver disease or cirrhosis. IgA and IgE levels fall when alcohol consumption is reduced. The precise mechanisms responsible for these Ig changes, at present, are unclear.

Alcohol alters the synthesis and secretion of cytokines. In individuals who consume excess amounts of alcohol, serum levels of a range of proinflammatory (IL-6, IL-8, and IL-12) and anti-inflammatory (IL-10, IL-13) cytokines have been shown to be elevated. However, these cytokine elevations fell when the alcohol intake was stopped [66].

In trying to understand these alterations in cytokine profiles, *in vitro* studies have shown that exposure to alcohol results in an increased release of TNF-α by macrophages, NF-κB activation, and increased production of chemokines such as transforming growth factor-beta (TGF-β) [67]. However, the impact of alcohol is complex because in *in vitro* studies contradictory findings are documented, using concentrations of alcohol which represent a moderate level of consumption *in vivo*. Further studies are needed to understand the complex biological effects that alcohol has on host defences.

Vitamins

Introduction

Vitamins are organic molecules and are generally classified as being either fat soluble (vitamins A, D, E, K) or water soluble (Vitamin B and C groups including folic acid, B_{12}, B_1, B_2, B_3, B_6, pantothenic acid, and biotin). They are necessary for normal development and the maintenance of health. In order to do this they have specific effects on key metabolic processes, but it is not within the scope of this chapter to consider all of these effects. However, vitamins can have an important and biological impact on the immune system, albeit the understanding of this is incomplete. More is known about the effects of vitamins A, C, D, and E and these are outlined below.

Vitamin A

Innate immunity

Vitamin A is obtained from the diet either as retinols or β-carotene and is specifically involved in the control of cellular growth and differentiation. It also has significant effects on the immune system. Vitamin A deficiency has important biological effects on mucosal surfaces, especially in the eye, urinary tract and GIT, and the respiratory epithelium, inducing a reduction in the number of goblet cells which produce mucus. In addition, there is some evidence that IgA levels on the surfaces of epithelial cells are reduced if there is deficiency in this vitamin. This increases the potential for pathogens to translocate across epithelial surfaces, therefore predisposing to infection.

The effect of vitamin A on neutrophils is also important because lack of vitamin A not only interferes with normal development but also causes impairment in migration of these cells to sites of inflammation, together with their ability to ingest and destroy bacterial pathogens. There are similar effects on macrophages, with deficiency resulting in impairment of phagocytosis and bacterial destruction. However, macrophages will increase production of IL-12 and IFN-γ which results in more severe inflammation at any site where this is occurring [68]. In contrast, supplementation with vitamin A will result in an increased phagocytic activity of both macrophages and Kupffer cells, and increased production of ROSs in both neutrophils and monocytes [69].

Adaptive immunity

In terms of effects on lymphocytes, vitamin A has been considered to be necessary for both T and B lymphocytes homing to the GIT. More specifically, vitamin A appears to be necessary to control Th1 and Th2 responses and their homeostatic balance. For example, there may actually be an enhancement of Th1 responses (production of IL-2 and IFN-γ), leading to stimulated macrophage function and B cell development. In contrast, there is a decreased Th2 type response in vitamin A deficiency with a decreased production of IL-4, IL-5, and IL-10. Other effects of vitamin A deficiency include decreases in NK cell numbers and their lytic activity [70].

The effects of vitamin A on B cells are complex and of a variable nature. For example, some studies have demonstrated that vitamin A will enhance B cell proliferation, whereas others have shown the opposite effect with there being reduced B cell proliferation [70,71]. It seems likely, however, that these effects are controlled by different metabolites of vitamin A, which accounts for these differences. In terms of antibody production by B cells, vitamin A has important effects with respect to the type of antibody produced [72]. This is because Th1 and Th2 cytokines (vitamin A causing an enhancement of Th1 responses) regulate this. Th1 cytokines lead to production of IgG2 and IgG3. In contrast, the Th2 cytokine response suppresses the production of these antibodies but leads to the production of IgG1 [73].

In GALT, vitamin A is important in the regulation of IgA production through DCs and, although the mechanism is complex and not fully understood, this response requires the presence of either IL-5 or IL-6 [74]. More recently, a role has been suggested for NO in the regulation of IgA production at these sites. It has been recognized that vitamin A (retinoic acid) bound to its receptor activates a promoter leading to iNOS and NO production [75] and stimulates IgA secretion, both independent of and through T cells [70]. However, it is not only in antibody production but also in the trafficking of lymphocytes to the GALT that vitamin A plays an important role. Vitamin A (which is also produced by DCs in GALT) induces the expression of receptors on lymphocytes (e.g. integrin and CCRs), which are necessary for migration to the GIT [70].

Vitamin E

Vitamin E consists of a group of compounds that exhibit α-tocopherol activity and are commonly found in high amounts in oils derived from plant seeds (e.g. corn and rape), olives, and palms. The most important of these compounds are α-, β-, and γ-tocopherols (in corn oils) and tocotrienols (in palm oils) with the γ isoforms being the least abundant but most effective antioxidants. In addition to having important antioxidant effects, these compounds also have multiple effects on the immune system.

Studies of vitamin E supplementation have shown that there is a modulation of the bactericidal activities of neutrophils and macrophages, although the effects are variable and not clearly defined. For example, short-term supplementation with vitamin E appears to cause a reduction in these activities with a decrease in the production of ROSs (most likely the cause of the reduced bactericidal activity); this does not appear to occur if there is long-term supplementation [76]. In other studies, an enhanced phagocytosis was documented when vitamin E was supplemented. The mechanistic reasons for these observations have not, as yet, been clearly defined.

Vitamin E supplementation results in an increase in T lymphocyte numbers (but no effects on T cell subsets) and an increase in delayed type hypersensitivity reactions.

Lymphocyte proliferation in response to mitogenic stimulation (*in vitro*) is, in general, enhanced in studies of vitamin E supplementation [77]. However, this does depend on the type of mitogen used. Other studies have shown that supplementation does not affect circulating levels of immunoglobulins. The mechanisms underlying these effects of vitamin E are also unclear but some studies have suggested that it may exert its effects, at least in part, through an inhibition of NF-κB which is required for the transcription of many proteins that are involved in the oxidative/inflammatory stress response. In particular, it affects production of the proinflammatory cytokines and the COXs and LOXs that result in increased eicosanoid synthesis, and the expression of HSPs.

Vitamin D

Introduction

Vitamin D_3, the key form of vitamin D, is synthesized in the skin by the action of UV light on 7-dehydrocholesterol or ingested via the diet. It is then converted into 25 hydroxyvitamin D_3 in the liver and finally into the most active metabolite, 1,25-hydroxyvitamin D_3, by the enzyme 1-α-hydroxylase, which is located in the renal proximal tubule. Interestingly, this enzyme is also found in a variety of immune cells, including macrophages, and can produce substantial quantities, when stimulated by IFN-γ and LPS.

The physiological effects of vitamin D_3, mediated via its binding to a specific vitamin D receptor (VDR) in the nucleus, especially in relation to bone metabolism, is well understood. However, there are other effects which are only just being recognized. It has been known for some time that vitamin D is metabolized by cells of the immune system and can also affect their function which, in general, is of an inhibitory nature.

Innate immunity

Macrophages, and aspects of their function, are regulated by vitamin D in an inhibitory fashion. Vitamin D will not only prevent the differentiation of mononuclear precursors into DCs but also affects their survival and activation [78,79]. As a consequence, there is a reduced DC antigen presentation capacity and stimulation of T cell functions. Other effects of vitamin D on macrophages include a stimulation of production of PGE2 and reduction in the expression of MHC class II antigens [80]. There is also a reduction in the expression of other antigens, by DCs and other APCs, which further impairs T cell stimulation [81]. However, in contrast to these effects, vitamin D will stimulate macrophages to increase the production of cathelicidin (hCAP) which is a protein involved in lysosomal bacterial destruction [82].

Adaptive immunity

Vitamin D regulates T and B cell function and, specifically, will inhibit T cell proliferation [83]. It also reduces the activity and cytokine production by Th1 cells (e.g. reduced IFN-γ) while increasing Th2 cytokines (e.g. IL-4 and IL-5), and can suppress Th1 cell function by suppressing IL-12 synthesis and Th17 function by reducing the production of IL-6 and IL-23 [84]. At the molecular level, the potential for widespread effects of vitamin D on Th cells was illustrated by demonstrating that more than 100 genes were regulated by vitamin D, including those involved in NF-κB regulation and cytokine production [85]. In addition, vitamin D reduces the activity of $CD8^+$ CTLs and enhances the activity of nonspecific T cell suppressor activity [70].

B cell function is also affected directly by vitamin D; again, in an inhibitory way. Vitamin D will reduce B cell proliferation and differentiation, plasma cell differentiation, and IgG production [86]. Recent observations suggest that this vitamin may have important roles in prevention of certain neurological disorders, such as multiple sclerosis, and possibly the development of malignancies, but this needs to be verified by further studies.

Vitamin C

Vitamin C (ascorbic acid) is a powerful antioxidant which protects a range of intracellular molecules and cell membranes from oxidative damage and is usually deficient in the diets of a large section of the UK population. Like other vitamins it has other physiological effects which will not be discussed here. However, its potential for stimulating the immune system, particularly in relation to the common cold, has attracted much interest over the last 25 years. Despite this work and lack of proven benefit it does have effects on immunity which are deemed important.

As a result of its antioxidant properties, vitamin C also reduces the production of ROSs. This may be important in ensuring neutrophils function properly in conditions such as inflammation where there is an increase in production of ROSs, the oxidative burst that has an important bactericidal action. Under normal circumstances, vitamin C is required for normal neutrophil motility and there is some evidence to suggest that supplementation with vitamin C will increase the motility and metabolic activity of neutrophils further [87].

Studies examining the effects of vitamin C supplementation on circulating numbers of a variety of immune cells (e.g. neutrophils, NK cells, monocytes) have found no effect. In contrast, there appears to be an effect on the *in vitro* proliferative response of lymphocytes, as some studies have shown an enhanced response after 1 month's dietary supplementation with vitamin C [88]. There is, however, no effect on immunoglobulin production or circulating levels with vitamin C supplementation.

The combined actions of the water-soluble vitamin C and the lipid-soluble vitamin E are generally regarded as the most effective antioxidant combination for preventing ROS damage in the cytosol and membranes of mammalian cells and, consequently, as an effective mechanism for attenuating disease due to oxidative processes. However, although laboratory and animal studies support this suggestion, large-scale clinical supplementation studies have failed to endorse the role of antioxidant deficiencies in disease initiation. It is plausible, that in cancer patients, antioxidant supplementation could have beneficial effects in opposing the action of chemotherapeutic drugs, since they induce an increase in ROS formation. In people with latent disease, whether cancer or heart disease, supplementation with antioxidants might well be ineffective. This could explain the lack of any noticeable effect of antioxidants in supplementation trials where the outcome is usually changes in morbidity and mortality.

Clinical implications

This brief review of the effect of various components of the diet on a number of important aspects of the immune system emphasizes the pivotal role played by a balanced and optimal nutritional status in the maintenance of a satisfactory immune function. The situation in surgical patients is complicated by the possible up- or down-regulation of the immune and inflammatory responses by selective nutritional deficiencies or excesses. However, the evidence cited above suggests that a fundamental improvement in immune function can be achieved prior to surgery through nutritional interventions. Clearly, further studies are required to understand these effects and their interactions in relation to overall health and, in particular, in patients undergoing surgery with specific diseases and any concomitant comorbidity.

Studies of supplementation with a single key nutrient generally have not shown major clinical benefits. However, combinations of these nutrients, when used in certain clinical settings, have been shown in some cases to have significant clinical benefits.

Combinations of nutrients, most commonly based on L-arginine, n-3 LCPUFAs, and RNA, are commercially available and have been evaluated in randomized controlled trials. The patients studied have had various types of critical illnesses and the nutrients have usually been given after surgery for malignant disease (mainly upper or lower gastrointestinal cancers), major trauma, and major burns. If given postoperatively for several days, significant clinical benefits will occur in terms of reductions of infectious complications (e.g. wound infections, intra-abdominal sepsis) and a decreased hospital stay, although mortality is not altered [89–91]. The categories of patients for whom this is currently recommended are shown in Box 6.2. A full discussion of immunonutrition is beyond the scope of this chapter but further details can be found in the references cited and elsewhere in the book.

Summary and conclusions

Dysregulation of immune, metabolic, and inflammatory processes can occur in an individual when there is PEM or obesity. More specifically, the impact of certain dietary nutrients in modulating key aspects of inflammation, metabolic processes, and a variety of immune functions has been documented. However, the mechanisms underlying these effects have not, as yet, been fully clarified.

Box 6.2 Patient groups in whom immunonutritional support is recommended

- Patients about to undergo major intra-abdominal surgery and surgical resection of cancers
- Patients with ARDS
- Patients with mild sepsis (defined as an Apache II score <15)

Recommended by European Society of Parenteral and Enteral Nutrition (http://www.espen.org/Education/documents/ENICU.pdf)

Several specific nutrients are of particular relevance for surgical patients. Micronutrients play a key role in regulation of the immune system, wound healing, and antioxidant defence mechanisms. In addition, they also modulate numerous metabolic processes as they are important components of specific enzyme systems. Macronutrients, in particular amino acids and FAs, also have important effects. The key amino acids include L-arginine, L-glutamine, and the BCAAs; they have been shown to stimulate various aspects of immune, inflammatory, and metabolic functions.

FAs (saturated, MUFAs and the ω-3 and ω-6 LCPUFAs), can influence immune functions, particularly inflammatory processes in different, and often opposing, ways. The understanding of the molecular mechanisms underlying these actions is becoming better understood. Saturated FAs activate TLR4 and the stress-related NF-κB inflammatory cascade in immune cells and adipocytes. ω-3 LCPUFAs attenuate this pathway and reduce proinflammatory cytokine production and secretion and eicosanoid synthesis, as well as maintaining normal, healthy membrane function in cells and tissues.

However, nutritional supplementation with a single individual nutrient, while modifying immune function *in vitro* has, in general, not yet been shown to have clinical benefit *in vivo*. More promising is the possibility that ω-3 supplements may attenuate inflammatory diseases such as rheumatoid arthritis in certain individuals. Interestingly, combinations of amino acids, FAs, and micronutrients have been shown to elicit clinical benefits by reducing infectious complications in severely ill patients, together with a reduction in patient stay in the intensive care unit. These effects have important implications for the provision of health care worldwide.

Further elucidation of the way in which nutrition affects genes and their regulation will be crucial to a better understanding of how nutrients precisely impact on the immune system. This knowledge will lead to wider and more beneficial clinical applications of nutritional interventions in human diseases.

References

1. Chandra RK. Nutrition, immunity and infection: from basic knowledge of dietary manipulation of immune responses to practical application of ameliorating suffering and improving survival. *Proc Natl Acad Sci U S A* 1996; **93**: 14304–14307.
2. Chandra RK. Nutrition and the immune system: an introduction. *Am J Clin Nutr* 1997; **66**: 460S–463S.
3. Chandra RK. Protein-energy malnutrition and immunological responses. *J Nutr* 1992; **122**: 597–600.
4. Bastard J-P, Maachi M, Lagathu C *et al.* Recent advances in the relationship between obesity, inflammation and insulin resistance. *Eur Cytokine Netw* 2006; **17**: 4–12.
5. Lamas O, Marti A, Martinex JA. Obesity and immunocompetence. *Eur J Clin Nutr* 2002; **56**: S42–S45.
6. Iyer A, Fairlie DP, Prins JB, Hammock BD, Brown L. Inflammatory lipid mediators in adipocyte function and obesity. *Nat Rev Endocrinol* 2010; **6**: 71–82.
7. Isolauri E, Sutas Y, Arvilommi H, Salminen S. Probiotics: effects on immunity. *Am J Clin Nutr* 2001; **73**(Suppl): 440S–450S.

8. Bernet-Camard MF, Lievin V, Brasart D, Neeser JR, Servin AL, Hudault S. The human lactobacillus acidophilus strain LA1 secretes a nonbacteriocin antibacterial substance(s) active in vitro and in vivo. *Appl Environ Microbiol* 2007; **63**: 2747–2753.
9. Saier MH, Mansour NM. Probiotics and prebiotics on human health. *J Mol Microbiol Biotechnol* 2005; **10**: 22–25.
10. Ezendam J, van Loveren H. Probiotics: Immunomodulation and evaluation of safety and efficacy. *Nutrition Rev* 2006; **64**: 1–14.
11. Borchers AT, Selmi C, Meyers FJ, Keen KL, Gershwin ME. Probiotics and immunity. *J Gastroenterol* 2009; **44**: 26–46.
12. Minocha A. Probiotics and preventive health. *Nutr Clin Practice* 2009; **24**: 227–241.
13. Kaila M, Isolauri E, Soppi E, Virtanen E, Laine S, Arvilommi H. Enhancement of the circulating antibody secreting cell response in human diarrhea by a human lactobacillus strain. *Paed Res* 1992; **32**: 141–144.
14. Parkes GC, Sanderson JD, Whelan K. The mechanisms and efficacy of probiotics in the prevention of clostridium dificile-associated diarrhoea. *Lancer Infect Dis* 2009; **9**: 237–244.
15. Prasad AS. Zinc in human health:effect of zinc on immune cells. *Mol Med* 2008; **14**: 353–357.
16. Wintergerst ES, Maggini S, Hornig DH. Contribution of selected vitamins and trace elements to immune function. *Nutrition and Metabolism* 2007; **51**: 301–323.
17. King LE, Osatai-Ashtiani F, Fraler PJ. Apoptosis plays a distinct role in the loss of precursor lymphocytes during zinc deficiency in mice. *J Nutr* 2002; **132**: 974–979.
18. Powell SR. The antioxidant properties of zinc. *J Nutr* 2000; **130**: 1447S–1454S.
19. Failla ML. Trace elements and host defense: recent advances and continuing challenges. *J Nutr* 2003; **133**(suppl1): 1443S–1447S.
20. Prasad AS. Effects of zinc deficiency on Th1 and Th2 cytokine shifts. *J Infect Dis* 2000; **182**(Suppl): S62–S68.
21. Heyland DK, Jones N, Cvijanovich NZ, Wong H. Zinc supplementation in critically ill patients: a key pharmaconutrient? *JPEN* 2008; **32**: 509–519.
22. Arthur JR, McKenzie R, Beckett GJ. Selenium in the immune system. *J Nutr* 2003; **133**(Suppl 1): 1457S–1459S.
23. Hoffman PR, Berry MJ. The influence of selenium on immune responses. *Mol Nutr Food Res* 2008; **52**: 1273–1280.
24. Hawkes WC, Kelley DS, Taylor PC. The effects of dietary selenium on the immune system in healthy men. *Biol Trace Elements Res* 2001; **81**: 189–213.
25. Avenell A, Noble DW, Barr J, Engelhardt T. Selenium supplementation for critically ill adults. *Cochrane Database Syst Rev* 2007; 3: CD003703.DOI:10.1002/14651858.CD003703.pub2.
26. Klotz HO, Kroencke KD, Buchczyk DP, Sies H. Role of coper, zinc, selenium and tellurium in the cellular defense against oxidative and nitrosative stress. *J Nutr* 2003; **133**: 1448S–1451S.
27. Bonham M, O'Connor JM, Hannigan M, Strain JJ. The immune system as a physiological indicator of marginal copper status? *Br J Nutr* 2002; **87**: 393–403.
28. Kelly DS, Daudu PA, Taylor PC, Mackey BC, Turnlund JR. Effects of low copper diets on human immune response. *Am J Clin Nutr* 1995; **62**: 412–416.
29. Tam M, Gomez S, Gonzalez-Gross M, Marcos A. Possible roles of magnesium on the immune system. *Eur J Clin Nutr* 2003; **57**: 1193–1197.

30. Mooren FC, Golf SW, Volker K. Effect of magnesium on granulocyte function and on the exercise induced inflammatory response. *Magnesium Res* 2003; **16**: 49–58.
31. Kuvibidila S, Baliga S. Role of iron in immunity and infection. In: Calder PC, Field LJ, Gill HS (eds). *Nutrition and immune function*. CABI Publishing, Wallingford, Oxon, 2002, pp. 209–228.
32. Weiss G. Iron and immunity: a double-edged sword. *Eur J Clin Invest* 2002; **32**(suppl): 70–78.
33. Heys SD, Park KGM, Garlick PJ, Eremin O. Nutrition and malignancy: implications for surgical practice. *Br J Surg*, 1992; **79**: 614–623.
34. Heys SD, Gough DB, Khan L, Eremin O. Nutritional pharmacology and malignant disease: a therapeutic modality in patients with cancer? *Br J Surg* 1996; **83**: 608–619.
35. Roth E. Immune cells and modulation by amino acids. *Clin Nutr* 2007; **26**: 535–544.
36. Pollheimer J, Zellner M, Elliasen MM *et al.* Increased susceptibility of glutamine-depleted monocytes to fever-range hyperthermia. The role of 70-kDa heat shock protein. *Ann Surg* 2005; **241**: 349–355.
37. Heys SD, Broom J, Eremin O. L-Arginine: biochemistry and basic biology. In: Eremin O (ed). *L-Arginine: biological aspects and clinical application*. RG Landes, Austin, TX, 1997, pp. 1–25.
38. Wu G, Bazer FW, Davis TA *et al.* Arginine metabolism in growth, health and disease. *Amino Acids* 2009; **37**: 153–168.
39. Brittenden J, Heys SD, Eremin O. Immunological properties of L-arginine. In: Eremin O (ed). *L-Arginine: biological aspects and clinical application*. RG Landes, Austin, TX, 1997, pp. 1–25.
40. Brittenden J, Heys SD, Ross J, Park KG, Eremin O. Natural cytotoxicity in breast cancer patients receiving neoadjuvant chemotherapy: effects of L-arginine supplementation. *Eur J Surg Oncol* 1994; **20**: 467–472.
41. Peranzoni E, Marigo I, Dolcetti L *et al.* Role of arginine metabolism in immunity and immunopathology. *Immunobiology* 2008; **212**: 795–812.
42. Calder PC. Branched-chain amino acids and immunity. *J Nutr* 2006; **136**: 288S–293S.
43. Negro M, Giardina S, Marzani B, Marzatico F. Branched-chain amino acid supplementation does not enhance athletic performance but affects muscle recovery and the immune system. *J Sports Med Phys Fitness* 2008; **48**: 347–351.
44. Petro TM, Bhattacharjee JK. Effect of dietary essential amino acid limitations on susceptibility to Salmonella typhimurium and the effect upon humoral and cellular immune responses in mice. *Infect Immun* 1981; **32**: 251–259.
45. Cerra FB, Mazuski JE, Chute E *et al.* Branched chain metabolic support. A prospective, randomized, double-blind trial in surgical stress. *Ann Surg* 1984; **199**: 286–291.
46. Grimble RF. The effects of sulphur amino acid intake on immune function in humans. *J Nutr* 2006; **136**: 1660S–1665S.
47. Herzenberg LA, De Rosa SC, Dubs JG *et al.* Glutathione deficiency is associated with impaired survival in HIV disease. *Proc Natl Acad Sci U S A* 1997; **94**: 1967–1972.
48. Zapolska-Downa D, Naruszewicz M. Propionate reduces the cytokine-induced VCAM-1 and ICAM 1 expression by inhibiting nuclear factor k-B (NF-κB) activation. *J Physiol Pharmacol* 2009; **60**: 123–131.
49. Shi H, Kokoeva MV, Inouye K, Tzameli I, Yin H, Flier JS. TLR4 links innate immunity and fatty acid-induced insulin resistance. *J Clin Invest* 2006; **116**: 3015–3025.

50. Lee JY, Sohn KH, Rhee SH, Hwang D. Saturated fatty acids but not unsaturated fatty acids induce the expression of cyclooxygenase2 mediated through Toll-like receptor 4. *J Biol Chem* 2001; **276**: 16683–16689.
51. Kopp A, Gross P, Falk W *et al.* Fatty acids as metabolic mediators in innate immunity. *Eur J Clin Invest* 2009; **39**: 924–933.
52. Puertollano MA, Puertollano E, Alvarez de Cienfuegos G, de Pablo MA. Significance of olive oil in the host immune resistance to infection. *Br J Nutr* 2007; **98** (Suppl 1): S54–58.
53. Yakoob P. Monounsaturated fatty acids and immune function. *Eur J Clin Nutr* 2002; **56**: S9–S13.
54. Calder PC. Polyunsaturated fatty acids and inflammation. *Biochem Soc Trans* 2005; **33**: 423–427.
55. Calder PC. Polyunsaturated fatty acids, inflammatory processes and inflammatory bowel disease. *Mol Nutr Food Res* 2008; **52**: 885–897.
56. Wahle KWJ, Heys SD, Rotondo D. Conjugated linoleic acids (CLAs): Are they beneficial or detrimental to health? *Progr Lipid Res* 2004; **43**: 553–587.
57. Singer P, Shapiro H, Theilla M, Singer J, Cohen J. Anti-inflammatory properties of omega-3 fatty acids in critical illness: novel mechanisms and an integrative perspective. *Intensive. Care Med* 2008: **34**; 1580–1592.
58. Lee JY, Plakidas A, Lee WH, Heikkinen A, Chanmugam P, Bray G, Hwang D. Differential modulation of Toll-like receptors by fatty acids: preferential inhibition by n-3 polyunsaturated fatty acids. *J Lipid Res* 2003: **44**; 479–486.
59. Chapkin RS, Kim W, Lupton JR, McMurray DN. Dietary docosahexaenoic and eicosapentaenoic acid: emerging mediators of inflammation. *Prostgl Leukotr Essent Fatty Acids* 2009; **81**: 187–191.
60. Calder PC. Long-chain n-3 fatty acids and inflammation: potential application in surgical and trauma patients. *Brazil J Med Biol Res* 2003; **36**: 433–446.
61. Wanten GJA, Calder PC. Immune modulation by parenteral lipid emulsions. *Am J Clin Nutr* 2007; **85**: 1171–1184.
62. Calder PC. Immunonutrition in surgical and critically ill patients. *Br J Nutr* 2007; **98**: S133–S139.
63. Liang B, Wang S, Ye Y-J *et al.* Impact of postoperative omega-3 fatty acid supplemented parenteral nutrition on clinical outcomes and immunomodulations in colorectal cancer patients. *World J Gastroenterol* 2008; **14**: 2434–2439.
64. Okamoto Y, Okano K, Izuishi K, Usuki H, Wakabayashi H, Suzuki Y. Attenuation of the systemic inflammatory response and infections complications after gastrectomy with preoperative oral arginine and ω-3 fatty acids supplemented immunonutrition. *World J Surg* 2009; **33**: 1815–1821.
65. Diaz LE, Montero A, Gonzalez-Gross M, Vallejo AI, Romeo J, Marcos A. Influcence of alcohol consumption on immunological status: a review. *Eur J Clin Nutr* 2002; **56**(Suppl 3): S50–S53.
66. Dominguez-Santalla MJ, Vidal C, Vinuela J, Perez LF, Gonzalez-Qunitela A. Increased serum IgE in alcoholics: relationship with Th1/Th2 cytokine production by stimulated blood mononuclear cells. *Alcohol Clin Exp Res* 2001; **25**: 1198–1205.
67. Szabo G, Mandrekar P, Oak S, Mayerle J. Effect of ethanol on inflammatory responses. *Pancreatology* 2007; **7**: 115–123.
68. Stephensen CB. Vitamin A, infection, and immune function. *Ann Rev Nutr* 2001; **21**: 167–192.

69. Hoglen NC, Abril EA, Sauer JM *et al.* Modulation of Kupffer cell and peripheral blood monocyte activity by in vivo treatment of rats with all-trans-retinol. *Liver* 1997; **17**: 157–165.

70. Mora JR, Iwata M, von Andrian UH. Vitamin effects on the immune system: vitamins A and D take centre stage. *Nat Rev Immunol* 2008; **8**: 685–698.

71. Ballow M, Xiang S, Wang W, Brodsky L. The effects of retinoic acid on immunoglobulin synthesis: role of interleukin 6. *J Clin Immunol* 1996; **16**: 171–179.

72. Ertesvag A, Aasheim HC, Naderi S, Blomhoff HK. Vitamin A potentiates CpG-mediated memory B-cell proliferation and differentiation: involvement of early activation of p38MAPK. *Blood* 2007; **109**: 3865–3872.

73. Mora JR. Homing imprinting and immunomodulation in the gut: role of dendritic cells and retinoid. *Inflamm Bowel Dis* 2008; **14**: 275–289.

74. Mora JR, Iwata M, Eksteen B *et al.* Generation of gut-homing IgA-secreting B cells by intestinal dendritic cells. *Science* 2006; **314**: 1157–1160.

75. Zou F, Liu Y, Liu L *et al.* Retinoic acid activates human inducible nitric oxide synthase gene through binding of RARalpha/RXRalpha heterodimer to a novel retinoic acid response element in the promoter. *Biochem Biophys Res Commun* 2007; **355**: 494–500.

76. Webb AL, Villamor E. Update: effects of antioxidant and non-antioxidant vitamin supplementation on immune function. *Nutr Rev* 2007; **65**: 181–217.

77. Lee CY, Man-Fan Wan J. Vitamin E supplementation improves cell-mediated immunity and oxidative stress of Asian men and women. *J Nutr* 2000; **130**: 2932–2937.

78. Griffin MD, Lutz WH, Phan VA, Bachman LA, McKean DJ, Kumar R. Potent inhibition of dendritic cell differentiation and maturation by vitamin D analogs. *Biochem Biophys Res Commun* 2000; **270**: 701–708.

79. Piemonti L, Monti P, Sironi M, *et al.* Vitamin D3 affects differentiation, maturation and function of human monocyte-dervied dendritic cells. *J Immunol* 2000; **164**: 4443–4451.

80. Cantorna MT, Mahon BD. Mounting evidence for vitamin D as an environmental factor affecting autoimmune disease prevalence. *Exp Biol Med* 2004; **229**: 1136–1142.

81. van Etten E, Mathieu C. Immunoregulation by 1,25-dihydroxyvitamin D3; basic concepts. *J Steroid Biochem Mol Biol* 2005; **97**: 93–101.

82. Gombart AF, Borregaard N, Koeffler HP. Human cathelicidin antimicrobial peptide (CAMP) gene is a direct target of the vitamin D receptor and is strongly upregulated in myeloid cells by 1,25-dihydroxyvitamin D3. *FASEB J* 2005; **19**: 1067–1077.

83. Boonstra A, Barrat FJ, Crain C, Heath VL, Savelkoul HF, O'Garra A. 1-alpha, 25-dihydroxyvitamin D3 has a direct effect on naive $CD4^+$ T cells to enhance the development of Th2 cells. *J Immunol* 2001; **167**: 4974–4980.

84. Daniel C, Sartory NA, Zahn N, Radeke HH, Stein JM. Immune modulatory treatment of trinitrobenzene suphonic acid colitis with calcitrol is associated with a change of T helper (Th)1/Th17 to a Th2 and regulatory T cell profile. *J Pharmacol Exp Ther* 2008; **324**: 23–33.

85. Mahon BD, Wittke A, Weaver V, Cantorna MT. The targets of vitamin D depend on the differentiation and activation status of CD4 positive T cells. *J Cell Biochem* 2003; **89**: 922–932.

86. Chen S, Sims GP, Chen XX, Gu YY, Lipsky PE. Modulatory effects of 1,25-dihydroxyvitamin D3 on human B cell differentiation. *J Immunol* 2007; **179**: 1634–1647.

87. Volchegorskii IA, Vasil'kov AY. Effects of ascorbic acid on lipid peroxidation and functional state of neutrophils at the early period after transurethral resection of the prostate. *Bull Exp Biol Med* 2000; **130**: 516–518.

88. Kennes B, Dumont I, Brohee D, Hubert C, Neve P. Effect of vitamin C supplements on cell-mediated immunity in old people. *Gerontology* 1983; **29**: 305–310.
89. Heys SD, Walker LG, Smith IC, Eremin O. Enteral nutritional supplementation with key nutrients in patients with critical illness and cancer. A metaanalysis of randomised controlled clinical trials. *Ann Surg* 1999; **229**: 467–477.
90. Heyland DK, Novak F, Drover JW, Jain M, Su X, Suchner U. Should immunonutrition become routine in critically ill patients? *JAMA* 2001; **286**: 944–953.
91. Heys SD, Simpson WG. Surgical Nutrition. In: Paterson-Brown S (ed.) *Core topics in general and emergency surgery*. Saunders Elsevier, Philadelphia, 2009, pp. 309–330.

Chapter 7

Therapy and host defences

Mark Aloysius, Chandan Verma, and
Oleg Eremin

Key summary points

- Surgery, anaesthesia (volatile agents, e.g. halothane), and related drugs (e.g. opioids) have a variable detrimental effect on the innate and adaptive immune systems. The severity of tissue damage determines the nature and extent of the cytokines (e.g. IL-1, IL-6, TNF-α, IFN-γ) released and resultant impact on wound healing and postoperative rehabilitation.
- Patients who undergo a splenectomy are at a significant risk of developing infections, especially when due to encapsulated bacterial organisms, and should be vaccinated with a polyvalent vaccine and be considered for long-term use of prophylactic antibiotics.
- Allogeneic blood transfusions are immunosuppressive (e.g. transplantation, Crohn's disease). Humoral factors in blood up-regulate Tregs. Multiple transfusions increase risk of sepsis postoperatively and long-term tumour recurrence in cancer patients.
- Conventional cancer treatments, like radiotherapy and chemotherapy, are immunosuppressive affecting both innate and adaptive immunity and therefore need to be used judiciously in the already immunocompromised cancer patient. Chemotherapy-induced release of IL-2, IL-6, IL-10, and IFN-γ mediates some of the toxicity associated with chemotherapy.
- Evidence is emerging, however, that aspects of the beneficial effects of anticancer drugs are due to important modulation of host defences (e.g. reduction of Tregs with low-dose cyclophosphamide). Chemotherapy and radiotherapy may also lead to enhanced expression of TAAs in tumours and release of new antigenic peptides, thereby, enhancing humoral and cellular anticancer effects, as well as increasing the efficacy of apoptosis. Also, various agents have been shown to increase the level and activity of DCs both *in vivo* (gemcitabine) and *in vitro* (vincristine, paclitaxel). Late fibrosis with radiation is due to production of TGF-β. Low doses of ionizing radiation can upgrade expression of MHC, Fas (CD95), and adhesion molecules.

- Corticosteroids inhibit DC activity, suppress a wide range of Th1 and Th17 proinflammatory immune responses, up-regulate secretion of IL-10 and TGF-β, and amplify expansion of Tregs.
- DCs, macrophages, and B cells express receptors for oestrogen. Oestrogen deficiency enhances CMI and production of proinflammatory cytokines (IL-1, IL-6, TNF-α). Aromatase inhibitor therapy is associated with arthralgia, myalgia, and bone loss, and reduces Treg infiltration in breast cancers.
- Cytokines are proving to be useful anticancer agents in selective malignancies, albeit with some toxicity, e.g. IL-2 systemically for renal cancer and melanoma, selective limb perfusion with TNF-α for sarcoma and melanoma, and combinations of IFN-α with chemotherapy.
- Gene therapy and immunotherapeutic strategies are evolving and have shown some promise in cancer and autoimmune diseases. An important approach in immunotherapy is to pulse autologous DCs (isolated or *in situ*) with TAAs and peptides. Their efficacies have been limited and often short-lived.
- MABs and SMIs, targeted to specific membrane proteins and intracellular tyrosine kinases, respectively, are showing promise. MABs against growth factors, HER2/neu on tumour cells or VEGFRs in tumour vasculature, can inhibit breast cancer and colorectal cancer cell growth, respectively. CTLA-4 blockade with MABs in various metastatic cancers has shown partial responses but with significant morbidity (20% enterocolitis). MABs to specific inflammatory cytokines (e.g. TNF-α) can significantly improve outcome in rheumatoid arthritis, but with an increased risk of acquiring bacterial infections, including TB.

Introduction

Advances and developments in modern surgical practice have resulted in improved survival and enhanced quality of life. This is seen especially in the modern management of cancer. Unfortunately, a number of such treatments can be associated with significant morbidity, and even mortality in a small number of patients. Various factors contribute to this morbidity; inhibition or dysregulation of host defences is an important contributory factor in many of such patients, where the primary therapeutic strategy is not to intentionally disrupt or down-regulate the body's immune defences. However, it is now being appreciated that some of the beneficial effects seen with these modalities are due to both specific and broad-based modulations of host defences. Many drugs used in the intensive care setting are important for regulating the physiological homeostasis of critically ill patients. Some of these agents can suppress essential components of the host defences, predisposing to possible infections and delays in wound healing and tissue repair processes. Blood transfusion provides a crucial replacement fluid for the critically ill, shocked patient, following major trauma. However, it is now recognized that allogeneic transfused blood can have a significant detrimental effect on immunity, predisposing to infection in the early posttraumatic/postoperative phase, and in the long term can increase the risk of tumour recurrence following apparently curative surgery for cancer. Immune suppression, which is crucial in the transplant setting, to prevent donor organ rejection and induce graft tolerance, if used over a prolonged period of time can lead to the development of various cancers, in particular those with a viral aetiology such as lymphomas and squamous cell carcinoma of skin. Interfering, on a prolonged basis, with various proinflammatory mediators, in particular autoimmune disorders such as rheumatoid arthritis, has significantly reduced the progressive pathological destruction of tissues (e.g. joints). However, the long-term consequences on other aspects of health are unclear and are being carefully monitored.

Surgery and anaesthesia

Immunosuppressive aspects of surgery

Stress response to surgery

The body's acute-phase response to injury represents a complex interaction between neuroendocrine, metabolic, and immune systems. Tissue trauma, as a result of surgical incisions and tissue dissection, organ manipulation, and vascular compromise, very early stimulates innate immunity and its resultant inflammatory response. This response is believed to be proportional to the degree of the initial insult, trauma, and resultant tissue damage [1]. Inflammation is an early protective homeostatic immune response to injury. It is characterized by the initiation of proinflammatory mediator cascades (cytokines, chemokines, complement system), as a result of an early and prominent activation of innate immunity and major perturbation of neutrophil release and function. This is followed by the subsequent activation and modulation of cellular and humoral adaptive immune mechanisms [2]. The impact of trauma on the body defences and their homeostasis, through the release of pro- and anti-inflammatory mediators, is discussed comprehensively in Chapter 2.

The local environment at the site of injury (external or surgically induced), through the release of 'danger' or 'stress' signals (e.g. heat shock proteins [HSPs]) from damaged and necrotic cells, stimulates the pattern recognition receptors (PRRs) on polymorphonuclear leucocytes and monocytes-macrophages, inducing these to become activated and to produce and secrete a variety of proinflammatory cytokines—tumour necrosis factor-alpha (TNF-α), interleukin-1 (IL-1), IL-6, etc. The rapid and prompt activation of innate immunity results in the induction of the systemic inflammatory response syndrome (SIRS). This inflammatory response spreads rapidly and systemically, and its impact on the adaptive immune system is determined by the balance between proinflammatory and anti-inflammatory humoral and cell-mediated immune responses elicited. We have previously shown that surgically induced inflammatory immune responses can be attenuated by minimal access surgery in a study comparing minilaparatomy with full laparotomy in patients undergoing cholecystectomy [3].

Up-regulation of cytokine production marks the initiation of the acute phase reaction in response to injury, such as surgery [4,5]. Certain cytokines (IL-1, IL-6, TNF-α), which appear to be beneficial at low plasma levels as immune modulators, are associated with patient deterioration and mortality when present in large and uncontrolled quantities [6] (see Chapter 2).

IL-6 is one of the most studied cytokines in the context of the stress response to surgery. There is an increase in circulating levels of IL-6 within 1–3 hours of surgical tissue damage and the levels remain elevated for 2 to 3 days postoperatively [5]. Plasma concentrations of IL-6 correlate with duration of surgery, blood loss, and extent of tissue trauma [7]. Prolonged and excessive IL-6 elevations are associated with increased morbidity and mortality. Moreover, the degree of IL-6 elevation has been shown prospectively to predict subsequent clinical deterioration in patients and, in some studies, has been documented to be a predictor of mortality [8]. Human studies have shown systemic IL-6 levels to be lower in patients who undergo laparoscopic surgery on the abdomen, compared with those who have a standard laparotomy. Cholecystectomy is the most commonly used clinical model demonstrating the advantage of the laparoscopic approach on the basis of the postoperative IL-6 levels and postoperative rehabilitation [9,10].

Neutrophil and monocyte dysfunction in patients are known to predict postsurgical sepsis and mortality following major trauma [11]. The traditional abdominal laparotomy impairs a wide range of host defences, both innate and adaptive [12] (Table 7.1). Laparoscopic surgery appears to induce a smaller stress response to injury, resulting in a proportionally better preservation of the host's immunological function. Natural killer (NK) cell and lymphokine-activated killer (LAK) cell cytotoxicities are significantly inhibited in the perioperative period, following general anaesthesia and major abdominal surgery. Both these killer cells are regarded as innate immune cells and as key bridging components between innate and adaptive immunity (see Chapter 1). The critical impact of trauma and any resultant sepsis on innate immunity (and adaptive immunity) is discussed comprehensively in Chapters 2 and 5.

Lymphadenectomy

The pivotal role of loco-regional lymph nodes (LNs) in the development of immunity that could mediate the rejection of malignant tumours has been documented [14]. Animal studies have shown that excision of the immunization site 2 days after injections had little impact on the eventual development of systemic immunity, whereas draining LNs were required to be left *in situ* for 7–9 days after vaccination in order to immunize an animal to reject subsequent tumour challenges [15,16].

Table 7.1 Impairment of host defences (innate and adaptive) following laparotomy and major abdominal surgery

Monocyte-macrophage suppression	Neutrophil dysfunction	Lymphocyte changes
Impaired phagocytosis	Decreased reactive O_2 species production	Impaired delayed type hypersensitivity
Increased cytokine production	Decreased production of elastase and collagenase	Shift of Th:T suppressor ratio
Decreased HLA-DR expression	Diminished chemotaxis	Down-regulation of Th1 type cell function

Reproduced by kind permission from Novitsky YW, Litwin DE, Callery MP. The net immunologic advantage of laparoscopic surgery. Surg Endosc 2004;18:1411–19 [13].

Lymph node dissection is an integral part of the surgical resection for many solid tumours. It is important for long-term loco-regional control of the tumour and it allows prognostic evaluation through accurate staging and determination of the need for adjuvant therapy. Studies have demonstrated an immune reaction by tumour-infiltrating lymphocytes (TILs), which attests to an ongoing interaction between the tumour and systemic host defences [17]. The regional LNs constitute an important first line of immune defence, where the initial host anticancer response is initiated; they may also participate in inducing a local state of immunosuppression if the LNs contain metastatic tumour [18]. Therefore, in light of these findings, resection of loco-regional LNs (if tumour-free), may impair the regional immune response to the tumour. However, the establishment of progressive malignant disease in a tissue or organ may be interpreted as indicating a failure of loco-regional defences and surgical removal is likely to be of little anticancer therapeutic relevance (see Chapter 4).

Splenectomy

Patients who have undergone a splenectomy (e.g. due to traumatic injury) are at a significant risk of developing infections, because the spleen is the largest accumulation of lymphoid tissue in the body. Overwhelming postsplenectomy infection (OPSI) is a serious septic process and is associated with a high mortality rate (50–70%) [19]. Possible causes of OPSI include loss of splenic phagocytic function, decreasing serum immunoglobulin levels, suppression of lymphocyte reactivity, or alterations in the opsonin system [20,21]. Outside the spleen, polysaccharide antigens (encapsulated organisms) are poorly immunogenic in comparison with protein antigens. This contributes to polysaccharide-coated bacteria evading phagocytosis and the subsequent immune response [21]. Host defences against bacteria, therefore, are critically dependent on humoral immunity and production of type-specific antibodies (see Chapter 1). While liver Kupffer cells are able to remove most well-opsonized bacteria, encapsulated organisms resist antibody binding and are primarily removed by the spleen. Therefore, exposure of these patients to encapsulated organisms such as *Streptococcus pneumoniae*, *Neisseria meningitides*, *Haemophilus influenzae*, and *Streptococcus pyogenes* could result in fatal sepsis.

Vaccines are available for common encapsulated organisms and include a 23-valent pneumococcal polysaccharide vaccine, a 7-valent protein-conjugated pneumococcal vaccine, the *Haemophilus influenzae* type B vaccine, and the meningococcal vaccine [21]. A new 13-valent protein-conjugate pneumococcal vaccine has recently been licensed for use in the USA and UK. The polysaccharide-based pneumococcal vaccine is recommended for all adults at increased risk of pneumococcal infection and, in particular, for the asplenic patient [22]. The Centre for Disease Control and Prevention in the USA recommends revaccination every 6 years. The British Committee for Standards in Haematology recommends revaccination every 5–10 years for the prevention of OPSI [23,24]. A small percentage (5%) of postsplenectomy patients develop OPSI, despite vaccination after splenectomy [25]. Therefore, for elective splenectomy, the vaccine should be given at least 2 weeks before surgery to allow for adequate circulating antibody levels to be present when the spleen is absent [25].

Clinicians should be aware that these vaccines do not provide full protection and long-term antibiotic prophylaxis should also be considered for these patients.

Thymectomy

Thymectomy achieves remission of myasthenia gravis with the help of medication including steroids. This operation is carried out mainly in adults. This is because the thymus loses most of its functional capacity after adolescence, but does retain a small portion of its function during adulthood. This is shown in the decreasing size of the thymus with increasing age after adolescence. The role of the thymus prior to adolescence is to educate T cells to a specific response to antigens and to delete self-reactive T cells, thereby, promoting effective T cell immunity and preventing autoimmunity [26] (see Chapter 1). Removal of the thymus in an adult appears to have no overt effect on the immune system as its core functional role has been completed by then. However, thymectomy, for whatever reason, in a preadolescent individual may lead to serious autoimmunity through uncontrolled production and release of self-reactive T cells (see Chapter 8).

Immunosuppressive aspects of blood transfusion

Allogeneic blood transfusion has immunosuppressive effects as evidenced by pre-transplantation autologous blood transfusion with a resultant improvement in renal allograft survival [27] (see Chapter 3). Consistent with the beneficial effects of blood transfusion as an immunosuppressant is the reduced severity and recurrence of Crohn's disease following multiple blood transfusions [28]. In contrast to these beneficial effects of immunosuppression, detrimental immune regulatory effects of blood transfusion have been well documented, such as increased incidence of cancer recurrence [29–31] and increased risk of infection [32]. Interestingly, allogeneic packed red blood cells and plasma transfusions have been found to induce the proliferation of $CD4^+$ $CD25^+$ $Foxp3^+$ T regulatory cells (Tregs) [33]. However, this effect was abrogated if washed packed red cells were used for transfusion [33]. This implicates plasma factors and offers an explanation for the differential effects of blood transfusion seen in trauma (see Chapter 2), sepsis (see Chapter 5), cancer (see Chapter 4). and with autoimmune disease (see Chapter 8) (Figure 7.1).

Immunosuppressive aspects of anaesthetic agents and drugs

General anaesthetic agents

General anaesthetic agents have been shown to have a deleterious effect on the immune system in humans and animals (*in vitro* and *in vivo*), as outlined below.

Neutrophil dysfunction: Halothane has been shown to inhibit (reversibly) human neutrophil bactericidal activity *in vitro*; the mechanism of inhibition is attributable to a deleterious effect of halothane on the oxidative killing activity of neutrophils [34]. Other studies have also suggested inhibition of reactive oxygen species (ROSs) production by activated neutrophils; this was also seen with enflurane, isoflurane, and sevoflurane [35,36].

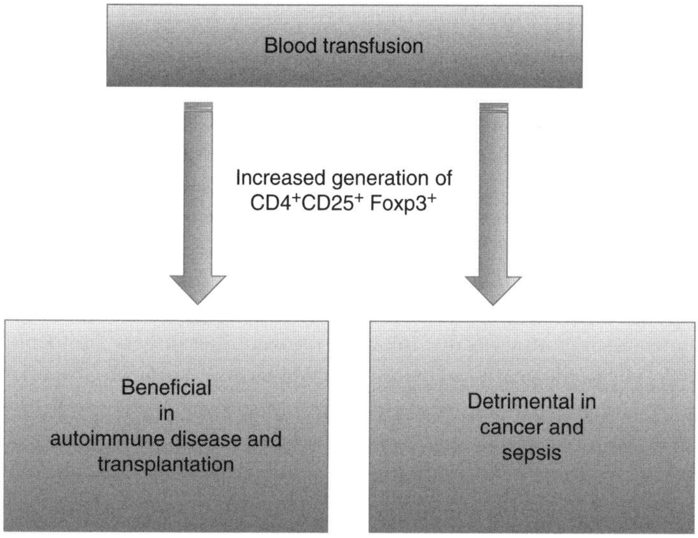

Fig. 7.1 Differential effects of blood transfusion on autoimmune disease, transplantation, cancer, and sepsis, mediated by Tregs.

Monocyte and macrophage dysfunction: In animals, halothane inhibits the intra-alveolar recruitment of macrophages in response to influenza virus infection [37]. Isoflurane is known to decrease the phagocytic capacity of human alveolar macrophages during surgery [38]. An *in vivo* animal study, involving the generation of endotoxaemia in rats, showed that the inhalation of isoflurane reduced the release of the proinflammatory cytokine IL-1 [39].

Natural killer cell dysfunction: NK cells are an important component of innate immunity and are believed to be important in the elimination of tumour cells in the early stages of tumour initiation and growth (see Chapters 1 and 4). Decreased NK cell function during the perioperative period is associated with an increased risk of mortality in patients with cancer [40,41]. Volatile anaesthetics, such as halothane and enflurane, reversibly inhibited NK cell activity in a dose-dependent manner *in vitro* [42]. The effect was transient and following removal of NK cells from exposure to the volatile anaesthetics, full recovery of NK cell activity was documented [42].

T and B lymphocyte dysfunction: Exposure to halothane impairs the secretion of interferon-gamma (IFN-γ) by lymphocytes. Other volatile anaesthetics (sevoflurane, isoflurane, and enflurane) also suppress the release of IL-1 and TNF-α [43]. Impairment of lymphocyte function by these anaesthetic agents reduces the capacity of these cells to target microorganisms and tumour cells. The intravenous short-acting anaesthetic agent propofol has been shown to inhibit B cell function and to favour a T helper 1 (Th1) $CD4^+$ T cell response, which may be beneficial in an immune compromised host [44].

Regional and local anaesthetic agents

Surgery-related increases in serum cortisol are attenuated by extradural analgesia. Afferent neural blockade induced by extradural anaesthesia can decrease intraoperative and postoperative neuroendocrine stress responses [45]. The decreased lymphocyte proliferation and lymphokine production seen in patients under general anaesthesia were not seen in patients undergoing extradural anaesthesia [46]. In addition, spinal anaesthesia prevented the depression of mitogen-induced lymphocyte proliferation *in vitro* in patients undergoing general anaesthesia for prostate surgery [47]. Thus, the combination of regional anaesthesia with general anaesthesia may help to blunt the perioperative immunosuppression. This approach has been employed by some colorectal surgeons using the 'enhanced recovery after surgery' protocols [48,49]. This is currently in the process of being evaluated by other surgical subspecialties.

Opioids

In vivo studies in animals have demonstrated that morphine inhibits the proliferation and differentiation of macrophage progenitor cells [50], phagocytosis by monocytes and macrophages [51], and IL-10 and IL-12 production by monocytes and macrophages [52]. These impairments were documented in peritoneal, alveolar, and splenic macrophages, indicating a general down-regulation of innate immunity. It appears from these studies that morphine impairs host defences. This may be important in the management of the critically ill patient and the risk of developing infectious complications (see Chapters 2 and 5). Furthermore, *in vivo* administration of morphine to volunteers impaired spontaneous and cytokine-induced NK cell activity [53].

Chemotherapy, corticosteroids, radiotherapy, and hormonal therapy

Introduction

Chemotherapy and radiotherapy are important therapeutic modalities in the management of patients with malignant disease. However, chemotherapy and radiotherapy are able to either suppress or enhance the host's immune system, depending on the type of agent used and the dosage and scheduling employed. Therefore, the term 'immune modulation' is more appropriate when describing their effects on the immune system.

Immune modulation by chemotherapy

Several of the cancer chemotherapeutic agents that are currently in use are also used as immunosuppressants for the treatment of severe systemic autoimmune diseases (see Chapter 8). Cancer drugs inhibit globally or selectively the functions of both the innate and adaptive immune systems [54,55].

A large body of evidence also suggests that some cytotoxic compounds promote specific anticancer immune responses that contribute to the therapeutic effects of conventional therapy [54,55]. This is outlined in Table 7.2.

Chemotherapy, by damaging/stressing malignant cells, induces the release of 'danger' signals (e.g. HSPs), which then activate antigen presenting cells (APCs) and other cells

Table 7.2 Anticancer immune activation induced by chemotherapeutic agents

Agent	Immune activation
Cyclophosphamide (low dose), gemcitabine, taxanes	Reduction in circulating Tregs
Vincristine, vinblastine, paclitaxel, methotrexate	Activation of DCs (CD40, CD80, CD83)
Cisplatin, 5-fluorouracil, 5-aza-2′-deoxycitidine	Up-regulation of FasL and HLAs in tumours
Gemcitabine, antivascular flavonoids	Increased tumour homing by lymphocytes
Gemcitabine	Generation of T cell help (cross-presentation)
Alkylating agents, antimetabolites	Maintainence of tumour-lytic T cell clonotypes
Gemcitabine	Enhancement of CD14$^+$ DC precursor proliferation

Based on data from Baxevanis et al. [54] and Zitvogen et al. [55]

of the innate immune system via their PRRs and cause the release of proinflammatory cytokines. Chemotherapy-induced death of cancer cells can cause the release of immunogenic antigens (cell fragments, proteins, and peptides), which result in a cell-mediated immune response to the tumour, augmented by the concurrent cytokines released by cells of the innate immune system [56,57].

Cytokine production and secretion associated with chemotherapeutic drug therapy mediates the development of various side effects (e.g. lethargy, weakness, myalgia), including psychobehavioural alterations, during and after treatment. Paclitaxel can mimic the effects of lipopolysaccharide (LPS), a ligand for Toll-like receptor (TLR)-4 expressed on innate immune cells. Treatment with the taxanes paclitaxel or docetaxel has been reported to increase the levels of IL-2, IL-6, IFN-γ, and granulocyte-macrophage-colony stimulating factor (GM-CSF), and to decrease the level of IL-1 and TNF-α in women with advanced breast cancer who responded to treatment [58]. Adjuvant and neoadjuvant treatment of women with breast cancer with paclitaxel also increased serum levels of IL-6, IL-8, and IL-10, and these changes correlated with joint pain and flu-like symptoms [59]. Some drugs may increase the production of cytokines by the expansion of immune cells, which are involved in anticancer mechanisms. Treatment with gemcitabine (an antimetabolite) increased the numbers of IFN-producing T cells and activated CD69$^+$ cells in patients with pancreatic cancer [60]. Bleomycin (cytotoxic antibiotic), used to treat testicular cancer and Hodgkin's lymphoma, is associated with pulmonary toxicity and, occasionally, with fatal pulmonary fibrosis. In animal models of bleomycin-induced lung fibrosis, transforming growth factor beta-1 (TGF-β1) (a profibrotic cytokine) and other proinflammatory cytokines (IL-1, IL-6, and TNF) have been implicated [61].

Lutsiak *et al.* documented that low metronomic doses of cyclophosphamide (an alkylating drug) caused a substantial reduction in the number and function of Tregs by down-regulating the expression of key functional markers of Tregs, namely Foxp3 and glucocorticoid-induced TNF-receptor-related protein [62]. Low-dose cyclophosphamide has been shown to selectively kill Tregs in humans and mice without affecting T effector cells [63]. In animals, low-dose cyclophosphamide induces a Th2/Th1 shift in the cytokine profile produced. It also enhances immunity by preferentially depleting $CD8^+$ lymphoid resident DCs, which diminishes Treg suppression [64]. The effects of cyclophosphamide on Tregs and cyclophosphamide-stimulated type I IFN production might account for the augmented antibody responses and the persistence of memory T cells [65]. All these effects contribute to the eradication of immunogenic tumours in synergy with specific immunotherapies [66]. Combining low-dose cyclophosphamide with active immunotherapy is an attractive strategy. Our group has shown recently that favourable clinical responses are seen in patients with prostate cancer with low levels of circulating Tregs, and undergoing vaccination [67].

Dendritic cells (DCs) are specialized and key APCs, found in most tissues of the body and essential for initiating and developing an effective cell-mediated immune response (see Chapter 1). *In vitro* studies with various drugs (vincristine, vinblastine, paclitaxel, methotrexate) added at low, noncytotoxic doses increased expression of CD40, CD80, CD 83, and enhanced the ability of DCs to stimulate allogeneic T lymphocytes [68]. However, ifosphamide (DNA-alkylating agent) depletes DC intracellular glutathione in human DCs, impairing their functional activity. Recent evidence suggests that radiotherapy and chemotherapy can enhance anticancer immune responses by enhancing engulfment and processing of apoptotic bodies by DCs through translocation of calreticulin to the plasma membrane and the release of high-mobility group box 1 (HMGB-1) protein [69]. Also, in patients with pancreatic cancer, treatment with gemcitabine-induced proliferation of $CD14^+$ monocyte precursors of DCs as well as myeloid ($CD11c^+$) and plasmacytoid ($CD123^+$) DCs [70] (Table 7.2). In an animal tumour model gemcitabine (given in a dose equivalent to that used in humans) significantly reduced the number of myeloid suppressor cells ($CD11b^+$) in the spleens of animals bearing large tumours but with no reduction of $CD4^+$T, $CD8^+$T, NK or B cells and enhancing antitumour immune activity [71].

There have been several clinical trials in the last 10 years combining the immune-modulating effects of chemotherapy with various forms of immunotherapy [54,72]. Many of these studies have shown encouraging results, albeit only transiently because of the advanced stages of the cancers treated [54,72]. There is, therefore, a need to investigate the efficacy of such treatments in low-volume early-stage disease in order to demonstrate clinically durable tumour regression.

Immune modulation by corticosteroids

Corticosteroids are hormones which are produced in the adrenal cortex. They are involved in stress; immune responses; regulation of inflammation; carbohydrate, and protein metabolism; and regulation of blood electrolyte levels. They have been used in a range of disease states (asthma, allergies, inflammations, autoimmune diseases). Early studies on the effects of corticosteroids on cell-mediated immunity (CMI) suggested they suppressed wide-ranging aspects of cell-mediated immune responses [73].

Glucocorticoids have been shown to suppress the Th1 proinflammatory immune response [74] with a resultant shift towards the Th2 anti-inflammatory immune

Table 7.3 Immune dysfunction induced by steroids

Inhibition		Augmentation	
Cellular	Cytokine	Cellular	Cytokine
DCs	Th1	$CD4^+$ Th2	IL-10
$CD8^+$ T cells	Th17	Tregs	TGF-β
$CD4^+$ Th1	IL-12		Th2

response [75]. In giant cell arteritis, glucocorticoids suppressed Th17 but not the Th1 production of cytokines [76]. Corticosteroids may also enhance the production of TGF-β and suppress the Th1 response, both of which are believed to be detrimental to cancer patients [54,55] (Table 7.3) (see Chapter 4). Recent evidence has shown that glucocorticoids amplified IL-2-induced selective expression of $CD4^+$ $CD25^+$ Fox $p3^+$ Tregs *in vivo* and suppressed graft-versus-host disease in an animal model [77].

The effects of corticosteroids on other subpopulations of cells involved in innate immunity (e.g. NK cells, γδ T cells) and humoral immunity (B cells) is poorly established and requires further investigation (see Chapter 1 for comprehensive discussion of these cells).

Immune modulation by radiotherapy

Systemic or whole-body radiotherapy is known to be lymphoablative and results in neutropenia, thrombocytopenia, and anaemia. However, localized radiation, besides its direct cytotoxic properties on tumour cells, mediates a number of pathobiological effects on cells and tissues, some of which may stimulate an immune response.

Low doses of ionizing radiation up-regulate the expression of major histocompatibility complex (MHC) class I molecules, tumour-associated antigens (TAAs: carcinoembryonic antigen and mucin 1) and CD95 (also known as Fas) by tumour cells [78]. Adhesion molecules on endothelial cells may also be up-regulated [79], thereby, boosting antitumour $CD8^+$ T cell activity [80] and T cell trafficking towards the irradiated tumour sites [81].

Local irradiation of the primary tumour can reduce the size of the metastases that are located at distant sites. This is referred to as the *abscopal effect*, and is believed to be mediated by the immune system. Interestingly, irradiation enhances tumour antigenicity by modulating the repertoire of tumour-derived peptides that are presented to the immune system [82]. Firstly, radiotherapy enhances the degradation of existing proteins, increasing the intracellular pool of peptides for MHC class I presentation. Secondly, activation of the molecular target of rapamycin (mTOR) in irradiated tumour cells stimulates protein translation and increases peptide production. Thirdly, radiotherapy stimulates the synthesis of new proteins and, possibly, antigenic peptides, which can be presented for recognition by different T cell repertoires [82]. Moreover, potent synergistic effects against established tumours by passively transferred $CD8^+$ cytotoxic T lymphocytes (CTLs) [78] or TLR-9 ligands and ionizing radiation have been reported [82].

Radiotherapy can lead to release of cytokines in various tissues, and cytokines are associated with the development of late radiation damage that can occur in irradiated normal tissues months or years after treatment [83]. TGF-β has a crucial role in the initiation, development, and persistence of radiation-induced fibrosis, and circulating levels of TGF-β1 predict radiation-induced lung damage [84]. The TGF-β1 allele is associated with increased circulating levels of TGF-β1 and radiation-induced damage in normal tissues in women with early breast cancer [85].

Immune modulation by hormonal therapy

Aromatase inhibitors, which further reduce the already low levels of oestrogen in the plasma and tissues of postmenopausal women, are frequently used as adjuvant hormonal treatment in postmenopausal women with breast cancer. Treatment can be associated with arthralgia (joint pain) and bone loss, sometimes leading to discontinuation of treatment. Various immune cells (such as DCs, macrophages, and B cells) express oestrogen receptors and oestrogen can influence their activity [86]. Oestrogen down-regulates cell-mediated immune responses and promotes humoral immune responses. Oestrogen deficiency, on the other hand, increases cell-mediated immune responses and the production of proinflammatory cytokines such as IL-1, IL-6, and TNF-α [87]. These cytokines may mediate the arthralgia and inflammatory changes in joints associated with aromatase inhibitors.

A recent study has demonstrated a significant reduction of tumour-infiltrating Tregs in patients with breast cancer receiving primary therapy with letrozole; another possible beneficial result with aromatase inhibitors [88].

Immune-enhancing cytokine therapy

Introduction

Most cytokines are associated with unacceptably high levels of toxicity, which precludes their widespread use in humans. There are currently only a few cytokines (IL-2, TNF-α, and IFN-α) approved for systemic use in patients. IFN-γ has been shown to be very effective in certain rare conditions—chronic granulomatous disease (CGD) and severe malignant osteopetrosis.

Interleukin-2

In addition to being an excellent agent for increasing lymphocyte numbers and activity for adoptive immunotherapy, IL-2 has been used therapeutically in advanced malignancies. Initial efforts focused on the systemic infusion of IL-2 *in vivo* to stimulate anticancer CMI. This was based on experiments in murine tumour models demonstrating that direct infusion of IL-2 had significant beneficial antitumour effects [89,90]. Clinically, IL-2 is now approved for treating renal cell carcinoma and melanoma in North America and the European Union. Modest but statistically significant response rates have been documented in clinical trials [91–95].

Despite the initial enthusiasm for the use of IL-2 and impressive preclinical data that indicated potential antitumour efficacy, overt long-term clinical benefits were seen only in a limited number of patients with renal cell carcinoma and malignant melanoma. In addition to the lack of consistently high efficacy and clinical response rate, a major factor limiting the use of recombinant (r) human (h) IL-2 is its toxicity, particularly at high doses and if given intravenously. These toxicities include hypotension, vascular leak, and respiratory insufficiency [95]. Less severe but nonetheless treatment-limiting side effects have been demonstrated. Therefore, the systemic use of rhIL-2 has to be balanced between the morbidity of treatment and the likely patient benefit.

Tumour necrosis factor-alpha

TNF-α has been used in a number of phase I and II clinical trials against a variety of human tumours [96–98]. There are three key mechanisms by which TNF-α can eradicate tumours [99]. Firstly, it has direct cytolytic activity against tumour cells. Secondly, it can kill tumours by selectively destroying tumour neovasculature and causing haemorrhagic necrosis [100,101]. Thirdly, it can stimulate CMI against tumour cells. Therefore, it possesses potent antitumour activities.

Most clinical trials have been unsuccessful as a result of the serious systemic toxicity associated with TNF-α. Because of the side effects, such as hypotension, vascular leak, fever, and neurotoxicity, an effective antitumour dose cannot be achieved in most cases [101]. Humans can only tolerate less than 2% of the dose necessary to cause tumour regression in mice [101]. However, if TNF-α can be localized to certain organs or compartments of the body and an effective dose delivered, it is then effective in destroying human malignancies [102,103]. A good example is the use of TNF-α in treating osteosarcomas and metastatic melanomas in limbs by isolated limb perfusion with TNF-α [104].

Interferon-alpha

Studies using adjuvant IFNs with chemotherapy have shown significant improvement in response over that of chemotherapy alone. This therapeutic combination, called biochemotherapy, typically consists of chemotherapy together with IL-2 and IFN-α [105]. Biochemotherapy has increased overall response rates by 36–66% among patients with metastatic melanoma [105]. Long-term complete response rates of 10% have been obtained in several studies with biochemotherapy, compared with less than 2% with chemotherapy alone [105].

Flu-like symptoms occur in most patients (>75%) treated with IFNs, including fever, chills, headache, malaise, myalgia, and arthralgia [106]. Injection site reactions occur in 10–15% of cases, and include necrotic lesions and cellulitis [107].

Gene therapy

Gene therapy is the insertion of genes into an individual's cells and tissues to treat a disease, such as cancer or a hereditary disorder in which a deleterious mutant allele is replaced with a functional one. Although the biotechnology is still in its infancy, it has been used with some selective success.

When used to deliver therapeutic cytokines, the advantages of such local gene delivery approaches are: (1) the ability to generate locally high concentrations of cytokines,

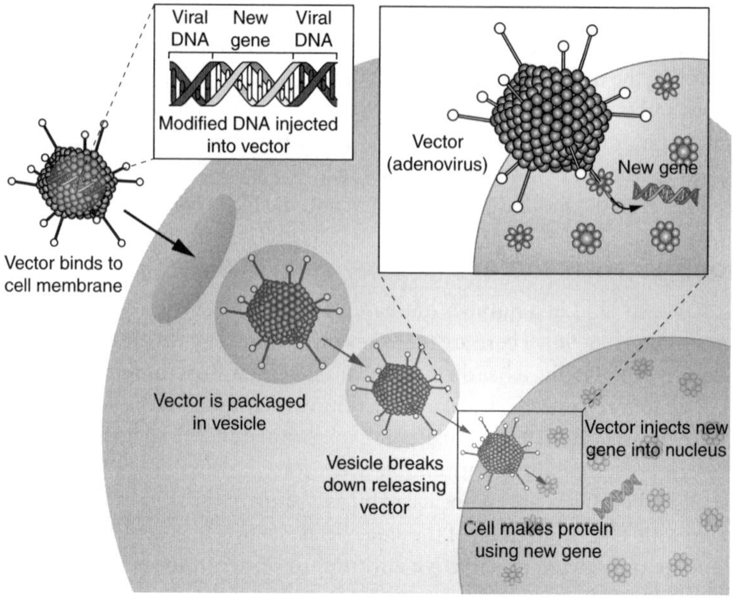

Fig. 7.2 Gene therapy using an adenovirus vector. A new gene is inserted into an adenovirus vector, which is used to introduce the modified DNA into a human cell. If the treatment is successful, the new gene will make a functional protein.

similar to the body's own responses against foreign antigens; (2) the ability to provide sustained high levels of cytokines with paracrine effects that activate the immune system. Many different gene therapy vectors have been used for the delivery of tumour cytokine therapy. A large variety of viral and nonviral vectors have been adopted for delivery of gene therapy experimentally. Among the ones that have been used to deliver cytokines are murine retrovirus vectors, human or feline lentiviral vectors, adenoviral and adeno-associated virus vectors, herpes simplex virus, and vaccinia virus vectors, fowlpox virus, Semliki forest virus, and naked plasmid DNA virus vectors in combination with 'gene guns' [108]. Currently, there is no consensus on the optimal vector to use for cancer gene therapy. Figure 7.2 schematically outlines the principles underlying gene therapy (see Chapter 9).

Evidence is emerging that with local injections of adenoviral vectors these are not localized to the site of injection. Intratumoural injections have been shown to spread locally and disseminate systemically. The resultant immune response against the vectors and the elevated levels of circulating cytokines, can induce toxic side effects in the host [109]. Therefore, to ensure maximum efficacy and minimal toxicity of gene therapy in cancer, cytokine expression has to be limited to the tumour mass.

In cancer treatment, regardless of the vector used, there are chiefly three gene therapy delivery approaches:

- The direct injection of the gene therapy vectors into the tumour mass or at the periphery of the tumour.

- The implantation of *ex vivo* cytokine-modified autologous or allogeneic fibroblasts, stem cells, or other normal cell types into or in the vicinity of the tumour mass.
- The use of *ex vivo* modified autologous or allogeneic lethally irradiated tumour cells as vaccines. Various immunostimulatory cytokine genes are transduced into tumour cells, which are subsequently made harmless through irradiation to become cancer vaccines [110].

A large number of cytokine genes have been evaluated in preclinical studies and clinical trials for their antitumour efficacy. However, the most successful, to date, has been the vaccine comprising tumour cells that are gene-modified and irradiated to secrete GM-CSF [111–113]. Many clinical trials with GVAX vaccine have been completed and others are ongoing in various solid and haematological malignancies such as prostate, lung, and pancreatic cancers, leukaemia, and myeloma [111–113]. Results, to date, are encouraging and have been carried out mostly in patients with advanced malignancies who have failed conventional therapies.

Immunotherapy

Vaccination

The principles underlying vaccination are discussed in detail in Chapter 1. Immunotherapies with cancer vaccines are designed to boost the anticancer immune responses, specific to a particular tumour and leading to its elimination. Traditionally, vaccines for infectious diseases have been preventive in nature. Cancer vaccines differ, however, in that they are given, for the most part, after the malignancy has become established. Favourable clinical responses have been observed, albeit these have been modest (10–20%), usually transient, and limited to selected tumour types (e.g. melanoma, renal and prostate cancers) (see Chapter 4).

One of the best approaches so far is the 'DC' vaccine. The function of DCs is to act as sentinel or surveillance cells detecting and interacting with foreign peptides (e.g. from bacteria or viruses), and using these to induce the immune system to mount peptide-specific cell-mediated or humoral responses. The ability of DCs to take up, process, and re-express foreign antigens can be adopted to produce cancer vaccines (see Chapter 1). DC precursors can be isolated from blood by leucophoresis. Activated and partially mature DCs are generated by *in vitro* culture (in a Good Manufacturing Practice facility). These activated DCs are then exposed to TAAs or tumour extracts in *in vitro* culture and finally reintroduced into the body as a vaccine. The resulting DCs can educate the immune system to respond to the peptides expressed on the TAAs, generating CTLs which home to the cancer cell milieu, and lyse the cancer cells expressing the TAA peptides. Recent approaches have harnessed the Langerhans cells (sentinel DCs), resident in skin and which are very effective for this purpose, if primed with the optimal combination of immunological adjuvants (see Chapters 1 and 4).

Data are emerging suggesting a beneficial effect associated with the use of vaccination protocols combined with selective anticancer chemotherapeutic drugs. Trials of such combinations are being carried out (e.g. gemcitabine and vaccination with human telomerase reverse transcriptase).

Monoclonal antibodies and small molecule inhibitors

Humanized or mixed monoclonal antibodies (MABs) are currently being used in various diseases. Chapter 1 discusses the general principles underlying their uses and potential benefits in humans. In rheumatoid arthritis a range of MABs is being used, as exemplified by infliximab. There is good evidence for efficacy but with an increased risk of bacterial infection and tuberculosis (TB).

Anti-TNF-α treatment with MABs (fully human or chimeric) has been approved by NICE (the National Institute for Health and Clinical Excellence) for use in the UK in the chronic arthritides, such as rheumatoid arthritis and ankylosing spondylitis. Infliximab has been shown to be effective in inducing complete remissions in patients with early rheumatoid arthritis [114]. However, these agents not only block TNF but also interfere with aspects of innate and adaptive immunity—reduced phagocytosis, reduction of IFN-γ secretion, and up-regulation of Tregs [115]. The consequences of this prolonged suppression of proinflammatory mediators are enhanced incidence of bacterial infections, including TB.

Immunotherapy and vaccination (including the use of MABs) are discussed in more detail in Chapters 1, 4, and 8. Immunesuppressive therapy for preventing rejection of transplanted organs is discussed comprehensively in Chapter 3. Chapter 5 discusses the findings, to date, of MAB therapy trials in patients with sepsis.

In cancer, MABs have made a major impact on the diagnostic pathway and with small-molecular inhibitors, (SMIs) have shown important therapeutic benefits in selected cancers, using a targeted approach (see Chapters 1 and 4). Protein kinases, which play a key role in regulating cell proliferation, differentiation, survival, and cell death, have been a focus of major research endeavours by the pharmaceutical industry and studies in patients with various solid cancers and haematological malignancies. It is worth noting that more than 150 protein kinases are involved in various other diseases apart from cancer, e.g. the arthritides, cardiovascular disorders, and neurodegenerative diseases. An ever-increasing number of MABs have been produced for clinical use, with a major emphasis on controlling the malignant process by disrupting cell growth control mechanisms (epidermal growth factor receptors—HER2/neu, EGFR), and angiogenesis and disruption of tumour blood supply (vascular endothelial growth factor receptors—VEGFR1–3). The efficacy is variable, with major benefit in the use of trastuzumab in HER2$^+$ overexpressed breast cancers with mild and acceptable side effects, but cardiac toxicity in combination with anthracyclines is well documented. A range of adverse skin reactions and gastrointestinal disturbances have been recorded; with bevacizumab in colorectal cancer, gastrointestinal haemorrhage, perforation, and fistula formation are serious and well-documented side effects [116]. CTLA-4 blockade with MABs has been carried out in patients with a range of metastatic cancers. Partial responses have been reported but have been associated with significant autoimmune side effects (20% enterocolitis and colectomy in some cases, due to inability to control the colitis) [117].

Recent reports in metastatic melanoma have reported antitumour efficacy (tumour necrosis, prominent CD8$^+$ CTLs, and reduced Tregs) in patients vaccinated with GVAX and subsequent infusions of CTLA-4 blocking MABs, with acceptable morbidity [118]. Therapeutic antibodies are playing an important role in treating certain autoimmune disorders, such as rheumatoid arthritis, Crohn's disease, plaque psoriasis (anti-TNF, CD20-specific), and specific malignancies—breast cancer, bowel cancer, lung cancer, non-Hodgkin's lymphoma (anti-HER2, anti-VEGFA, CD20-specific) [119,120].

Summary and conclusions

Surgery, anaesthetic agents, opioids, and blood transfusion in the critical care setting, as well as corticosteroids, have been shown to have a detrimental effect on the host's immune system. Chemotherapy depletes cells involved in innate and adoptive immunity. Chemotherapy, however, does not invariably cause immune suppression, but can induce selective immune activation of host defences, depending on the chemotherapeutic agents, doses, and regimens used. Such therapies have been shown to have enhanced beneficial effects when combined with immunotherapy. At present, precise evidence is lacking about the exact mechanisms responsible for the chemotherapy-mediated potentiation of anticancer immune responsiveness. Reduction of Tregs and activation of DCs are two likely mechanisms. Systemic cytokine therapy is emerging as an effective treatment but its use is limited by serious toxicity in the host. However, selective, high-dose agents (e.g. TNF-α) in limb perfusion show promise. Gene-mediated cytokine therapy is being piloted in patients with some antitumour-specific benefit and with acceptable toxicity. Immunotherapy to modulate systemic inflammation in trauma and sepsis is still very much at an investigative stage, with little overt benefit, to date. In autoimmune diseases (e.g. rheumatoid arthritis) promising results are being obtained with anti-TNF-α MAB therapy. Immune-enhancing therapies for cancer (e.g. vaccination with DCs pulsed with TAAs) are currently being evaluated in clinical studies. A number of MABs and SMIs are showing promise in the cancer setting.

References

1. Davies MG, Hagen PO. Systemic inflammatory response syndrome. *Br J Surg.* 1997; **84**: 920–935.
2. Hackam DJ, Rotstein OD. Host response to laparoscopic surgery: mechanisms and clinical correlates. *Can J Surg.* 1998; **41**: 103–111.
3. Bruce DM, Smith M, Walker CB *et al.* Minimal access surgery for cholelithiasis induces an attenuated acute phase response. *Am J Surg* 1999; **178**: 232–234.
4. Vittimberga FJ Jr, Foley DP, Meyers WC, Callery MP. Laparoscopic surgery and the systemic immune response. *Ann Surg* 1998; **227**: 326–334.
5. Biffl WL, Moore EE, Moore FA, Peterson VM. Interleukin-6 in the injured patient. Marker of injury or mediator of inflammation? *Ann Surg.* 1996; **224**: 647–664.
6. Rixen D, Siegel JH, Abu-Salih A, Bertolini M, Panagakos F, Espina N. Physiologic state severity classification as an indicator of posttrauma cytokine response. *Shock* 1995; **4**: 27–38.
7. Schwenk W, Jacobi C, Mansmann U, Bohm B, Muller JM. Inflammatory response after laparoscopic and conventional colorectal resections—results of a prospective randomized trial. *Langenbecks Arch Surg* 2000; **385**: 2–9.
8. Baigrie RJ, Lamont PM, Kwiatkowski D, Dallman MJ, Morris PJ. Systemic cytokine response after major surgery. *Br J Surg* 1992; **79**: 757–760.

9. Maruszynski M, Pojda Z. Interleukin 6 (IL-6) levels in the monitoring of surgical trauma. A comparison of serum IL-6 concentrations in patients treated by cholecystectomy via laparotomy or laparoscopy. *Surg Endosc* 1995; **9**: 882–885.
10. Joris J, Cigarini I, Legrand M *et al.* Metabolic and respiratory changes after cholecystectomy performed via laparotomy or laparoscopy. *Br J Anaesth* 1992; **69**: 341–345.
11. Polk HC Jr, George CD, Hershman MJ, Wellhausen SR, Cheadle WG. The capacity of serum to support neutrophil phagocytosis is a vital host defense mechanism in severely injured patients. *Ann Surg* 1988; **207**: 686–692.
12. Deehan DJ, Heys SD, Ashby J, Eremin O. Interleukin-2 (IL-2) augments host cellular immune reactivity in the perioperative period in patients with malignant disease. *Eur J Surg Oncol.* 1995; **21**: 16–22.
13. Novitsky YW, Litwin DE, Callery MP. The net immunologic advantage of laparoscopic surgery. *Surg Endosc* 2004; **18**: 1411–1419.
14. Shu S, Cochran AJ, Huang R-R, Morton DL, Maecker HT. Immune responses in the draining lymph nodes against cancer: Implications for immunotherapy. *Cancer Metast Rev* 2006; **25**: 233–242.
15. Hanna MG, Jr., Bucana CD, Pollack VA. Immunological stimulation in situ: the acute and chronic inflammatory responses in the induction of tumor immunity. *Contemp Top Immunobiol* 1980; **10**: 267–296.
16. Stephenson KR, Perry-Lalley D, Griffith KD, Shu S, Chang AE. Development of antitumor reactivity in regional draining lymph nodes from tumor-immunized and tumor-bearing murine hosts. *Surgery* 1989; **105**: 523–528.
17. Aloysius M, Takhar A, Robins R, Eremin O. Dendritic cell biology, dysfunction and immunotherapy in gastrointestinal cancers. *Surgeon* 2006; **4**: 195–210.
18. Shu S, Cochran AJ, Huang RR, Morton DL, Maecker HT. Immune responses in the draining lymph nodes against cancer: implications for immunotherapy. *Cancer Metast Rev* 2006; **25**: 233–242.
19. Lynch AM, Kapila R. Overwhelming postsplenectomy infection. *Infect Dis Clin North Am* 1996; **10**: 693–707.
20. Machesky KK, Cushing RD. Overwhelming postsplenectomy infection in a patient with penicillin-resistant *Streptococcus pneumoniae. Arch Fam Med* 1998; **7**: 178–180.
21. Shatz DV. Vaccination considerations in the asplenic patient. *Expert Rev Vaccines.* 2005; **4**: 27–34.
22. Musher DM, Ceasar H, Kojic EM *et al.* Administration of protein-conjugate pneumococcal vaccine to patients who have invasive disease after splenectomy despite their having received 23-valent pneumococcal polysaccharide vaccine. *J Infect Dis* 2005; **191**: 1063–1067.
23. Whitney CG. Preventing pneumococcal disease. ACIP recommends pneumococcal polysaccharide vaccine for all adults age > or = 65. *Geriatrics* 2003; **58**: 20–2, 5.
24. Davies JM, Barnes R, Milligan D. Update of guidelines for the prevention and treatment of infection in patients with an absent or dysfunctional spleen. *Clin Med* 2002; **2**: 440–443.
25. Jockovich M, Mendenhall NP, Sombeck MD, Talbert JL, Copeland EM 3rd, Bland KI. Long-term complications of laparotomy in Hodgkin's disease. *Ann Surg* 1994; **219**: 615–21; discussion 21–4.
26. Jiang H, Chess L. Chapter 2: how the immune system achieves self-nonself discrimination during adaptive immunity. *Adv Immunol* 2009; **102**: 95–133.

27. Opelz G, Sengar DP, Mickey MR, Terasaki PI. Effect of blood transfusions on subsequent kidney transplants. *Transplant Proc* 1973; **5**: 253–259.
28. Peters WR, Fry RD, Fleshman JW, Kodner IJ. Multiple blood transfusions reduce the recurrence rate of Crohn's disease. *Dis Colon Rectum* 1989; **32**: 749–753.
29. Amato A, Pescatori M. Perioperative blood transfusions for the recurrence of colorectal cancer. *Cochrane Database Syst Rev*. 2006; **1**: CD005033.
30. Amato AC, Pescatori M. Effect of perioperative blood transfusions on recurrence of colorectal cancer: meta-analysis stratified on risk factors. *Dis Colon Rectum* 1998; **41**: 570–585.
31. Busch OR, Marquet RL, Hop WC, Jeekel J. Colorectal cancer recurrence and perioperative blood transfusions: a critical reappraisal. *Semin Surg Oncol* 1994; **10**: 195–199.
32. Chang H, Hall GA, Geerts WH, Greenwood C, McLeod RS, Sher GD. Allogeneic red blood cell transfusion is an independent risk factor for the development of postoperative bacterial infection. *Vox Sang* 2000; **78**: 13–18.
33. Baumgartner JM, Silliman CC, Moore EE, Banerjee A, McCarter MD. Stored red blood cell transfusion induces regulatory T cells. *J Am Coll Surg* 2009; **208**: 110–119.
34. Hu G, Salem MR, Crystal GJ. Isoflurane prevents platelets from enhancing neutrophil-induced coronary endothelial dysfunction. *Anesth Analg* 2005; **101**: 1261–1268.
35. Nakagawara M, Takeshige K, Takamatsu J, Takahashi S, Yoshitake J, Minakami S. Inhibition of superoxide production and $Ca2^+$ mobilization in human neutrophils by halothane, enflurane, and isoflurane. *Anesthesiology* 1986; **64**: 4–12.
36. Frohlich D, Rothe G, Schwall B *et al.* Effects of volatile anaesthetics on human neutrophil oxidative response to the bacterial peptide FMLP. *Br J Anaesth* 1997; **78**: 718–723.
37. Tait AR, Davidson BA, Johnson KJ, Remick DG, Knight PR. Halothane inhibits the intraalveolar recruitment of neutrophils, lymphocytes, and macrophages in response to influenza virus infection in mice. *Anesth Analg* 1993; **76**: 1106–1113.
38. Kotani N, Hashimoto H, Sessler DI *et al.* Intraoperative modulation of alveolar macrophage function during isoflurane and propofol anesthesia. *Anesthesiology* 1998; **89**: 1125–1132.
39. Boost KA, Flondor M, Hofstetter C *et al.* The beta-adrenoceptor antagonist propranolol counteracts anti-inflammatory effects of isoflurane in rat endotoxemia. *Acta Anaesthesiol Scand* 2007; **51**: 900–908.
40. Tartter PI, Steinberg B, Barron DM, Martinelli G. The prognostic significance of natural killer cytotoxicity in patients with colorectal cancer. *Arch Surg* 1987; **122**: 1264–1268.
41. Schantz SP, Brown BW, Lira E, Taylor DL, Beddingfield N. Evidence for the role of natural immunity in the control of metastatic spread of head and neck cancer. *Cancer Immunol Immunother* 1987; **25**: 141–148.
42. Woods GM, Griffiths DM. Reversible inhibition of natural killer cell activity by volatile anaesthetic agents in vitro. *Br J Anaesth.* 1986; **58**: 535–539.
43. Mitsuhata H, Shimizu R, Yokoyama MM. Suppressive effects of volatile anesthetics on cytokine release in human peripheral blood mononuclear cells. *Int J Immunopharmacol* 1995; **17**: 529–534.
44. Salo M, Pirttikangas CO, Pulkki K. Effects of propofol emulsion and thiopentone on T helper cell type-1/type-2 balance in vitro. *Anaesthesia* 1997; **52**: 341–344.
45. Kehlet H. Manipulation of the metabolic response in clinical practice. *World J Surg* 2000; **24**: 690–695.
46. Hole A, Unsgaard G. The effect of epidural and general anaesthesia on lymphocyte functions during and after major orthopaedic surgery. *Acta Anaesthesiol Scand* 1983; **27**: 135–141.

47. Whelan P, Morris PJ. Immunological responsiveness after transurethral resection of the prostate: general versus spinal anaesthetic. *Clin Exp Immunol* 1982; **48**: 611–618.
48. Fearon KC, Ljungqvist O, Von Meyenfeldt M *et al.* Enhanced recovery after surgery: a consensus review of clinical care for patients undergoing colonic resection. *Clin Nutr* 2005; **24**: 466–477.
49. Fearon KC, Luff R. The nutritional management of surgical patients: enhanced recovery after surgery. *Proc Nutr Soc* 2003; **62**: 807–811.
50. Roy S, Ramakrishnan S, Loh HH, Lee NM. Chronic morphine treatment selectively suppresses macrophage colony formation in bone marrow. *Eur J Pharmacol* 1991; **195**: 359–363.
51. Eisenstein TK, Hilburger ME. Opioid modulation of immune responses: effects on phagocyte and lymphoid cell populations. *J Neuroimmunol* 1998; **83**: 36–44.
52. Sacerdote P, Limiroli E, Gaspani L. Experimental evidence for immunomodulatory effects of opioids. *Adv Exp Med Biol* 2003; **521**: 106–116.
53. Yeager MP, Colacchio TA, Yu CT *et al.* Morphine inhibits spontaneous and cytokine-enhanced natural killer cell cytotoxicity in volunteers. *Anesthesiology* 1995; **83**: 500–508.
54. Baxevanis CN, Perez SA, Papamichail M. Combinatorial treatments including vaccines, chemotherapy and monoclonal antibodies for cancer therapy. *Cancer Immunol Immunother* 2009; **58**: 317–324.
55. Zitvogel L, Apetoh L, Ghiringhelli F, Kroemer G. Immunological aspects of cancer chemotherapy. *Nat Rev Immunol.* 2008 Jan; **8**(1): 59–73.
56. Shurin GV, Tourkova IL, Kaneno R, Shurin MR. Chemotherapeutic agents in noncytotoxic concentrations increase antigen presentation by dendritic cells via an IL-12-dependent mechanism. *J Immunol* 2009; **183**: 137–144.
57. Liu WM, Fowler DW, Smith P, Dalgleish AG. Pre-treatment with chemotherapy can enhance the antigenicity and immunogenicity of tumours by promoting adaptive immune responses. *Br J Cancer* 2010; **102**: 115–123.
58. Tsavaris N, Kosmas C, Vadiaka M, Kanelopoulos P, Boulamatsis D. Immune changes in patients with advanced breast cancer undergoing chemotherapy with taxanes. *Br J Cancer* 2002; **87**: 21–27.
59. Pusztai L, Mendoza TR, Reuben JM, *et al.* Changes in plasma levels of inflammatory cytokines in response to paclitaxel chemotherapy. *Cytokine* 2004; **25**: 94–102.
60. Plate JM, Plate AE, Shott S, Bograd S, Harris JE. Effect of gemcitabine on immune cells in subjects with adenocarcinoma of the pancreas. *Cancer Immunol Immunother.* 2005 Sep; **54**(9): 915–925.
61. Tabata C, Tabata R, Kadokawa Y *et al.* Thalidomide prevents bleomycin-induced pulmonary fibrosis in mice. *J Immunol* 2007; **179**: 708–714.
62. Lutsiak ME, Semnani RT, De Pascalis R, Kashmiri SV, Schlom J, Sabzevari H. Inhibition of CD4$^{(+)}$25^{+} T regulatory cell function implicated in enhanced immune response by low-dose cyclophosphamide. *Blood* 2005; **105**: 2862–2868.
63. Ghiringhelli F, Larmonier N, Schmitt E *et al.* CD4^{+}CD25^{+} regulatory T cells suppress tumor immunity but are sensitive to cyclophosphamide which allows immunotherapy of established tumors to be curative. *Eur J Immunol* 2004; **34**: 336–344.
64. Nakahara T, Uchi H, Lesokhin AM *et al.* Cyclophosphamide enhances immunity by modulating the balance of dendritic cell subsets in lymphoid organs. *Blood* 2010; **115**: 4384–4392.

65. Schiavoni G, Mattei F, Di Pucchio T *et al.* Cyclophosphamide induces type I interferon and augments the number of CD44(hi) T lymphocytes in mice: implications for strategies of chemoimmunotherapy of cancer. *Blood* 2000; **95**: 2024–2030.

66. Emens LA, Jaffee EM. Leveraging the activity of tumor vaccines with cytotoxic chemotherapy. *Cancer Res* 2005; **65**: 8059–8064.

67. Aloysius MM, Mc Kechnie AJ, Robins RA *et al.* Generation in vivo of peptide-specific cytotoxic T cells and presence of regulatory T cells during vaccination with hTERT (class I and II) peptide-pulsed DCs. *J Transl Med.* 2009 Mar 19; **7**(1): 18–46.

68. Kaneno R, Shurin GV, Tourkova IL, Shurin MR. Chemomodulation of human dendritic cell function by antineoplastic agents in low noncytotoxic concentrations. *J Transl Med* 2009; **7**: 58–68.

69. Locher C, Rusakiewicz S, Tesnière A, *et al.* Witch hunt against tumor cells enhanced by dendritic cells. *Ann N Y Acad Sci.* 2009 Sep; **1174**: 51–60.

70. Soeda A, Morita-Hoshi Y, Makiyama H *et al.* Regular dose of gemcitabine induces an increase in $CD14^+$ monocytes and $CD11c^+$ dendritic cells in patients with advanced pancreatic cancer. *Jpn J Clin Oncol* 2009; **39**: 797–806.

71. Suzuki E, Kapoor V, Jassar AS, Kaiser LR, Albelda SM. Gemcitabine selectively eliminates splenic Gr-1+/CD11b+ myeloid suppressor cells in tumor-bearing animals and enhances antitumor immune activity. *Clin Cancer Res* 2005; **11**: 6713–6721.

72. Zhang T, Herlyn D. Combination of active specific immunotherapy or adoptive antibody or lymphocyte immunotherapy with chemotherapy in the treatment of cancer. *Cancer Immunol Immunother* 2009; **58**: 475–492.

73. Langhoff E, Ladefoged J, Dickmeiss E. The immunosuppressive potency of various steroids on peripheral blood lymphocytes, T cells, NK and K cells. *Int J Immunopharmacol* 1985; **7**: 483–489.

74. Schleimer RP, Jacques A, Shin HS, Lichtenstein LM, Plaut M. Inhibition of T cell-mediated cytotoxicity by anti-inflammatory steroids. *J Immunol* 1984; **132**: 266–271.

75. Franchimont D, Galon J, Gadina M *et al.* Inhibition of Th1 immune response by glucocorticoids: dexamethasone selectively inhibits IL-12-induced Stat4 phosphorylation in T lymphocytes. *J Immunol* 2000; **164**: 1768–1774.

76. Deng J, Younge BR, Olshen RA, Goronzy JJ, Weyand CM. Th17 and Th1 T-cell responses in giant cell arteritis. *Circulation* 2010; **121**: 906–915.

77. Xie Y, Wu M, Song R *et al.* A glucocorticoid amplifies IL-2-induced selective expansion of $CD4(^+)CD25(^+)FOXP3(^+)$ regulatory T cells in vivo and suppresses graft-versus-host disease after allogeneic lymphocyte transplantation. *Acta Biochim Biophys Sin (Shanghai)* 2009; **41**: 781–791.

78. Hareyama M, Imai K, Ban T *et al.* Effect of radiation on the expression of carcinoembryonic antigen on the membranes of human gastric adenocarcinoma cells—immunological study using monoclonal antibodies. *Nippon Igaku Hoshasen Gakkai Zasshi* 1988; **48**: 1572–1574.

79. Gaugler MH, Squiban C, van der Meeren A, Bertho JM, Vandamme M, Mouthon MA. Late and persistent up-regulation of intercellular adhesion molecule-1 (ICAM-1) expression by ionizing radiation in human endothelial cells in vitro. *Int J Radiat Biol* 1997; **72**: 201–209.

80. Garnett CT, Palena C, Chakraborty M, Tsang KY, Schlom J, Hodge JW. Sublethal irradiation of human tumor cells modulates phenotype resulting in enhanced killing by cytotoxic T lymphocytes. *Cancer Res* 2004; **64**: 7985–7994.

81. Lugade AA, Moran JP, Gerber SA, Rose RC, Frelinger JG, Lord EM. Local radiation therapy of B16 melanoma tumors increases the generation of tumor antigen-specific effector cells that traffic to the tumor. *J Immunol* 2005; **174**: 7516–7523.
82. Reits EA, Hodge JW, Herberts CA *et al.* Radiation modulates the peptide repertoire, enhances MHC class I expression, and induces successful antitumor immunotherapy. *J Exp Med* 2006; **203**: 1259–1271.
83. Muller K, Meineke V. Radiation-induced alterations in cytokine production by skin cells. *Exp Hematol* 2007; **35**(4 Suppl 1): 96–104.
84. Madani I, De Ruyck K, Goeminne H, De Neve W, Thierens H, Van Meerbeeck J. Predicting risk of radiation-induced lung injury. *J Thorac Oncol.* 2007 Sep; **2**(9): 864–874.
85. Andreassen CN, Alsner J, Overgaard J *et al.* TGFB1 polymorphisms are associated with risk of late normal tissue complications in the breast after radiotherapy for early breast cancer. *Radiother Oncol* 2005; **75**: 18–21.
86. Nalbandian G, Kovats S. Understanding sex biases in immunity: effects of estrogen on the differentiation and function of antigen-presenting cells. *Immunol Res* 2005; **31**: 91–106.
87. Generali D, Bates G, Berruti A *et al.* Immunomodulation of FOXP3$^+$ regulatory T cells by the aromatase inhibitor letrozole in breast cancer patients. *Clin Cancer Res* 2009; **15**: 1046–1051.
88. Carlsten H. Immune responses and bone loss: the estrogen connection. *Immunol Rev* 2005; **208**: 194–206.
89. Rosenberg SA, Mule JJ, Spiess PJ, Reichert CM, Schwarz SL. Regression of established pulmonary metastases and subcutaneous tumor mediated by the systemic administration of high-dose recombinant interleukin 2. *J Exp Med.* 1985 May 1; **161**(5): 1169–1188.
90. Lafreniere R, Rosenberg SA. Successful immunotherapy of murine experimental hepatic metastases with lymphokine-activated killer cells and recombinant interleukin 2. *Cancer Res.* 1985; **45**: 3735–3741.
91. Rosenberg SA, Lotze MT, Yang JC *et al.* Experience with the use of high-dose interleukin-2 in the treatment of 652 cancer patients. *Ann Surg* 1989; **210**: 474–84; discussion 84–5.
92. Fyfe G, Fisher RI, Rosenberg SA, Sznol M, Parkinson DR, Louie AC. Results of treatment of 255 patients with metastatic renal cell carcinoma who received high-dose recombinant interleukin-2 therapy. *J Clin Oncol* 1995; **13**: 688–696.
93. Parkinson DR, Abrams JS, Wiernik PH *et al.* Interleukin-2 therapy in patients with metastatic malignant melanoma: a phase II study. *J Clin Oncol.* 1990 Oct; **8**(10): 1650–1656.
94. Keilholz U, Conradt C, Legha SS, *et al.* Results of interleukin-2-based treatment in advanced melanoma: a case record-based analysis of 631 patients. *J Clin Oncol* 1998; **16**: 2921–2929.
95. White RL, Jr., Schwartzentruber DJ, Guleria A *et al.* Cardiopulmonary toxicity of treatment with high dose interleukin-2 in 199 consecutive patients with metastatic melanoma or renal cell carcinoma. *Cancer* 1994; **74**: 3212–3222.
96. Kemeny N, Childs B, Larchian W, Rosado K, Kelsen D. A phase II trial of recombinant tumor necrosis factor in patients with advanced colorectal carcinoma. *Cancer* 1990; **66**: 659–663.
97. Figlin R, de Kernion J, Sarna J, Moldwer N, Saks S. Phase II study of recombinant tumor necrosis factor in patients with metastaic renal cell carcinoma and malignant melanoma. *Proc Am Soc Clin Oncol* 1988; **7**: 169.
98. Rhinehart J, Balcerzak S, Hersh M. Phase II trial of tumor necrosis factor in human sarcoma. *Proc Am Soc Clin Oncol* 1990; **9**: 317.

99. Fiers W. Tumor necrosis factor. Characterization at the molecular, cellular and in vivo level. *FEBS Lett* 1991; **285**: 199–212.

100. Manda T, Shimomura K, Mukumoto S *et al.* Recombinant human tumor necrosis factor-alpha: evidence of an indirect mode of antitumor activity. *Cancer Res* 1987; **47**: 3707–3711.

101. Gresser I, Woodrow D, Moss J, Maury C, Tavernier J, Fiers W. Toxic effects of recombinant tumor necrosis factor in suckling mice. Comparisons with interferon alpha/beta. *Am J Pathol* 1987; **128**: 13–18.

102. Mavligit G, Zukwiski A, Wallace S. Tumor regression after hepatic arterial infusion of recombinant tumor necrosis factor in patients with colon carcinoma metastatic to the liver. *Proc Am Soc Clin Oncol* 1990; **9**: 118.

103. Raeth U, Schmid H, Karck U, Kempeni J, Schlick E, Kaufmann M. Phase II trial of recombinant human necrosis factor in patients with malignant ascites from ovarian carcinomas and non-ovarian tumors with intraperitoneal spread. *Proc Am Soc Clin Oncol* 1991; **10**: 86.

104. Lienard D, Ewalenko P, Delmotte JJ, Renard N, Lejeune FJ. High-dose recombinant tumor necrosis factor alpha in combination with interferon-gamma and melphalan in isolation perfusion of the limbs for melanoma and sarcoma. *J Clin Oncol* 1992; **10**: 52–60.

105. Chowdhury S, Vaughan MM, Gore ME. New approaches to the systemic treatment of melanoma. *Cancer Treat Rev* 1999; **25**: 259–270.

106. Munschauer FE 3rd, Kinkel RP. Managing side effects of interferon-beta in patients with relapsing-remitting multiple sclerosis. *Clin Ther* 1997; **19**: 883–893.

107. Shah M, Jenis EH, Mookerjee BK *et al.* Interferon-alpha-associated focal segmental glomerulosclerosis with massive proteinuria in patients with chronic myeloid leukemia following high dose chemotherapy. *Cancer* 1998; **83**: 1938–1946.

108. Bouard D, Alazard-Dany D, Cosset FL. Viral vectors: from virology to transgene expression. *Br J Pharmacol* 2009; **157**: 153–165.

109. Varnavski AN, Calcedo R, Bove M, Gao G, Wilson JM. Evaluation of toxicity from high-dose systemic administration of recombinant adenovirus vector in vector-naive and pre-immunized mice. *Gene Ther* 2005; **12**: 427–436.

110. Deshmukh P, Glick RP, Lichtor T, Moser R, Cohen EP. Immunogene therapy with interleukin-2-secreting fibroblasts for intracerebrally metastasizing breast cancer in mice. *J Neurosurg* 2001; **94**: 287–292.

111. Dummer R. GVAX (Cell Genesys). *Curr Opin Investig Drugs* 2001; **2**: 844–848.

112. Nemunaitis J. Granulocyte-macrophage colony-stimulating factor gene-transfected autologous tumor cell vaccine: focus[correction to fcous] on non-small-cell lung cancer. *Clin Lung Cancer* 2003; **5**: 148–157.

113. Tani K, Azuma M, Nakazaki Y *et al.* Phase I study of autologous tumor vaccines transduced with the GM-CSF gene in four patients with stage IV renal cell cancer in Japan: clinical and immunological findings. *Mol Ther.* 2004 Oct; **10**(4): 799–816.

114. Breedveld FC, Emery P, Keystone E, *et al.* Infliximab in active early rheumatoid arthritis. *Ann Rheum Dis* 2004; **63**: 149–155.

115. Harris J, Keane J. How tumour necrosis factor blockers interfere with tuberculosis immunity. *Clin Exp Immunol* 2010; **161**: 1–9.

116. Giamas G, Man YL, Hirner H *et al.* Kinases as targets in the treatment of solid tumors. *Cell Signal* 2010; **22**: 984–1002.

117. Phan GQ, Weber JS, Sondak VK. CTLA-4 blockade with monoclonal antibodies in patients with metastatic cancer: surgical issues. *Ann Surg Oncol* 2008; **15**: 3014–3021.

118. Hodi FS. Overcoming immunological tolerance to melanoma: Targeting CTLA-4. *Asia Pac J Clin Oncol.* 2010; **6**(Suppl 1): S16–23.

119. Chan AC, Carter PJ. Therapeutic antibodies for autoimmunity and inflammation. *Nat Rev Immunol* 2010; **10**: 301–316.

120. Weiner LM, Surana R, Wang S. Monoclonal antibodies: versatile platforms for cancer immunotherapy. *Nat Rev Immunol* 2010; **10**: 317–327.

Chapter 8

Autoimmune disease and inflammatory disorders

Herb Sewell

Key summary points

- The specific unresponsiveness of the immune system against self molecules sometimes fails. This is associated with the genetic background (HLA alleles) of the individual as well as induction of aberrant innate and adaptive immune responses. Failure of immune regulatory cells (e.g. T regs) contributes to the development of autoimmunity.
- Autoimmune diseases cover a wide spectrum of entities some predominantly expressed within specific organ systems (OSA), particularly within the endocrine system. Other diseases are multisystemic (e.g. SLE, rheumatic diseases). Autoimmune diseases can be characterized by definition of autoreactive T cells and specific autoantibodies. The latter can be detrimental in some situations and by passive transfer, with the disease persisting until disappearance of the antibody.
- Examination of tissues in autoimmunity delineates the importance of inflammatory reactions (chronic inflammation) for induction and persistence of disease and the development of complications. The autoimmune and inflammatory components also provide targets for therapeutic modalities.
- Many autoantibodies are not detrimental but are useful biomarkers for contributing to diagnosis and, more limitedly, for monitoring disease and for assessing prognosis.
- Some autoantibodies are known to occur in individuals harbouring defined neoplasms, as part of a paraneoplastic syndrome. These antibodies have been implicated in the pathological manifestations and have been shown to have specificity for antigens in the tumours. Removal of the tumour, if possible, can often be shown to lead to a decline in the antibody levels over time. Early detection of the antibodies may predate clinical evidence of the tumour or signal its presence at an early stage of tumour growth.
- Increasing knowledge of the links between immune and inflammatory reactions is providing new insight into diseases of the GIT. Knowledge of interactions

induced by dietary molecules (potential antigens) and of the immune systems interaction with the GIT commensal flora is helping to explain coeliac and inflammatory bowel disease.

- The deeper understanding of innate immunity and the genes and molecules involved in its regulation has allowed the elucidation of the mechanisms underlying a relatively rare set of primary autoinflammatory diseases. These diseases are generally not associated with T or B cell immunity. Although rare, they may present with common clinical features to the surgeon; e.g. as an acute abdomen or an acute inflammatory swelling in various anatomical sites. Awareness of these diseases is essential and their management requires specialist input and long-term collaboration between medical specialists.
- Surgical interventions have long been linked, but with limited evidence, to the induction of autoimmunity and other inflammatory lesions/diseases. For induction of autoimmunity, biologically plausible mechanisms need to be considered together with evidence of autoreactive T cells and/or specific autoantibodies.

Introduction

Autoimmune reactions characterized by the presence of autoantibodies and autoreactive T cells can be demonstrated in a significant number of diseases. In some situations, such as following surgery, trauma, and infection, the autoreactive elements appear to be transient and of little clinical or pathophysiological relevance. Furthermore, sensitive immunoassays reveal that within the normal population many individuals have low levels of autoantibodies, particularly of the IgM class. These autoantibodies tend to be polyreactive and are believed to play important physiological roles in the removal of cell debris during cell turnover, and also in immune surveillance in detecting altered/stressed self-cells and contributing to their removal. In contrast, many major rheumatological, endocrinological, haematological, and hepatological disorders have autoimmune reactions which are clearly of major significance in the pathophysiology of the clinical disorders. In this chapter, limited aspects of autoimmune diseases are presented. They are not exhaustive but of direct clinical usefulness to specialists in surgical and associated practice. For further clinical details see 'Further reading'. Considerations of the aetiology of autoimmune disease and of practical assays to evaluate autoimmunity can be found in Chapters 1 and 9, respectively.

Inflammatory diseases of the intestinal tract—coeliac disease, Crohn's disease, and ulcerative colitis—are highlighted as entities which are encountered frequently in surgical practice. In these diseases, significant autoimmune reactions and responses to environmental factors, to which the host is normally tolerant, are considered central to the pathogenesis of these disorders. The immunological aspects of these diseases are becoming more relevant to clinicians.

Paraneoplastic syndromes often have associated autoimmune changes. The associated autoantibodies are helpful in supporting the diagnosis and have useful correlates with the varying types of cancers underlying or linked to the syndrome (see Chapter 4).

In recent years, much has been learnt about a group of relatively rare, genetically inherited autoinflammatory diseases. These diseases do not have associated autoantibodies or autoreactive T cells. They can present in paediatric or adult medical practice, and their associated inflammatory lesions can often result in these patients presenting to or being referred to surgeons for management of perceived surgical clinical entities. Awareness of these disorders is important because the diagnosis and management of these patients requires specialist medical and surgical input and long-term management.

Organ-specific autoimmunity

Organ-specific autoimmunity (OSA) exists in conditions where tolerance to self-antigens (which are expressed by and restricted to a particular organ) is abrogated and autoantibodies and autoreactive T cells can be demonstrated. In this situation of abnormal immune regulation, the autoreactive components, in some cases, can be shown to cause direct tissue damage and are termed *primary agents*. In other cases, they appear to be *secondary* and arise as a consequence of tissue damage. This distinction is becoming blurred with advancing knowledge. Some of the antibodies that used to be considered secondary can now be shown to mediate tissue-damaging reactions in their own right. In clinical practice, most of the evidence indicates that autoantibodies are of crucial importance in the induction of tissue damage and, accordingly, most emphasis is directed to detecting and monitoring autoantibodies rather than autoreactive T cells. Also, the assays for autoantibodies are much more straightforward than those required to detect autoreactive T cells (see Chapter 9).

OSA is largely associated with endocrinopathies and autoantibodies can be demonstrated against endocrine cells, their products, or the hormone receptors on target tissues. Measurements of these autoantibodies can prove useful in establishing or supporting the diagnosis and in monitoring disease activity, and in some cases the response to therapy. Common findings in patients with OSA are that the affected glands have a marked immune-inflammatory cell infiltrate. In some cases, the infiltrate is so abundant that the tissues may partly resemble a secondary lymphoid organ. Within the infiltrate can be demonstrated many activated T and B cells, some with documented autoimmune specificity. T and B cell clones have been isolated from such tissues and shown to have specificity for target self-antigens. Within the infiltrates are also found plasma cells secreting antibodies (including autoantibodies), and macrophages. The epithelial elements within the immune-inflammatory environment often express aberrantly large amounts of human leucocyte antigen (HLA) class II molecules. A common finding in OSA patients is a family history of autoimmune disorders. Relatives may have other endocrinopathies, e.g. involving the thyroid and adrenal glands or the pancreas; other relatives may present with an increased incidence of diseases such as coeliac disease. Also, there is linkage to an increased incidence of selective IgA primary antibody deficiency. The family history of association with OSA is believed to reflect increased associations of these diseases with particular linkages within the extended major histocompatability complex (MHC) region (see Chapters 1 and 3). Many organ-specific autoimmune diseases and systemic autoimmune diseases have associations with HLA molecules, in particular the HLA class II D region encoded antigens, as well as with HLA class I alleles.

Thyroid autoimmunity

Thyroid autoimmunity covers a spectrum of diseases ranging from autoimmune hyperthyroidism (Graves' disease), autoimmune thyroiditis (including Hashimoto's disease), atrophic thyroiditis (presenting as primary hypothyroidism), and others, including postpartum thyroiditis and de Quervain's disease (granulomatous thyroiditis). Graves' disease is the most common cause of presentation of thyrotoxicosis. It is associated with a smooth, diffusely enlarged thyroid gland and often with exophthalmos, which can cause significant morbidity. Graves' disease, in common with many autoimmune diseases, has a female preponderance (approximately 8:1) with a family history of autoimmunity and linkages to various HLA alleles. Autoantibodies have been established as the primary agents (mechanistically causing a type II hypersensitivity reaction) in Graves' disease. The main molecules inducing tissue damage are the thyroid stimulating antibodies. These are directed against the thyroid epithelial cell membrane and include antibodies which have specificity for and bind to the thyroid stimulating hormone receptor (TSHR). Historically, this antibody was called LATS (long-acting thyroid stimulator). The interaction with the TSHR results in continuous stimulation of the gland and increased secretion of thyroid hormones (T_3 and T_4), detectable in blood and usually linked with a depressed level of TSH (positive feedback). Other stimulating autoantibodies have been demonstrated that are responsible for promoting the growth of the gland. Ophthalmopathy is associated with specific autoantibody activity directed against antigens present in orbital tissues. Some of these antibodies have been shown to have marked cross-reactivity with antigens in thyroid tissue. The current evidence of these cross-reacting antigens for hyperthyroidism, and for the associated ophthalmopathy of Graves' disease, has significant implications for the surgical management of the disorder. It is postulated that total removal of the antigenic source (i.e. the thyroid gland) may arrest or induce remission of the eye disease. This is an area of ongoing medical/surgical discussion within the overall management protocol for patients with Graves' disease with significant ophthalmopathy. Total thyroidectomy has important surgical considerations regarding the risk of complications (e.g. damage to the recurrent laryngeal nerves and loss of parathyroid tissue). However, it ensures the removal of the antigenic source driving the autoimmunity-induced pathology. The postoperative thyroid status is managed by simple thyroid hormone replacement therapy with the possibility of improvement or, at worse, the stabilization of a serious eye disorder.

The abnormal antithyroid antibodies are mainly of the IgG class. This is significant, as these antibodies can cross the placenta and have been shown to cause neonatal hyperthyroidism. Awareness of this is important for the management of the newborn with the potential dangerous consequences of thyrotoxicosis, and its effects on the cardiovascular system and the baby's metabolism.

In common with other thyroid autoimmune disorders, other autoantibodies can be found in Graves' disease. These include autoantibodies to cytoplasmic organelles of the thyroid epithelial cells. The most useful autoantibodies in clinical practice are those directed to the microsome-associated peroxidase enzyme. These anti-thyroid peroxidase (anti-TPO) antibodies are found in up to 80% of patients with Graves' disease. Another commonly found autoantibody is that to thyroglobulin. Tests for anti-TPO are the most commonly used in clinical practice in supporting the diagnosis of Graves' disease. The IgG anti-TSHR autoantibody is not routinely assayed. Anti-TPO antibody is a good general marker of thyroid autoimmunity. Anti-TPO and antithyroglobulin antibodies are considered to be secondary antibodies, arising as a result of thyroid damage by the marked immune- inflammatory reaction. However, recent experimental evidence, particularly using anti-TPO antibodies, have shown that they may also be inducing tissue damage.

Hashimoto's (chronic) thyroiditis can present with a spectrum of clinical features ranging from initial hyperthyroidism or euthyroid state to subsequent hypothyroidism, the latter being the most common clinical presentation. Like Graves' disease, there is a female preponderance and a family history of the disorder. There are significant MHC associations with Hashimoto's disease, particularly with HLA class II alleles, namely HLA-DR5, -DR4 and -DR3. Patients with Hashimoto's disease presenting with hyperthyroidism need to be differentiated from Graves' disease. Testing for anti-TPO antibodies is helpful. Although both diseases have the antibody, the anti-TPO titres are very much higher in Hashimoto's disease than in Graves' disease,. Indeed, testing for anti-TPO and antithyroglobulin will usually show high titres of both antibodies in Hashimoto's disease, while antithyroglobulin antibodies are usually present in very low levels in Graves' disease.

The goitre found in Graves' and Hashimoto's disease has a varying degree of immune- inflammatory cell infiltrates, being more pronounced in the latter. Prominent lymphoid aggregates with germinal centres can be demonstrated within the enlarged thyroid. The marked increase of HLA class II molecules on the thyroid epithelial cells, together with the prominent infiltrates of $CD4^+$ and $CD8^+$ T cells, along with macrophages, monocytes, and plasma cells has been associated with increased local production of various cytokines including tumour necrosis factor-alpha (TNF-α), interferon-gamma (INF-γ), interleukin-1 (IL-1), and IL-6. The immune- inflammatory reactions between these various elements within the gland are seen as an amplification system resulting in very prominent glandular inflammation. Over time, the extensive immune inflammation leads to tissue destruction with glandular fibrosis and hypothyroidism. This is the likely natural history seen in the late presentation of patients with Hashimoto's disease. Similar pathological processes are responsible for the presentation of primary hypothyroidism (myxoedema) with a markedly fibrotic gland and little evidence of any remaining inflammatory infiltrate. The assumption is that the antecedent thyroiditis was not diagnosed or was subclinical. The chronic thyroiditis patients who may require surgery for cosmetic or other reasons and who have high titres of anti-TPO antibodies are believed to be likely to develop significant thyroid hypofunction. Accordingly, anti-TPO titres may be one important factor for the surgeon to consider with regard to the extent of thyroid resection undertaken.

In obstetric practice, cases of transient postpartum hypothyroidism, usually presenting within 6 months after delivery, are associated with increased levels of anti-TPO and antithyroglobulin antibodies. Most women improve spontaneously, but evidence indicates that those with high levels of anti-TPO antibodies are unlikely to go into remission. Hence the antibody assays may be useful in monitoring the outcome of the disorder.

Gastric autoimmunity and pernicious anaemia

Autoimmune gastritis, associated with low acid production, high serum gastrin levels, and autoantibodies to gastric parietal cells (GPCs) and intrinsic factor (IF), over time results in pernicious anaemia. The latter is considered to have an autoimmune origin. Also, patients with autoimmune gastritis commonly have thyroid autoantibodies in the circulation, although they are usually clinically euthyroid. Reciprocal findings have been demonstrated in patients with chronic thyroiditis with regard to the presence of antibodies to GPCs. This reflects the general finding that patients with a clinically expressed OSA can have autoantibodies to other organs without clinical disease in those organs. The tissue lesions in autoimmune gastritis are similar to that described for thyroid disease, with a strong immune-inflammatory infiltrate, eventually leading to chronic inflammation which, in turn, can lead to atrophic gastritis. The gastritis involves the GPC containing body of the stomach; parietal cells are important for producing IF. Long-standing autoimmune gastritis can result in intestinal metaplasia. Importantly, the disease has also been associated with an increased incidence of gastric carcinoma. This raises the interesting link between long-standing chronic inflammation and the induction of neoplasia (see Chapter 4).

Pernicious anaemia, which is considered the end result (over many years) of autoimmune gastritis, has no specific clinical profile. Patients can present with a sore tongue (25% of cases), general tiredness (>90%), or with the much more serious neurological features of subacute combined degeneration of the spinal cord (<5% of cases); all of these clinical disturbances are secondary to the acquired vitamin B_{12} deficiency. As in autoimmune gastritis, a useful immunological assay is the measurement of autoantibodies which are documented in over 90% of cases, but are of low specificity for pernicious anaemia. GPC autoantibodies occur in 50–80% of patients and are much more specific for pernicious anaemia. GPC antibodies are found in 2–20% of the older population, and are found in iron deficiency anaemia and in association with other autoimmune disorders. They can, therefore, be used as a clinical screening test. IF autoantibodies, particularly of the IgA class, are produced locally in the gastrointestinal tract (GIT). Within the gut lumen they form complexes with IF and interfere with the absorption of dietary vitamin B_{12}, which is complexed to IF. This prevents the IF–vitamin B_{12} complex being absorbed at its natural site within the terminal ileum, resulting in the development of megaloblastic anaemia and the clinical presentations alluded to above. IF autoantibodies rarely occur without overt or latent pernicious anaemia. Thus, it is a highly useful and specific test to establish the diagnosis or predict the development of pernicious anaemia. Measurement of autoantibodies to GPCs and IF is an especially useful and noninvasive procedure when the Schilling test is equivocal.

Systemic (non-organ-specific) autoimmunity

In systemic autoimmune disorders, autoantibodies and autoreactive T cells can be demonstrated with specificity for antigens which are distributed widely throughout various organs and tissues. The antigens are usually subcellular particles or are membrane-associated and may be secreted into the circulation. Many of the systemic autoimmune diseases show elements of abnormal immunological activity and of immune regulation (see Chapter 1). The autoantibodies detected are usually helpful in establishing the diagnosis and prognosis, although their role in the aetiology of the disorders is unclear.

Rheumatoid arthritis and seronegative arthritides

Rheumatoid arthritis (RA) affects approximately 1% of the adult population but can present at any age and involve any joint. Some extra-articular manifestations may present to surgeons in different specialties, without the classical joint and radiographic stigmata. Thus, chronic skin ulcers, carpel tunnel syndrome, episcleritis, oral ulcers, nerve root compressions, and lymphadenopathy may all be associated with RA. Immune serology can be an aid to diagnosis and of value in prognosis. Immunogenetic studies in patients, as with many other autoimmune diseases, have documented some significant linkages to the HLA system. In particular, there are significant associations with HLA class II alleles (e.g. DR4, DR1), the associations varying with different racial groups. Although RA is a multisystem disease, the major pathological tissue changes are located in the joints. Like other autoimmune diseases a marked immune-inflammatory cell infiltrate is present in the synovium; activated $CD4^+$ and $CD8^+$ T cells can be demonstrated, as well as macrophages and locally differentiated plasma cells. Vascular endothelial cells show marked activation. Analysis of local cytokine production indicates the presence of TNF-α, IL-1, and IL-6. The activated endothelial cells are responsible for the production of chemokines which further facilitates the influx of more inflammatory cells.

These findings are helpful in explaining the pathological mechanisms leading to the expression of the disease. Currently, there is evidence for type II, III, and IV hypersensitivity reactions being involved in the immunopathology of RA. Many autoantibodies have been defined including the classical IgM rheumatoid factor (RF); other specificities that have been demonstrated include low levels of antinuclear antibodies (ANAs) (commonly IgM class), antikeratins, antifillagrins and, importantly, anti-cyclic citrullinated peptide (anti-CCP). This last autoantibody has proven to be extremely useful clinically. Historically, RF has been demonstrated in up to 80% of patients, the highest titres being found in patients with significant extra-articular disease. However, it is important to note that RF is not a diagnostic test for RA. The anti-CCP antibodies, however, are proving to be most valuable and appear to be more specific markers of RA. Moreover, these antibodies can identify very early disease and are considered highly specific at any disease stage. Another useful and simple test to help in the management and monitoring of patients is detection of the acute-phase response C-reactive protein (CRP). Its level in blood tends to be elevated in active disease, but with effective therapy and control of the disease the CRP levels are reduced. It is a simple and useful marker to help monitor disease and its response to therapy.

Based on studies of biopsies from patients with RA and findings from organ cultures, as well as from experimental models, better insights into the underlying immune pathological mechanisms have led to significantly improved therapies. The characterization of key tissue-damaging cytokines and knowledge of their interactions with various receptor systems has led to the introduction of new biological agents into clinical practice. Used either alone or with established treatments, they are helping to markedly improve the management of this disease. The biological therapies, which have had a major impact on the management of RA, include the anti-TNF monoclonal antibodies (MABs), and, more recently, anti-IL-6 receptor (IL-6R) antibodies along with constructs such as the cytotoxic T lymphocyte antigen-4 (CTLA-4)–Ig fusion protein (see Chapter 1). Other biological agents are presently under investigation. Current evidence suggests that continued use of low-dose methotrexate gives additional benefits when used with these biological treatments. It is hoped that these newer therapies will avoid the need for the same level of surgical intervention regarding the replacement of damaged joints as has been the case historically. These new therapies appear to have major disease-modifying effects preventing the development of severe joint destruction, if introduced early in the disease. Indeed, some authorities are now advocating the use of early markers, such as the anti-CCP antibody test, which often is positive long before imaging investigations suggest the need for the introduction of biological therapy. The aim of treatment is to prevent irreversible tissue damage.

Anti-CCP and RF antibodies can be demonstrated in synovial joint fluid. They may contribute to local tissue damage, through type II and III hypersensitivity reactions, activating complement and stimulating more inflammatory cell ingress, cell activation, and cytokine production, thus, amplifying the local tissue-damaging reactions.

Seronegative athritides exclude cases associated with known infections and are characterized by the absence of RF and of anti-CCP antibodies. They include conditions such as ankylosing spondylitis, psoriatic and enteropathic arthritis, Reiters' and Behçet's syndromes, and rarer disorders such as relapsing polychondritis. The latter three conditions may present to ophthalmologists, ENT, and dental/oral surgeons, and some of the former to orthopaedic surgeons. Currently, there are no immunological tests of sufficient sensitivity and specificity that contribute meaningfully to clinical diagnosis with the possible exception of typing for the HLA-B27 antigens in suspected cases of ankylosing spondylitis. The association of HLA-B27 with ankylosing spondylitis is very strong and its occurrence in the white population is low. Thus, in suspected cases of ankylosing spondylitis without clear ultrasound or MRI findings, the absence of B27 makes the diagnosis very unlikely. Ankylosing spondylitis and psoriatic arthritis cases, including patients with severe plaque psoriasis, also show significant beneficial responses when treated with the newer biological agents, in particular anti-TNF MABs, as well as with the CTLA4-Ig fusion protein. Recently, very beneficial results have been obtained in the treatment of plaque psoriasis using MABs against anti-IL-12 and IL-23 (see Chapter 1).

Systemic lupus erythematosus and antiphospholipid syndrome

Systemic lupus erythematosus (SLE) is the prototype non-organ-specific autoimmune disorder which is associated with ANAs and, more specifically, with antibodies to double-stranded (native) DNA. These represent the two most definitive laboratory assays to assist in the diagnosis of SLE. SLE has protean manifestations and can present

Table 8.1 Clinical presentation and cumulative organ pathology in systemic lupus erythematosus

Clinical presentation	%	Organ involvement	%
Arthritis and arthralgia	62	Joint and/or muscle	>90
Skin lesions	~20	Skin	>90
Thrombocytopaenic purpura and haemolytic anaemia; recurrent thrombophlebitis	~10	Blood	~60
Neuropsychiatric problems	~4–5	Brain	~60
Proteinuria		Kidney	~40
Pericarditis		Heart	~20

to any medical or surgical specialty. Table 8.1 shows clinical presentations in cumulative organ pathology in SLE. The multisystem nature of SLE, which typically affects young females, is illustrated in the table. Like other autoimmune diseases there is often a family history of other autoimmune diseases, and there are associations with various HLA antigens.

Table 8.1 reveals that skin involvement is frequent in SLE, and a biopsy can be diagnostic. Immunofluorescent staining of frozen sections shows granular deposits of immunoglobulins and complement components at the epidermal–dermal junction (the lupus band test). More than 70% of SLE patients have a 'positive' skin biopsy test.

SLE activity is evaluated by the sequential monitoring of the serum levels of complement components C3 and C4 and other complement breakdown/activation products. With active disease and substantial organ involvement, C3 and C4 are detected at subnormal levels as a result of their consumption by immune complexes (antigens and autoantibodies) and activation of the complement system (see Chapter 1). With diminished disease activity the C3 and C4 serum levels return toward the normal range. The levels of complement products are more sensitive than the erythrocyte sedimentation rate (ESR) or sequential ANA or DNA antibody levels in monitoring disease activity.

In contrast to RA, measurements of CRP level are not an indicator of disease activity in SLE. Interestingly, in some difficult clinical situations it can be helpful as it is elevated in early RA, but is normal or marginally changed in early SLE. The biological basis for this difference is unclear as both are potent immune-inflammatory disorders. There is a suggestion that some of the acute-phase responsive elements in SLE, including that associated with the macrophage–monocyte systems, may be compromised.

There is research evidence linking the onset of SLE to mechanisms of abnormalities or failure in apoptotic pathways. For instance, the failure to remove apoptotic cells and the subsequent degeneration of such cells may release autoantigens that can stimulate autoreactive responses. Additionally, experiments have shown that sunlight can itself induce excess formation of apoptotic complexes, which could trigger immune responses. Importantly, molecules such as DNA, which have long been considered inert, have now been shown, if they associate with certain internal danger signals (alarmins) such as high-mobility group box-1 (HMGB-1) protein (see Chapter 1), to become antigenic and stimulate autoantibody responses. Better understanding of immune mechanisms in SLE has led to significant improvements in therapy, beyond the broad-based use of steroids and immune suppressants such as azathioprine and cyclophosphamide. There is now a range of other therapeutics available to the clinician including, agents with significant anti-T cell effects, such as calcineurin blockers, ciclosporin, tacrolimus, and mycophenalate mofetil (see Chapter 3) and, more recently, the use of the anti-CD20 MAB. The evidence for the efficacy of the latter is variable, but ongoing clinical trials should clarify the matter. Recent phase III clinical trials have shown that the use of MABs against the cytokine BAF (B cell activating factor) is apparently proving efficacious in the management of SLE.

Apart from the use of autoantibodies in diagnosis it is important to remember certain other specificities, such as autoantibodies to extractable nuclear antigens (ENAs). Amongst the subtypes of ENAs are antibodies to antigens termed Ro (SS-As) and (SS-Bs) La. These are important because they belong to the IgG class and, as in thyroid autoimmunity, they can cross the placenta and have been associated in the newborn with congenital complete heart block (due to damage to the foetal conducting system); they have also been associated with neonatal SLE.

Paediatric chronic arthritis

In the investigation of chronic arthritis in children, which may be due to many disorders, including infections, juvenile RA (JRA), juvenile ankylosing spondylitis (JAS), and the varying forms of juvenile chronic arthritis (JCA), the paediatric physician and surgeon should find the measurement of RF and ANAs particularly useful. The JCA group, according to some authorities, includes cases (~10%) which behave like adult RA, and the presence of RF and/or anti-CCP antibody confirms the diagnosis. Such children have a form of RA which tends to progress to severe joint destruction and have associated extra-articular complications, such as vasculitis. Early diagnosis contributes to more efficient clinical management. JAS (~15% of cases) behaves similarly to the adult disease and the association of and testing for the HLA-B27 antigen is equally relevant. The remaining forms of JCA include the systemic disorder (synonymous with Still's disease), the pauciarticular, and the polyarticular disease. Children in the pauciarticular group who have positive ANAs appear to have a greatly increased risk of developing chronic iridocyclitis. The measurement of CRP is useful in the monitoring of disease activity in cases of childhood non-infection-associated arthritis.

Currently, some of the newer biological agents are being used in the management of children with paediatric JCA and Still's disease. In association with methotrexate, rituximab (anti-CD20) and anti-IL-6 receptor MAB therapies are being used.

Antiphospholipid antibody syndrome

Antiphospholipid antibody (APA) syndrome can present to different surgical and medical specialties. Patients can have very varied disorders, the underlying pathology being associated with increased thrombotic events, either on the arterial or venous side. Suspicion of APA syndrome may be triggered in patients with a history of recurrent deep vein thrombosis or pulmonary embolism; recurrent miscarriages; or premature stroke or multi-infarct dementia; particularly in younger patients and without obvious risk factors; severe vasculitis also occurs. APA syndrome may be associated with known connective tissue diseases such as SLE and it may present with rare diseases such as Sneddon's disease or the Budd–Chiari syndrome. The key test to help in establishing the diagnosis of the APA syndrome is detection of cardiolipin antibodies—these are known to represent a subset of APAs. The other important test that should be carried out is for the so-called lupus anticoagulant assay. Lupus anticoagulants are autoantibodies that interfere with the clotting process and are usually detected by the prolongation of activated partial thromboplastin time (APTT) *in vitro*. Although this test shows the antibodies prolong clotting *in vitro*, paradoxically, the problem for the patient *in vivo* is one of excess clotting.

An additional useful test for the APA syndrome is the detection of anti-β_2-glycoprotein 1 (β2-GP1) antibodies. β2-GP1 is a cofactor involved in the APA reaction.

The APA syndrome, when detected without a known disease or associated autoimmune disease, is said to be the primary syndrome. When the diagnostic autoantibodies occur within the setting of an established disease, it is referred to as the secondary syndrome. Whether this represents a true distinction or purely a factor of time before the full expression of the disease is a matter of continuing debate. It is important that women with SLE who are planning to become pregnant should be screened for anticardiolipin antibodies and lupus anticoagulant. As well, as indicated above, they should be tested for SS-As and SS-Bs antibodies.

Wegener's granulomatous disease and Churg–Strauss syndrome

Wegener's granulomatous disease (WGD) and Churg–Strauss syndrome (CSS) are multisystem vasculitic diseases. The inflammatory response affecting the blood vessels may be of primary (of unknown aetiology e.g. WGD and CSS) or of secondary causes, associated with infections, malignancy, drugs, autoimmune diseases (such as SLE), or secondary to inflammatory bowel disease.

The vasculitides tend to be classified histologically, based on the size and type of blood vessel involved. Accordingly, the most important diagnostic test is often the biopsy of an affected organ. Among the known primary vasculitic diseases affecting arteries of medium size are WGD and CSS, where immunological investigations can prove helpful in diagnosis, in monitoring therapy, and in assessing prognosis. Particularly helpful are the antineutrophil cytoplasmic antibodies (ANCAs) which are strongly associated with WGD and CSS. Other vasculitides involving medium arteries include Buerger's disease, Kawasaki's syndrome, polyarteritis nodosa, and lymphomatoid granulomatosis; these are generally negative for ANCAs.

WGD is of unknown aetiology, although some reports have suggested it can be triggered by infection. It occurs in two forms, systemic and limited. The systemic disease often has severe renal involvement, usually in the form of a necrotizing glomerulonephritis. The systemic and limited forms both tend to involve the upper respiratory tract. The limited form of the disease may present as sinusitis or as otitis; there may be nasal crusting with ulceration and bleeding, and the nasal cartilage may become eroded; a severe problem can occur with subglottic stenosis. The granulomatous lesions can also erode into main arteries. Lung lesions of WGD can be mistaken for tumours. The key immunological test for ANCAs is performed by incubating patients sera on preparations of alcohol-fixed human neutrophils. The antibodies bind to widely dispersed antigens within the cytoplasmic granules of the cells (see Chapter 9). Detailed biochemical analyses have established that ANCAs found with two main patterns on stained neutrophils—cytoplasmically dispersed (C-ANCA) peripherally or surrounding the nucleus (P-ANCA)—have specificity for particular enzymes/antigens. C-ANCA is directed to a proteinase 3(PR3) molecule whilst P-ANCA is mainly to a myeloperoxidase (MPO) antigen. Solid-phase assays are used to define these anti-enzyme specificities after the screening assays on neutrophil preparations. Diagnostically important C-ANCA is confirmed by a positive anti-PR3 test. The anti-PR3 specificity is strongly associated with the diagnosis of WGD. Anti-MPO antibodies confirm important P-ANCA positivity and are found associated with microscopic polyangiitis and distinguishes that disorder from WGD. These correlates are not absolute. Additionally, P-ANCAs are being detected which are not of the MPO specificity but relate to other minor but different targets detected in solid-phase antigen assays. Their diagnostic usefulness is still being evaluated in conditions such as inflammatory bowel disease.

ANCAs (with successful treatment of the disease) can be shown to decline over time, although they are not the best assays for monitoring disease activity. Standard indices, such as CRP and ESR, are more useful markers for disease activity. However, in patients with WGD in remission, if ANCA titres are rising (even without obvious clinical disease), they are a useful predictor of likely relapse for such patients.

CSS is considered by some authorities to be a subset of polyarteritis nodosa. The vasculitic inflammation may involve the GIT, the patients presenting with rectal bleeding or symptoms of inflammatory bowel disease. The disease may involve the respiratory tract, particularly the sinuses and the upper airways; there may be neurological involvement with mononeuritis multiplex. Not unusually, CSS patients may present with severe asthma; the diagnosis is confirmed by biopsy, demonstrating medium-artery-associated vasculitis. Testing for ANCAs suggests that up to two-thirds of such patients are positive for P-ANCA with anti-MPO specificity; a small group may be C-ANCA anti-PR3 positive.

The usefulness of ANCA testing should not be underestimated; the severe vasculitic processes underlying these diseases results in patients presenting to different medical and surgical specialties. A simple assay for ANCAs, and for the specific anti-PR3 and anti-MPO antibodies, is most helpful within this clinical setting.

Overview of autoantibodies in clinical practice

Organ-specific and non-organ-specific autoimmune diseases are often presented as two distinct groups but, in reality, the clinical and laboratory evidence indicate that they are often part of a spectrum of autoimmune disorders.

Table 8.2 summarizes a selection of autoantibody tests which may prove useful in varying aspects of surgical practice. For example, a fairly rapid onset of ascites and deepening jaundice in the older patient is one of the presentations of primary biliary cirrhosis.

Table 8.2 Tests for selected autoantibodies*

Test	Normal range	Report	Interpretation
ANAs	Negative (but very low titre IgG often found in 'normals')	Negative or positive titre IgG class Staining pattern	Negative ANA virtually excludes SLE Speckled ANA suggestive of mixed connective tissue disease Nucleolar ANA suggestive of scleroderma
ACAs	Negative	Negative or positive	Suggestive of scleroderma, especially the CREST variant Many patients present with idiopathic Raynauds
Anti-Ro antibodies (SS-As) (Ro/La are small protein antigens found in the nucleus and cytoplasm of cells)	Negative	Negative or positive	Especially useful in SLE presenting with prominent photosensitive cutaneous lupus; Sjögren's syndome Ro positive lupus has been described in the ANA negative SLE groups Anti-Ro: useful in the investigation of patients with a history of recurrent spontaneous miscarriages
Anti-La antibodies (SS-Bs)	Negative	Negative or positive	Primary Sjögren's syndrome positive in 10% of SLE. La antibodies usually found together with Ro antibodies. Ro and La antibodies have been found in almost all mothers and infants with neonatal lupus syndrome
RF	Units and normal ranges will be quoted by laboratories with respect to their system of analysis		Useful in differential diagnosis of connective tissue disorders
Anti-CCP antibodies	Units and normal ranges will be quoted by laboratories with respect to their system of analysis	Negative or positive	Anti-CCP: specific marker for RA RF is not diagnostic for RA
AMAs	Negative	Negative or positive titre	Strong positive associated with primary biliary cirrhosis
Anti-phospholipid and anti-cardiolipin antibodies	Determined by the laboratory	Positive ELISA units	Associated with thrombotic disease–small and large vessels As part of SLE syndrome with the lupus anticoagulant A discrete phospholipid syndrome
Anti-SMAs	Negative (but SMA, of low positivity often found with viral infection)	Negative or positive	Strong positive association with chronic active hepatitis.

(continued)

Table 8.2 Tests for selected autoantibodies* *(continued)*

Test	Normal range	Report	Interpretation
Anti-thyroid antibodies Anti-thyroglobulin antibodies Anti-TPO antibodies	Different laboratories will quote their established normal ranges	Titre	Useful in the differential diagnosis of a goitre High titre; found in over 90% of cases of autoimmune thyroiditis Low titre; found in 30% of Graves' disease and about 10% of adenocarcinomas
GPC antibodies	Negative	Negative or positive	Associated with atrophic gastritis; found in >90% of cases of pernicious anaemia and 40% of cases of gastric atrophy. Found in 30% of patients with autoimmune thyroid disease. GPC antibodies may be the first indication of an autoimmune organ specific disorder, e.g. in the investigation of a macrocytosis of red blood cells
IF antibodies	Negative	Negative or positive	Occurs in >70% of pernicious anaemia cases. More specific for pernicious anaemia than GPC antibodies
Skin antibodies: epidermal (basement membrane) and intercellular cement (desmosomal)	Negative	Negative or positive	Useful in differential diagnosis of bullous eruptions
Antibodies to adrenal cortex	Negative	Negative or positive	Positive in about 65% of cases of idiopathic adrenal insufficiency
Skeletal muscle antibodies	Negative	Negative or positive	Found in 40–50% of patients with MG (especially with thymoma). Anti-acetylcholine receptor antibody more sensitive and specific for MG.
ANCAs	Negative	Negative or positive with pattern: C-ANCA or P-ANCA	Very useful in differential diagnosis of vasculitides; positive in WGD, microscopic polyangitis, and related disorders

ACAs, anticentromere antibodies; AMAs, antimitochondrial antibodies; ANAs, antinuclear antibodies; ANCAs, antineutrophil cytoplasmic antibodies; CSS, Churg–Strauss syndrome; GPC, gastric parietal cell; IF, intrinsic factor; MG, myasthenia gravis; RA, rheumatoid arthritis; RF, rheumatoid factor; SLE, systemic lupus erythematosus; SMA, smooth muscle antibodies; WGD, Wegener's granulomatous disease.

*The autoantibodies listed have varying degrees of clinical usefulness and discriminatory value in diagnosis and management. Information should be obtained by discussion with the consultant immunologist or other trained specialist personnel regarding uncertainty about tests, their interpretation, and disease relevance.

The findings of high serum levels of antimitochondrial autoantibody together with high levels of serum IgM (~80% of cases) rapidly establishes the correct diagnosis. Consultation with a clinical immunologist or other relevant personnel should ensure the most efficacious use of such autoantibody investigations.

Paraneoplastic syndromes and autoimmunity

Paraneoplastic syndromes are often associated with underlying malignant disease and are characterized by findings of autoantibodies in blood (see Chapter 4). These antibodies often induce or are associated with clinical neurological disorders. Experimental data has demonstrated that many of the autoantibodies have specificity for particular tumour-associated antigens, in particular, antigens that are also found within neural tissues. Mechanistically, antibodies to the tumour antigens have been shown to cross-react with antigens found in neural tissues. The patient's immune system in responding to the tumour-associated antigens also responds against neural tissues expressing such antigens. The binding of the autoantibodies may either directly impair the function of the neurological tissue and/or may recruit effector mechanisms, such as complement activation and/or antibody-dependent cellular cytotoxicity, resulting in destruction or impairment of the function of the neurological tissue. Clinically, a presentation suggestive of a paraneoplastic syndrome (and, importantly, the findings of the presence of autoantibodies) should indicate the need to investigate the possibility of an underlying malignancy. Importantly, the autoantibodies may be detected long before the cancer is suspected, or may indicate an existing occult malignancy not readily found by standard imaging techniques.

The cancers most often associated with paraneoplastic syndromes are small-cell lung carcinoma, breast cancer, ovarian cancer, and, less commonly, thymoma, Hodgkin's lymphoma, and non-Hodgkin's lymphoma. Table 8.3 summarizes some of the best-known autoantibodies associated with the paraneoplastic syndrome and correspondingly involved cancers. By definition, many of these syndromes, because of the focus on the nervous system, present to neurologists. However, other specialists should have a high index of suspicion in particular clinical settings. These essentially cross-reacting anti-tumour-antigen-directed autoantibodies are rarely found in healthy individuals, or indeed in cancer patients who do not have the neurological dysfunction.

It must be remembered that paraneoplastic syndromes and their associated antibodies are much less common then direct metastatic involvement by the cancer and treatment-related neurological complications. However, they are important because they can cause severe morbidity and premature mortality. The paraneoplastic syndromes are important examples of how an autoimmune response directed against a tumour antigen can lead to significant pathology in the nervous system due to cross-reactivity with antigens found associated with neural tissues.

Gastrointestinal and inflammatory diseases

Coeliac disease

Coeliac disease is a multifactorial (genetic and environmental) autoimmune disorder with a strong inheritable component, linked to genes within the MHC class II region

Table 8.3 Some autoantibodies documented with paraneoplastic syndrome and associated cancers

Autoantibody	Clinical presentation	Associated cancer
Anti-HU (ANNA-1)	Encephalomyelitis Peripheral neuropathy	SCLC
Anti-Ri (ANNA-2)	Ocular signs Cerebellar or spinal cord dysfunction	Breast cancer and SCLC; less commonly bladder and cervical cancer.
Anti-Yo	Cerebellar degeneration Ataxia Sensorimotor neuropathy	Breast or gynaecological tumours SCLC and Hodgkin's lymphoma
Antiamphiphysin	Neurological	Breast cancer or SCLC
Anti-voltage-gated calcium channel antibodies	Myasthenic syndrome (not classical myasthenia gravis which is associated with acetylcholine receptor antibodies)	LEMS associated with SCLC.

ANNA, antineuronal nuclear antibody; LEMS, Lambert–Eaton myasthenic syndrome; SCLC, small cell lung cancer.

and to other genes outside the MHC. It is triggered by a well-defined environmental factor in food (protein gluten), found in wheat, barley, and other foods. The immune-inflammatory lesion of coeliac disease, which mainly affects the small intestine, is characterized by a marked infiltrate of lymphocytes, macrophages, plasma cells, and antigen presenting cells (APCs), with a small number of polymorphs. The early inflammatory lesion is also characterized by increases in intraepithelial lymphocytes and crypt hyperplasia, followed later by the loss of villous architecture (leading to villous atrophy). Coeliac disease can present at any age from infancy to old age. Although the GIT features predominate, the disease can also have significant extraintestinal manifestations. Coeliac disease can often be asymptomatic and may need to be considered in the differential diagnosis of patients shown to have anaemia or in children lagging in their developmental milestones (failure to thrive).

Excellent immune serological tests (see below) with high sensitivity and specificity, used in epidemiological screening studies, indicate a high prevalence of the disease. Varying studies have indicated a prevalence of 0.5–1% in white populations (USA and UK). Very low prevalence is found in some racial groups, such as Africans and Chinese. This appears to be due to lack of known permissive HLA susceptibility-linked class II alleles in these populations.

Coeliac disease, with its known environmental trigger (gluten), has well-defined linkages to HLA class II, in particular HLA-DR3 or -DR4 and even stronger linkages to HLA-DQ region alleles: DQ2 (~90%) and DQ8 (~7%). There is a breakdown of tolerance to a key autoantigen now known to be a ubiquitous enzyme called tissue transglutaminase (tTG). Elements of aberrant innate and adaptive immunity have been described in coeliac disease, with most data coming from studies of adaptive immunity. The latter have identified specific peptide sequences from gluten that bind to HLA-DQ2 and DQ8 on dendritic cells (DCs) and other APCs in the gut lamina propria. These cells stimulate local gluten specific CD4$^+$ $\alpha\beta$ T cell receptor$^+$ ($\alpha\beta$TCR$^+$) T cells. Such cells have been cloned from surgical specimens and shown *in vitro* to have these binding specificities. The resulting T helper 1 (Th1) cytokine responses include release of IFN-γ which contributes to the type IV hypersensitivity inflammatory response that is seen in the small intestine. This localized inflammation contributes to the intestinal villous atrophy characteristic of the disease. tTG is known to contribute to the pathogenesis of the disease by its deamination enzyme reaction (changes glutamine in the gluten peptide to glutamic acid). These changes in charge effects increase the binding strength of the peptides to the grooves of HLA-DQ2 and -DQ8, thus enhancing APC presentation to the CD4$^+$ T cells. B cells, in turn responding to tTG with help from T cells, produce anti-tTG antibodies (IgA and IgG class). It is speculated that the complexing of tTG with gliadin (a protein in gluten) facilitates epitope spreading, one of the mechanisms invoked in the development of autoimmune responses (see Chapter 1). How or if the anti-tTG antibodies contribute directly to the underlying GIT tissue damage or dysfunction is still unclear. However, these antibodies have been detected in the skin of patients with dermatitis herpetiformis and in central nervous system tissues of coeliac patients with ataxia. Assays for anti-tTG antibodies are extremely useful in confirming the diagnosis of coeliac disease and for monitoring patient's compliance with a gluten-free diet.

Some evidence indicates a role for unconventional intraepithelial lymphocytes (IELs) (see Chapter 1). IELs can recognize molecules induced on stressed (e.g. by inflammation) epithelial cells such as MICA/B (see Chapter 1), using non-TCR molecules similar to those found on natural killer/natural killer T (NK/NK T) cells, such as NKG2D. Recognition of stressed cells by IELs results in cell activation and secretion of cytokines—IL-15, IL-17 and IFN-γ. The cytokines produced *in situ* further aggravate epithelial disruption and increase the ingress of food antigens, including gluten, to the subepithelial spaces. This disruption of the epithelial barrier with increased ingress of antigens, together with epithelial cell production of cytokines and chemokines, is believed to increase the immune- inflammatory reactions and the downstream adaptive immune responses described within the lamina propria.

As in other autoimmune diseases, there is a strong family history of autoimmunity. Additionally, patients may have autoantibodies for other organ-specific diseases, e.g. type 1 diabetes or thyroid disease, without overt clinical evidence of these diseases. In some situations, however, over a period of time they may develop these diseases. Coeliac disease is also linked to an increased incidence of selective IgA primary antibody deficiency and to atopy. Thus, patients should be screened for these immune serological markers. Less commonly, some nonautoimmune disorders such as Down's syndrome and more rarely neurological (cerebellar) syndromes are linked to coeliac disease. Recent genome-wide association studies (GWASs) using single nucleotide polymorphism (SNP) analysis have started to demonstrated genetic linkages outside the extended MHC region. These studies show linkage to the occurrence of coeliac disease with type 1 diabetes and with other associations, including linkage to the genes for the cytokines IL- 2 and IL-21.

Because of the varied nature of presenting signs and symptoms and wide age range, clinicians should be aware of the diagnosis and tests for coeliac disease in patients presenting with diverse clinical symptoms and profiles. These include diarrhoea, constipation, abdominal pain and/or distension, nausea and vomiting, recurrent mouth ulcers, indeterminate arthritis and arthralgia; in children with failure to thrive or dental enamel hypoplasia of the permanent teeth; and in women with infertility problems. The blistering skin disease dermatitis herpetiformis is strongly associated with coeliac disease. Skin biopsy shows IgA deposition in the dermal papillae. Serology may also be positive for anti-tTG in these patients. The skin disease often responds to a gluten-free diet but additional therapy may be needed.

Coeliac disease is often diagnosed very late. Because of the increased incidence in patients with IgA deficiency (some studies suggest up to 10%) in relevant settings (no serum IgA) testing for IgG anti-tTG should be carried out (see Chapter 9). An assay using primate tissue for detection of an antibody called endomysial antibody is also highly specific for coeliac disease. However, this assay, in many laboratories, has been replaced by assays for anti-tTG antibodies. The endomysial antigen is known to share cross-reacting determinants with tTG. The 'gold standard' for diagnosis is still endoscopic biopsy of the distal duodenum although some authorities, particularly in the paediatric setting, may proceed with patient management based on clinical findings and laboratory results, including positive antibody serology. Coeliac disease patients on long-term treatment with a gluten-free diet often demonstrate reductions in titres of anti-tTG antibodies; in some cases becoming negative. Noncompliance with the diet is noted by increases in antibody levels in blood. Long-standing, poorly treated disease is associated with an increased incidence of non-Hodgkin's lymphoma—of T cell type associated with the gut-associated lymphoid tissue (GALT). There is also an increased incidence of osteomalacia and rickets due to vitamin D deficiency, and osteoporosis associated with prolonged malabsorption.

Crohn's disease and ulcerative colitis

Crohn's disease and ulcerative colitis, collectively termed inflammatory bowel disease (IBD), are chronic inflammatory diseases of the intestine with significant innate and adaptive immune dysfunction. The latter is believed to involve inappropriate biological immune responses to intestinal microbes in a genetically susceptible host. Some investigators consider IBD to be an autoimmune disorder with excessive inflammatory responses against the host's own (self) gut microbial population. Current data suggest that T regulatory cells (Tregs) and immune suppressive cytokines, such as IL-10 and transforming growth factor-beta (TGF-β), in the gut environment play a significant part in maintaining homeostasis of the host with its accompanying gut microorganisms and resultant good health (see Chapter 1). Immunological, cell biological, and molecular genetic studies including GWAS, together with model systems (*ex vivo* and *in vivo*), are producing detailed insights into the mechanisms underlying Crohn's disease and ulcerative colitis. These studies are suggesting new therapeutic options to improve current management. Highlighted below are some of the more recent findings.

The inflammatory lesions of Crohn's disease, which comprise infiltrates of innate and adaptive immune cells in the lamina propria, involve predominantly the ileum and the colon but can affect any part of the GIT. The inflammation is often transmural and granulomatous. By contrast, the inflammation of ulcerative colitis is typically confined to the mucosa involving the rectum or in some cases the whole colon. In both diseases, it is assumed that immune tolerance to gut microbes and possibly to other dietary antigens has broken down and resulted in a cycle of self-amplifying immune- inflammatory reactions. A complex series of interactions of the GIT epithelial lining cells, their associated goblet and Paneth cells, along with subepithelial and lamina propria cell populations, all contribute to the maintenance of intestinal homeostasis and tolerance. The epithelial barrier function of tight junctions and paracellular spaces prevents intestinal microbes from entering into the lamina propria and beyond. It is recognized that epithelial cell membrane and intracellurally located pattern recognition receptors (PRRs)—Toll-like receptors (TLRs) and NOD-like receptors (NLRs)—help to maintain basal signalling by recognition of luminal microbial pathogen-associated molecular patterns (PAMPs) (see Chapter 1). This basal signalling is assumed to facilitate lamina propria reactions such as the activation of subsets of DCs which produce immune suppressive molecules such as IL-10 and TGF-β. IL-10 is known to have broad suppressive actions on T and B cells and on macrophages and other cell types. These cytokines are also known to favour the emergence in the GALT of Tregs, which in turn help to control the effector T cell reactivity in the gut. Thus, there is a balance amongst the Th1, Th2, and Th17 effector responses. The GALT also favours the expression in the lamina propria of plasma cells committed to the production of the dominant antibodies of the IgA class. Retinoic acid (a derivative of vitamin A) is known to be a key molecule, favouring the emergence of IgA antibodies and the immune suppressive cytokines in the GALT. Secretory IgA, along with mucus produced by goblet cells and antimicrobial peptides from Paneth cells, prevent microbial adherence to the epithelial lining and induction of GIT immune reactivity.

If this balance between the microbes, epithelium, and lamina propria function is perturbed then tissue-damaging chronic inflammatory lesions can occur; this is well documented in several animal model systems. Studies of IBD models have indicated that dysregulation of intestinal $CD4^+$ T cell subgroups contributes to intense and persistent inflammation. Experiments have shown excessive $CD4^+$ Th17 responses linked to augmenting IL-23 activity (IL-23 is a cytokine produced by inflammation-driven lamina propria DCs and APCs—see Chapter 1). The DCs in IBD models are stimulated by TNF-α, IL-1, and IFN-γ produced by the infiltrates of innate and adaptive immune cells. The mouse model systems clearly indicate that intestinal microbes are needed for the development of IBD. They have delineated the roles of cytokines such as IL-1, IL-12, IL-23, and TNF-α in the pathogenesis of IBD. The role of microbes in initiating human IBD is less well established. Recent findings from clinical, pathological, immunological, and genetic studies have suggested some clear associations with human IBD, particularly with regards to dysregulated cytokine production and activity.

GWAS and SNP analysis have established certain significant associations with IBD and polymorphisms in genes for NLRs. These have been clearly linked to Crohn's disease in some populations, although not to ulcerative colitis. Thus, nucleotide-binding domain 2 (NOD2) homozygous polymorphisms confers an increased risk of an individual developing Crohn's disease. NOD2s function as intracellular PRRs, detecting bacterial PAMPs. In the intestinal environment, NOD2 activation of the signalling molecules NF-κB and MAP kinase is believed to down-regulate proinflammatory cytokines (see Chapter 1). This contrasts with NF-κB and MAP kinase activation in leucocytes which induce proinflammatory cytokines. NOD2 polymorphisms appear to interrupt the epithelial suppressive function, thus favouring inflammation. NOD2 polymorphisms, however, are not in themselves sufficient to induce IBD. Also, NOD2 association is not found in ulcerative colitis. Recently, studies of rare families with severe forms of early-onset IBD have confirmed a key role for IL-10. The investigations demonstrated homozygous, recessive loss of function mutations in the receptors for IL-10. The findings support in humans the functional immune suppressive role of IL-10 in the pathogenesis of IBD. Clearly, nonfunctional IL-10 is not the cause of most cases of IBD. However, its balance with other cytokines within the inflammatory lesions in the GALT may be crucial.

Extensive, well-controlled, and statistically powered GWAS have recently identified some significant new associations with Crohn's disease and ulcerative colitis or segregations with each disease separately. Associations which increase disease risk have been found with polymorphisms of autophagy genes and with genes involved in adaptive immunity (IL-23R, IL-10, IL-12, and STAT3). Also, associations are found with molecules of innate immunity (confirmation of NOD2, cytokine gene for IL-27). IL-27 is produced by DCs and has recently been shown to inhibit the development of $CD4^+$ $CD25^+$ $FoxP3^+$ Tregs. Tregs are thought to be key factors in suppressing excessive inflammation in the GALT and assisting in maintaining homeostasis in the GIT. Also, IL-27, apart from inhibiting the development of Tregs, has been shown to assist the differentiation of $CD4^+$ Th1, IFN-γ secreting cells which favour proinflammatory reactions.

The role of inflammation, and as a target for therapy of IBD, is well recognized by the use of anti-inflammatory drugs such as aminosalicylate and steroids. However, a better understanding of the mechanisms of IBD has encouraged more specific targeted therapies. The introduction of anti-TNF MABs has proved to be very effective, particularly in Crohn's disease. TNF plays multiple roles in innate and adaptive immunity affecting the responses of DCs, NK cells, T and B cells, and macrophages. Over time, anti-TNF therapy can lose its efficacy, underlying the pleotropic cytokine activities in IBD and significant degree of redundancy.

Based on the mechanistic understanding of much of the immune- inflammatory reactions in IBD, ongoing investigations are pursuing new therapies. Antibodies against the IL-23/IL-12 pathway are being studied. Clinical efficacy has been established in Crohn's disease (and also in severe psoriasis—a linked autoimmune disease in Crohn's disease patients). Other therapies include the use of anti-integrin antibodies that restrict leucocyte infiltration into the gut. Populations of gut homing leucocytes (T and B cells and eosinophils) use their α_4/β_7 cell surface molecules to engage the mucosal addressin cell adhesion molecule 1 (MADCAM1) expressed on the high endothelial venules in the GALT, enhancing selective entry (see Chapter 1).

The relative segregation of these integrin ligand interactions in the GALT makes for an attractive target, at least in principle. Attempts are being made to increase the presence of the immunosuppressive cytokine IL-10 in the GALT of IBD patients. Trials are currently ongoing. Optimizing the means, route, and form of delivery of IL-10 will be important parameters in these studies. Other studies are attempting to 'reset' the GALT immune response and microbial balance, with the aim of re-establishing immune tolerance and homeostasis by using commensal and/or probiotic microbes.

Recent studies suggest that the cytokine IL-21 (produced by subpopulations of $CD4^+$ T cells in the lamina propria) is a key driver of innate and adaptive immune cells, and may provide a new immunotherapeutic target similar to TNF in the management of IBD.

The pathophysiology of IBD can be summarized as follows. Microbes are considered as key players in the onset and perpetuation of the inflammation in IBD. Normally, immune responses to intestinal microbes are tightly regulated, providing an effective hyporesponsiveness to gut microbes (tolerance) as well as to other antigens in the diet. This hyporesponsiveness is, in part, due to an anti-inflammatory response, mediated by APCs secreting immunosuppressive cytokines. Additionally, innate immune responses mediated via gut epithelial cells ensure the maintenance of an immunosuppressive microenvironment. Disturbance of these homeostatic interactions, associated with dysregulated innate and adaptive immunity in the genetically susceptible host, incites tissue-damaging intestinal inflammation, much of which is cytokine driven. Molecules produced by and indicative of inflammatory reactions of intestinal epithelial and lamina propria cells, such as the protein calprotectin (detectable in faeces), are contributing to the noninvasive diagnosis of IBD.

Autoinflammatory diseases

Autoinflammatory diseases are characterized by recurrent, often unprovoked, inflammation, with patients presenting with a fever. The diseases have historically been called periodic fever syndromes. They also present with signs and symptoms of a generalized acute inflammatory disorder skin rashes and oedema, arthralgia, etc. They are best considered as disorders of innate immunity; there is little or no evidence of significant autoimmunity with absence of pathological autoantibodies and autoreactive T cells. Autoinflammatory diseases have mainly been characterized as genetic or hereditary conditions due to various underlying mechanisms, often associated with gene mutations. These tend to be linked to perturbations in the regulation of cellular targets such as inflammasomes with resulting dysregulated production of proinflammatory cytokines such as IL-1, IL-6, and IL-18. The inflammasomes, which are normally recruited by TLRs and NLRs in the host physiological reactions to PAMPs and damage-associated molecular patterns (DAMPs), facilitate antipathogen protective inflammatory responses (see Chapter 1). However, in some of these hereditary diseases, activation of inflammasomes is uncontrolled and leads to undesirable and unprovoked periodic clinical inflammation.

The autoinflammatory diseases have been classified in varying ways—clinicopathologically, by molecular and physiological mechanisms. They can be defined by inappropriate activation, via inflammasomes, of the cytokines of the IL-1 superfamily. They may be considered as IL-1 activation disorders; some can mechanistically be considered as NF-κB activation syndromes and others as protein misfolding disorders. Dysregulation of cytokine signalling and inappropriate macrophage activation syndromes provides yet another explanation of some of the clinical syndromes. Currently, however, the clinical description of autoinflammatory diseases remain the most commonly encountered in medical practice. The clinical nomenclature includes TNF receptor-associated periodic fever syndromes (TRAPS), hyperimmunoglobulin D and periodic fever syndrome (HIDS), familial Mediterranean fever (FMF), cryopyrin-associated period fever syndromes (CAPS), familial cold autoinflammatory syndrome (FCAS), Muckle–Wells syndrome (MWS), and neonatal onset multisystem inflammatory disease (NOMID), and a few other very rare conditions.

TRAPS patients have an autosomal dominant disease characterized by recurrent, but irregular, intervals of fever and they often present early in life. Patients with TRAPS present with signs of inflammation affecting many organs and tissues, including episodes of abdominal pain (presenting with an acute abdomen to surgeons). Skin rashes, pleurisy, arthritis, myalgia, and also nephrotic syndrome, linked to the development of amyloidosis, are also seen in the disease. There is usually a strong family history. Genetic and immunological studies have defined multiple mutations in the TNF receptor genes which link to different molecular mechanisms associated with the disease—receptor shedding, protein misfolding, etc. Blood analyses of TRAPS patients indicate increased levels of acute-phase proteins. Monitoring reveals increased levels of IL-1 and IL-6. Therapy is directed at controlling the acute inflammation with nonspecific agents such as steroids. Newer biological therapies have been introduced, including the use of the anti-TNF etanercept. Patients' symptoms can be exacerbated by infliximab and adalimumab, but significant efficacy is seen in some patients. Other biological therapies are being investigated, notably anakinra, which has proved effective also in the CAPS group of autoinflammatory conditions.

FMF is an autosomal recessive disease presenting more frequently in certain populations residing in the Mediterranean region. Like TRAPS, it can present at any age with irregular, recurrent attacks of fever and inflammation affecting various sites, including the abdomen. Inappropriate surgical procedures have been performed in such patients. The target gene (*MEFV*) for FMF has been described, and causative mutations documented. Therapy with colchicine is effective in the majority of cases. Various biological therapies, including anti-TNF agents, have been used in patients with a poor response to colchicine, again with variable outcomes.

HIDS is an autosomal recessive autoinflammatory disease presenting with fever, often with lymphadenopathy and acute onset of severe abdominal clinical features—pain, diarrhoea, and vomiting. Skin rashes are common. The disease gene has been noted to be the *MVK* gene; it is not associated directly with the raised levels of IgD. Interestingly, recent research on IgD shows this to be an immunoglobulin that links innate immunity and the inflammatory response, and can cause significant increases in TNF and IL-1. IgD binds to basophils via an Fc receptor and stimulates these cells to secrete cytokines and other inflammatory mediators. Why IgD is increased in HIDS is still unclear. IgD with specificity for microbes encountered within the respiratory tract has been shown to mediate induction of proinflammatory cytokines.

CAPS, which are autosomal dominant diseases, include FCAS, MWS, and NOMID. They are part of a clinical spectrum, all having mutations in the *C1AS1* gene encoding cryopyrin. Mutations in the gene lead to dysregulation in inflammasome activation causing excessive production of IL-1. In the mildest disorder (FCAS), symptoms only develop on exposure to cold. The most severe form (NOMID) presents shortly after birth with chronic inflammation, urticaria, aseptic meningitis, arthalgia, sensorineural deafness, and uveitis. Amyloidosis is a feature of both MWS and NOMID. These conditions have been shown to respond substantially to IL-1 blockade by biological agents. The initial studies looked at anakinra, but newer IL-1-related therapies are now being evaluated.

In summary, patients with autoinflammatory diseases may rarely present to surgeons. If the diagnosis is suspected, after appropriate conservative management, there needs to be close collaboration with clinicians and clinical scientists experienced in the diagnosis (genetic and serological) and management of such patients. Their management will require intensive interaction with family members. Patients require long-term management, including monitoring and using preventative strategies to avoid complications such as the development of amyloidosis.

Surgical interventions and autoimmune inflammation

Surgical procedures have been linked for decades to the development of autoimmune inflammation in some patients. A few of these linkages are well founded and are supported by the demonstration of autoreactive antibodies and T cells after surgery. The associations are strengthened by the latent period after surgery and before the development of autoreactivity, consistent with the development of adaptive immune responses. Such immune responses have been documented following surgical procedures that have resulted in the release of sequestered antigens, such as those associated with the lens protein of the eye and with cardiac antigens. The latter occurs in the postpericardial injury syndrome (Dressler's syndrome). In this condition, prospective studies, collecting serum samples before cardiotomy and over several weeks after surgery, have clearly demonstrated the induction and increasing titres of antibody, followed subsequently by the disappearance of the anticardiac autoantibodies. In some patients, the autoimmune response appears secondary (not inducing tissue damage) but in others it can be associated with clinical myocardial disturbances in conduction and contractile function. Those cases may require medical supportive therapy over a period of time. The syndrome generally resolves over several weeks to months. Not only must the cardiac self-antigens be recognized by T cells, but there also must be appropriate additional signals to induce autoantibody formation and persistence. Additionally, there needs to be persistence of the antigen(s) to lead to a protracted autoimmune disease (see Chapter 1).

Apart from examples associated with sequestered antigens, many claims of surgery-induced autoimmunity or autoimmune disease need to be considered with caution. There are long-standing assertions that the use of silicone products in breast augmentation or in ophthalmological surgery have led to the development of autoimmune diseases such as scleroderma and SLE. These assertions have not been supported by expert reviews over many years, including reviews conducted by the US Food and Drug Administration (FDA). Undoubtedly, in some cases, autoantibodies characteristic of these diseases have been demonstrated as well as clinical disease. However, in the case of silicone breast implants, this is occurring on a particular patient background, namely women who have an increased incidence of autoimmune diseases such as SLE and scleroderma. It has not been convincingly established that there is an increased incidence of these diseases, compared with a controlled population. Further surveillance and monitoring is required. Other documented occurrences of postsurgical autoimmunity are the well-founded cases of thyroid autoimmunity following surgery for Cushing's disease. It is suggested that the hypercortisolism associated with Cushing's suppressed an occult underlying thyroid inflammation. However, following surgery and over a period of time the thyroiditis evolves as the endogenous cortisol levels fall. Other situations where autoimmunity apparently develops following surgery need to exclude patients' medications, especially those known to be associated with the induction of systemic autoimmunity.

Historically, there have been several case reports which have described the development of coeliac disease as a consequence of abdominal surgery. However, serological screening for autoantibodies (see above) has shown that the prevalence of coeliac disease (overt and occult) is much higher than previously thought (1:200 to 1:1000). Moreover, it is now recognized that patients with undiagnosed coeliac disease may be subjected to unnecessary appendicectomies.

Undoubtedly, vigilance needs to be continued in this area of autoimmunity following surgery. Some recent reports have documented the development of clinical myasthenia gravis (with positive anti-acetylacholine receptor and anti-MuSK antibodies) post-thoracotomy for coronary artery bypass surgery. Investigations are suggesting that damage to the thymus gland at the time of surgery may contribute to this association.

Major surgery leads to the induction of increased levels of innate immune acute-phase proteins and of proinflammatory cytokines and chemokines, as well as, in some situations, the release of sequestered self-antigens. Clearly, this could provide the requisite signals (1–3) for inducing autoimmunity (see Chapter 1). However, for such responses to persist and induce a long-term autoimmune disease would require the necessary genetic susceptibility in the patient as well as a persisting source of autoantigens. Additionally, the dominance of effector tissue-damaging T cells and autoantibodies, uncontrolled by biological regulators such as T regs and immune-suppressive cytokines, would be required. The convergence of all these requirements in the patient undergoing surgery is likely to be uncommon. Clinically significant autoimmunity, as a primary consequence of surgical interventions, is a most uncommon occurrence and not a major clinical problem.

Summary and conclusions

Autoimmune and autoinflammatory diseases range from common (RA and thyroiditis) to rare entities (FMF and TRAPS). However, the pathophysiological disturbances they cause increase the likelihood that they may present or be referred to surgical specialists, at some time in the natural history of the disease. Clinicians need to have an understanding of the aetiology and of the possible mechanisms underlying these diseases, and how this knowledge base is shaping and influencing management (including newer biological therapies). Additionally, the overview of these disorders strongly indicates the need for collaborative working and interactions to ensure optimal management for patients and opportunities to advance knowledge in these interesting areas of medicine and essential immunology.

Further reading

Textbooks

Chapel H, Haeney M, Misbah S, Snowden N. *Essentials of clinical immunology* (5th edn). Wiley-Blackwell, Chichester, 2006.

Spickett G. *Oxford handbook of clinical immunology and allergy* (2nd edn). Oxford University Press, Oxford, 2006.

Reviews

Cho JH. The genetics and immunopathogenesis of inflammatory bowel disease. *Nat Rev Immunol* 2008; **8**: 458–466.

Dalmau J, Rosenfeld MR. Paraneoplastic syndromes of the CNS. *Lancet Neurol*, 2008; **7**: 327–340.

Di Sabatino A, Corazza GR. Coeliac disease. *Lancet* 2009; **373**: 1480–1493.

Kaser A, Zeissig S, Blumberg RS. Inflammatory bowel disease. *Annu Rev Immunol* 2010; **28**: 573–621.

Ryan JG, Goldbach-Mansky R. The spectrum of autoinflammatory diseases: recent bench to bedside observations. *Curr Opin Rheumatol* 2008; **20**: 66–75.

Chapter 9

Principles of immunological assays and molecular technologies

Herb Sewell, Paddy Tighe, and Adrian Robins

Key summary points

- Immunological assays are very variable and are widely used in medicine. Some tests are essential for diagnosis or monitoring disease, others are playing major roles in clinical and translational research.
- Immunological assays exploit the precise *specificity* of individual antibody molecules recognizing and binding to antigens. The antibody–antigen complex bound in cells or tissue sites, on a solid phase matrix, or in solution, can be detected by using systems that amplify the initial reaction, thus, increasing *sensitivity* of detection. The amplification systems often involve other antibody species (antiglobulin, anti-immunoglobulin) directed at the initial antibody in the complex. The amplified reactions can be demonstrated (read out) by various systems which link molecules usually to the antibody molecules within the reaction. The linker molecules may be fluorescent compounds, enzymes, radio-isotopes, etc. They can be visualized using UV, light, and, less commonly, electron microscopic systems. A major detection system used is flow cytometry.
- Sensitive immunological assays are employed as an aid in the detection of tumour markers; they are mainly used in monitoring disease progression and in assessing prognosis. Currently, they have very limited applications in primary diagnosis of tumours and are not used in screening of unselected populations. This is because many markers can be induced nonspecifically, e.g. by inflammatory conditions. Some tests are being developed to help in the early diagnosis of cancer in at-risk/high-risk groups (family history, environmental exposure).
- Deficiencies of the immune system, disease-inducing reactions of immunopathology (type I–IV hypersensitivity), and clinical translational research into the immune system all require analysis of components of the immune system itself. This is to assist in the clinical diagnosis and management of a wide range of diseases, as well as to provide new insights into disease processes. The cellular elements of innate and adaptive immunity, the soluble cytokines and chemokines and the antibodies produced by B cells for humoral immunity can be tested

and be evaluated *in vitro*, *ex vivo* and, in limited ways, *in vivo*. *In vivo* tests include the skin prick test for type I hypersensitivity diagnosis, delayed hypersensitivity, and patch testing for diagnosis of type IV cell-mediated hypersensitivity.

- Technological advances in flow cytometry, the introduction of multiplex assays (multiple tests performed on a finite sample) have accelerated the use of biomarkers to assist in diagnosis and clinical research. Antibody and protein microarrays used in robotic fluid-handling technologies have developed rapidly in research laboratories, and are now being exploited in the clinical setting. The assays are very precise, sensitive, and diverse in testing but very highly specific.
- Sequencing of the human genome has accelerated a range of major postgenomic technologies (the 'omics'). Sophisticated information technology and computer science has developed in parallel to handle the vast amount of information generated from postgenomic technologies. New ways of integrating information from biological reactions together with information technology has led to the emergence of systems biology/medicine. The systems approaches permit the study of dynamic integrated networks, associated with physiological and pathological processes.
- Human gene therapy, to correct defective genes implicated in a range of immune system diseases (especially monogenic disorders) and in cancers, is being carefully developed with some notable successes. Technological advances continue into delivery systems (vectors) that are needed to overcome some of the barriers to gene therapy, not least the immune system itself. More complex and common multigene-associated diseases are proving more challenging. Stem cell therapy, using embryonic-derived or induced pluripotential stem cells or other types of reprogrammed cells is indicating significant promise in a range of common diseases and in transplantation.

Introduction

Immunological assays have been shown to be very useful in both patient management and clinical research. Surgeons should have a working knowledge of the principles of the standard assays and of newer developments which may contribute to the practise and scientific understanding of surgery. Outlined below are selected immunological assays, together with aspects of modern cellular and molecular technologies.

Tumour markers

Background

Cancer is essentially a genetic disorder caused by multistage events, associated with environmental insults and with alterations and disruptions in the molecular milieu within the cell, which ultimately contribute to the emergence and establishment of the cancer phenotype (see Chapter 4). This phenotype differs from normal cellular counterparts, in particular, by the possession of either unique tumour-specific antigens (TSAs), or more commonly, by aberrant expression of normal gene products—differentiation and functional molecules—which are termed tumour-associated antigens (TAAs). The increased expression of these antigens in malignant tissues or their secretion into body fluids by tumour cells can be detected by immunological assays.

A wide range of monoclonal (and some polyclonal) antibodies have been generated with defined specificity for tumour-associated markers. Their reaction with TSAs or TAAs is revealed by various detection systems, including immunohistochemical (immunocytochemical) methods, on tissue sections, smears and cells in suspension (the latter using flow cytometry), and by solid- and fluid-phase assays such as the enzyme-linked immunoabsorbent assay (ELISA) and radio-immunoassay (RIA).

The immunological assays to be described are used in helping to establish a diagnosis of cancer and to predict prognosis, as well as to monitor the response to therapy in patients with malignant disease.

Principles of techniques and monoclonal antibodies

Köhler and Milstein in 1975 [1] described the method of generating potentially limitless quantities of highly specific antibodies to antigens of choice, by fusing *in vitro* an antibody-secreting B cell (to provide specificity of the antibody) with a cultured malignant B cell line (to provide continuous production of antibody) to produce an antibody-secreting 'immortalized' hybridoma. The latter was grown in selective medium, able to support the growth of hybrid cells but not the unfused lymphocytes or tumour cells. Their hybridization method has been employed by various scientists and clinicians to generate numerous monoclonal antibodies (MABs) with specificity for many TAAs (see Figure 9.1). MABs have exquisite specificity as they react with only a single antigenic determinant (an *epitope*) of complex antigens.

Mouse MABs continue to play major and distinctive roles in diagnostic procedures; their use as therapeutic agents has been shown to be more limited (see Chapters 1 and 7). The breakthrough technologies developed by Greg Winter and colleagues from 1986 onwards have allowed the production of humanized mouse and fully human MABs, which are now used therapeutically in a wide range of diseases (see Chapter 1, 'HIV, AIDS, and the surgeon'; Chapter 7).

Immunohistochemical techniques

Various sensitive detection systems are employed to demonstrate (visualize) the binding of monoclonal (or polyclonal) antibodies to tumour antigens. The techniques are known by many abbreviations such as PAP (peroxidase–antigen–peroxidase), APAAP (alkaline phosphatase–anti-alkaline phosphatase), IFA (indirect fluorescent antibody), and ABC (avidin–biotin complex). The principles of these techniques are illustrated in Figure 9.2. Substrates containing tumour cells or extracts (processed to preserve the integrity of antigens) are reacted with defined MABs. The binding of the latter is demonstrated by the use of stepwise procedures, whereby a second or subsequent antibody with an attached 'label' is used.

Immunohistological methods, using only a one-stage reaction (direct)—directly labelled MABs—are often too insensitive and too expensive for routine use. Many of

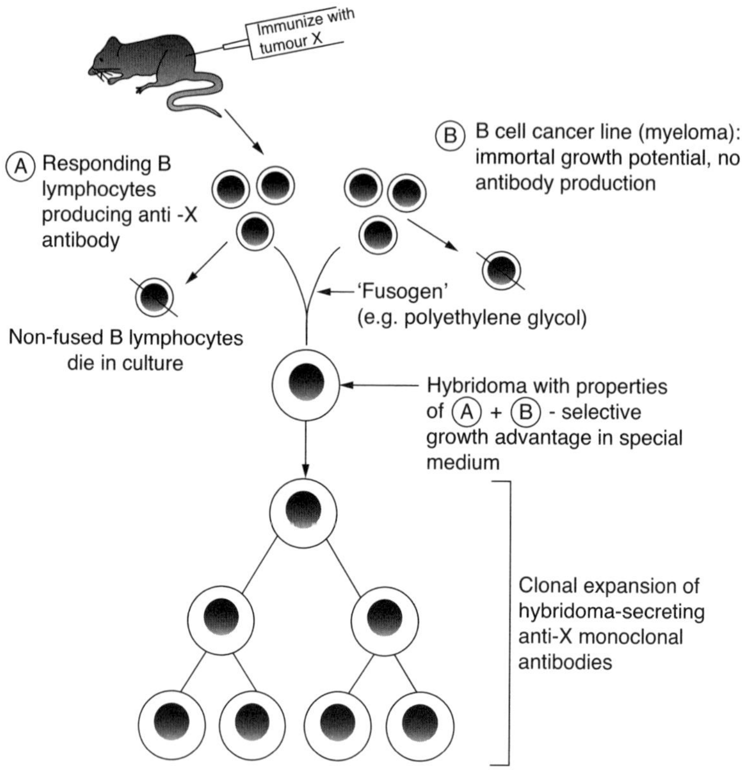

Fig. 9.1 Principle of monoclonal antibody (MAB) production. The B lymphocytes from the immunized animal produce antitumour antibodies. The myeloma cancer cells, when fused with the B cells, confer the genetic information for infinite growth (immortalization). The immunoglobulin-secreting B lymphocytes confer on the hybrid the ability to produce antibody. A special tissue culture medium is used which enables the hybridoma to grow and proliferate but results in the death of the unfused B lymphocytes (A) and myeloma cells (B). The secreted MAB is harvested from the supernatant.

the multistep immunohistochemical staining techniques have now been completely automated.

The multiple stages in the techniques increase substantially the signal for detection and, thus, the sensitivity of the technique. The 'labels' used may be enzymes (e.g. peroxidase, alkaline phosphatase) which are exposed to a substrate (usually an organic chemical); the enzyme–substrate reaction results in the deposition of a visible colour product in the vicinity of the tumour antigen–MAB reaction complex. Other labels, such as fluorescein, are excited by light (UV or visible) and, in turn, emit light of a wavelength detectable by a microscope with appropriate optics or by photodetection systems within recording equipment, such as flow cytometers (see below).

Like most laboratory methods, immunohistochemical methods require attention to methodology, controls (positive and negative), reagent quality assurance, and trained

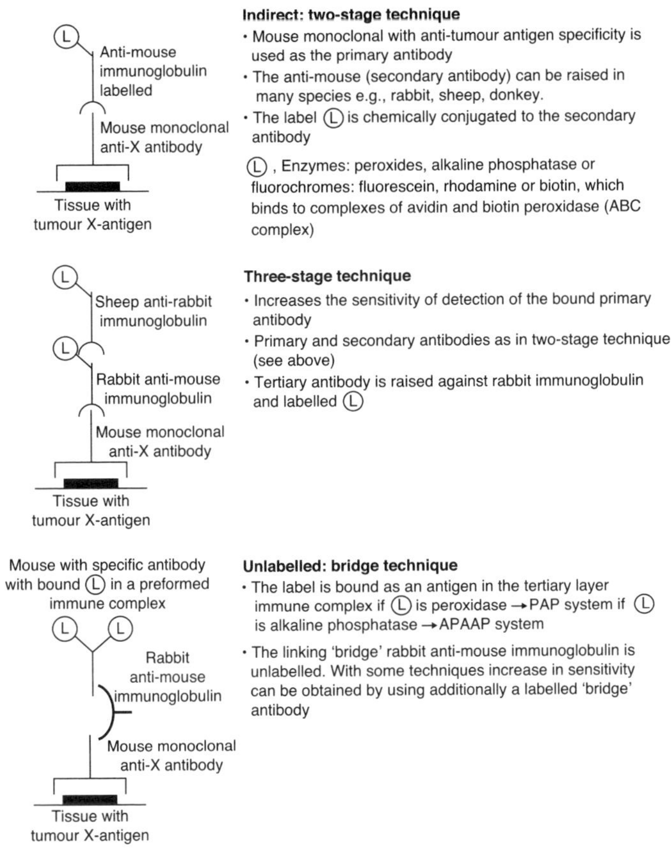

Fig. 9.2 Imunohistochemical techniques used in monoclonal antibody detection of tumour antigens/markers. If (L) is a peroxidase enzyme, a chemical substrate (diaminobenzidine) is added and results in deposition of an insoluble brown product. If (L) is a fluorochrome, the tissue is examined in a UV fluorescent microscope. Enzyme (L) labels have advantages over fluorochromes, e.g. tissue reactions are visible with a light microscope and a permanent preparation is available.

expertise in the interpretation of the immunohistochemical results. mmunohistochemical methods are mainly qualitative or at best semiquantitative.

ELISA and RIA techniques

ELISAs employ many similar methods to the immunohistochemical techniques, but are designed to detect free molecules in solution (Figure 9.3). In the detection of TAAs in blood and other body fluids, ELISA techniques are based on linking the antibody to the solid phase. If a patient's serum sample contains the antigen, it reacts with the bound antibody. The presence of the antigen is revealed by another reaction with antibody with specificity for that antigen, followed by an enzyme-labelled antiglobulin.

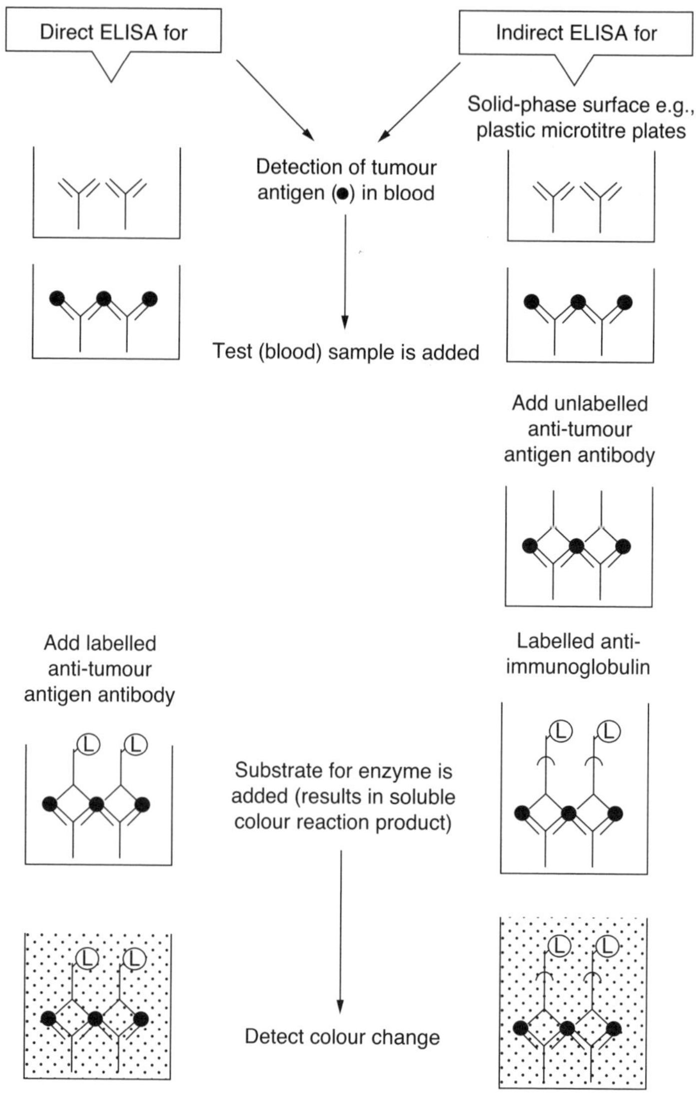

Fig. 9.3 ELISA techniques used to detect and quantitate tumour antigens in fluids. Y, antibody specific for tumour antigen (•)—bound or adsorbed to solid phase; •, tumour antigen/marker-secreted and present in body fluids (blood, synovial fluid, etc); L, enzyme (e.g. peroxidase)—(a) linked to a second tumour antigen (•) specific antibody in the direct ELISA; (b) linked to an anti-immunoglobulin (i.e. anti-anti-tumour immunoglobulin) in the indirect ELISA. This is a more sensitive technique (can detect tumour antigen in ng/mL in blood).

The enzyme is reacted with a substrate, generating a fluid-phase colour reaction product. The final reaction product can be read manually or more rapidly and efficiently by automated spectrophotometry (ELISA readers). By the incorporation of various standards (e.g. dilutions of antigen and suitable controls) the amounts of tumour antigen in any sample can be accurately quantitated.

Well-known ELISA assays are used to quantitate antigens, such as carcinoembryonic antigen (CEA), CA125, and CA19–9 which are carbohydrate-associated antigens secreted by and associated with various tumours (see below).

RIAs are used in similar situations to ELISAs but the indicator systems are based on the emission of various radionuclides linked to antigens or antibodies (e.g. ^{125}I, ^{131}I, ^{3}H). Many laboratories have moved from RIA to ELISA systems, thus, avoiding the use of isotopes and their attendant problems. Many ELISA systems are of a sensitivity comparable with the ranges detected by RIA.

Flow cytometry

Flow cytometry (see 'Flow cytometry: current practice and future developments', below) has been used extensively to help establish the diagnosis and cellular origin of different leukaemias and lymphomas and to analyse cytological preparations (washings and aspirates) from carcinomas (e.g. thyroid, cervical, and bladder cancers). Also, documentation of the DNA content of various solid tumours—breast, thyroid, bladder, and non-Hodgkin's lymphoma—have been obtained by flow cytometry and correlated with the degree of malignancy on histological evaluation and with prognosis on patient follow-up.

Tumour marker assays in laboratory practice

For markedly dedifferentiated (anaplastic) tumours, it can be difficult to characterize them precisely and establish their tissue of origin using standard histologic methods. A simple panel of MABs has proved extremely valuable in this situation. The antibodies used are directed against intermediate filaments (IFs), which are proteins that constitute a major part of the cell cytoskeleton. Different cell types, even when malignant, maintain their characteristic IFs. Thus, normal epithelial cells and their corresponding tumours (carcinomas) possess the IF *cytokeratin*, muscle cells contain *desmin*, mesenchymal cells *vimentin*, and neural cells *neurofilaments*. Table 9.1 summarizes the pattern of activity found using a panel of MABs to IFs in the diagnosis of anaplastic cancers. Table 9.2 illustrates some tumour markers and appropriate assays used in clinical laboratory practice.

Over several decades, various research laboratories have documented the occurrence of autoantibodies with specificity for TAAs in the blood of patients with different cancers. The role of such autoantibodies in the aetiopathology of the cancers is unclear. Nevertheless, the autoantibodies have been studied as potential biomarkers to assist in cancer diagnosis, monitoring of response to therapy and for prognosis. Recently published data have demonstrated that a relatively small panel of TAAs, used in solid-phase assays (e.g. ELISA), have the ability to be bound by autoantibody in the sera of cancer patients and can be used as a diagnostic signal for detection of early-stage

Table 9.1 Monoclonal antibody specificities and immunohistochemical reactivity

Anaplastic tumour type	IF[a] cytokeratin	IF desmin	IF vimentin	LCA[b]	IF neurofilament
Carcinoma	+	–	– (+)	–	–
Lymphoma	–	–	+ (–)	+	–
Melanoma	–	–	+	–	–
Neural tumours	–	–	–	–	+
Rhabdomyosarcoma	–	+	+	–	–
Leiomyosarcoma	–	+	–	–	–
Ewing	–	–	+	–	–

[a]IF, intermediate filament.
[b]Leucocyte common antigen (LCA or CD45) is not an IF; it is a macromolecular protein restricted to leucocytes.

solid tumours, such as lung and breast cancers [2]. Such autoantibody based tests to detect early cancer, if proven to be reproducible, sensitive, and specific with appropriate clinical predictive value, will add to the growing biomarker armamentarium.

Assessment of immune responsiveness

Qualitative, quantitative and functional assays of lymphocytes and phagocytes *in vitro* and *in vivo* provide an opportunity to characterize an individual's state of immune responsiveness. The assays include:

in vitro counts and analysis of total T, B, and T cell subsets of lymphocytes

in vitro functional assays of T and B cell responses to antigens and mitogens; these assays are commonly referred to as proliferation assays

in vivo functional tests of T cells as manifested by delayed type hypersensitivity (DTH) reactions in skin tests

in vitro assays of functional cytotoxicity tests for natural killer (NK) and lymphokine-activated killer (LAK) cell activity.

Methods for *in vitro* counts include definition of cell surface and, in some situations, intracellular protein molecules collectively termed *lymphocyte markers*. Additionally, tests are carried out for other markers which correlate with functions such as lymphocyte activation and phagocyte cell migration. These markers include human leucocyte antigen (HLA)-DR, interleukin-2 (IL-2) receptor, and markers for integrins such as those of the CD18 family. In some specialist laboratories intracellular identification of cytokines and chemokines is done as part of in-depth clinical investigation of patients or for research purposes. These assays are collectively referred to as *cellular/immune phenotyping*. They are dependent on the availability of a wide range of MABs to various cell markers, especially to cluster of differentiation (CD) antigens (see Chapter 1). Specialist laboratories also use immune phenotyping to characterize and assist in identifying the abnormal cells involved in leukaemias and lymphomas. Currently,

Table 9.2 Tumour-associated markers and immunological assays

	Tumour-associated marker/antigen	Tumour	Assay	Comment
1	IFs	See Table 9.1	Immunohistology	Additional antibodies may contribute to further characterization of anaplastic tumours
2	CEA	Colonic and other gastrointestinal tumours	Tissue: immunohistology Serum: ELISA/RIA	Pre- and postsurgical monitoring of serum CEA in patients with known colonic cancer
3	CA19–9	Gastrointestinal tumours	Tissue: immunohistology Serum: ELISA/RIA	Not specific for a particular cancer. Serum assays show some selectivity in detecting pancreatic cancer
	CA125	Ovarian cancer-associated	Tissue: immunohistology Serum: ELISA/RIA	Serum ELISA for CA 125 is good for monitoring ovarian cancer patients. Tissue does not react with mucinous ovarian tumours, found in other carcinomas
	CA15–3	Breast cancer	Tissue: immunohistology Serum: ELISA/RIA	Not specific for breast cancer
4	Placental alkaline phosphatase	Seminoma and some carcinomas	Tissue: immunohistology Serum: ELISA/RIA	Good marker for seminoma metastases Positive in some ovarian cancers ELISA/RIA used to monitor seminoma patients Antibody also useful in radionuclide 'imaging' techniques *in vivo*
5	p97–melanoma-associated antigen	Malignant melanoma	Tissue: immunohistology	Positive in pigmented and amelanotic melanoma. Useful in defining metastases with occult primary
6	GFAP	Brain tumours	Tissue: immunohistology	Useful in distinguishing glial tumours from metastases in the brain from non-CNS sites.
7	AFP	Hepatoma, malignant testicular tumours	Tissue: immunohistology Serum: ELISA/RIA	Very useful for serum monitoring of patients with tumours, and following therapy

(*Continued*)

Table 9.2 Tumour-associated markers and immunological assays (*continued*)

Tumour-associated marker/antigen	Tumour	Assay	Comment
8 hCG	Trophoblastic tumours, gestational choriocarcinoma, testicular and ovarian tumours	Tissue: immunohistology Serum: ELISA/RIA	Serology used pre-and postsurgery and for patient monitoring
9 Thyroglobulin	Thyroid tumours (papillary, follicular and anaplastic)	Tissue: immunohistology Serum: ELISA/RIA	Pre- and postsurgical serology
10 PSA	Prostatic cancer	Tissue: immunohistology Serum: ELISA/RIA	Local tissue invasion: differentiates bladder from prostate cancer Serology ELISA: antigen increased in metastatic disease
11 Oestrogen receptor protein	Breast cancer (ovarian cancer)	Tissue: immunohistology Tissue homogenate: ligand-binding assay, RIA	Prognostic; influences therapy decisions
12 CD antigens (panels of monoclonals; see Chapter 1)	T/B cell lineage and null leukaemias and lymphomas	Tissue: immunohistology Cells in suspension: flow cytometry	Diagnosis/subtyping: prognostic monitoring of cells for remission, relapse status
13 κ and λ staining	B cell tumours	Tissue: immunohistology Cells in suspension: flow cytometry	Defining monoclonality (neoplastic nature) of B cell populations
14 Immunoglobulins, monoclonal proteins	Multiple myeloma, other plasma cell dyscrasias	Tissue: smears Biopsies: immunohistology Serum: electrophoresis Cells: flow cytometry	Staining for κ and λ light chains often reveals the monoclonal (neoplastic) nature of B lineage proliferations
15 Ectopic hormones (e.g. ACTH, ADH)	Lung tumours, oat cell carcinoma	Tissue: immunohistology Serum: ELISA/RIA	Can be used to evaluate response to therapy

AFP, alpha-fetoprotein; CA, carbohydrate-associated antigen; CEA, carcinoembryonic antigen; CNS, central nervous system; ELISA, enzyme-linked immunosorbent assay; GFAP, glial fibrillary acid protein; hCG, human chorionic gonadotrophin; IF, intermediate filament; PSA, prostate specific antigen; RIA, radioimmunoassay.

most of these immune phenotyping tests are done mainly by using high-quality flow cytometry (see 'Flow cytometry: current practice and future developments', below) operated by skilled personnel.

Cellular immunity (adaptive and innate)

Quantitative and qualitative analysis

Quantitative and qualitative analysis of lymphocytes (lymphocyte phenotyping) involves counting total T, B, and T subset lymphocyte populations. Quantification of the lymphoid populations is useful in: (1) the monitoring of HIV infection (see Chapter 1); (2) the investigation of other immune deficiency states suspected from a clinical history of persistent, recurrent, serious or unusual infections; (3) the determination of the type of cells involved in a probable lymphoproliferative malignancy; (4) the establishment of whether a persistent blood lymphocytosis is benign or malignant (e.g. normal B cells in blood have approximately 50% positive κ- and 50% positive λ-bearing cells; in contrast, malignant B cell proliferations are monoclonal and usually only one light chain is detected); and (5) monitoring the effects of using therapeutic biological agents (see Chapter 1).

Quantification is performed using samples of fresh anticoagulated blood or partially purified mononuclear cell populations obtained by density gradient sedimentation. Analysis of whole blood samples is preferred for accurate determination of absolute counts of specific lymphocyte subsets, for example $CD4^+$ T cells in HIV. More complex functional analyses evaluate mononuclear cell populations. The blood is diluted with phosphate buffered saline and layered over a suitable dense separation substance such as Ficoll-Isopaque (SG 1.077) and centrifuged (450*g* for 30 min). Blood cells move differentially through such a separation medium and mononuclear cells, comprising mainly lymphocytes (with some monocytes), collect at the interface of the gradient and the upper plasma layer. Red blood cells (RBCs) and granulocytes form a pellet at the bottom of the centrifuge tube. Whole blood or partially purified cells are incubated with MABs to various T and B cell-associated CD antigens (e.g. CD3, CD4, CD8, CD19; see Chapter 1) and to more specific markers, e.g. antigen-specific T and B cell receptors—TCR, αβ, γδ, and BCR-surface membrane immunoglobulin (SmIg)—on the lymphocytes (see Chapter 1). T cell activation is inferred by analysis for expression of markers such as CD69 and IL-2 receptor (IL-2R), and by the expression of HLA-DR on T cells. In contrast to T cells, B cells constitutively express HLA-DR The binding of the MABs is revealed by incubation with anti-mouse antibody reagents which are labelled with enzymes (see Figure 9.2) or more routinely with fluorescent probes.

The labelled cells are quantified by automation, e.g. flow cytometry (see below) and expressed as percentages and absolute counts relative to the total lymphocyte count and by use of established normal ranges.

In vitro functional assays

T and B lymphocyte activation following reaction to antigens (soluble or cell-associated) or mitogens (see Chapter 1) results in many biochemical (signal transduction)

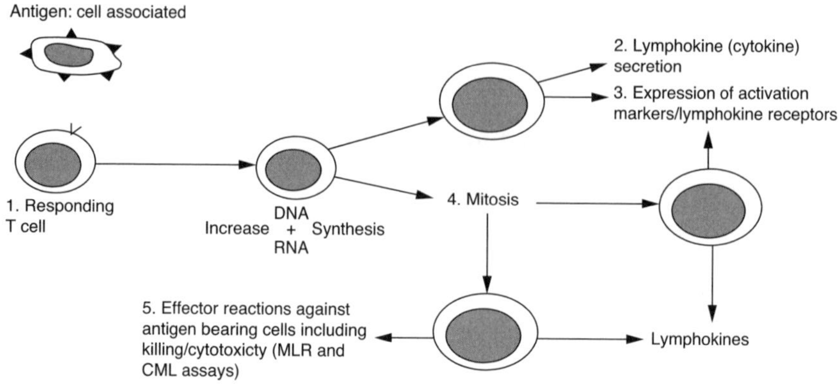

Fig. 9.4 Measurable consequences of T cell reaction to 'non-self' antigens on a cell. CML, cell-mediated lymphotoxicity; MLR, mixed lymphocyte reaction.

and cellular events involving cell synthesis of DNA/RNA, secretion of cytokines, and expression of activation markers, such as CD69 and CD25 (the α chain of IL 2R) and resultant cell mitosis. *In vitro* functional assays of T lymphocytes are useful: (1) In the investigation of a possible deficiency of cell-mediated immunity (CMI), including that associated with HIV infection; (2) as part of the documentation of a potential recipient's reactivity to donor cell-associated antigens which may result in acute allograft rejection. The classical *in vitro* mixed lymphocyte reaction (MLR) (also called mixed lymphocyte culture, MLC) and cell-mediated lympholysis (CML) assays are useful correlates of *in vivo* events in transplantation rejection (see Chapter 3).

Figure 9.4 indicates T cell recognition, activation and some subsequent events which follow antigen recognition. The numbered events (1–5) can be assayed as follows:

1) DNA/RNA synthesis can be measured by incorporation of radiolabelled nucleotide precursors in the cultures of responding lymphocytes and stimulatory cells. The antigen-bearing stimulatory cells are rendered nonresponsive before mixing with the lymphocytes by irradiation or the use of drugs (mitomycin C). If the lymphocytes respond to the stimulatory cells they will undergo blast transformation and cell division and incorporate the radiolabelled nucleotide precursors (e.g. tritiated (^{3}H-) thymidine) into their newly synthesized DNA, which is detected by measuring the disintegrations emitted per unit time in a beta counter. Detection of the earliest responses in T cell responses, namely the detection of specific T cells responding to peptide–MHC complexes, was revolutionized in the mid 1990s with the emergence of MHC tetramer technology (see below).
2) The responding T lymphocytes may secrete IL-2 or interferon-gamma (IFN-γ) which can be measured by ELISA, RIA, or bioassays in which known *in vitro* cell lines (Jurkat) respond to the addition of cytokines by growth and proliferation. Flow cytometry techniques using permeabilized and subsequently fixed cells together with anticytokine MABs have proved useful for demonstrating intracellular cytokines. This complements the ELISA and other bioassays which ultimately demonstrate the secretion and function of the cytokine.

3) Responding T cells can be documented by their expression of activation markers CD69, CD25, or HLA-DR molecules. These can be quantitated by direct or indirect immunocytochemical methods, manually or (much more commonly and rigorously) by flow cytometry.
4) The mitotic events of the responding T cells can be documented by counting the exponential increase in cells, or by radioactive tracing of incorporated isotopically labelled DNA precursor molecules. These approaches are commonly employed in the MLR test, where inactivated (irradiated or pretreated with mitomycin C) donor blood lymphocytes are incubated with normal recipient blood lymphocytes. If the recipient's cells possess significant anti-donor cell reactivity it is demonstrated by increased cell uptake of ^{3}H-thymidine and/or increased cell mitosis. Such a positive MLR would tend to indicate a heightened probability of graft rejection *in vivo*. A variant of this assay is the mixed lymphocyte tumour cell reaction (MLTR), where the stimulatory cells are autologous or allogeneic tumour cells (isolated from tumours, cell lines). Flow cytometry developments using dyes such as CFSE (see 'Flow cytometry: current practice and future developments', below) have proved to be a very sensitive methodology for detection of cell mitotic events with the additional bonus of use of nonradioactive material.
5) A further assay (CML) documents the killing of viable donor stimulatory cells (labelled with chromium -51[^{51}Cr]), following incubation (4–24 hours) with recipient's lymphocytes (activated CD8^{+}T killer cells). MLR and CML are used to estimate presensitization and histocompatibility in clinical transplantation (see Chapter 3). Cellular assays are time consuming and require careful setting up with appropriate controls. Assays are usually set up in triplicates and each reaction uses the lowest number of cells, e.g. 5×10^{4} cells per well or tube in 0.2–0.5 mL of tissue culture medium. Flow cytometric methods are now adding to or superseding some of these assays, avoiding the use of radioisotopes.
6) Major histocompatability complex (MHC) tetramer technology was developed in the mid 1990s [3]. It has allowed the enumeration, initially of antigen/peptide-specific CD8^{+} T cells and subsequently, CD4^{+} T cells, responding to peptide/antigen complexed to HLA class I and II molecules, respectively. MHC tetramers are generated *in vitro* as complexes of four genetically engineered MHC molecules linked with a specific peptide with a bound fluorochrome. Tetramers are used to detect specific T cells in whole blood or in partially purified peripheral blood lymphocytes (PBLs) by flow cytometry (see Chapter 4). The technology has now extended to using CD1d tetramers to detect cells such as the subsets of NK T cells. The technology has been used to precisely monitor specific CD8^{+} T cell responses in infections associated with HIV, Epstein–Barr virus (EBV), cytomegalovirus (CMV), and other viruses. Detection of specific CD8^{+} and CD4^{+} T cells in cancer, autoimmune diseases, and transplantation rejection can be readily obtained using MHC tetramers. This technology has proven to be highly specific and sensitive, e.g. detecting down to 1 in 5000 specific CD8^{+} T cells in whole blood [4]. MHC tetramer technology is being used to define and monitor individuals being vaccinated with respect to specific T cell

responses. This technology has revolutionized our capacity to identify specific T cells recognizing precise peptide–HLA complexes.

In vitro, the possible antitumour cell killing abilities of innate immune mononuclear cells (Chapter 1) can be documented by cytotoxicity assays, using well-defined target cell lines. Human NK cell activity is demonstrated using the target cell line K562; LAK cell killing is monitored using the Daudi cell line, which is resistant to NK lytic activity. When LAK activity is present, then killing of both K562 and Daudi is clearly demonstrable.

The target cells, which are in suspension, are labelled with ^{51}Cr and incubated with the test effector mononuclear cells at defined target/effector cell ratios. Centrifugation before incubation at 37 °C for 4 hours ensures intimate contact and subsequent interaction following the incubation; culture supernatants are collected and isotope emission (^{51}Cr) is measured in a gamma counter. The ^{51}Cr, which labels the cytosol proteins in the living cells is released into the supernatant following cell membrane damage and osmotic lysis of target cells. Thus, counts of radioactivity in the supernatant and the target cells, relative to various controls, give a measure of the effector cell cytoxicity. *In vitro* LAK activity can be generated by incubating NK cells, or mononuclear cell preparations, with IL-2 for 2–3 days. Certain MABs (CD16 and CD56), are used in immunocytochemical assays to phenotypically define and quantitate NK and LAK cells (which are $CD3^-$, $CD56^+$, $CD16^+$). Flow cytometric analyses for perforin (damage and pore formation in cells) and granzyme (lytic granules released into cells through pores and causing intracellular damage) for documenting these cell cytotoxic functions are replacing radio-isotope-based methods with the attendant advantages.

In vivo assays of CMI–DTH skin test

Injection of standard 'recall' antigens (i.e. antigens to which an individual has been exposed to in the past and therefore possesses the appropriate memory T cells) into the dermal layers of the skin results in activation of the specific memory T cells, secretion of cytokines, and attraction of other T lymphocytes and macrophages–monocytes into the skin site, resulting in a classical DTH skin reaction. The latter consists of redness, oedema, and swelling, of variable size, some 48–72 hours after antigen injection. This test gives an overall analysis of an individual's T cell immune competence, i.e. from the earliest TCR–antigen recognition to the generation of the effector cells and associated reactions. Commercial preparations of sterile 'recall' antigens, derived from microbial extracts—mumps virus, antigens of streptococci (streptokinase/streptodornase), and antigens of fungi (*Candida, Trichophyton*)—are employed at standard doses. The antigens and controls are injected intradermally (e.g. 0.1 mL of a defined preparation into the injection sites) or applied using multiple small puncture needles and are read at 48–72 hours to document the extent of the characteristic erythematous–indurated lesion.

Assessment of neutrophils and monocytes

Assays of phagocyte cell function

Phagocytic cells (neutrophil polymorphs and mononuclear phagocytes) play crucial roles in the engulfment and killing of bacteria and fungi and in the removal of damaged tissue within the body (see Chapter 1). In order to do this, they must be able to locate, recognize, ingest, and subsequently destroy/digest the offending pathogens via the action of lysosomal enzymes. A key event for phagocyte function is for the cells to move from the intravascular site via selectin and integrin interactions, which allows the cells to bind to the endothelium and then to leave the vessel to localize at the site of microbial invasion.

Defects in the phagocytic ability of patients' cells or in the capacity of patients' sera to facilitate the opsonization of particles via complement, can be examined in 'crossover' studies. In these assays, the cells are incubated with particles, such as yeast cells, which activate the alternative complement pathway directly. Suitable phagocytic particles include latex beads, or RBCs coated with immunoglobulin with or without complement components; yeasts; or bacteria. Following incubation and ingestion the cells are usually fixed and stained to optimize counting.

Primary immune deficiencies, associated with genetic mutations of molecules involved in cell adhesion, have been described, in particular, the so-called leucocyte adhesion deficiency syndromes (see Chapter 1). A simple test that aids in the diagnosis of this defect in phagocyte function is to use phenotypic cell marker analysis for the expression of integrin molecules, such as CD18, by flow cytometry. Other primary genetic deficiencies of phagocyte cell functions are relatively rare. Included in this category is chronic granulomatous disease (CGD), in which there is defective intracellular killing of (otherwise normally) engulfed bacteria or fungi, due to failure of the cells to produce reactive oxygen intermediates. Another rare disease is Chediak–Higashi syndrome, in which lysosomal abnormalities within phagocytes predispose to pyogenic infections which can prove fatal. A disease called 'lazy leucocyte syndrome' is characterized by defective neutrophil chemotactic responses.

More common than rare primary genetic phagocyte diseases are secondary defects in phagocyte function, which may result from infection, malnutrition, burns, or trauma (see Chapters 2, 5, and 6). It should also be noted that deficient phagocyte function *in vivo* may be a consequence of defective production and inadequate levels of opsonins. These latter molecules bind to particles to be phagocytosed and to receptors on phagocytic cells, thereby acting as a bridge between the two (e.g. IgG, C3b, and C-reactive protein).

Absolute numbers of circulating neutrophils and monocytes are readily determined from total and differential white blood cell counts. As with tests of T CMI, assays of phagocytic cell function are in general difficult to perform and labour-intensive. Like the former assays, they should be done only if the clinical features indicate immune deficiency. Neutrophils are separated from anticoagulated whole blood by centrifuging on Ficoll-Hypaque; they are obtained from the centrifuged pellet (RBCs and granulocytes) after hypo-osmotic lysis of the erythrocytes and removal of the RBC ghosts. Monocytes, on the other hand, are separated from lymphocytes, both isolated at the Ficoll–plasma interface, by their capacity to adhere to glass or plastic surfaces from which the latter can be subsequently removed. Sophisticated flow cytometry (see 'Flow cytometry: current practice and future developments', below) with the ability to analyse, sort, and collect different cell populations from whole blood, has made cellular assays much more amenable to analysis.

Assays of chemotaxis

The capacity of a patient's neutrophils or monocytes to respond to standard chemotactic stimuli (e.g. casein, or the synthetic peptide f-Met-Leu-Phe) can be determined by placing the cells suspended in medium on one side of a chamber ('Boyden' chamber) separated by a thin membrane (either polycarbonate or nitrocellulose membranes may be used) from the medium containing the chemotactic stimulus (Figure 9.5). After incubation at 37° C for 1–3 hours, the membrane is stained and examined microscopically to establish the extent of cell migration (distance migrated or number of cells reaching the lower surface) towards the chemoattractant. Incorporation of normal control standards is essential in all these cellular assays.

Killing of bacteria

Standard assays of intracellular killing (e.g. *Staphylococcus aureus*) involve incubation of the cells with live organisms followed by removal of noningested bacteria by centrifugation, then release (by osmotic lysis of the phagocytes) and subsequent culture of the viable organisms. The number of viable organisms is related inversely to the extent of intracellular killing.

Particle ingestion by phagocytic cells induces a respiratory burst which can be quantified by the intracellular reduction of yellow nitroblue tetrazolium (NBT) dye to insoluble blue crystals which can be counted under the light microscope or extracted and quantified spectrophotometrically. A widely available screening test which assesses total function is the *activated NBT test*, in which phagocytes are first primed with a standard amount of bacterial endotoxin. These assays for metabolic functions of phagocytes are now routinely analysed using flow cytometry (with dyes such as dihydrorhodamine) which can define the defects qualitatively and, importantly, also quantitatively. The latter is important when family studies for carrier status are under investigation in genetic diseases such as CGD.

Humoral immunity

Qualitative and quantitative immunoglobulin assays

The detection, analysis, and measurement of immunoglobulins present in plasma or other body fluids depend on their physicochemical and immunochemical properties as proteins. Immunoglobulin (Ig) abnormalities *per se*, or more commonly, other pathological conditions affecting the cells (plasma cells) that produce Igs, occur in a variety of conditions including immunodeficiency states, infections, lymphoproliferative disorders, liver disease, autoimmune disorders, and chronic inflammation. Detectable abnormalities of Igs include the following:

- Absolute increase/decrease in the concentration of one of the five Ig classes
- Excessive production of a homogeneous (monoclonal) Ig (which may indicate multiple myeloma)
- Excessive production of free Ig light chains (κ, λ, or both)
- Increased production of polymeric Igs
- Production of 'cryoglobulins'—Igs or other serum proteins which come out of solution at temperatures below 37° C.

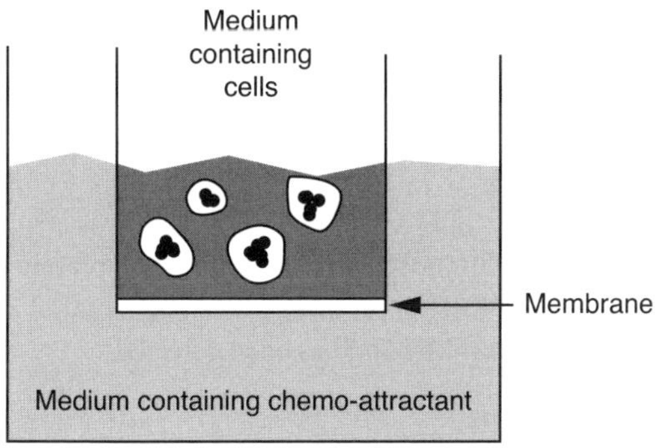

Fig. 9.5 Schematic diagram of chamber used for testing neutrophil or monocyte chemoattractant ability.

Qualitative investigations

The initial screening test of fresh sera for possible Ig abnormalities is *serum protein electrophoresis*, which is usually conducted using a cellulose acetate membrane ('strip') as the support medium. A normal serum sample is always run under the same conditions. Following the deposition of samples at the cathodal end of the membrane and the application of an electric current for 45 minutes, the membrane is removed from the electrophoresis tank and the protein bands visualized using an appropriate dye, e.g. Coomassie blue or nigrosin. Normal serum separates into prealbumin, albumin, and five globulin bands, the most cathodal of which is the broad gamma (γ)-globulin band formed by the Igs. The principal value of this screening test is in the detection of excessive production of homogeneous Ig, which is visualized by discrete monoclonal bands (M-bands), usually in the γ-globulin region. Whenever the M-band is detected or suspected, the serum is subjected to *immunoelectrophoresis* to ascertain the monoclonal nature of the Ig. The principle of this test is similar to serum protein electrophoresis, but agar gel is used as the support medium and serum is placed in wells punched in the agar. Following electrophoretic separation of the proteins, troughs are carefully cut between the wells, parallel to the axis of migration, and filled with antisera specific to the Ig classes or light chain (κ or λ) isotypes. Proteins reacting with these antisera are precipitated (after 12–24 hours) within the agar, and subsequently stained; nonprecipitated proteins are removed by washing.

An alternative approach to the typing of monoclonal Igs, which has the advantage of speed and sensitivity, is *immunofixation*. In this assay, membranes presoaked in specific antisera are overlaid onto the electrophoresed sample (cellulose acetate or agar gel) with protein precipitation (immunofixation) occurring within 2 hours. Whenever serum cryoglobulins are suspected, blood sampling, clotting, and serum separation must take place at 37°C. Thereafter, the serum is maintained at 4°C for 24–48 hours, after which any resulting precipitate is centrifuged and washed at 4°C. Redissolving of the precipitate (at 37°C) is followed by immunoelectrophoresis or immunofixation. Cryoglobulins may be monoclonal (myeloma) or mixed macroglobulin proteins (usually IgM–IgG complexes) associated in the latter instance with chronic inflammatory or autoimmune diseases.

Minute free quantities of Ig light chains are present in the urine of all normal individuals. Abnormal levels of heterogeneous free light chains are encountered in conditions associated with increased Ig production, whereas free monoclonal light chains (Bence Jones proteins) are encountered in cases of myelomatosis. Routine investigation of suspected Bence Jones proteins first requires concentration of the urine (e.g. by ultrafiltration), followed by cellulose acetate electrophoresis and then immunoelectrophoresis or immunofixation to confirm the presence of either monoclonal κ or λ free light chains. Analysis of urine is deemed essential in myeloma and in any other condition in which an M-band has been detected.

Quantitative investigations

Measurements of serum Igs are essential in cases of suspected immune deficiency, in patients with severe or repeated infections, and in lymphoproliferative disease. They may also prove helpful in the diagnosis of a variety of other conditions, including liver disease and autoimmune disorders. Each laboratory establishes its own normal population ranges, according to in-house methods and standards. The basis of the most convenient and commonly used assay (single radial immunodiffusion) is immunoprecipitation, i.e. the formation of precipitates when antigen (Ig) and appropriate precipitating antibody are present in optimal proportions.

In the single radial immunodiffusion assay, precipitating (usually polyclonal) antibody directed specifically against the heavy chain of the Ig class to be measured is mixed with molten agar and the resulting mixture poured on to a glass or plastic plate. After the agar gel has set, a series of holes is punched in it to which samples of test or control serums (or other body fluids) are added. Commercial plates based on this principle for the measurement of either Igs or certain complement components (e.g. C3, C4), are readily available.

As the antigen (Ig) diffuses radially from the well, a precipitin ring or 'halo' is formed at the distance where optimal proportions of antigen and antibody are achieved. The concentration of antigen is directly related to the square of the ring diameter. Unknown samples are determined by reference to a calibration curve constructed using three reference antigen standards. This method is convenient for small numbers of samples and is comparatively sensitive and reliable, although results are not usually read before 48 hours.

Functional antibody tests

Testing for functional antibodies (FABs) against defined microbial antigens is an important assay in the investigation of patients with suspected immune deficiency. FABs are detected by ELISA-based assays looking for preformed antibodies which reflect the individual's encounter with antigens or appropriate vaccinations in the past. In some clinical situations patients are immunized with microbial antigens (these are nonviable, nonreplicating vaccines). The individual's responses are analysed some 3–4 weeks after immunization, reflecting the time required to develop a good adaptive immune response. Testing for antibody function is important for suspected primary or secondary immune deficiencies. The importance of FABs has become even more apparent when it is realized that certain individuals, who have normal levels of serum Igs (measured as proteins), actually lack the ability to produce specific antibodies. This is apparent when these individuals are immunized and tested for antibody production. The antibodies commonly tested for are those to pneumococcal antigens, *Haemophilus influenza* type B (Hib), and tetanus toxoid. Specific antiviral antibodies can also be investigated. When patients are immunized to detect their immune responsiveness or function, their pre- and postimmunization blood samples are ascertained in the same assay.

Tests for FABs can be variable and lack some of the precision found with other immunological assays. Difficulties that arise include the definition of what is considered a protective level of antibodies. Also, there are other technical issues which require that FAB testing must be done as part of a good quality assurance scheme and utilizing national/international agreed standards.

Antibodies to microorganisms

Detection of antimicrobial antibodies is used in the diagnosis of infection, in the investigation of immune deficiency (as above) and in determining the response to vaccination with microorganisms (e.g. polio virus) or their products (e.g. tetanus toxoid). With respect to bacterial infections, the main immunological techniques for antibody detection are: (1) direct or indirect (Coombs) agglutination of suspensions of bacteria; (2) precipitation of soluble antigen by antibody in agar; (3) complement fixation, using rabbit antibody-coated sheep RBCs as the indicator system—absence of haemolysis indicates complement fixation, due to an initial reaction of antibody in the patient's serum with the original (bacterial) antigen; (4) immunofluorescence—reaction of serum antibody with the antigen (organism) in smears is detected by a fluorescein-labelled anti-human Ig antibody using UV microscopy; (5) RIA or ELISA—antibody in patient's serum is detected by binding of anti-human Ig labelled with either a radio-isotope (most often ^{125}I) or an enzyme (e.g. horseradish peroxidase or alkaline phosphatase) which produces a colour change in the presence of the appropriate substrate (see 'Immunohistochemical techniques', above).

A similar spectrum of assays (3–5 above) is available for serological detection of virus-specific antibodies. More sensitive assays, such as RIA and ELISA, especially those which detect virus-specific IgM, are replacing the classical complement fixation test. In addition, antibodies to the many viruses which agglutinate RBCs can be detected by haemagglutination inhibition. Antiviral antibodies can also be detected by neutralization of viral cytopathic effects on cultured cells (viral neutralization test).

Antibodies to nonreplicating antigens detected in allergy

The tests used to detect and quantify antibodies to noninvasive antigens, such as grass pollen, fungal antigens, or food allergens, depend on: (1) the type of immune (hypersensitivity) reaction elicited by the antigen, and (2) the class of Ig mediating the response.

For immediate (type I) hypersensitivity (see Chapter 1) the intradermal skin prick test, performed on the forearm using a panel of allergens, is useful in establishing that an IgE-mediated response is involved and in identifying the offending allergen(s) from the antigen panel. These tests are of value in the investigation of extrinsic asthma, hay fever, and anaphylactic reactions to various substances (latex, drugs, and anaesthetics—see Chapter1). The *in vitro* test for type I reactions uses serum where levels of IgE are extremely low and antigen-specific IgE antibodies must be detected by a highly sensitive assay such as the radio-allergosorbent test (RAST). This test is identical to a standard RIA, except that the antigen (allergen) is coated on to (covalently bound) cellulose discs rather than a plate, resulting in very high sensitivity. Test serum (containing IgE antibodies) is added, then unbound protein washed away, and the bound antibody is detected by a radiolabelled anti-IgE. Other test systems use enzyme labels rather than isotopes.

Assessment of complement

Complement (C) (see Chapter 1, 'Complement system of proteins') is one of the major effector systems of innate immunity and also the system that is recruited by humoral immune reactions to deal with antigen elimination. Individuals who have defects in their complement system have various disease syndromes. Tests of complement measure the functional activity of the system using antibody-coated RBCs as targets (i.e. the antigen–antibody complex). The activated complement proteins result in the lysis of the RBCs, associated with the terminal components C8 and C9. The classical pathway of complement activation can be assessed functionally in an assay referred to as CH100 (complement haemolysis 100) test or also as CH50 (complement haemolysis 50) test. Additionally, testing for the alternative pathway of complement activation is done via an AP100 (alternate pathway 100) or an AP50 (alternate pathway 50) test. If these functional tests result in no detectable lysis of RBCs then that is indicative of a global deficiency of the complement pathway, associated with a genetic lesion in one of its components. Further analyses can be done by immunochemical measurements of all of the individual components within the complement system to precisely define the level of the deficiency. Defects in early, mid, and late components relate to various clinical diseases/syndromes (see Chapter 1).

Total functional complement activity can be detected at low level in severe immune-complex diseases, such as very active systemic lupus erythematous (SLE). It is very low, but not absent, as in the rare genetic complement deficiency disorders. ELISA and RIA assays are used for detection of complement activation products. The immunochemical measurement of C3, C4, and C1 inhibitor protein (see Chapter1) (and other components) is made possible by the use of specific antisera, using simple tests such as radial immunodiffusion or autoanalyser technology.

Assessment of cytokines

Introduction

Cytokines are key signalling molecules involved in innate and adaptive immunity. They play essential roles in the inflammatory response and are central regulators of fundamental processes such as haematopoesis and apoptosis (see Chapter 1). Assessment of cytokines is used in clinical and basic research. Currently, such analyses have a limited role in patient diagnosis and management, but they will contribute more in the clinical arena in due course.

Cytokines can be assessed at the genetic or molecular level (DNA/mRNA), as proteins intracellularly, as secreted molecules in the extracellular milieu/fluid phase, or by their binding to receptors on target cells. Cytokines can thus be assayed in the fluid phase (blood and bodily secretions, e.g. saliva, tears) and in cells or tissue samples, including biopsies or organ cultures, or within mixed populations of cells in whole blood. Cytokine assessments may be correlated with disease burden, disease activity, or response to therapy. They can be used to assess responses to vaccines or recall responses to infections. Analysis of tissue biopsies for cytokine production can delineate cells and possible hierarchies of cytokine cascades involved in disease *in vivo*.

Growth in knowledge of the functions of T and B lymphocytes and their subsets has been enhanced by assessment of cytokines, used in the delineation of T cell effector subsets and their contribution to disease. Thus, assessments of effector subsets such as Th1, Th2, and Th17 can be readily carried out. Analysis of cytokines in biopsy tissues from patients with autoimmune diseases or with cancer have provided vital information in guiding some immunotherapeutic strategies based upon targets that have arisen from such analyses. The use of therapeutic biologicals such as MABs and fusion proteins (see Chapter 1, 'HIV, AIDS, and the surgeon') has developed from key information obtained from assessing the *in vivo* role of cytokines. A great deal of research exploring cancer cell interactions with the cellular microenvironment is using assessment of *in situ* cytokine production. Along with the assessment of cytokines it is also important to test for cytokine receptors, which may be cell-associated or detected as shed proteins in the fluid phase. Such receptor analyses also inform pathophysiological understanding of diseases.

Cytokine assays

There are many types of cytokine assays, all with their various strengths and weaknesses. Common assays in use include the following:

- Measurement of soluble cytokine or cytokine receptors in blood and other body fluids or in culture supernatants. These assays most often use anticytokine antibodies (polyclonals or monoclonals), ensuring high specificity and high sensitivity. Common assays are based on ELISA and RIA techniques. These assays measure cytokines or their receptors as proteins, but do not provide information about their biological functions. Competing molecules in the solutions or on cells associated with the fluid may have anticytokine actions which may, in part, confound the true titres of the cytokine detected in solution. Recently, cytokine assays based on capture antibodies immobilized on beads or microarrays are coming into use (see 'Antibodies and protein microarrays', below). These methods have the advantage of working with small sample volumes, and allow multiple cytokines to be detected simultaneously.
- Bioassays complement the deficiencies of the ELISA and RIA systems. They mainly consist of cell lines which express receptors for the cytokine being assessed. On binding the cytokine the cell line will undergo functional activities indicative of binding, signalling, and cellular genetic and biological responses (proliferation, activation, etc.). A well used bioassay is for IL-2, which binds to the cell line CTLL-2.

The binding induces cell activation and proliferation, which can be monitored by radio-isotope techniques or by flow cytometric analysis. However, bioassays lack precise molecular specificity (this is inferred). On the other hand, antibody inhibition studies can be used to define the specificity of the interaction of the cytokine with the cell and its receptor. Bioassays of many cytokines are more complex than their antibody-based counterparts, requiring the maintenance of many cell lines and constant monitoring to ensure that these lines maintain their fidelity.

- Cytokine production by populations of cells (e.g. B cells, T cells, monocytes, etc.), due to either constitutive or stimulated production of cytokines, can be sensitively and specifically assessed by multiparametric flow cytometry (see below). Stimulated or constitutively produced cytokines can be retained within the cell by agents such as brefeldin A, which block secretion without affecting synthesis of the cytokine. Detection of the cytokine will require cell fixation and permeabilization as a prerequisite for intracellular cytokine analysis. Alternatively, secreted cytokines can be captured at the surface of the secreting cell, allowing identification and separation of viable cytokine secreting cells. Also, the secreted cytokines may be captured by immobilized antibodies on a surface and visualized by enzyme-linked antibodies in ELISPOT assays (see below). These techniques demonstrate the cytokine *in situ* as a protein but do not describe its biological activity.
- Molecular techniques using real time reverse transcriptase-polymerase chain reaction (RT-PCR) and mRNA-based extraction techniques can be used to evaluate cytokines in tissues or from defined cell populations. *In situ* hybridization techniques are used to define the tissue or cellular origin of cytokine-producing cells. Less sensitive antibody-based immunocytochemical stains can also demonstrate cytokine production and intracellular sources within tissue specimens. These molecular and antibody assays do not inform on cytokine secretion, binding, or biological activity.

Thus, all of the major cytokine assays have their strengths and weaknesses. Depending on the investigation or research questions being asked, more than one type of assay may be required. Researchers will often choose complementary assays. Problems associated with inherent differences in the levels of cytokines produced by cells may dictate, in the main, the assay to be used. For instance, detection of abundant IL-2 produced by immune T cells contrasts with much lower levels of the production of IL-4 or IL-17 produced by different T cell subsets. The sensitivity of the assays may dictate which is best for specific cytokines in particular situations.

Recent developments in cytokine assessment have tried to address the problem of analysis of the complex mixture of cytokines that are produced *in vivo* and at the site of disease expression. Two important assays should be noted:

1) The use of *microarray systems*, sometimes called *biochip arrays* (see 'Multiplex and planar assays', below): These technologies may be DNA-based, protein, or antibody arrays. This system enables the simultaneous assessment of multiple cytokines (e.g. 12–20 different cytokines) from a single patient sample. This global analysis provides greater insight into physiological and pathologically relevant processes such as the balance of proinflammatory (IL-1, IL-6, TNF-α) versus anti-inflammatory (IL-10, TGF-β) cytokines in a disease process. Such information may inform therapeutic

strategies and also give far greater insights into the complexity of the disease process.

2) The use of *ELISPOT* assays: These assays have been used for some time in basic research. They usually combine prior cell stimulation before assessment of cytokine production. ELISPOT allows assessment of cytokines produced by single cells secreted in the vicinity of the cell. The assays are usually interpreted in semi-solid media or on fixed postassay membranes. ELISPOT is being used in clinical practice, for instance to assay a subject's immunity or response to bacteria (e.g. mycobacteria). The patient's mononuclear cells, including antigen-presenting cells (APCs) and T cells, can be pulsed with antigen extracts of microbes, which when properly presented by the APCs, stimulate the primed T cells to produce the cytokines. In the case of mycobacterial antigens, IFN-γ is a key signature molecule which is secreted by and is located in the vicinity of the cytokine-producing T cells in the assay medium. The presence of the secreted IFN-γ is demonstrated by the use of labelled anti-IFN-γ antibodies. The reaction site is seen as a spot on a membrane. ELISPOT assays are also used in vaccine studies to monitor responses.

In the field of clinical immunology the only routine mandatory use of cytokine and/or cytokine receptor assessment is in the investigation of patients with possible deficiency of IL-12/IL-23/IFN-γ cytokine and/or cytokine receptor abnormalities. Patients with nonfunctional mutations in these molecules are prone to serious recurrent or persistent infections with intracellular microbes (see Chapter 1). Assessment of patients' immunity or current infection status with mycobacterial organisms is being explored by use of commercially available ELISPOT assays. Initial clinical data suggests such testing may supplant the Mantoux skin test in some situations. The assay is also being used to evaluate patients receiving biological immunotherapies (e.g. for rheumatoid arthritis and other disorders), particularly using anti-TNF MABs. Such patients are now known to have an increased risk of developing mycobacterial infection (new or reactivated). Beyond these limited clinical applications, the assessment of cytokines remains predominantly in the realm of clinical or basic research.

Flow cytometry: current practice and future developments

Flow cytometry is a widely used methodology in immunology, but also has many applications in other fields, especially cell biology. The principle of the approach is to analyse single cells using fluorescent labels or probes. By performing this analysis on large numbers of cells rapidly in a flow system, it becomes possible to characterize complex heterogeneous cell populations. The presentation of each individual cell for analysis is achieved by a fluidic system, in which the suspension of cells to be analysed is injected into the centre of a constant laminar stream of sheath fluid, which draws the sample down into a narrower and narrower stream, until the width of the sample stream is similar to the cell diameter. In this way, cells can be passed individually through a specific point. In the design illustrated in Figure 9.6, this interrogation point is within a quartz flow cell; in other designs, the cells are interrogated as the stream emerges from a fine nozzle tip. This continuous flow of cells can be very rapid, allowing thousands of individual cells to be analysed per second.

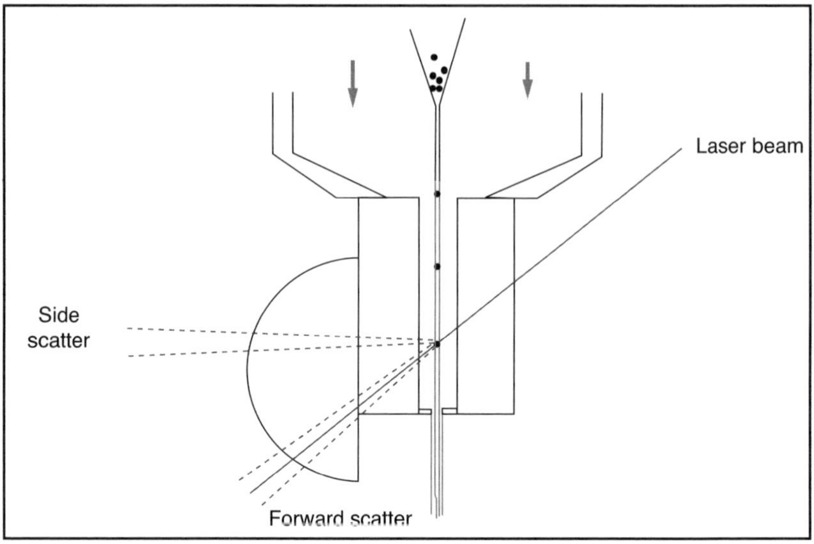

Fig. 9.6 An example of a flow cytometer flow cell analysis (see text for details of technique).

Interrogation of the individual cells requires a very bright, focused, and preferably monochromatic light source. In almost all flow cytometers, this is achieved using a laser. The most commonly used laser in flow cytometry is an argon ion laser, which produces a strong blue output at 488 nm. Interestingly, important information can be obtained about each cell from the blue light that simply bounces off it. This scattered blue light is usually measured in the same direction as the laser (forward or narrow angle scatter), and at a wide angle to the laser (side scatter or 90° scatter), as shown in Figure 9.7. Forward scatter is strongly related to cell size, whereas side scatter is strongly influenced by intracellular structures.

The blue laser light also excites fluorescence, e.g. the green fluorescence of fluorescein, and this label was the first to be used extensively in immunology. Antibodies can be labelled with fluorescein using its isothiocyanate derivative (FITC), and the binding of the FITC-labelled antibody detected by the green fluorescence stimulated by the blue laser light. This fluorescence is captured electronically by a photomultiplier tube, which converts the flash of green light emitted by a FITC-labelled cell as it passes through the laser beam into an electrical pulse. The size of this pulse is proportional to the total amount of fluorescein on that particular cell. This information is captured by converting the electrical pulse from the photomultiplier tube into digital form (analogue to digital conversion), so that it can be recorded in a computer file.

The flow cytometer does not just measure the green fluorescence of fluorescein. Over the years, various fluorochromes suitable for labelling antibodies have been developed. In parallel, there has been an ever-increasing diversity of MABs available for use as probes, and the capacity of computer systems to capture and store the data generated. The great benefit of flow cytometry comes from measuring each of these

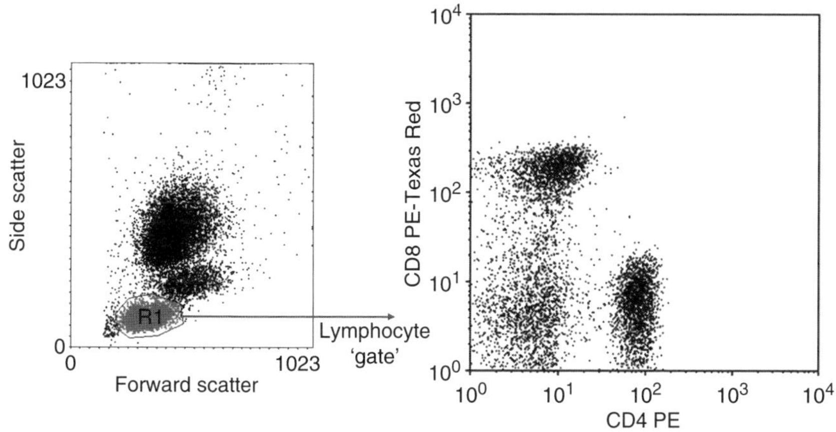

Fig. 9.7 Analysis of human peripheral blood leucocytes. Forward scatter (FS lin) and side scatter (SS lin) allows identification of the main leucocyte subsets. An example of 'gating' is shown, where the distribution of CD4 and CD8 staining is shown only for cells in the R1 region, defined as the lymphocyte gate (see also colour plate section).

fluorescent labels independently, as well as the scattered blue light referred to above. This is achieved by splitting the light that each cell emits as it passes through the laser beam into its constituent colours, and measuring each with its own photomultiplier tube. This light splitting is performed by an array of dichroic mirrors, each of which is designed to reflect or transmit light in specific wavelength ranges, together with band-pass filters, which exclude residual light of the 'wrong' colour.

A fluorochrome that is widely used is phycoerythrin (PE), a protein derived from marine algae—one of many energy-capturing algae proteins called phycobilirubins. PE is excited by blue light and emits yellow/green fluorescence, well separated from that of fluorescein. Additional fluorochromes, preferably with longer Stokes shift (the difference between excitation and emission wavelengths), have been introduced with what are known as *tandem conjugates*. This approach takes a protein fluorochrome such as PE, and links to it a second small-molecule fluorochrome, such as Texas Red. The effect of this is that the energy of the blue light absorbed by the PE is not emitted as yellow/green fluorescence, but is passed on to the Texas Red, which emits it as longer-wavelength (orange) fluorescence. This PE–Texas Red tandem is also known as ECD. Other tandem conjugates of PE with Cy5 and Cy7 are in wide use, with fluorescences in the deep red and infrared respectively. The range of available fluorochromes has also been increased by using additional lasers on the flow cytometer. Probably the next most common flow cytometer laser is the red (633 nm) helium/neon laser, which excites a range of both small-molecule fluorochromes (e.g. Alexa647) and phycobilirubins such as allophycocyanin (APPC), which is also used to make tandem fluorochromes such as APPC-Cy7.

In order to display and analyse the information recorded for each cell in a complex population, the data can be plotted in a variety of formats. The simplest is known as a *single-parameter histogram*, where the distribution of one of the measured fluorescence values is plotted. More information is displayed by *dual-parameter plots*, most commonly the *dotplot* (Figure 9.7). Although these plots show the coexpression of two measurements, further strategies are required to explore the relationships between multiple measurements made on each cell. Most flow cytometers allow the measurement of at least two scatter parameters and 5 colours, with the most sophisticated allowing many more (up to 18 colours). The simplest approach to this problem is to use 'gating' to define a cell population of interest by employing forward and side scatter (a lymphocyte gate is shown in Figure 9.7). The subsequent plot of other measurements (in this case CD4 and CD8 antibody staining) only includes cells with the defined scatter characteristics of lymphocytes.

Information gained by multiparameter analysis demonstrates that there are lymphocyte populations expressing CD4 only, CD8 only, and neither CD4 nor CD8, but almost no cells expressing both CD4 and CD8. Gating is not restricted to scatter parameters, and gates can be combined, so that for example in Figure 9.7, a further gate could be defined by a region surrounding the $CD4^+$ cells, and a further plot of measurements made in other colours could then be gated on both the 'lymphocyte' and 'CD4' gates.

Some flow cytometers are equipped to sort individual cells using criteria derived from the analysis. This is achieved by breaking the fluid emerging from the flow cell into reproducible droplets using an ultrasonic vibrating transducer attached to the flow cell. If a cell passing through the laser meets set sort criteria, then at the critical moment when the drop of fluid that contains that cell is about to break off from the stream, the stream is momentarily charged, so that the drop containing the selected cell is charged. This charged drop is then deflected by charged plates, and may be collected in a tube. Positive or negative charge may be applied to the stream, allowing two selected subpopulations to be sorted simultaneously. The sorting may also be programmed to put specific numbers of selected cells into the wells of microplates. The whole procedure may be done under aseptic conditions, allowing the selected cells to be cultured in further experiments. The speed of this process is determined by the rate at which drops can be generated from the stream. In many sorters this is 20 000–30 000 per second, allowing sort rates of around 5000 cells/second.

Measuring cell surface antigen expression, which allows the enumeration of important lymphocyte subsets, is an important application of flow cytometry, exemplified by the determination of absolute $CD4^+$ T cell counts in HIV infection. However, other flow cytometric methodologies have become widely used, including the analysis of cell proliferation by dye dilution, and intracellular cytokine analysis.

The principle of *dye dilution analysis* is that cells are labelled at the beginning of the experiment with a fluorescent label that binds irreversibly to long-lived proteins in the cell. If the cell does not divide, the fluorescence will remain bright. If the cell does divide, the fluorescent label will be distributed between the daughter cells, each having half the fluorescence of the parent. This process continues, with cells that have divided twice having a quarter of the fluorescence of the parent cell, three divisions giving one eight of the fluorescence, and so on. These populations of dividing cells with successively halving fluorescence levels can be identified on the flow cytometer, as illustrated in Figure 9.8. The fluorescent label that has been used most extensively for dye dilution

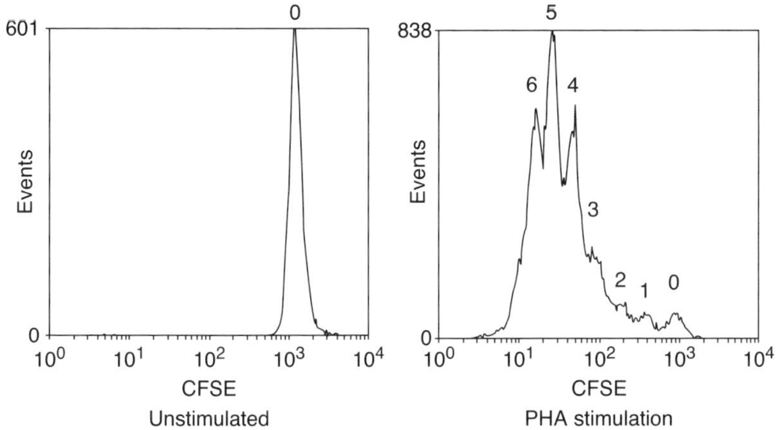

Fig. 9.8 An example of proliferation by dye dilution, using cells labelled with carboxyfluorescein diacetate succinimidal ester (CFSE). In the left panel, labelled blood mononuclear cells were cultured without stimulation, and the cells remain in a single brightly fluorescent peak. In the right panel, the cells were stimulated with phytohaemagglutinin (PHA), a plant lectin that stimulates the proliferation of the majority of the cells. Succeeding peaks of lower fluorescence reflect populations that have undergone successive cell divisions, with some cells having undergone six divisions in this example.

proliferation analysis is carboxyfluorescein diacetate succinimidal ester (CFDA-SE), often abbreviated to CFSE.

The CFSE method avoids the use of radioactive isotopes, and has the advantage that proliferation can be related to other functional and phenotypic markers measured in the flow cytometer. This is illustrated in Figure 9.9, where cells have been stimulated to proliferate using a bacterial superantigen, staph enterotoxin B. After the proliferation phase (7 days), the cells were restimulated for 4 hours in the presence of brefeldin A, then fixed, permeabilized, and stained with antibodies to INF-γ, CD69 (an early activation marker), CD4, and CD8.

Current developments are providing more powerful analysis capabilities, with the increasing availability of new fluorochromes. Analysis is being facilitated by fully digital data capture, allowing more accurate compensation spillover of fluorescence between fluorochromes. This becomes significant as more excitation wavelengths become available with developments in solid-state lasers, and fluorochromes excited by UV, violet, and green lasers are added to those excited by the conventional blue and red lasers. New fluorochromes include nanocrystals that can be tuned to emit narrow bands of fluorescence; these are excited by UV and violet lasers. A wider range of fluorescent proteins is becoming available, and these can be used to detect specific gene expression. Green fluorescent protein (GFP) was the first of these, but many variants have now been isolated giving the possibility of monitoring multiple gene activities simultaneously, at the single cell level. Green laser excitation is valuable for analysis of the longer-wavelength fluorescent proteins. When all these advances are combined, the modern flow cytometer can measure 18 colours simultaneously, and is capable of sorting cells at rates up to 70 000/second.

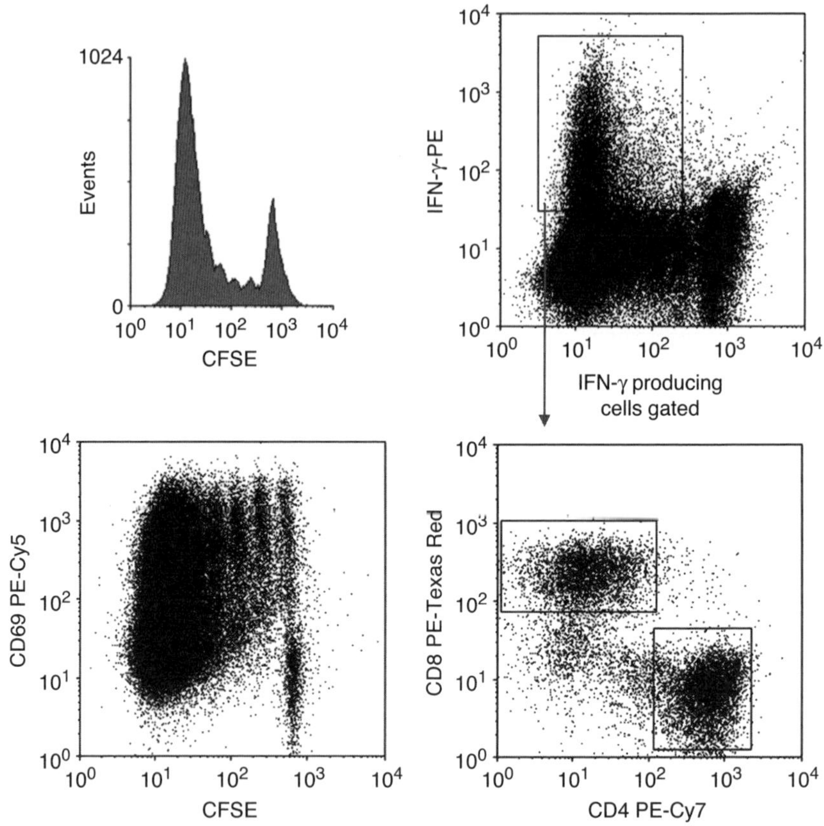

Fig. 9.9 An example of combining intracellular staining for cytokine with CFSE proliferation and cell surface markers. Gating on the interferon-producing cells that have proliferated shows that both $CD4^+$ and $CD8^+$ cells have responded. The CD69 plot shows the loss of this early activation marker as proliferation proceeds. CFSE, carboxyfluorescein diacetate succinimidal ester.

Detection of autoantibodies

Introduction

Testing for autoantibodies (see Chapter 8) is usually performed using the following assays: immunofluorescence, haemagglutination and other particle agglutination, immunodiffusion, counter immunoelectrophoresis, immunoprecipitation, immunoblotting, RIAs, and ELISA-based assays.

Immunofluorescence techniques

Direct

In this method fluorescein-conjugated antisera (anti-human Ig and complement) are added directly to surgical biopsy specimens (e.g. skin and renal biopsies), to demonstrate *in vivo* bound autoantibodies and activated or deposited complement components. Such assays are used in the differential diagnosis of skin lesions associated with autoimmune bullous skin disease and other diseases (e.g. SLE, Goodpasture's sysndrome).

Indirect

This method employs substrates (tissues) of animal or human origin which contain the relevant autoantigens. Patients' sera (primary layer in Figure 9.2) are incubated with the substrate and any circulating autoantibodies bind to their respective tissue autoantigens. Following repeated washings to remove unreacted serum proteins, the presence of bound autoantibodies is revealed by a secondary layer (Figure 9.2) consisting of serum containing fluorescein-labelled anti-human Ig. Controls (positive and negative) are included in the assays and the distribution of the staining patterns, in relation to tissue cell type and anatomic locations, is determined. For indirect methods many autoantigens, especially those associated with non-organ-specific autoimmunity (e.g. nucleic acids, smooth muscle, and mitochondrial antigens), are not species specific—hence, substrates such as rat and mouse tissues can be used. Substrates (commonly fresh material) are snap frozen in liquid nitrogen, and sectioned on cryostats resulting in optimal antigen preservation. Other autoantigens (Chapter 8), especially for organ-specific autoantibodies, are much more species specific; human surgical or early postmortem tissue, or closely related primate substrates, have to be used. The use of human tissue is highly regulated, with informed consent and robust governance procedures in place. In Europe and North America, laboratories are required by law to work to these regulations. In recent years, definition of the important autoantigens in organ-specific and systemic autoimmunity has resulted in moves away from the use of tissue substrates to ELISA-based systems, using purified or in some cases recombinant antigens.

Agglutination assays

Haemagglutination and other agglutination assays use RBCs (of various species coated with antigens) as indicator particles, to detect various autoantibodies (e.g. antithyroglobulin and microsomal antibodies) in autoimmune thyroid diseases. The antigens are chemically crosslinked to the RBC membrane. Incubation with several dilutions of the patient's serum is performed; if autoantibodies are present they induce agglutination (clumping) of the RBCs which can be readily seen in a microtitre plate. In some assays, such as the historical Rose–Waaler test for detecting classical IgM rheumatoid factor (RF), the RBCs (to which are bound subagglutinating doses of IgG anti-RBC antibodies) are used as the antigen carrier. There has been a move away from using RBCs for RF detection with the introduction of particle agglutination (e.g. using latex and gelatine) which provides more stable systems than the use of RBCs. The RF in a patient's serum interacts mainly with the Fc region of the IgG, resulting in agglutination of the red cells. As outlined in Chapter 8, testing for RF is now being superseded by ELISA-based test systems for anti-CCP antibodies, which appear to be much more informative in the diagnosis and management of rheumatoid arthritis.

In vivo generated pathological anti-RBC antibodies, as found in autoimmune haemolytic anaemias, are demonstrated by the classic direct and indirect Coombs tests.

The endpoint of haemagglutination assays can be quantified and expressed as a titre (degree of RBC lysis or particle agglutination), or with respect to national/international standards and international units. Laboratories will quote a range of values for interpreting such autoantibody assays.

ELISA assays

There is an ever-increasing use of ELISA technology for the detection of autoantibodies. These usually represent highly sensitive systems and care has to be taken to ensure they retain specificity for disease diagnosis. Increasingly, ELISAs are replacing tissue-based analysis. For instance, anti-tissue transglutaminase antibodies are replacing the use of primate tissue and/or human umbilical cord tissue in tests for coeliac disease (see Chapter 8). Other important areas for ELISA technology are the detection of various antinuclear antibodies (ANAs) and the antibodies to so-called extractable nuclear antigen and to double-stranded DNA. Other techniques used less commonly in autoantibody detection include counter immunoelectrophoresis, which is a sensitive assay used in the detailed characterization of certain autoantigens. Undoubtedly, there will soon be sensitive multiple autoantibody testing using antibody microarray systems, which should help in the clinical arena. Newer assays, based on technologies such as multiplex and planar assays, as well as refined western blotting techniques (see below), are likely to make positive contributions.

Multiplex and planar assays

Introduction

The ELISA has become a mainstay of both research and diagnostic antibody and antigen detection methods. However, the ability to scale assays or achieve multiple tests with a finite sample becomes a limiting factor, due to the reagent volumes and costs involved in performing a single assay per well of a 96-well plate, and the cost of automation to process increasing numbers of ELISA plates. The continuing and accelerating discovery of soluble biomarkers associated with complex diseases, and the desire for more informed diagnosis by examination of these markers, is driving the development of multianalyte assays. Multiplexed assays offer substantial benefits for diagnostics: multiple parameters measured per sample with lower overall sample requirements, improved scalability, and often simplified processing. The logical extension of multiplexing into the realm of antibody and protein microarrays and microfluidic devices is the automation of their processing and analysis. This is bringing the era of point-of-care diagnostics and disease screening ever nearer.

Line immunoassays

Line immunoassays (LIAs) are an established multiplexing approach for antigen, antibody and, with modification, DNA detection, offering a moderate scale of multiplexing and relatively simple processing. Detection of autoantibodies requires the purified

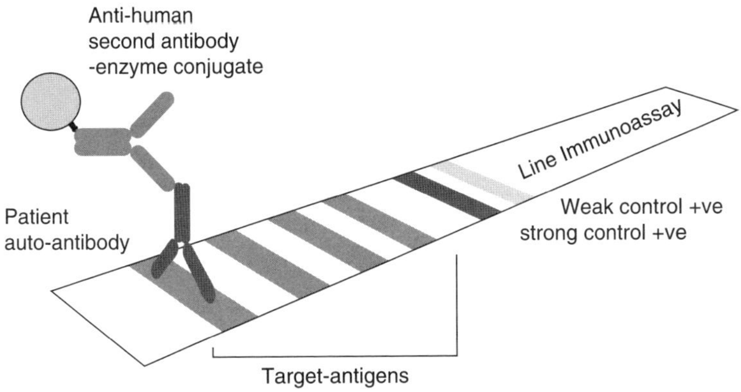

Fig. 9.10 Diagramatic representation of a multiplexing line immunoassay detecting autoantibodies. Coloured lines represent specific autoantigens applied to the assay strip. Detectable colour would only develop where antibody is bound to the surface and detected with the second antibody conjugate. Controls for patient sample addition and functioning of the detection system are also included to ensure good quality control.

or recombinant antigens to be immobilized as discrete lines across a narrow (~5 mm) strip of supporting material (usually nitrocellulose backed by a flexible plastic or glass slide). Multiple antigens and control targets can be accommodated on one strip with defined locations. The assay is then done similarly to an ELISA, by sequentially immersing and washing the strip in blocking agents, diluted patient sample, anti-human second antibody–enzyme conjugate, and finally colorimetric detection reagent (Figure 9.10). Lines detected on the strip are interpreted as specific autoantibody responses. Prime examples of such technology include LIAs for antibodies to extractable nuclear antigens (ANAs/ENAs) where 10 or more separate antigens (both nuclear and cytoplasmic) are present on one strip, spanning autoantigens associated with SLE, mixed connective tissue disease, diffuse scleroderma, polymyositis, and other autoimmune conditions (see Chapter 8).

Bead immunoassays

Bead immunoassays take multiplexed analysis to a further level of sophistication. The basic premise is similar to ELISA or LIA: immobilized antibody or antigen is used to capture cognate target from the solution phase, then the captured molecule is detected by an appropriate second antibody, usually by fluorescence for bead immunoassays. The key difference is that the solid substrate for each immobilized molecule are microscopic plastic beads (commonly 1–5 μm in size). Each bead set is specific for a single target molecule, and is differentiated by two colours of fluorescence, integral to the plastic bead. Ten levels of fluorescence intensity in each colour allows the production of a 10×10 array of fluorescently differentiated bead sets, when analysed for both fluorescent colours. Such assays are now commonly available for research use for cytokine and chemokine detection, intracellular signalling pathway analysis, etc., although routine clinical diagnostic use is still minimal.

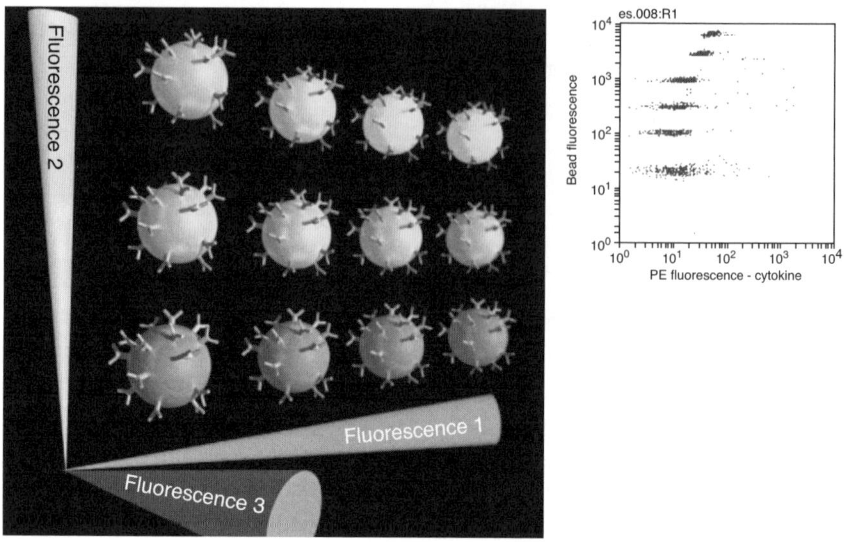

Fig. 9.11 Principle of the bead immunoassay. One bead here represents many thousands of identically coloured beads in a real assay. Each defined mixture of fluorescence 1 and 2 within a bead set allows separation of different bead sets in two dimensions. Each bead set is coated in a different specific antibody. Once target antigen is bound (not shown) a second specific antibody, labelled with fluorescence 3, is bound to each target molecule. Thus, each cluster of beads can be identified and the level of fluorescence 3 on the beads indicates the level of antigen present in the sample, which can be compared with a standard curve for quantification. The insert plot shows actual results from a 6-plex assay (see also colour plate section).

The multiplexed assay is achieved by mixing unique bead sets (~5000 or more beads per set), each coated to detect a single type of capture molecule and with defined bead fluorescence in both colours. This mixture is then added to a small sample (20–50 μL plasma or serum) and the target molecules are captured on the specific beads during incubation. After washing, a mixture of appropriate second antibodies, labelled uniformly with a third fluorescent dye, is added to the beads. Subsequently, all three fluorescence levels are measured for each bead in the mixture, giving a three-dimensional space where intensity of the first two colours separates the bead sets (and hence the specific analysis associated with each bead set) and the third colour provides quantification of the detectable signal for each assay (Figure 9.11). Acquiring many thousands of readings per bead set provides robust statistical measurements. The whole assay is performed in a 96-well plate, allowing 80 or more samples and a multiplexed standard curve per assay plate. Data acquisition through a flow cytometer or dedicated reader is essential, and often provides easy automation of the entire plate sampling process.

Multiplexed bead immunoassays are becoming more widespread for research use, and are beginning to enter the clinical diagnostics market with assays for detecting

ANA antibodies for autoimmune disease diagnosis and assays for diagnosis of antibody responses to viral pathogens such as EBV, HIV, herpes simplex virus (HSV), and mumps, measles and rubella (MMR). Issues relating to the scope of multiplexing, such as antibody cross-reactivities when extensively multiplexing in solution, limit the plexing currently available to approximately 20–30-fold antibody-based assays. Further work, identifying increasingly compatible antibody sets, will allow this limit to be extended considerably.

Antibodies and protein microarrays

Advances in robotic liquid handling technology over the past two decades present the possibility of extending the concept of the LIAs to spatially arrange many hundreds or even thousands of antibodies or antigens in regular grid patterns on a solid support. The microscopic precision of such robots generates protein spots (features) in the 50–150 μm diameter range, separated by similar distances. Thus, several hundred features can be encompassed with ease in the area of a single ELISA well, or many thousands of features on a microscope slide. A wide range of commercially available antibody and protein chips are now available for research use.

These protein microarrays have a great potential to provide a step-change in assay multiplexing and diagnostic/prognostic capabilities. For complex diseases, the analysis of many biomarkers may be required to accurately diagnose, screen, and provide therapeutic options and monitoring. The scope of target features on an array is limited only by availability of the target proteins allowing many biomarkers to be resolved. Commercial examples containing several hundred antibodies are available, and experimental microarrays containing many thousands of samples from cellular fractionations have been made to enable autoantigen discovery methods.

The quantity of antigen or antibody required to generate a feature on the array is within the 50–300 pL range, providing efficient use of resources on a scale previously unheard of.

Detection methods mirror those used for ELISAs or LIAs (colorimetric) and flow cytometry or bead immunoassays (fluorescence), but reagents are a small fraction of those used in ELISAs, minimizing assay costs. Recent application of biophysical methods, such as surface plasmon resonance (SPR), to enable detection of unlabelled interacting biomolecules on solid supports suggests that label-free detection will become an attractive detection method for such arrays. Microfluidic liquid handling techniques applied to such arrays will allow automation on unprecedented scales, while reducing operator skill levels. Point-of-care diagnostics and community screening programmes will greatly benefit from these ongoing developments.

Protein and antibody array technology has been rapidly adopted for studying cancer markers. By 2001, examples had been published demonstrating the potential of antibody arrays to identify protein expression patterns, such as those associated with oral cavity squamous cell carcinomas, profiling of TAAs, such as epidermal growth factor receptor (EGFR)/ErbB2 across tumour types, and, more recently, detection of pancreatic cancer by serum profiling [5]. Other noncancer examples include identifying biomarkers of graft-versus-host disease, serum viral antigen detection, and wide-ranging use for assessment of inflammatory cytokines and chemokines. Reverse-phase

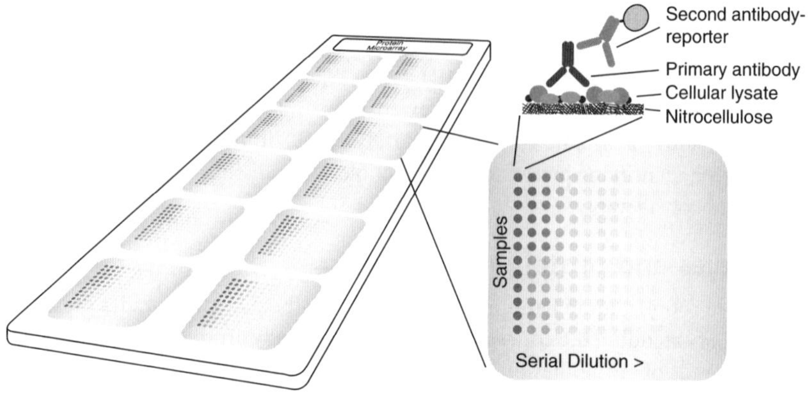

Fig. 9.12 Protein lysate array (reverse-phase protein array, RPPA) shown after development of the signal. RPPA can be used to examine samples for many proteins in both qualitative, and as shown here, quantitative applications. Serial dilutions of lysed tissue, cell, or body fluid samples, replicated on to each of the binding surfaces, are probes with well-defined antibodies to target proteins. The dilution curve obtained after detection of the bound antibody allows calculation of the level of each protein assayed within each sample.

protein arrays (Figure 9.12) have been used with similar success, including differentiation of signalling pathway alterations across cancer cell lines and cells undergoing stimulation with antigens, protein phosphorylation patterns associated with metastatic ovarian carcinoma, and mapping of the specificity of anticitrullinated protein autoantibodies in rheumatoid arthritis.

Postgenomic technologies

Introduction

The landmark publication of the sequence of the whole human genome in 2003 can be seen as heralding the postgenomic era and associated technologies to underpin the exploitation of genomic knowledge in medicine and science. Postgenomic technologies (PGTs) facilitate studies of genes and their encoded proteins in ways hitherto unknown and have driven forward significant innovation. PGTs and their influence on new research areas can be seen in a broad range of activities. These include single nucleotide polymorphism (SNP) analysis, sequencing of whole genomes of many species, bioinformatics, microarray studies, proteomics, metabolomics, pharmacogenomics and systems biology, rational drug design, population genomics using genome-wide association studies (GWASs), and gene therapy. PGTs are making major contributions to the advancement of basic scientific research. Beneficial medical outcomes are expected by way of earlier diagnosis and better tailored treatments for individual patients, together with enhancement in prediction of disease and beneficial outcomes. PGTs provide state-of-the-art tools for the analysis of complex biological systems in an integrated and more holistic manner than has previously been possible. Outlined below are some selected key PGTs, with an overview of the technological

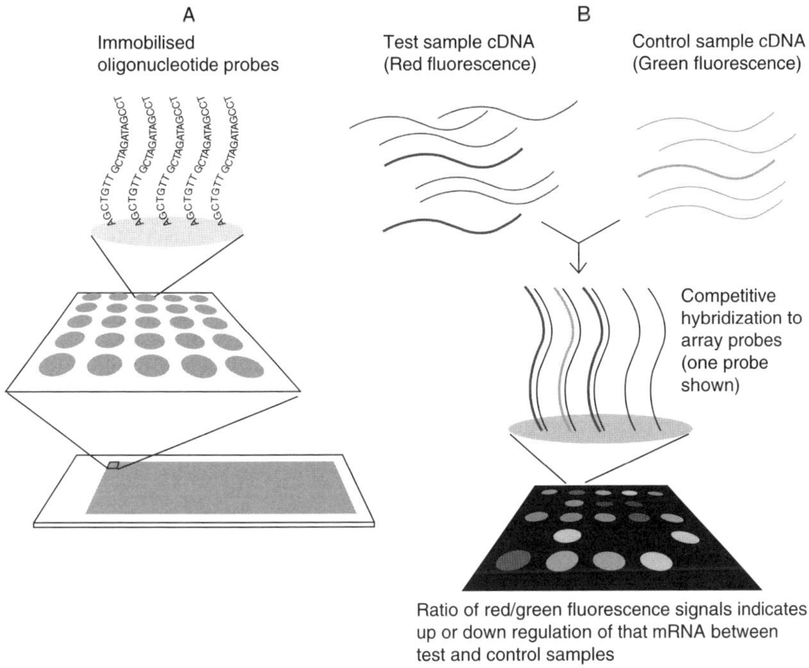

Fig. 9.13 Principle of a dual-colour comparative transcriptome analysis. (A) Gene (mRNA) specific oligonucleotide probes are arrayed in extremely dense arrays across the surface of a solid support. (B) mRNA samples from a control sample (cells or tissue) are converted to cDNA, labelled with a fluorescent dye (shown in green). Test sample cDNA is labelled with a different dye (shown in red). Hybridization of equal quantities of each sample to the array results in proportional binding of cDNAs from both samples, if present. Quantification of each fluorescence bound to a probe feature allows comparison of gene expression between the samples (see also colour plate section).

principles and their contribution to the rapidly changing and expanding areas of biomedical research.

Transcriptomics

The sequencing and analysis of the human genome has provided an unprecedented level of detail regarding both the total number of genes in the genome and the structure of these genes. This basic data has enabled existing technologies, such as oligonucleotide synthesis and microarray robotics, to be fully harnessed to study the expressed genome at the level of messenger (m)RNAs, otherwise known as the *transcriptome*. Examination of the messenger mRNA content within a cell or tissue informs, but does not categorically imply, the presence of protein for each detected expressed gene. Thus, transcriptomics or expression analysis can only give insight into yet another layer of cellular regulation, but represents a fundamentally important step forward in examining the differences between cells under a wide range of conditions.

Using oligonucleotide microarrays encompassing probes for all known and predicted genes, comprehensive screening for gene expression became a reality. From this point, comparative analyses (see Figure 9.13) have provided remarkable insight across a wide range of topics, including between normal and tumour cells, activated and quiescent cells of the immune system, cells in the presence and absence of therapeutic drugs, and developmental and differentiation stages of innumerable cell types. Increasingly, such analyses are enabling identification of new biomarkers for a host of complex diseases. So extensive are the datasets generated by transcriptome analysis that specific databases, including the Gene Expression Omnibus (Geo: NCBI, USA) and Array Express (EBI, UK), host search data from many tens of thousands of experiments.

Continued development of novel applications of DNA microarrays has provided the ability to study genes targeted by specific transcription factor binding (chromosome immunoprecipitation on a DNA chip, termed ChIP-on-Chip), translational activity of a mRNA (through examination of cellular mRNAs after fractionation by polysome loading), alternative transcript splicing analysis, and detection of both large-scale genome alterations (array-comparative genomic hybridization, CGH) and minute differences in genome sequence across populations (SNPs), which will be discussed more fully in 'Principles of newer molecular technologies and therapeutic approaches', below.

DNA sequencing technology has undergone a paradigm shift since 2005, with the introduction of multiple methodologies allowing extensively parallel DNA fragment sequencing. Reading many millions of small fragments of DNA allows for total outputs in excess of 100 Gb (10^{11} bases) per run. Such capabilities not only offer the possibility of personal genome sequencing, but transcriptome analysis of unparalleled detail.

Proteomics

Proteomics, a term first coined in the late 1990s, describes the study of proteins on a large scale and incorporates the gamut of analyses: protein structure, function, expression, regulation, degradation, modification, and interaction with both other proteins and other biomolecules. As such, proteomics is a generalized tool to discover how biological systems function, far beyond the level of the genome and transcriptome. The scope of the challenge ranges from understanding individual proteins to protein–protein interactions through to the dynamics of biological pathways, such as signalling from surface receptors, up to the interactions ongoing within whole cells and between cells and tissues. The genome map and transcriptome provide the blueprint and basic data (the sequence of every potential protein within the genome) to aid the proteomics revolution. The rapid development of protein mass spectrometry (MSpec) as a highly sensitive tool for identifying proteins provided the key methodologies of high-throughput proteomic research. MSpec for peptide identification offers, at its simplest, a means to accurately measure the mass of a peptide fragment derived from one or more proteins in a mixture. The method employed is termed MALDI-TOF (matrix-assisted, laser desorbed/ionized, time-of-flight) MSpec. Essentially, the peptides are ionized, using a laser beam to vaporize and simultaneously ionize them from a matrix material. The ionized peptides are then accelerated down a flight tube towards a mass detector. Ions travel according to their mass to charge ratio (*m/z*). Thus, with equal charge, a large ion will travel more slowly than a small ion. Although complex, the resultant data can provide accurate estimates of peptide masses.

Peptide fragments for MSpec are most often generated by purposeful digestion of the protein sample by trypsin, a protease with a very well characterized cleavage specificity (immediately C-terminal to lysine or arginine amino acids, but not if either is directly followed by proline). Thus, tryptic digestion fragments can be predicted from existing database entries for either DNA or protein sequences. This allows for the mass of the fragments to be calculated accurately (to at least two decimal places, incorporating known isotopic ratios) and provides a unique peptide 'fingerprint' for each protein. Any new peptide masses derived from a sample can thus be compared with a database of predicted tryptic fragments, and matched to existing proteins. Naturally occurring peptides present within biological fluids also offer a 'target-rich' environment for MSpec analysis, enabling the generation of peptide profiles which can be compared between samples, patients, treatments, etc., without direct need for absolute identification of the component peptide identities. Pattern recognition software can then be used to identify differences associated with the condition being studied.

In more complex forms of MSpec (termed MS-MS or tandem MSpec) the exact sequence of individual peptides within a mixture can be determined. This is achieved using instruments which can be tuned to select specific peptides from a mixture (quadrupole analysers), along with methods for randomly breaking up the peptide into smaller fragments. Linked mass analysis of these fragments in a TOF analyser allows the deduction of the original peptide sequence from the contributing subpeptides.

Proteomics research of all kinds provides many types of data which is rapidly assimilated into modern systems biology, as an integrative discipline using computational tools to build associative networks and give biological context to data spanning the 'omics'

In a clinical context, MSpec is an increasingly powerful technique. Clinical proteomics offers the potential for disease biomarker discovery, especially when allied with ever more complex molecular methodologies for separating and isolating proteins and protein complexes from biological material. Such biomarkers present exciting opportunities for enhanced diagnostic sensitivity, patient stratification, personalization of therapeutic regimens, and disease monitoring.

Metabolomics

The *metabolome* represents the entire set of small-molecule compounds, involved as intermediates in metabolic and signalling pathways, enzyme cofactors, by-products, and secondary metabolites, which are present within and released by the examined biological entity (cell or organism). Estimates of the size of the human metabolome vary widely, from several thousands to tens of thousands of diverse small molecules. The terms metabolomics, and the largely synonymous term metabonomics, refer to the comprehensive, quantitative study of this incredibly dynamic aspect of molecular biology. It could be argued that metabolomics is the most ancient of the 'omics', dating back many centuries to the examination of urine colour, smell, and taste as indicators of health and disease. Targeted analysis of specific metabolites in serum and urine is now embedded within routine clinical laboratory practice: for example, assessing liver, kidney, thyroid, and other organ function through the quantification of metabolites, breakdown products, and hormones such as creatinine, bilirubin, and thyroxine. Standard analyses currently extend to many defined small molecules associated with specific biochemical pathways.

Finding metabolic markers associated with complex diseases, such as cancer, autoimmunity, and neurological disorders, is a highly active field of study. Herein lies the challenge of comprehensive clinical diagnostic metabolomics: almost any differences between individuals in genetic make-up and environment, from diet through to exercise, trauma, drug abuse, infection, inflammation, and cancer, alter the metabolome and leave evidence within it. Identifying those changes that are of value in predicting, diagnosing, and assessing therapeutic responses for a specific clinical condition is extremely complex, as day-to-day activity of the metabolome causes significant noise within the system.

No single analysis methodology can currently encompass all metabolites, because of their extreme diversity. It is, therefore, not surprising that MSpec and nuclear magnetic resonance (NMR) spectroscopy are proving to be the most widely accepted analytical techniques for such studies. Cancer studies have swiftly taken on board these developments, with examples of multiple choline metabolites having diagnostic potential in breast, prostate, and brain tumour patients, and alterations in a variety of metabolites of amino acids, fatty acids, and other compounds being detected and reflecting tumour responses during the course of therapeutic interventions. As the metabolome is further defined, metabolic intermediates in serum, sputum, and urine may once again have us looking, albeit in a more sophisticated way, at the colour of urine to aid diagnosis and prognosis.

Principles of newer molecular technologies and therapeutic approaches

Genome-wide association studies

GWASs are the culmination of many years of work into mapping variations in the human genome [6]. The principle underlying GWASs is that variations in allele frequency for polymorphic DNA markers between patients with a specific disease or characteristic and controls will differentiate genomic locations which are influential in that disease or in those characteristics. This began with the identification of restriction fragment length polymorphisms (RFLPs) and repeated DNA sequences in the genome (minisatellites) as useful identity markers, applied in a technique termed 'DNA fingerprinting' in the early 1980s, This work was extended with great effect through population profiling with other abundant repeated short DNA sequences (microsatellites). The utility of SNPs for genetic comparison in support of disease associations was realized with the publication of the human genome in early 2003 and the discovery of approximately 1.5 million SNPs. This number now exceeds 20 million reported SNPs (dbSNP, January 2010). Individually, SNPs have a relatively low information content, each representing a change in just one base pair of DNA. However, the density of SNPs across chromosomes provides a collective information content far in excess of any other polymorphic DNA reporter. That said, many SNPs are at extremely low frequency in a population (far below 1%), or exist within recombination hotspots—in either case, limiting their utility.

SNPs are amenable to detection by many molecular methods, including DNA hybridization techniques, where individual SNPs can be differentiated on the basis of their ability to hybridize perfectly to a complementary oligonucleotide probe sequence, but not to a similar probe with the alternative SNP base complement present. As SNP numbers grow, the technology has grown accordingly to culminate in the detection of millions of SNPs on a single microarray. This has become an essential technology of GWASs, especially since current estimates suggest that 500 000 to 1 000 000 SNPs are required for comprehensive coverage by GWASs. GWASs are also highly dependent on having sufficiently large numbers (thousands) of sampled genomes, from both control and patient samples, to provide statistical rigour to the associations inferred. High-throughput methods have therefore become the norm, as has the use of highly specialized software to perform the resultant analysis.

A landmark publication, highlighting both the immediate utility and future promise of GWASs, was the result of a study from the Wellcome Trust Case Control Consortium (WTCCC) in 2007, identifying new genetic loci and confirming existing loci associated with autoimmune diseases. More recent studies, with much larger datasets from WTCCC and other consortia, have discovered loci associated with many disease states, including prostate cancer, Parkinson's disease, Crohn's disease, and Alzheimer's disease.

Bioinformatics and systems biology in medicine

The vast amount of information generated from the PGTs (see above) has driven developments in the science of bioinformatics—a science built on the application of advanced information technology and computer science to create and handle large databases and computational and statistical algorithms to manage the analysis of complex, large biological datasets. Additionally, sophisticated mathematical modelling techniques are used in theoretical systems to advance understanding and support predictive models amenable to experimentation. Bioinformatics provides the tools to enhance our understanding of biological processes [7].

Major areas of application of bioinformatics relate to gene sequences and protein alignments, prediction of gene expression, and protein structure, and also include protein–protein interactions. Bioinformatics underpins the development of systems biology which involves the integrated and holistic analysis of complex connections in cellular processes. Systems biology allows the study of dynamic networks, including signal transduction pathways, gene regulatory, and metabolic networks, all giving insights not attainable by classical reductionist science—the science that dominated 20th century biological and immunological research.

The study of interacting networks has allowed new insights (termed *emergent properties*) into diseases that hitherto were not predicted. The essential features of modern systems biology relies on quantitative and global measurements of changes in all genes, mRNA, protein, and metabolites and the integration of such data to give new insight into disease processes. Accordingly, the systems biology approach has led to interdisciplinary researchers and teams applying the approach to address problems in wide areas of medicine. Major targets include the analysis of cancer genomes, host–pathogen interactions, and GWASs of multigenic disorders (e.g. diabetes, hypertension), the aim being to achieve a better understanding of the dynamics of normal physiological and abnormal pathological processes to enhance diagnosis, therapy, and prevention of disease.

The generation of personalized genome sequences in various patient groups is envisaged as leading to better predictive individualized and preventative medical practice. Indeed, a recent published study has illustrated the usefulness of an 'integrated analysis of a complete human genome in a clinical context' [8]. New diagnostics, based on rapid analysis of multiple parameters, should enhance presymptomatic diagnosis. Additionally, patient stratification based on data from a systems approach is being used to better direct appropriate therapy; thus, personalized medicine is becoming a reality.

Drug development and molecular diagnostics are already benefiting from the application of bioinformatics and systems biology approaches. This has led to the refinement of chronic inflammatory/immune disorders (e.g. rheumatoid arthritis and SLE), cardiovascular diseases, and psychiatric disorders. Patients' susceptibility to these diseases is being better defined using GWASs and patient stratification.

Bioinformatics and systems biology has been used recently to stratify patients with rheumatoid arthritis who are being treated with the newer biologicals (e.g. anti-IL-6R MABs and CTLA4-Ig fusion proteins) (see Chapters 1 and 8). Recently, the systems biology approach, linked to extended MHC haplotypes and to increased numbers of associated SNPs, has made it possible to better tailor the use of particular biologicals in specific subsets of patients and enhance their efficacy.

Molecular diagnostic tools are already yielding clinical benefits by defining low, medium, and high risk of recurrence in certain cancers. In breast cancer such tests are already being used in clinical practice to guide treatment strategies. Another example of the benefit and potential usefulness of these technologies is full genome sequencing of individual patient's cancers. Rather than defining SNPs, researchers in the USA reported in 2010 on the usefulness of mapping an individual's genetic variations in large segments of tumour DNA associated with gene rearrangements. Such variations were shown to act as a genetic fingerprint for that individual and their particular tumour. This facilitates a highly specific biomarker to track that patient's cancer, based on the recognition that many cancers shed their genetic material into blood, which is detectable by sensitive techniques. Preliminary studies of patients with bowel and breast cancers have established that this approach is highly sensitive and exquisitely specific, providing clinically more useful information than routine imaging. This type of molecular genetic fingerprinting has been successful in the management of a limited number of leukaemias and lymphomas.

In medical science, modelling of virus–host interactions, integrated interrogation of multiple signal transduction pathways, and the sequencing of cancer genomes are already yielding findings of new genes and mechanisms associated with pathophysiological disturbances.

The advances linked to bioinformatics and systems biology in medicine will synergize with but not replace well-established clinical associations—the influence of age, gender, and environmental factors (critical factors in the development and expression of disease).

Gene therapy

Human gene therapy to correct defective genes implicated in disease development holds great promise. The precise definition of genetic mutations in a range of diseases, from common cancers to rare primary immune deficiencies and to inheritable genetic disorders, has provided the stimulus for various gene therapy approaches [9]. Methods to correct defective genes include the random insertion of a normal gene into a recipient's genome to replace the nonfunctional gene. This has been used clinically in the area of single-gene defects such as in patients with SCID (X-linked and ADA deficiency—see Chapter 1). Other, less common, gene therapy approaches have used homologous recombination, endeavouring to directly swap the abnormal gene with the therapeutic DNA in a very targeted approach. Yet other approaches have been directed at *in vivo* repair of the diseased gene through selective reverse mutation or by *in situ* regulation of gene function, using small interfering RNA constructs.

The transfer of genes has most often been done by incorporation of the therapeutic DNA into a viral vector. Viruses are exploited for their evolutionary ability to colonize the genetic apparatus of human cells. Commonly used (nonpathogenic) viral vectors include those from retroviruses, adenoviruses, and herpesvirus (see Chapter 7). Each has particular advantages for differing gene therapy protocols. Retroviruses readily copy RNA into double-stranded DNA which integrates into the chromosomes of target host cells. Adenoviruses readily infect epithelial lining cells of the respiratory and intestinal tract and other gut-associated lymphoid tissue (GALT) sites. Accordingly, adenoviral vectors were the obvious choice in attempts at gene therapy for diseases such as cystic fibrosis. Herpesvirus type 1 vectors give preferential targeting of neural tissue (the virus is neurotropic) and have been used in gene therapy studies of brain tumours. Two major gene therapy methods are considered: somatic and germ-line therapy. The former introduces the therapeutic DNA to normal body tissues and cells, whereas germ-line therapy introduces genes into sex (germ) cells capable of producing eggs or spermatozoa. By definition, germ-line therapy changes the genome and the changes are inheritable in offspring and transmittable from there onwards. Somatic gene therapy is widely supported internationally, but many countries have a moratorium on germ-line therapy. There is ongoing ethical discussion on these matters worldwide.

Clinical experience of using somatic gene therapy has had a mixed outcome since the earliest trials in the 1990s. The target diseases have been monogenic disorders and the most used vectors have been retroviral and adenoviral. Early studies treating some forms of SCID were successful and greatly celebrated. By the late 1990s, and into the early 21st century, gene therapy sustained significant setbacks, because of the death of patients or the development of unexpected disease directly attributable to the therapy. A patient participating in a gene therapy study which delivered a corrective gene in an adenoviral vector to liver cells died from multiple organ failure. This was attributed to his immune system developing an excessive response (cytokine storm) against the viral vector. Indeed, the human antiviral response has also proved problematic, though not lethal, in other studies, the immune response militating against any subsequent attempts to repeat the therapy. In some studies of somatic gene therapy, the gene is introduced into stem cells which have the ability for long-term renewal of cells expressing the corrected gene. This is not always possible, hence the need for the procedure to be repeated at various time points. However, in 2002 children with X-linked SCID, who had been treated successfully with a retroviral gene construct containing a normal common γ-chain gene, subsequently developed leukaemia-like disorders. Investigative analyses demonstrated that the random insertion into the genome of the retroviral vectors had precipitated the genetic events leading to the leukaemia; the retrovirus was inserted next to leukaemogenetic elements that switched on deleterious functions. The effect on gene therapy of these adverse events was two-fold. First, there was an agreed international moratorium for a time while investigation of the incidents proceeded. Secondly, added impetus was given to finding safer vector systems for delivery of therapeutic genes. Currently, the moratorium on gene therapy has been eased, with trials proceeding under very tight regulation. There are also promising new delivery systems using nanotechnology, with genes enveloped in nanoparticles to target specific cancer cells. Yet other delivery systems use combinations of liposomes and nanoparticles. These delivery systems bypass the problem of the human immune response as the vectors are nonimmunogenic (nonantigenic). The short-lived nature of some gene therapies (where the therapeutic gene is not in self-renewing cells) required repeat procedures; this is now more feasible with these nonmicrobial vectors.

There have been recent reports of successful examples of gene therapy, including the treatment of patients with inherited types of blindness (Leber's congenital amaurosis), caused by a single abnormal gene. Successful outcomes have also been reported in patients with acute myeloid leukaemia. Other studies involve genetic engineering of patients' lymphocytes to enhance their anti-cancer-cell function, suicide genes introduced into cancer cells to deliver a very targeted toxin directly to such cells (see Chapters 4 and 7). Thus, with safer constructs and consideration of the risk benefit, gene therapy will target a single or very limited number of aberrant genes. The challenge of multigene disorders, associated with very common diseases (e.g. cardiovascular, neurodegenerative, and endocrine) remains formidable.

Stem cell therapy

In contrast to gene therapy, the use of stem cells is considered a highly feasible route towards the treatment of a range of human multigene disorders, including Parkinson's disease, diabetes, and cardiovascular disease. Much research is ongoing using predominantly embryonic-derived stem cells (ability to give rise to many different specialized cell types), as well as reprogrammed adult stem cells [10].

Stem cell therapy has a long history of successful use in humans (albeit in limited areas), most noteworthy being adult stem cells in bone marrow transplants and, more latterly, peripheral blood and umbilical cord blood stem cells. These have proved highly successful in treating haematological malignancies, some primary immune deficiencies and, lately, some cases of severe immune inflammatory disorders. Another interesting area where stem cells have been found and are readily isolated is that associated with dental tissues. Within the dental pulp and in the soft surrounding periodontal tissues, dental and oral stem cells can be isolated and these have been shown to have the ability to differentiate into all types of mature dental elements. This raises the potential for novel treatments for dental diseases such as caries (tooth decay), traumatic tooth loss, and severe destructive periodontitis, and for craniofacial disease and surgery. Whether the easily accessible dental stem cells have the potential to differentiate into tissue types outside the oral cavity is the subject of ongoing research.

The use of embryonic stem cells, however, is the subject of continuing, active ethical debate. The use of such cells will never be acceptable to some individuals, whereas others support their use within tightly regulated settings. Fully differentiated adult cells had been considered unusable for many decades until seminal work in the 1990s, using the technique of somatic cell nuclear transfer (SCNT), showed that adult cells could be reprogrammed. SCNT (used in part in the successful cloning of Dolly the sheep) involved the removal of the nucleus from an adult somatic cell and its transfer to a previously enucleated egg cell. The recipient cell was then manipulated, originally using an electrical current, with the result that the somatic nucleus and the genes within it were reprogrammed and behaved like stem cells. Such cells re-expressed a significant amount of 'stemness'. They were able to differentiate in a manner similar to embryonic pluripotent stem cells. These derived adult cells have been called *induced pluripotent stem cells* (iPSCs). Many of the ethical concerns associated with using embryonic cells are avoided using iPSCs.

The technique of SCNT is cumbersome, inefficient, and unpredictable. Recently, researchers have been able to define a limited number of genes (3–4) encoding transcription factors which, when transfected into the nucleus of adult cells, could result in their reprogramming as iPSCs. Such cells have been successfully used in a range of animal model systems. Donor-derived iPSCs are attractive therapeutic targets, as their inherent histocompatibility would favour autologous use of generated tissues or possibly organs without the need for immunosuppression. However, caution is necessary because some experimental model systems have indicated the potential of transplanted iPSCs to develop and behave *in situ* like tumour cells. It is necessary to continue working with embryonic stem cells, as well as with adult cell-derived iPSCs, to delineate safe and efficacious therapy. Another recent research finding using mouse cells has unequivocally demonstrated that cell reprogramming can be achieved directly—a process termed *cell transdifferentiation*. Using gene transfer for three or four lineage-specific transcription factors, it was possible to directly convert fibroblasts into functional excitatory neurons [11]. This direct route of transdifferentiation is attractive in enhancing therapeutic options for central nervous system disorders. However, matters such as scalability, long-term maintenance, and functioning of transferred genes, as well as safety, will all need thorough study.

Summary and conclusions

Scientific discoveries continue to flow from the study of immunology and knowledge of the immune system, coupled with rapid advances in cellular, molecular biological, biophysical, and genetic technologies along with information technology. These advances are making major impacts on diagnostic procedures and on translational biomedical research, as well as providing novel therapeutic approaches for a range of diseases. The exquisite specificity of antibodies and T cells, the availability of recombinant molecules (antibodies and cytokines), and increasingly sensitive assays, allows unparalleled multiparametric and multiplex analyses of human bodily fluids, single cells, and complex tissues *in vitro*, *ex vivo*, and to some extent *in vivo*. Assays developed from the PGTs have turned the concept of personalized genomes and use of systems medicine into a reality. This is facilitating more individualized diagnosis with risk assessment and stratification of disease using novel biomarkers, as well as signalling the potential for more targeted therapeutics using pharmocogenetics and biological therapies.

Cellular and molecular developments in the derivation and manipulation of genes and stem cells, along with advances in areas such as nanotechnology and tissue engineering, are pointing the way towards newer management procedures for a range of multigenic and relatively intractable diseases. Therapy using reprogrammed stem cells is likely to emerge in some areas of clinical practice within the next decade. Moreover, the area of regenerative medicine using such cells combined with innovative tissue engineering to possibly generate complex tissues in the laboratory, will certainly impact on some areas of surgical practice.

The principles of immunological assays and molecular technologies outlined in this chapter provides optimism for use of newer modalities, using biomarkers and systems medicine. These will enhance the management of a range of human diseases and disorders associated with cancer, transplantation, neurodegeneration, destructive inflammation, and infections. The challenges remain formidable, but the horizons to success are discernible and perhaps are not too distant.

References

1. Kohler G, Milstein C. Continuous cultures of fused cells secreting antibody of predefined specificity. *Nature* 1975; **256**: 495–497.
2. Murray A, Chapman CJ, Healey G *et al.* Technical validation of an autoantibody test for lung cancer. *Ann Oncol* 2010; **21**: 1687–1693.
3. Altman JD, Moss PH, Goulder PJ *et al.* Phenotypic analysis of antigen-specific T lymphocytes. *Science* 1996; **274**: 94–96.
4. Ogg GS, McMichael AJ. HLA-peptide tetrameric complexes. *Curr Opin Immunol* 1998; **10**: 393–396.
5. Knezevic V, Leethanakul C, Bichsel VE *et al.* Proteomic profiling of the cancer microenvironment by antibody arrays; *Proteomics* 2001; **1**: 1271–1278.
6. Kruglyak L. The road to genome-wide association studies. *Nat Rev Genet* 2008; **9**: 314–318.
7. Auffray C, Chen Z, Hood L. Systems medicine: the future of medical genomics and healthcare. *Genome Med* 2009; **1**: 2.
8. Asheley EA, Butte AJ, Wheeler MT *et al.* Clinical assessment incorporating a personal genome. *Lancet* 2010; **375**: 1525–1535.
9. Gene Therapy Review: http://www.genetherapyreview.com/default.html.
10. Takahashi K, Yamanaka S. Induction of pluripotent stem cells from mouse embryonic and adult fibroblast cultures by defined factors. *Cell* 2006; **126**: 663–676.
11. Vierbuchen T, Ostermeirer A, Pang ZP *et al.* Direct conversion of fibroblasts to functional neurons by defined factors. *Nature* 2010; **463**: 1035–1041.

Glossary

Acquired tolerance: Immunological state consisting of the inability (acquired) of an individual to respond to a particular antigen.

Activation marker: Molecule expressed on the cell surface indicating activation of the cell (e.g. IL-2 receptor).

Acute-phase response: Enhanced rates of liver synthesis of certain serum proteins (e.g. CRP, fibrinogen, and most of the complement components) during inflammation which rapidly protect the host against microorganisms. The acute-phase response is induced by agents such as IL-1, IL-6, and TNF-α, and is an important part of the innate immune response.

Adaptive immunity: The immunity mediated by T and B lymphocytes, characterized by exquisite specificity for antigen and immunological memory for the subsequent encounter of the antigen.

ADCC (**antibody-dependent cellular cytotoxicity**): A cytotoxic reaction in which Fc receptor-bearing cells recognize target cells coated with specific antibodies. Cells that mediate ADCC have been called killer (K) cells and are composed of a heterogeneous group of cells, including NK cells, monocytes, and eosinophils.

Adhesion molecules: Molecules found on cell surfaces that promote adhesive interactions between cells or with the extracellular matrix. Molecules such as integrins and selectins, found on most leucocytes, play major roles in cell migration and activation in immune responses.

Adaptor proteins: Are key bridging molecules involved in the signal transduction pathways within lymphocytes.

Adjuvant: Substance that enhances, nonspecifically, the immune response to an antigen. An adjuvant is usually administered with antigen, but may also be given before or after administration of the antigen (e.g. Freund's adjuvant). Adjuvants promote APC accumulation and expression of costimulatory molecules(CD80/86) and production of cytokines at sites of administration.

Affinity: A measure of the binding strength between two molecules (e.g. an antigenic determinant and an antibody-combining site).

Affinity maturation: Results from somatic mutation of Ig genes and selective survival of some B cells which produce antibodies with increased affinity for an antigen.

AIDS (**acquired immunodeficiency syndrome**)**:** Form of immunodeficiency resulting from infection with a lymphocytotropic virus (HIV). HIV infection can cause profound lymphopenia, primarily of $CD4^+$ T lymphocytes. Affected individuals are extremely susceptible to opportunistic infections and certain malignancies.

Agglutination: Clumping of particulate antigens (e.g. red blood cells, bacteria) by antibodies. Agglutination may be observed grossly or microscopically, and may be used as a test to detect the presence of and/or measure the level of antigen or antibody.

AIRE: The transcription factor protein produced by the autoimmune regulator (*AIRE*) gene. It facilitates the expression of peripheral tissue antigens within the thymus to promote negative selection (deletion) of T cells specific for those antigens.

Allele: Alternative form of a gene at a particular genetic locus.

Allelic exclusion: Expression in a single cell, of only one allele at a particular locus. Allelic exclusion is characteristic of the expression of Ig genes.

Allergen: Antigen that induces allergy. Common environmental allergens are globular proteins in pollens, animal danders, insect venoms, and various foods.

Allergy: Altered immune reactivity to commonly encountered environmental antigens. Allergy is regarded as a form of atopy and mechanistically is described as type I hypersensitivity (Gell and Coombs classification). Allergen-induced crosslinking of IgE on mast cells and basophils can activate and trigger the release of cell products which induce the allergic response.

Alloantigen: Antigen found only in some members of a species, e.g. blood group substances, HLA antigens. Alloantigens are produced by polymorphic genes.

Allogeneic: Referring to genetic variants within a species.

Allograft: Graft to a genetically different member of the same species. Allografts are rejected mainly by virtue of an immunological response of T lymphocytes to histocompatibility antigens.

Allotype: The protein product of an allele that may be detected as an antigen by another member of the same species.

Alternative pathway of complement: One of three possible mechanisms (the others being the classical and the lectin pathways) for the activation of C3 in complement activation.

ANA (antinuclear antibodies): Antibody to DNA, RNA, histone, or nonhistone proteins found in the serum of individuals, particularly those with certain autoimmune diseases.

Anaphylatoxin: Complement peptides (C3a, C4a, and C5a) which cause mast cell degranulation, smooth muscle contraction, and neutrophil chemotaxis, thus promoting acute inflammation.

Anaphylaxis: An antigen-specific immune reaction mediated primarily by IgE, which results in vasodilation and constriction of smooth muscles, including those of the bronchus, and which may result, in extreme cases, in the death of the individual.

Anergy: Absence of an expected immune response. This term is used in clinical medicine to describe the diminished delayed-type hypersensitivity (DTH) found in some disease states. Anergy is usually demonstrated by skin tests with ubiquitous antigens. Anergy in clones of T and B lymphocytes is considered as one of the mechanisms for maintaining immunologic tolerance to self antigens.

Antibody (Ab): Protein that is produced by B lymphocytes in response to stimulation by antigen and that reacts specifically with that antigen.

Antigen (Ag): A molecule which reacts with antibody.

Antigen presentation: The process by which certain cells (e.g. DCs, macrophages) display peptide antigens bound to the HLA molecules on their cell surfaces in a form recognizable by T lymphocytes.

Antigenic determinant: Portion of an antigen that makes contact with a particular antibody or TCR. Most proteins probably have many determinants but, because of steric interference, only a limited number of antibodies can bind to the antigen at any one time.

Anti-idiotypic antibodies: Antibodies which react with the antigenic determinants (idiotypes) on the V (variable) region of other antibodies. Because anti-idiotypes can bind to antigen receptors on T and B cells they can, in some situations, be efficient antigen mimics in stimulating these cells.

APCs (antigen-presenting cells): A variety of cell type which displays peptides in association with HLA molecules on the cell surface and can activate specific T cells (signal 1). APCs also provide other costimulatory molecules (signal 2) and additional signals (cytokines—signal 3) to optimize T cell activation, proliferation, and differentiation.

Apoptosis: A genetically programmed cell death process, characterized by DNA cleavage and nuclear fragmentation, along with cell membrane blebbing. Apoptotic cells are phagocytosed without inducing tissue inflammation. Apoptosis is important in lymphocyte development and selection in central lymphoid organs and in regulation of the immune response to antigens. It is a key process in the maintenance of immunological tolerance and the maintenance of lymphocyte homeostasis after proliferative immune responses.

Arthus reaction: Antibody-mediated hypersensitivity reaction characterized by oedematous, haemorrhagic lesions of the skin. Occurs on introduction of antigen into an individual with pre-existing circulating IgG antibodies. The Arthus reaction is an experimental model of immune complex disease (type III hypersensitivity).

Atopy: The clinical manifestation, in a genetically susceptible individual, of type I hypersensitivity reactions, including eczema, asthma, and rhinitis, due to IgE antibodies. Approximately 10% of the population manifests some form of atopy.

Autoantibody: Antibody that reacts with an antigen that is a normal constituent of the tissues of the individual forming the antibody.

Autoantigen: Normal constituent of the tissues of an individual that induces and reacts with an autoantibody.

Autoimmunity: Condition whereby antibodies or T lymphocytes are reactive with antigenic determinants of self.

Autologous: Part of the same individual. The term is used to describe self antigens or grafts taken from and returned to the same individual.

Autosome: Chromosome other than the X or Y sex chromosome.

Azathioprine: Derivative of mercaptopurine, widely used in the treatment of malignant disease and for immunosuppression.

B lymphocyte: Lymphocyte that produces Ig. B cells constitute about half of all lymphocytes. In lymph nodes, B lymphocytes are localized mainly in the follicles, whereas, T lymphocytes are found in the paracortex. Distinguished from T cells by the presence of smIg and CR2 and by constitutive expression of MHC-encoded class II HLA-DR molecules (not found on resting T cells).

β_2M (β_2-microglobulin): A monomorphic polypeptide which constitutes part of some membrane proteins, and is noncovalently linked with the MHC class I molecular complex.

BCG (bacillus Calmette–Guérin): An attenuated strain of bovine *Mycobacterium tuberculosis*; used as a vaccine to protect against tuberculosis (and leprosy). It is named after the two Frenchmen who first cultivated the organism.

Bence Jones protein: Protein in urine of patients with multiple myeloma that precipitates when heated to 45–60° C, and re-dissolves on further heating. It is the light chain of the myeloma protein found in the serum of the same patient. Named after the 19th century English physician Henry Bence Jones.

Bursa of Fabricius: A lymphoepithelial organ found at the junction of the hind gut and cloaca in birds which is the site of B cell generation and maturation.

C1–C9: Components of the complement pathway which are responsible for mediating inflammatory reactions, opsonization of particles and cell lysis.

C1q: Subcomponent of the C1 complex that binds to Ig and, thereby, initiates complement activation by the classical pathway.

C1r: One of two serine esterases that are part of the C1 complex, the other being C1s.

C3a and C5a: Small peptides split from the parent molecules during complement activation which act directly on phagocytes (especially neutrophils) to stimulate chemotaxis and the respiratory burst. Both (especially C5a) have chemotactic properties and increase vascular permeability.

C4: Fourth component of complement which reacts in sequence following fixation of C1 to antigen–antibody complexes.

CEA (carcinoembryonic antigen): Glycoprotein antigen on the membrane of epithelial cells of the gastrointestinal tract and structures derived from the primitive gut. CEA is present in large amounts on colorectal carcinoma cells and in lesser amounts on normal foetal colon cells.

CD (cluster of differentiation): Antigenic determinant, often on cell surface molecules of leucocytes, platelets, and other cells, that is detected by Mabs.

CDR (complementarity-determining region): Segment of a variable region containing amino acid residues that determines antigen-binding specificity. Residues in CDRs often make contact with antigen.

Chemiluminescence: Generation of light by a chemical reaction used in the study of phagocytosis. Light is emitted from oxidants generated in neutrophils and monocytes during the respiratory burst that occurs with phagocytosis.

Chemotaxis: Reorientation and directional migration of cells in response to concentration gradients of certain chemical stimuli.

Chimerism: The coexistence of cells from genetically different individuals in one body.

Class I, II, and III antigens: The three major classes of molecules coded within the major histocompatibility complex (MHC). Class I molecules have one MHC-encoded peptide associated with β_2-microglobulin. Class II molecules have two MHC-encoded peptides which are noncovalently associated; class III molecules include complement components.

Clonal selection: The fundamental basis of lymphocyte activation in which antigen selectively stimulates only those cells which express receptors for it to divide and differentiate.

Clone: A family of cells or organisms having a genetically identical constitution, i.e. cells derived from a single individual by asexual multiplication.

CMI (cell-mediated immunity): Immunological reactions initiated by T lymphocytes and mediated by effector T lymphocytes and macrophages.

Complement: A group of serum proteins involved in the control of inflammation, the activation of phagocytes, and the lytic attack on cell membranes. The system can be activated by interaction with the adaptive immune system (classical pathway) or by the alternative pathway and lectin pathway of innate immunity.

Constant regions (C domains): The relatively invariant parts of Ig heavy and light chains and the α, β, γ, and δ chains of the TCR.

Coombs (antiglobulin) test: Method for detecting the deposition of IgG antibodies or complement on red blood cells or for detecting the presence of circulating IgG antibodies reactive against red blood cells.

CRP (C-reactive protein): One of the acute-phase proteins, synthesized in the liver and released into the circulation as the result of trauma/inflammation.

Cryoglobulin: Ig that precipitates when it is cooled below 37° C. Cryoglobulins are not found in normal serum but occur in certain diseases.

CSFs (colony-stimulating factors): A group of cytokines which control the differentiation of haematopoietic stem cells.

CTL (cytotoxic T lymphocyte): T lymphocyte that kills other cells (via perforin and granzyme).

Ciclosporin: A fungal metabolite (cyclic peptide) which selectively inhibits early events in $CD4^+$ T cell activation and lymphokine production.

Cytokines: A generic term for soluble molecules which mediate interactions between cells.

Cytolysis: Killing of target cells by damage to their surface membranes and release of their intracellular contents.

Cytophilic: Having a propensity to bind to cells.

Cytoskeleton: Network of different types of protein filaments present in the cytoplasm of eukaryotic cells. They serve as a scaffold or framework for other cell constituents and are essential for maintaining shape, internal organization, and motility of the cell.

Cytostatic: Having the ability to stop cell growth and proliferation.

Cytotoxic: Having the ability to kill cells.

Degranulation: Exocytosis of granules from cells such as mast cells and basophils.

Dendritic cells (DCs): APCs in lymph nodes, spleen and (at low levels) in blood.

DTH (delayed type hypersensitivity): This term includes the delayed skin reactions associated with type IV (cell-mediated) hypersensitivity.

EBV (Epstein–Barr virus): Causal agent of Burkitt's lymphoma and infectious mononucleosis, which has the ability to transform human B cells into stable cell lines.

Effector cells: A functional concept which, in context, means those lymphocytes or phagocytes which produce the end effect.

ELISA (enzyme-linked immunosorbent assay): Method for detecting antigens or antibodies utilizing solid-phase enzyme–substrate reactions.

Endocytosis: Uptake by cells of materials from the extracellular fluid by means of vesicles formed from the plasma membrane. There are two types of endocytosis—receptor-mediated and fluid-phase endocytosis (pinocytosis).

Endosomes: Intracellular vesicles formed in the process of endocytosis.

Endotoxin: Synonym for heat-stable LPSs, associated with the outer membranes of Gram-negative bacteria.

Epitope: A single antigenic determinant. In functional terms, it is the portion of an antigen which combines with the antibody paratope.

Exocytosis: Process whereby the contents of intracellular vesicles are released into the external environment.

Exon: Segment of an interrupted gene or primary RNA transcript that is represented in mature RNA.

Fab fragment: The part of an antibody molecule which contains the antigen-combining site, consisting of a light chain and part of a heavy chain.

Factor B: Heat-labile protein of the alternative pathway of complement, which binds to C3b.

Factor D: Serine protease of the alternative pathway of complement which cleaves factor B.

FACS (fluorescence-activated cell sorter): Machine which rapidly analyses the size and fluorescence intensity of single cells stained with specific, fluorescent antibodies. The cells can then be sorted using these parameters.

Fc: The portion of an antibody that is responsible for binding to antibody receptors on cells and the C1q component of complement.

Fc receptor: Receptor for the Fc portion of Ig.

FDCs (follicular dendritic cells): Cells located in the follicles of lymph node and spleen characterized by the presence of many thin cytoplasmic extensions between closely packed B lymphocytes.

Follicle: Structure in lymphoid tissues characterized by loosely packed lymphocytes and APCs. Follicles are found in the superficial cortex of lymph nodes and the splenic white pulp, and contain mainly B cells. Unstimulated lymph nodes contain primary follicles, which develop into expanded, secondary follicles after antigen stimulation.

Foxp3: A transcription factor required for the generation of natural regulatory T cells (rTregs), its presence is a key marker for identifying such cells.

GATA3: The transcription factor associated with the differentiation of Th2 from naive (Th0) T cells.

Genotype: Genetic constitution in an organism; not all of it is expressed in the individual.

Germinal centre: Region of rapidly proliferating cells seen in the centre of some secondary lymphoid follicles.

Graft-versus-host disease: Condition caused by allogeneic donor lymphocyte reactions against host tissue in an immunologically compromised recipient.

Granulocyte: White blood cell of myeloid lineage, characterized by a nucleus composed of distinct lobes that are connected by thin strands of chromatin. Also called polymorphonuclear leucocyte (PMNL).

Graves' disease: Autoimmune disease that results in hyperthyroidism. Patients may have an IgG autoantibody (known as long-acting thyroid stimulator, LATS) to the thyroid-stimulating hormone (TSH) receptor.

GWAS (genome-wide association studies): Studies of genetic variation across the whole human genome that are designed to identify genetic association with defined traits, or the presence or absence of a disease.

HAART (highly active antiretroviral treatment): The combination typically of three or more antiviral drugs taken in combination to treat patients with HIV/AIDS. HAART treatment is recognized as effective in keeping the patient's HIV viral load at low levels, thus, preserving the immune system.

Haplotype: A set of genetic determinants located on a single chromosome.

Hapten: A small molecule which can act as an epitope but is incapable, by itself, of eliciting an antibody response.

Heavy chain: Larger polypeptide chain in an Ig molecule.

Heterodimer: Protein composed of two different chains.

Histocompatibility: The ability of an individual to accept grafts from another individual.

HIV (human immunodeficiency virus): Retrovirus that causes AIDS and related disorders. The virus infects mainly T lymphocytes of the $CD4^+$ subset in which the virus can be latent or lytic. HIV also infects $CD4^+$ mononuclear phagocytes.

HLA (human leucocyte antigen): The human MHC encoded and expressed molecules; first described in leucocytes.

Humanized antibody: Defines a recombinant molecule composed of the antigen binding sites from a mouse monoclonal linked to the constant region domains of a human Ig. These humanized antibodies are in common usage to treat tumours, inflammatory and autoimmune disorders.

Humoral: Pertaining to the extracellular fluids including the serum and lymph.

Hybridoma: Cell line created *in vitro* by fusion of two different cells, one a lymphocyte and the other a tumour cell (myeloma).

Hypersensitivity: An immune response to a previously encountered antigen which occurs in an exaggerated or inappropriate form—four types described.

Type I (immediate) hypersensitivity is manifested within minutes of exposure to antigen and is dependent on the binding of antigen to IgE on the surface of mast cells and basophils and the degranulation of these cells (e.g. allergic asthma, hay fever).

Type II (antibody-mediated) hypersensitivity is caused by antibody reacting with cell surface antigens which sensitizes the cells for ADCC by killer (K) cells or lysis by complement (e.g. destruction of red blood cells in transfusion reactions).

Type III (immune complex-mediated) hypersensitivity is due to the deposition of antigen-antibody complexes in tissues and blood vessels, the activation of complement with consequent attraction of polymorphs resulting in tissue damage (e.g. extrinsic allergic alveolitis).

Type IV (delayed or cell-mediated) hypersensitivity is mediated by antigen-sensitized T cells which, following contact with antigen, release lymphokines. These attract and activate macrophages, causing tissue damage.

Hypervariable regions: The most variable areas (in amino acid sequences) of the V domains of Ig and TCR chains. These regions are clustered at the distal portion of the V domain and contribute to the antigen-binding site.

I-CAM1 (intercellular adhesion molecule 1): Cell surface glycoprotein found on endothelial, dendritic and many other cell types and which is the ligand for lymphocyte function-associated antigen-1 (LFA-1) which is present on T cells.

Idiotope: A single antigenic determinant on an antibody V region.

Idiotype: The antigenic characteristic of the V region of an antibody.

IFNs (interferons): A group of mediators which increase the resistance of cells to viral infection, and act as cytokines. There are three types: IFN-α and IFN-β, produced by leucocytes and fibroblasts, and IFN-γ, produced by activated T cells and NK cells, which can activate macrophages in innate and adaptive (CMI) immune responses. It also modulates other immune responses and enhances NK cell activity.

Immune complex: The product of an antigen–antibody reaction which may also contain complement components.

Immune surveillance: Concept that the immune system eliminates cells that express aberrant or neoantigens as a result of cell stressors, somatic mutation, or the action of carcinogens.

Immunoelectrophoresis: Technique combining electrophoresis and immunodiffusion. It is usually carried out in a gel medium, such as agar. Thus, antigens are characterized by both electrophoretic mobility and antigenic properties. The technique is very effective in identifying components in complex mixtures.

Immunofixation: Technique for detecting specific antigens in a complex mixture of proteins that have been separated by electrophoresis. After electrophoresis, the gel is flooded with antibodies, washed to remove soluble antigens and antibodies, and then stained to detect antigen–antibody precipitates.

Immunofluorescence: Technique used to identify particular antigen microscopically in tissues or on cells by the binding of a fluorescent antibody conjugate.

Immunoglobulin (Ig): Protein that has antibody activity.

Inflammation: The physiological process which can be generated and exploited by innate and adaptive immunity to combat infection. It involves attraction, accumulation, and activation of leucocytes and plasma proteins at the site of damage (e.g. by infection, toxin, or cell injury). The changes in the local vasculature help to define the characteristics of tissue inflammation. Inflammation serves an evolutionary protective function, preventing infection and promoting tissue repair. Uncontrolled, maladaptive, and persistent chronic inflammation can cause severe tissue damage, and disease.

Innate immunity: Use of pre-existing mechanisms present within an organism to protect against infections and tissue damage. Innate responses are rapid (minutes to hours) and react in essentially identical ways to repeat infections or trauma (there is no immunological memory—in contrast to the slower-acting adaptive immunity). Innate immunity includes epithelial lining cells and their functions, phagocytic cells, NK cells, complement system, chemokines, and cytokines. Elements of innate immunity regulate and coordinate activities of cells and products of adaptive immunity.

Integrins: Glycoproteins on cell membranes that act as receptors for extracellular matrix glycoproteins, blood proteins, and other cell surface glycoproteins. Integrins serve, in general, as transmembrane links between extracellular ligands and the cells' cytoskeleton. They facilitate cell migration in embryos, wound healing, phagocytosis, and target cell killing.

Interdigitating dendritic cells (IDCs): These are located in the T cell area of lymph nodes, and express HLA class II molecules; they are highly active in presenting antigen to Th cells. They are thought to be most important in the development of contact (delayed) type IV hypersensitivity reactions.

Interleukins (ILs): A group of molecules (cytokines) secreted mainly by leucocytes and involved in signalling between cells of the immune system. ILs induce growth and differentiation of lymphocytes and pluripotential haematopietic stem cells. The numerical suffix indicates a structurally defined cytokine, e.g. IL-2, IL-12.

Introns: Gene segments which lie between the exons. They do not encode protein but contain sequences important in gene control and the process of recombination.

Isotype: Refers to genetic variation within a family of proteins or peptides such that every member of the species will have each isotype of the family represented in its genome (e.g. Ig classes).

J chain: Monomorphic polypeptide present in and required for the polymerization of polymeric IgA and IgM.

K (killer) cells: A group of cells (predominant amongst which are NK cells) which are able to destroy their targets by ADCC and which bear Fc receptors.

Kinases: Enzymes that add phosphate groups to certain amino acids (particularly tyrosine) of proteins. Protein kinases of lymphocytes are involved in signal transduction and activation of transcription factors.

Knockout mice: Are animals with targeted disruption of one or more genes. Knockouts have proved invaluable in defining the precise roles of encoded cytokines, receptors, and signalling molecules in immune responses.

K562: Cell line from a patient with chronic myelogenous leukaemia, commonly used as target in *in vitro* assays of natural killer (NK) cell activity.

LAK (lymphokines-activated killer) cells: Cytotoxic lymphocytes with a wide repertoire of cellular targets, generated by interaction with IL-2.

Langerhans cells: APCs of the skin which emigrate to local lymph nodes to become mature DCs; they are very active in presenting antigen to T cells. They have a characteristic racket-shaped granule called the Birbeck granule, and are rich in HLA class II molecules.

LATS (long-acting thyroid stimulator): *See* Graves' disease.

Leukotrienes: A collection of metabolites of arachidonic acid produced by the lipooxygenase pathway, generating mediators of acute inflammation and other substances important in hypersensitivity.

LFAs (leucocyte functional antigens): A group of three molecules (LFA1–3) which mediate intercellular adhesion between leucocytes and other cells in a nonspecific manner.

LGLs (large granular lymphocytes): A group of morphologically defined (azurophilic granules) lymphocytes, containing the majority of NK cell activity.

Light chain: Small polypeptide chain in a heterodimer. As used by immunologists, the term usually refers to the light chain of an Ig molecule.

Loci: The positions on a chromosome at which a particular gene is found.

LPS (lipopolysaccharide): A polyclonal B cell mitogen in mice which induces Ig secretion. It is derived from the cell wall of Gram-negative bacteria and is recognized by certain TLRs (e.g. TLR4 in humans).

Lymphoblast: Large cell of lymphocyte lineage that contains a nucleolus and synthesizes DNA.

Lymphoid: Referring to lymphocytes or to tissues that contain large accumulations of lymphocytes.

Lymphokine: A generic term for cytokine molecules which are involved in signalling between cells of the immune system and are produced by lymphocytes.

Lysosomes: Enzyme containing organelles present in cells; in macrophages, important in the breakdown and digestion of phagocytosed material.

Lysozyme (muramidase): An enzyme which digests a bond in the cell wall proteoglycan of some Gram-positive bacteria.

Mabs (monoclonal antibodies): Antibodies produced by a single clone and which are homogeneous.

Mantoux test: Test for cell-mediated immunity (CMI) to tuberculosis in which tuberculin is injected intradermally.

MDP (muramyl dipeptide): The smallest adjuvant active part of the BCG extractable from the cell wall.

MHC (major histocompatibility complex): A genetic region found in all mammals whose products are primarily responsible for functional signalling between lymphocytes and cells expressing antigen. MHC-encoded molecules are also involved in the rejection of grafts between individuals.

Microglial cells: Itinerant phagocytes of the brain.

Mitogens: Molecules which induce polyclonal differentiation and division (mitosis) of cells. A few are commonly used to induce lymphocyte subset activation and transformation, e.g. LPS, PHA, CON A, PWM.

MLR (mixed lymphocyte reaction): A technique for typing or measuring the interaction between cells *in vitro*, in which lymphocytes from different individuals are cocultured. If the cells differ they are stimulated to undergo blast transformation and to divide. The T lymphocytes react against the MHC class I determinants on the surface of the other population.

Myeloma: Plasma cell tumour produced from cells of the B cell lineage, which secretes Ig, of limited clonality.

Neoantigen: Newly expressed antigenic determinant. Occurs as a result of conformational change in a protein, cell transformation, complex formation of two or more molecules, or cleavage of a molecule.

NK (natural killer) cells: A group of lymphocytes of innate immunity (predominantly Fc receptor-bearing LGL) which have the intrinsic ability to recognize and destroy some virally infected cells and various tumour cells (MHC independent) to which the individual has not previously been sensitized. NK cells secrete IFNγ and activate phagocytes. NK cell functions are regulated by families of cell surface inhibitory and stimulatory receptors.

NF-κB (nuclear factor–kappa B): A family of transcription factor proteins important for the activation of many genes in both adaptive and innate immunity.

Oncofoetal antigens: Antigens normally expressed in foetal life which reappear in tumours and may be secreted into the circulation.

Oncogene: Gene that brings about or contributes to the neoplastic transformation of cells, e.g. c-*erb*, K-*ras*, c-*myc*.

Opportunistic infection: Infections that occur mainly in patients with defects in CMI.

Opsonins: Molecules which bind both to particles to be phagocytosed and to receptors on phagocytic cells, so acting as a bridge between the two, e.g. IgG, C3b, and CRP.

Opsonization: This occurs when particles, microorganisms, or immune complexes become coated with molecules which make them more easily phagocytosed, i.e. coated with opsonins.

Peyer's patches: Collections of lymphocytes in the wall of the small intestine which appear macroscopically as pale patches on the gut wall. They contain B and T cell areas along with APCs and may have germinal centres. Immune responses can be generated to ingested antigen in these sites.

PGT (postgenomic technologies): Analytical approaches and platform technologies which took great leaps forward, or in some cases became achievable, as a result of the sequencing of the human and other genomes. Such technologies include large-scale proteomics, metabolomics, functional and comparative genomics, transcriptomics, and associated other 'omic technologies.

Phagocytosis: The process by which cells engulf material and enclose it within a vacuole (phagosome) in the cytoplasm.

Phenotype: The expressed characteristics of an individual; it depends on the genotype and how the genes are expressed.

Phosphatases: Enzymes that remove phosphate groups from amino acids of proteins. Lymphocyte phosphatases, such as calcineurin, regulate the activity of transcription factors and cell signalling.

Plasma cell: An antibody-producing B lymphocyte which has reached the end of its differentiation pathway.

Pluripotent stem cell: An undifferentiated bone marrow-derived cell. Characteristically, it divides continuously to generate additional stem cells able to differentiate into many lineages of different cells. The bone marrow stem cell can give rise to lymphoid, erthyroid, and myeloid cells. Experimentally-induced pluripotential stem cells (iPSc) have been generated by techniques using transfection of a few key genes for transcription factors into differentiated cells, inducing their reversion to iPSc.

Polyclonal activator: Substance that stimulates T and B lymphocytes, regardless of their antigen specificity.

Polyclonal antibodies: Antibodies derived from many different clones of antibody-forming cells, all of which react with particular antigenic determinants. Immunization usually results in a polyclonal antibody response.

Polymorphonuclear granulocyte: Cells recognizable by their multilobed nuclei and numerous cytoplasmic granules. They constitute the majority of blood leucocytes.

Properdin: Protein of the alternative complement pathway. It binds to the alternative pathway C3 convertase (C3bBb) and stabilizes it.

RAST (radioallergosorbent test): A specialized form of RIA for detecting antigen-specific IgE, in which antigen is covalently coupled to cellulose discs. Antigen-specific IgE binding to the disc is detected using radiolabelled anti-IgE.

Reactive oxygen species (ROS): Very reactive metabolites of oxygen which are produced by activated phagocytes. ROSs, such as the superoxide anion, hydrogen peroxide, and the hydroxyl radical, damage phagocytosed microbes. Uncontrolled or excessive release of ROSs can promote tissue damaging inflammatory responses.

Recall antigens: Antigens of common microbial pathogens that are used in skin testing for delayed hypersensitivity (e.g. *Candida albicans*, PPD, streptokinase–streptodornase, mumps antigens).

Recombinant proteins: The product of the process by which genetic information is rearranged during meiosis, called recombination. This process also occurs during the somatic rearrangements of DNA which occur in the formation of genes encoding antibody molecules and T cell antigen receptors. The term is also used to describe the genetically engineered proteins generated *in vitro* using isolated DNA and various expression systems.

Regulatory T cells (Tregs): Cells that regulate the activation and/or effector functions of other lymphocytes. They are considered important for the maintenance of self immune tolerance. The nT regs, which are generated in and exit from the thymus, express the transcription factor Foxp3 and are commonly $CD4^+$ and $CD25^+$ cells. Regulatory T cells induced in the peripheral (secondary) lymphoid system have a more heterogeneous phenotype.

Reticuloendothelial cells: Long-lived phagocytic cells distributed throughout the organs of the body. They are derived from bone marrow stem cells and most have been shown to have receptors for the Fc region of Ig and activated C3. Their function is to scavenge antigenic particles and debris. Some of them have the ability to present antigen to lymphocytes.

Rheumatoid factor (RF): Autoantibody to IgG or IgA, usually of the IgM class, found most frequently in serum of patients with rheumatoid arthritis.

RIA (radioimmunoassay): Includes a variety of techniques which use radiolabelled reagents to detect antigen or antibody. Antibody may be detected using plates sensitized with antigen. Test antibody is applied and this is detected by the addition of a radiolabelled ligand specific for that antibody. The amount of ligand bound to the plate is proportional to the amount of test antibody.

Serotype: Antigenic variant within a bacterial species identified using antibodies to surface antigenic determinants of the variants.

siRNA (small interfering RNA): Small double-stranded RNA molecules, generated endogenously or synthesized, which can act as regulators of genes within cells. Their interfering effects, by binding to complementary sequences in target mRNAs, result in target degradation and prevents expression of the gene-encoded protein and function. A subset of particularly small endogenous siRNA (usually <20 nucleotides) is called microRNA.

SNPs (single nucleotide polymorphisms): DNA polymorphisms that involve a single base change at a particular position in a DNA sequence. The human genome sequence and SNP consortia studies indicate that there are approximately 10 million SNPs across the genome. Most SNPs represent normal human diversity, but a proportion are linked to susceptibility to disease, as is commonly investigated in GWAS studies.

Somatic mutation: A process occurring during B cell maturation and affecting the antibody gene region, which permits refinement of antibody specificity.

Superantigens: Proteins (many of microbial origin) that bind to and activate all T cells within an individual that express a particular set or family of the Vβ part of the TCR. The nonpolymorphic residues of HLA class II molecules on APCs bind to parts of the superantigen (without any antigen processing), thus, facilitating the superantigen presentation and binding to the TCR. Superantigen activity is implicated in several human diseases, including toxic shock syndrome (linked to *Staphylococcus aureus* superantigen).

Suppressor cells: A subpopulation of cells, mainly T cells, which act to reduce the immune responses of other T or B cells. Suppression may be antigen-specific, idiotype-specific, or nonspecific in different circumstances. Many suppressor T cell activities are now attributed to Tregs.

Syngeneic: Strains of animals produced by repeated inbreeding so that each pair of autosomes within an individual is identical.

Systems biology: A holistic approach that permits the study of dynamic integrated networks associated with physiological and pathological processes. It allows integration of information from such processes together with powerful information technology in interdisciplinary studies. It is providing new avenues toward disease diagnosis and management, for drug development, and to exploit the potential for personalized medicine using personal genome sequences.

TCR (T cell antigen receptor complex): Protein on the surface of T cells that specifically recognizes HLA molecules encoded by the MHC genes, either alone or in association with foreign peptide antigens. In the cell membrane, the TCR is composed of the antigen-specific T cell receptor molecule (Ti) and is closely associated with the CD3 complex, which mediates signal transduction when the TCR is engaged. Ti consists of two distinct, membrane-embedded polypeptide heterodimer chains, either α/β or γ/δ.

T-bet: A transcription factor of the T-box family that promotes the differentiation of Th1 cells from naive (ThO) T cells.

Tetramer technology: Allows the recognition, enumeration, and isolation of T cells via their TCRs reacting specifically with peptide–HLA complexes generated *in vitro* as multimeric complexes (tetramers). HLA class I, class II, and CDId tetramers are used to detect, respectively, specific $CD8^+$, $CD4^+$, and unconventional T cells. The unconventional T cells recognize glycolipid antigens presented by the nonclassical MHC class I CDI molecule in contrast to peptides seen by $CD4^+$ and $CD8^+$ T cells.

T lymphocyte: Cell that matures in the thymus and is responsible for CMI and the regulation of growth and differentiation of other immune-competent cells (e.g. B cells, mononuclear phagocytes). Mature T cells can be divided into two major subsets that differ broadly in function on the basis of surface antigenic determinants: (1) $CD4^+$ (mainly helper T cells); (2) $CD8^+$ (mainly cytotoxic T cells).

Th1: A functional subset of $CD4^+$ Th cells, characterized by T-bet expression, and that secrete a particular set of cytokines, including the signature molecule IFN-γ. Th1 are key cells that stimulate phagocyte defences against intracellular microbes.

Th2: A functional subset of $CD4^{+}$ Th cells, characterized by expression of the GATA-3 transcription factor and that secrete a range of cytokines including the signature molecule IL-4. The principle role of Th2 cells is in the promotion of IgE and eosinophil/mast cell reactions and the reciprocal down regulation of Th1 responses.

Th17: A functional subset of $CD4^{+}$ helper T cells, characterized by expression of the RORγ transcription factor and that secretes a range of cytokines, including the signature molecule IL-17. Th17 responses generate protective immunity against certain microbial (especially extracellular) infections; they are also implicated in significant inflammation and pathology associated with autoimmune responses.

TNF (tumour necrosis factor): Cytokine released by activated macrophages which induces leucocytosis, fever, weight loss, the acute-phase reaction, and necrosis of some tumours. TNF-α (cachectin) and TNF-β (lymphotoxin) are homologous proteins, having approximately 30% amino acid identity; they bind to the same receptor and share biological activities.

Tolerance: A state of specific immunological unresponsiveness.

Toll-like receptor (TLRs): Families of molecules expressed by many cells, as cell surface, endosomal and other intracellular receptors. TLRs function as pattern recognition receptors (PRRs) for many different pathogen-associated molecular patterns (PAMPs), as well as for some self aberrantly expressed molecules as danger-associated molecular patterns (DAMPs). TLRs are linked to various signal transduction pathways and activate genes that promote inflammation and processes to resist microbial invasion.

Transgenic organism: Organism carrying and usually expressing an exogenous gene in its genome. In mice, the gene is usually introduced by microinjection of a recently fertilized egg.

Transformation: Morphological changes in a lymphocyte associated with the onset of division (blast transformation). Also denotes the conversion of cells in culture to a state of unrestrained growth (malignant transformation).

Tumour-infiltrating lymphocytes (TILs): Lymphocytes defined in and isolated from inflammatory infiltrates in and around tumours. TILs are enriched with tumour-associated $CD8^{+}$ CTLs, NK cells, and Tregs. They are used in experimental cancer treatments, often following *in vitro* expansion using high concentrations of cytokines (e.g. IL-2) before reinfusion into patients.

V domains: The *N*-terminal domains of antibody heavy and light chains and the α, β, γ, and δ chains of the TCR which vary between different clones and form the antigen-binding site.

Xenogeneic: Referring to interspecies antigenic differences.

Xenograft: Graft to a member of a different species. Xenografts are usually rapidly rejected by antibodies and cytotoxic T lymphocytes to histocompatibility antigens.

Zidovudine (3-azido-3-deoxythymidine, AZT): Analogue of thymidine that inhibits reverse transcriptase. It was the first drug specifically licensed for the treatment of HIV/AIDS.

Index

Locators in *italic* refer to figures/tables
Locators for headings which also have subheadings refer to general aspects of that topic